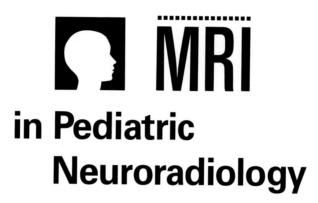

MRI
in Pediatric
Neuroradiology

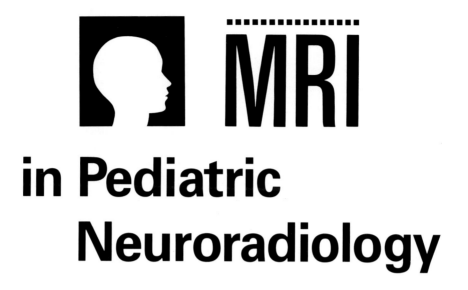

in Pediatric Neuroradiology

Samuel M. Wolpert, M.B., B.Ch.
Chief of Neuroradiology
New England Medical Center Hospitals
Tufts University School of Medicine
Boston, Massachusetts

Patrick D. Barnes, M.D.
Associate Neuroradiologist
Children's Hospital
Harvard Medical School
Boston, Massachusetts

with 1199 illustrations

Mosby Year Book

St. Louis Baltimore Boston Chicago London Philadelphia Sydney Toronto

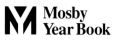

Mosby
Year Book
Dedicated to Publishing Excellence

Editor: Anne S. Patterson
Assistant Editors: Dana Battaglia
 Maura Leib
Project Manager: Patricia Tannian
Production Editor: John Casey
Book and Cover Design: Julie Taugner

Printed in the United States of America.

Mosby–Year Book, Inc.
11830 Westline Industrial Drive
St. Louis, Missouri 63146

Library of Congress Cataloging in Publication Data
Wolpert, Samuel M., 1930-
    MRI in pediatric neuroradiology / Samuel M. Wolpert, Patrick D.
Barnes.
       p.   cm.
    Includes bibliographical references and index.
    ISBN 0-8016-5370-3
    1. Central nervous system—Magnetic resonance imaging.   2. Central
nervous system—Imaging.   3. Pediatric diagnostic imaging.
    4. Pediatric neurology.   I. Barnes, Patrick D. II. Title.
    [DNLM: 1. Brain Diseases—diagnosis.   2. Brain Diseases—in
infancy & childhood.   3. Magnetic Resonance Imaging.   4.   Spinal
Diseases—diagnosis.   5. Spinal Diseases—in infancy & childhood.
WS 340 W866m]
RJ488.5.M3W65   1992
618.92′8047548—dc20
DNLM/DLC   91-38961
for Library of Congress   CIP

92 93 94 95 96 CL/MY/MY 9 8 7 6 5 4 3 2 1

To my mentor, friend, and colleague,
the late Dr. Mannie M. Schechter,
a giant in the field of neuroradiology.
Samuel M. Wolpert

To my family
Donna, Tammy, Shay, Amy, and Lauren
To my parents
Ruby F. Barnes and Harry E. Barnes, M.D.
To my teachers
Sidney Traub, M.D., Bob Eaton, M.D., Dan Galloway, M.D. (deceased),
Jean Vanhoutte, M.D., Teresa Stacy, M.D., Roy Strand, M.D.,
Ken Fellows, M.D., and John A. Kirkpatrick, Jr., M.D.
To the children and their families
Their courage and faith
Patrick D. Barnes

Contributors

Mary L. Anderson, M.D.

Instructor in Radiology
Tufts University School of Medicine
Staff Neuroradiologist
Assistant in Radiology
New England Medical Center Hospitals
Boston, Massachusetts

Edward M. Kaye, M.D.

Assistant Professor of Pediatrics and Neurology
Tufts University School of Medicine
Chief, Section Neurometabolic Diseases
Department of Pediatrics
New England Medical Center Hospitals
Boston, Massachusetts

Richard P. Klucznik, M.D.

Staff Neuroradiologist
Wilford Hall Medical Center
Lackland Air Force Base
San Antonio, Texas

Bruce R. Korf, M.D., Ph.D

Assistant Professor of Neurology
Harvard Medical School
Director of Clinical Genetics Program
Department of Genetics
Children's Hospital
Boston, Massachusetts

William J. Kupsky, M.D.

Instructor of Neuropathology
Harvard Medical School
Neuropathologist
Children's Hospital
Boston, Massachusetts

Robert V. Mulkern, Ph.D

Instructor of Radiology
Harvard Medical School
MR Physicist
The Children's Hospital
Boston, Massachusetts

Jane C. Share, M.D.

Instructor in Radiology
Harvard Medical School
Associate Radiologist
Children's Hospital
Boston, Massachusetts

Roy D. Strand, M.D.

Associate Professor in Radiology
Harvard Medical School
Associate Neuroradiologist
Children's Hospital
Boston, Massachusetts

David K. Urion, M.D.

Assistant Professor in Neurology
Harvard Medical School
Pediatric Neurologist
Director of Learning Disabilities/Behavorial
   Neurology Program
Department of Neurology
Children's Hospital
Boston, Massachusetts

Foreword

It is a pleasure to be associated with this text, *MRI in Pediatric Neuroradiology*. I have had the great good fortune over the past 15 years of knowing Drs. Barnes and Wolpert and of attending their lectures and conferences at Children's Hospital in Boston. Dr. Wolpert has been a frequent visiting speaker at the neurology, neurosurgical, and neuroradiology conferences; Dr. Barnes and Dr. Roy D. Strand have given a course in pediatric neuroradiology with emphasis on MRI to the staff, fellows, residents, and students each year for the past 4 years. The material in this text is so well organized and so lucidly presented because of these formal oral presentations. Consultants in neurology have been used in the preparation of some chapters to enhance clinical applicability.

For someone raised with ventricular air and opaque intracranial arteries and veins, the exquisite anatomy and physiology made possible by MRI is overwhelming. I have the further feeling that this text, when rewritten in 5 years, will be even more specific, anatomically, physiologically, and diagnostically. Despite the title, other modes for imaging are discussed in some detail, particularly ultrasonography and computed tomography.

The first chapter concerns physical and biological principles of magnetic resonance imaging. This is written with Dr. Robert Mulkern, an MR scientist. The *n*, the *m*, and the *r* in nuclear magnetic resonance are discussed in a way that brings these difficult concepts to life. The biomechanisms are then elucidated, and finally, techniques, guidelines, and diagnostic sensitivity and specificity of the magnetic resonance examination are described. Immediately following, the clinical principles of pediatric neuroradiology are presented in Chapter 2. This chapter includes an analysis of ultrasonography, computed tomography, and magnetic resonance imaging in relation to the signs and symptoms of diseases of the central nervous system in childhood, a chapter that will be interesting to the clinician as well as the neuroradiologist.

Chapters 3 to 8 are concerned with imaging of the brain. There is a comprehensive discussion of developmental disorders of the brain as well as metabolic and degenerative disorders, intracranial inflammatory processes, vascular diseases, hemorrhages, and trauma. The lists of diseases are comprehensive, and the discussion is full of clinical and imaging "pearls." Cranial and intracranial neoplasms are elucidated in Chapter 7, which is extremely well organized and illustrated. The tumors are presented according to their location in the cerebral hemisphere, followed by those that occur near the third ventricle and those that are found in the posterior fossa. In addition, parameningeal and metastatic tumors are included. Finally in this group are the neurocutaneous syndromes. Their names are already familiar, and the discussion of each, that is, inheritance, clinical presentation, associated disorders, and imaging is so lucidly presented that one has little excuse for not remembering them in detail.

Chapters 9 and 10 are concerned with imaging of the spine. They include appropriate discussions of osseous dysplasias involving the spine and skull, mucopolysaccharidoses, certain chromosomal disorders such as Down's syndrome, and a comprehensive presentation of the neurenteric continuum. The final chapter has to do with acquired disorders of the spine and the neuraxis; it examines spinal trauma, neoplastic disease, and inflammatory diseases.

The bibliography for each section is very appropriate. I am impressed by the comprehensiveness of this text. It will have great appeal to the clinician interested in neurological disorders in children as well as to those in training and practice in radiology and specifically in pediatric neuroradiology as a frequently consulted resource and reference.

John A. Kirkpatrick, Jr., M.D.
Radiologist-in-Chief
Children's Hospital
Professor of Radiology
Harvard Medical School
Boston, Massachusetts

Preface

To those of us involved in pediatric neuroradiology this book represents a preoccupation and a fascination with a topic that extends back to our training as fledgling neuroradiology fellows. Pediatric neuroradiology is a challenge, not only because of the inherent difficulties in obtaining state-of-the-art studies in a population whose basic inclination is to move that part of the body being examined, but also because the topic entails and demands a detailed knowledge of a structure—the central nervous system—*in development*. Since development is the key to many of the diagnostic challenges inherent in pediatric neuroradiology, solving the dual problems of the moving infant or child and the developing central nervous system leads to a unique satisfaction.

The preeminence of MRI for the investigation of pediatric diseases of the head and spine has stimulated our attempts to gather and display the role of this new technology in a comprehensible manner. We have tried to be inclusive, without being exhaustive, in mentioning most if not all central nervous system (CNS) diseases causing imaging abnormalities occurring in infants and children. This is a book on MRI, but many sick children are not amenable to MRI because of their fragility. The use of ultrasound in such infants is appropriate and alluded to in this text. Similarly, CT is still extremely useful and in many instances negates the need for MRI. Here again we have attempted to refer to the current use of CT in pediatric CNS disease without going into detail. The rapid advancement of the field of MRI necessitated that this text keep pace with current knowledge, a responsibility we have attempted to discharge with, we hope, a successful outcome. We are aware that this text may be outdated before it sees the light of day. We apologize for any lack of timeliness.

This book represents a beneficial collaboration from two perspectives: one from a full-time academic neuroradiologist with a significant pediatric experience as part of a larger adult practice (SMW), the other from a full-time academic pediatric neuroradiologist (PDB). Our experience extends from the era of traditional neuroradiology into the modern era of major technological advances.

We address this book to our colleagues involved in the pediatric neurosciences—neurologists, neurosurgeons, and neuroradiologists. We also hope the text is suitable for ophthalmologists, otorhinolaryngologists and head and neck surgeons, orthopedic surgeons, endocrinologists, pediatric radiologists, and neonatologists. Generalists in radiology who are fortunate to see and diagnose pediatric problems in their daily practice, as well as pediatricians and physicians in adolescent medicine, may also benefit from this book. Finally, we address this book to our trainees—fellows, residents, and interns in all the disciplines of medicine—who deal with sick children with CNS disease. We hope we have succeeded.

Samuel M. Wolpert
Patrick D. Barnes

Acknowledgments

Thanks are due to many people for this publication. First, my secretary Nancy Wysocki for typing and manuscript preparation; Michael Wood, Ph.D., for help in the development of the MR sequences, and Eileen Marr, MRI Coordinator, and her staff for the MR images; Drs. Roy McCauley and Deborah ter Meulen for assistance with the ultrasound images in Chapters 3 and 6 and Martha Pacetti, R.N., for her pediatric nursing assistance. Dr. Robert E. Paul has provided the foresight to bring MRI to the New England Medical Center Hospitals. Mr. Edward Cohen and Russell Soule have provided the administrative support to make MRI a viable clinical entity. My thanks also to Anne Patterson, Executive Editor, for her continued support and encouragement, and to John Casey, Senior Production Editor, for his editorial assistance at Mosby–Year Book, Inc.

Samuel M. Wolpert

I thank the following individuals at The Children's Hospital, Boston, who have made important contributions to the production of this text. Virginia Grove, project coordination and principal manuscript preparation; Jan Sucher and Elaine Donnelly, manuscript preparation; Don Sucher, photography; Steven Moskowitz, medical illustrations, Chapter 1; Miriam Geller, M.S., medical literature surveys; Carolyn Pickett, R.T.R., MR Supervisor; Mary Ann Chin, R.T.R, CT supervisor; the MR and CT technologists and nursing staff; Jim Brewer, image preparation; Rita Teele, M.D., for assistance with Chapter 2; James Meyer, M.D. (currently at Children's Hospital of Philadelphia) for assistance with Chapters 1 and 7. I also wish to thank my co-author, Samuel Wolpert, M.D., as well as Anne Patterson, Executive Editor, Dana Battaglia, Editorial Assistant, and John Casey, Senior Production Editor, Mosby–Year Book, Inc.

I am grateful also for the assistance provided by the radiologic technologists and administrative staff at The Children's Hospital of Oklahoma, the Oklahoma MR Center, the Department of Radiological Sciences, the University of Oklahoma Health Sciences Center, and the Oklahoma Diagnostic Imaging Center, Oklahoma City, Oklahoma. Special appreciation is expressed to Patrick Lester, M.D., formerly Radiologist-in-Chief, City of Faith Hospital, Tulsa, Oklahoma, and John R. Prince, Ph.D., Scientific Director, the Oklahoma MR Center, Oklahoma City, Oklahoma, both of whom worked diligently with me in the early development of MR imaging for pediatric use in that region of the country. I also acknowledge the leadership of Donald Halverstadt, M.D., formerly Chief Executive Officer, in bringing the MRI technology to the Oklahoma Teaching Hospitals and providing John R. Prince and myself the opportunity to develop the concept of a centralized special imaging facility and establish the Oklahoma MR Center in honor of Sidney P. Traub, M.D., Chairman of the Department of Radiological Sciences. Special recognition is also extended to G. W. "Butch" Schoenhals, M.D., Don Rhinehart, M.D., and Michael Polley, M.D., for their leadership in establishing the Oklahoma Diagnostic Imaging Center and affording Dan Galloway, M.D., Kenneth Wegner, M.E., and myself the privilege of implementing the CT and MR imaging programs to serve that community. Also I am grateful for the assistance provided by Timothy Tytle, M.D., in the preparation of the spine trauma section of Chapter 10.

Finally, I am grateful to John A. Kirkpatrick, Jr., M.D., for his valued contribution to this text and for his sustained stewardship in bringing MR imaging to The Children's Hospital, Boston, and also to Keith Strauss, M.Sc., Director of Physics and Engineering, Stephen Rizzo, Facilities Planning, Carolyn Pickett, R.T.R., MR technologic supervisor, Robert Mulkern, Ph.D., MR Physicist, Catharyn Gildesgame, Department Administrator, Linda Poznauskis, Technical Director, Eileen Schumacher, R.N. and Mary Pothier, R.N., Nursing Division, and Mark Rockoff, M.D., Anethesiology, who worked steadfastly with Fred Hoffer, M.D., and myself to implement the MR program.

Patrick D. Barnes

Contents

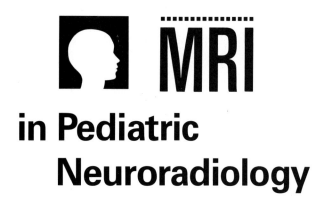

in Pediatric Neuroradiology

PART ONE

Basic Principles of Pediatric Neuroradiology

1 · Physical and Biological Principles of Magnetic Resonance Imaging

Patrick D. Barnes
Robert V. Mulkern

NMR and MRI

Nuclear magnetic resonance (NMR) is the science[1,2,11] behind the clinical magnetic resonance imaging (MRI)[5,8,12] and spectroscopic (MRS)[3,4] technologies (Fig. 1-1) for analyzing anatomy and chemistry in human health and disease. NMR is based on the concept that microscopic nuclear (N) magnets (for example, hydrogen) of human tissues align and spin at the Larmor frequency within the static main magnetic (M) field of the MRI system, are anatomically localized by the gradient (M) coils, and coherently interact with the radiofrequency (RF) coil to produce energy exchange or resonance (R), all to generate images reflecting normal and abnormal tissue states.[5,9] The NMR process takes place at the lower end (nonionizing radiofrequency range) of the electromagnetic spectrum[5] and represents the first successful employment of "natural" communication between medical imaging technology and human biology. Like its radiology-based counterpart, computer tomography (CT), MR is a computer-assisted, cross-sectional (tomographic, or slice), and matrix (two-dimensional digital display), technology that provides images of three-dimensional tissue volume elements, or voxels[10] (Fig. 1-2).

The basic conceptual components just outlined are developed further in the following sections to provide a practical technical and clinical foundation for the effective use of MRI in pediatric and adolescent neuroradiology.

References and additional readings are listed at the end of certain sections to provide more in-depth information concerning adjunctive imaging techniques, contrast agents, artifacts and implants, and spectroscopy.

THE *N* OF NMR: THE NUCLEI

Certain atomic nuclei (N) possess intrinsic spin (rotation along an axis). Those that contain an odd number of protons, neutrons, or both act as magnets; their spinning charge produces a magnetic field with orientation along the axis of spin, forming north and south poles.[2,5] Magnets are vector quantities, having magnitude (field strength) and direction (polarization). Hydrogen (H1), which contains a single proton (+ 1 charge), is the most abundant and strongest of the magnetically active nuclear species (Fig. 1-3), making up greater than 90% of human tissues (primarily water $-OH_2$, lipid $-CH_2$, and so on). Under the relatively weak, external magnetic influence of the earth's gravity, the H1 microscopic magnets (microvectors) contained within tissue voxels spin with random orientations (Fig. 1-4). The magnetic behavior (frequency of spin expressed in megahertz [MHz]) of a nuclear species in the presence of an external magnetic field (units of field strength expressed in tesla [T]) is described by its gyromagnetic ratio (γ)[2,5]; for example, for hydrogen, $\gamma = 42.58$ MHz/T.

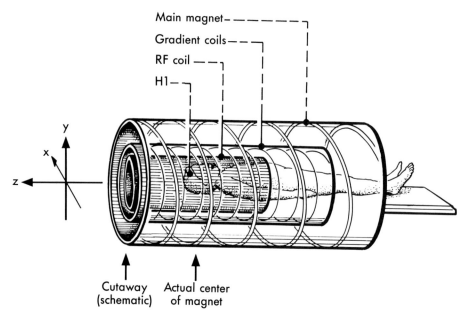

Fig. 1-1   The basic components of the NMR process and MRI system including the H1 *n*uclear magnets of human tissues, the main *m*agnetic field and the gradient *m*agnetic fields, and the radiofrequency *(RF)* coil.

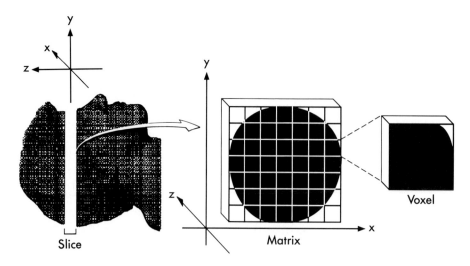

Fig. 1-2   Digital image display in MRI. MRI is a slice and matrix technology with the voxel representing the smallest distinct unit of tissue volume as the basis for intensity and contrast display.

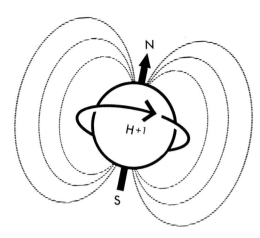

Fig. 1-3 The hydrogen micromagnet. The *N* in NMR, the H1 *n*uclear micromagnet or microvector with specific magnetic behavior described by the gyromagnetic ratio (γ).

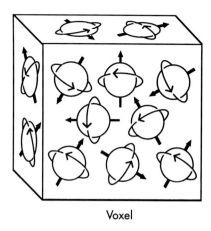

Voxel

Fig. 1-4 Voxel H1 microvectors. The H1 microvectors within tissue voxels spin with random orientations under the influence of gravity only.

THE *M* OF NMR: THE MAIN MAGNETIC FIELD

There are two major components to the *M* in NMR,[5,9] the main magnetic field (discussed in this section) and the gradient magnetic fields (covered in a later section). The main magnetic field (β_o) is a static (unchanging and homogeneous as possible) magnetic field many times the strength of earth's gravity. The β_o (with field strength expressed in tesla, units of magnetic induction) may be provided by large permanent magnets (for example, iron core) or electromagnets (resistive or superconducting). The electromagnet consists of conductor coils (see Fig. 1-1) carrying electric current that induces a magnetic field (Faraday's Law*) along the longitudinal axis (z) of the magnet. Permanent and resistive magnets produce fields of low to intermediate strength (up to approximately 0.3 T), with the field strength of the permanent magnet limited by the magnetic susceptibility (ability to become magnetized) and the magnetic capacity (ability to maintain the magnetic field) of the component material (for example, iron), as well as the weight of the permanent magnet. The field strength of the resistive magnet is limited by the resistance to current flow (heat capacity) of the wire coils. Superconducting magnet coils are composed of special alloys (niobium-titanium), which when supercooled to near-absolute zero within a cryostat of liquid helium (and also liquid nitrogen) essentially lose electrical resistance (superconducting state). Superconducting magnets, therefore, can generate much stronger and more homogeneous magnetic fields (for example, 0.5 to 1.5 T). Higher field strength generates stronger MR signals[6] more efficiently; in addition, external field homogeneity is critical because the MRI process is based on uniform internal magnetic field differences set

up by the gradients for signal encoding. Ideally this encoding should not be obscured by random background (artificial) nonuniformities or inhomogeneities of the external field.

When the patient, the source of the H1 nuclear protons (the *N* in NMR), is placed within the magnet the micromagnets of the patient's tissue voxels (Fig. 1-5) begin to precess (wobble as a spinning top does under gravity influence) along the longitudinal axis (z) of the main field at a rate or frequency (ω_o) characteristic for the nuclear species (H1) according to the Larmor equation[2,5] $\omega_o = \gamma\beta_o$, the product of the gyromagnetic ratio (γ) and the field strength of the external magnetic field (β_o). For example, the Larmor frequency of precession (ω_o) characteristic for H1 (γ = 42.58 MHz/T) in a field (β_o) of 1.5 T is $\omega_o = \gamma\beta_o$ = (42.58 MHz/T) × (1.5 T) = 64 MHz. The hydrogen protons then precess at a rate of 64 MHz, or 64 million cycles (hertz) per second. For a field of 0.3 T, the Larmor frequency is 12.8 MHz; for β_o = 0.5 T, ω_o = 21.3 MHz; for β_o 1.0 T, ω_o = 42.6 MHz.

During this process the H1 proton microvectors reorient themselves, or align along the z-axis of the main magnetic field, either in the north pole (+z) direction, representing a stable lower energy state, or in the opposite, south pole direction (−z), a relatively unstable higher energy state. The H1 microvectors do not align exactly parallel to the z-axis, but rather they align at an angle (θ) because of the torque interaction between the stronger main field and the weaker proton fields, much like that of gravity on a spinning top — the state of precession[2,5] (wobble), also referred to as spin. Furthermore the microvectors are spinning (precessing) with random vector positions (spin phase [ϕ]) for each individual spin orbit (Fig. 1-5). After a brief period more protons are aligned +z than −z, resulting in a net longitudinal magnetization (M_z) vector[2,5] (Fig. 1-6, *A*). When the maximum level of M_z is achieved (usually requiring only a few seconds after placing the patient in the

---

*An electric current within a conductor coil induces a magnetic field perpendicular to the direction of current flow. The converse is also true, that a changing magnetic field induces an electric current within an available conductor coil.

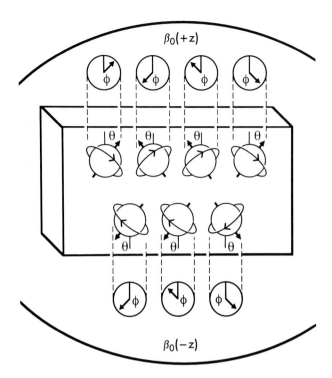

Fig. 1-5 Voxel H1 microvectors within β_o. Within the main magnetic field (β_o) the voxel H1 microvectors align with β_o (+z > −z) with the same spin frequencies (ω_o) and angles (θ) relative to z-axis but with random phases (ϕ).

magnet), the *equilibrium* state (M_o) is reached, which represents the highest level of tissue magnetization for that particular voxel tissue.[2,5,12] In summary, all the H1 protons within the main magnetic field (β_o) at M_z or M_o precess at the same characteristic spin frequency (ω_o) as determined by the Larmor equation ($\omega_o = \gamma\beta_o$), align (+z > −z) at an angle (θ), but with random orbit positions or spin phases (ϕ).

THE *R* OF NMR: RADIOFREQUENCY COIL AND RESONANCE

With the patient (the *N* in NMR) positioned within the magnet (the *M* in NMR) and the equilibrium state (M_o) achieved, a radiofrequency *(RF)* coil,[5,9] encircling (as with a volume head or body coil) or lying tangentially to (as with a surface spine coil) a specified region of interest (ROI) of voxel H1s, is activated (see Fig. 1-1). The RF coil, oriented perpendicularly (in the xy plane) to the longitudinal (z) axis of the main magnet and carrying a specific electric current, transmits secondary magnetic field (β_1) pulses (Faraday's Law) at the characteristic frequency (ω_o) for H1(γ) at the field strength (β_o)—64 MHz at 1.5 T—again according to the Larmor equation, $\omega_o = \gamma\beta_o$. As a result energy is transferred *(excitation* state) to the precessing protons producing transition of protons (resonance condition in quantum mechanic theory) from the lower energy state (+z alignment) to the higher energy state (−z alignment). During the excitation state the voxel H1 microvectors

become focused by the transmitter RF pulses (saturation) and achieve the same spin phases (ϕ) (phase coherence) along with the same spin frequencies ω_o and spin angles (θ) to form a single precessing *macro*scopic magnetization vector[2,5,12] (Fig. 1-6, *B*). This macrovector is deflected 90° by the transmitter RF excitation pulse and spirals into the transverse (xy) plane of the RF coil (Fig. 1-6, *B* and *C*), thus producing transverse magnetization (M_{xy}).[2,5]

When the RF coil is instantaneously switched from transmitter to receiver function (and tuned to the Larmor frequency, ω_o), the momentarily free-precessing macrovector (precessing at ω_o under the influence of the main field [β_o], but free of the transmitter RF pulses [β_1]) induces a voltage (Faraday's Law) in the receiver RF coil (Fig. 1-6, *D*) that is then transformed into the MR signal. This process is known as NMR: *n*uclear (H1 nuclear protons, [γ]) *m*agnetic (main magnet, [β_o]) *r*esonance (RF, β_1 at ω_o = $\gamma\beta_o$). Only RF electromagnetic pulses at the characteristic Larmor frequency will result in the resonance condition and produce the MR signal.

The generated MR signal derived from the free-precessing macrovector has an amplitude (intensity) that progressively decreases (decays) over a short time, and is known as the free induction decay, or FID[2] (Fig. 1-6, *D*). The initial maximum amplitude (intensity) of the FID is directly proportional to the magnitude of the voxel free-precessing macrovector, which in turn is directly related to the proton density and T1 relaxation time. The duration of the FID (decrease in signal over time) reflects the longevity of the free-precessing macrovector, which is related to the T2* and T2 relaxation times. The very brief duration of the FID (usually only a few milliseconds, msec) results from rapid breakdown of the voxel free-precessing macrovector (Fig. 1-6, *C* and *D*) caused by the loss of phase coherence[2] of the component H1 microvectors (proton dephasing) in the xy plane. Therefore, with progressive loss of the macrovector relationship to the RF receiver coil, loss of transverse magnetization (M_{xy}) occurs. The loss of M_{xy} is known as transverse relaxation[2,5] and occurs at the same time that the microvectors realign with the main field (β_o) and regain M_z, which is known as longitudinal relaxation.[2,5] This *relaxation* state results in reversal of the original energy transition with energy release (again, the resonance condition).

The rapid proton dephasing and very brief FID result primarily from external field inhomogeneities (random, disorderly variations in the main field, $\Delta\beta_o$) imposed on and dominating over preexisting, natural intrinsic tissue field variations (variations of intravoxel fields, $\Delta\beta_v$). As a result much wider variations in voxel tissue spin frequencies ($\Delta\omega_v$) and spin phases ($\Delta\phi_v$) occur with artificial acceleration of spin dephasing and loss of a coherent MR signal at the FID time T2*. This usually makes image production by FID impractical. As a partial solution, one or more 180°-refocusing RF pulses (Fig. 1-7) at the characteristic Larmor frequency (ω_o) are applied shortly after the FID within the xy plane to momentarily rephase (to the same ϕ_v)

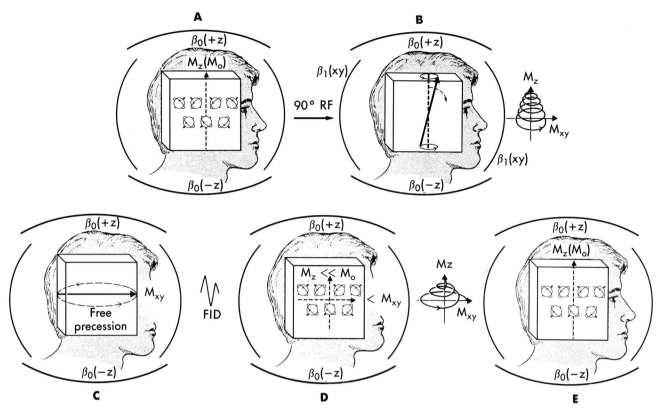

Fig. 1-6   Spin echo—90° RF excitation/relaxation. **A,** The equilibrium state exists when the tissue voxel H1 *micro*vectors (same ω_os and θs but random ϕs) preferentially align ($+z > -z$) with the β_o to produce net longitudinal magnetization (M_z), with M_o representing the maximum level. **B,** The excitation state is produced when RF transmitter coil pulses [β_1 (xy)] at ω_o focus the *micro*vectors (same ω_os, θs, and ϕs) to form a single H1 *macro*vector, which is diverted (**B** and **C**) as a spiralling vector into the xy plane ($\theta = 90°$) resulting in transverse magnetization (M_{xy}). The free-precessing *macro*vector generates the free induction decay *(FID)* via the RF receiver coil while breaking down into component net vectors **(D)**, representing simultaneous recovery of longitudinal magnetization (*micro*vector realignment with β_o) toward the maximum level (M_o) as an increasing vertical vector ($M_z << M_o$), and the loss of transverse magnetization (*micro*vector dephasing) from the original level (M_{xy}) as a decreasing horizontal vector ($< M_{xy}$), while the precessing *macro*vector spirals back toward the original equilibrium **(E)** and the same *micro*vector ω_os and θs, but random ϕs.

the proton microvectors (dephased primarily by the $\Delta\beta_o$) and re-form the free-precessing macrovector, which in turn reinduces receiver coil voltage for NMR signal generation to produce an echo. This process is referred to as the spin echo technique.[2,5,12] The echoes represent the true intrinsic tissue transverse relaxation time, or T2, since the 180°-RF refocusing reverses the T2★ effects.

BASIC INTRINSIC PARAMETERS: PROTON DENSITY AND PROTON RELAXATION

After excitation (RF saturation of spins) and during relaxation (the process of returning toward equilibrium), the free-precessing voxel macrovector (FID or echo) responsible for the detectable MR signal (which can be generated only in the xy plane of the RF coil) and made up of coherently precessing microvectors (same spin frequencies, phases, and angles) rapidly breaks down into two component net vectors (M_z and M_{xy}) representing the two separate but simultaneous relaxation processes (Fig. 1-6, *D*). Lon-

gitudinal relaxation[5,12] is the recovery of longitudinal magnetization (M_z) (spin realignment along z), an increasing vertical net vector ($+z$) over time (usually requiring seconds). Transverse relaxation[5,12] is the loss, or decay, of transverse magnetization (M_{xy}) (spin dephasing in xy plane), a decreasing horizontal net vector ($-xy$) over time (usually on the order of milliseconds). The rate or time for recovery of M_z toward equilibrium (M_o) (Fig. 1-6, *E*) is determined by the rate of proton alignment (after the patient voxel H1s are originally placed within the magnet) or proton *re*alignment (following RF excitation) and is governed by and referred to as T1 (spin-lattice) relaxation time.[2,5,7,12] Depending on field strength (T1s are longer at higher field strength), the time required for recovery of 63% of the equilibrium value (maximum level of tissue magnetization) for a given tissue is designated as 1T1 (for example, cerebrospinal fluid (CSF) 2700 msec, fat 290 msec), 86% recovery as 2T1 (for example, CSF 5400 msec, fat 580 msec), 94% recovery as 3T1, 98% recovery as 4T1,

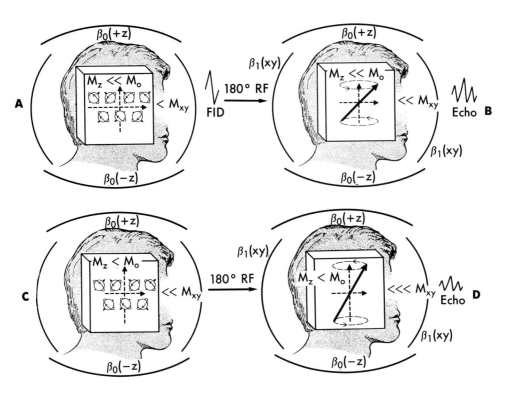

Fig. 1-7   Spin echo—180° RF refocusing. During relaxation (see Fig. 1-6, *D*) with generation of the FID and breakdown of the *macro*vector **(A)**, 180° RF transmitter coil pulses [β_1 (xy)] refocus the *micro*vectors (spin rephasing) to re-form the free-precessing *macro*vector **(B)**, which generates an echo representing $<< M_{xy}$. The re-formed *macro*vector again quickly breaks down **(C)**, but subsequent 180° RF pulses [β_1 (xy)] reestablish the *macro*vector **(D)** and generate a second echo ($<<< M_{xy}$). Notice that during this process there is progressive loss of M_{xy} with decreasing signal amplitude from FID to first echo to second echo at the same time that there is regrowth of M_z, all while the reappearing (refocused) free-precessing *macro*vector spirals back toward equilibrium.

and so forth, in a 1.5-T system (Table 1-1). The maximum level of longitudinal magnetization, M_o, the equilibrium value (100% recovery), obtained by way of T1 relaxation (usually greater than 4T1s), also known as saturation recovery (no RF in the spin system), is directly related to the number of resonating protons per tissue voxel (concentration) and is referred to as the proton (or spin) density (p).[2,5,7,12] For example, white matter has a p of 72% (Table 1-1).

The rate or time for decay of the transverse vector (loss of M_{xy} toward zero) is determined by the rate of proton dephasing (following excitation), that is, the rate of loss of microvector phase coherence in the xy plane, and thus the loss of the free-precessing macrovector (after 180°-RF rephasing and echo generation). This is referred to as T2 (spin-spin) relaxation time,[2,5,7,12] recalling that T2 actually refers to spin dephasing of the echo-generated macrovector and loss of M_{xy} caused by intrinsic tissue field variations, whereas T2* denotes external field variations as the primary cause of artificial spin dephasing of the initial (FID) and subsequent free-precessing macrovectors (echoes). Even

Table 1-1   MR tissue parameters and estimated relative values

Tissue	Proton density (%)*	T1(msec)	T2(msec)
Fat	100	290	60
Gray	84	520	95
White	72	380	85
CSF	100	2700	160

*Expressed as a percentage relative to the tissue with the highest proton density, for example, fat and water (100%).

though the T2*-FID effect may be partially reversed by one or more 180°-RF refocused echoes beyond the original FID, each subsequent echo is of progressively declining amplitude and duration (Fig. 1-7; also see Fig. 1-13), the rate of decline representing the true T2. The time required for loss of 63% of the original M_{xy} for a given tissue is designated as 1T2 (for example, CSF 160 msec, fat 60 msec, and so on), for 86% loss of M_{xy}, 2T2 (for example, CSF 320 msec, fat 120 msec, and so on), 94% loss as 3T2, 98% loss as 4T2, and so forth (Table 1-1). These three intrinsic tissue parameters (T1, p, and T2) are the most important determinants of MR signal brightness (voxel intensity) and contrast (intensity differences between voxels), especially for stationary (nonflowing) tissues.[5,8,12]

THE OTHER *M* OF NMR: THE GRADIENTS

The MR signal generated by the NMR process is spatially defined or encoded as to body region of interest (ROI) by way of the gradient (G) magnetic coils.[5,9,10,12] The gradient coils are superimposed on the static main magnetic field (β_o) in a three-dimensional array (Figs. 1-1 and 1-8) and apply rapidly but orderly changing (pulsed) magnetic fields sequentially along the x, y, and z axes of the main field. The gradients precisely define tissue volume elements (voxels) by slices and pixels (picture elements) arranged in rows and columns of a matrix within each slice[10] (Fig. 1-2). The operator-controlled, rapidly alternating gradient pulses (G_x, G_y, G_z) produce uniform incrementations, or steps ($\Delta\beta_o$), in the main magnetic field, and therefore, frequency steps or bands ($\Delta\omega_o$) along each axis according to the Larmor equation $\Delta\omega_o = \alpha\Delta\beta_o$ (Fig. 1-9).

The slice-selection gradient (Gs), along with the 90°- and 180°- RF pulses (Figs. 1-9 and 1-10, *A*) at the same frequency band ($\Delta\omega_o$), defines slice position, orientation (axial, coronal, sagittal, oblique, and so forth), and thickness (3 mm, 5 mm, 1 cm, and so on). With the patient supine in the magnet and surrounded by the RF and gradient coils (Fig. 1-1) and with the slice-selection gradient applied along the z-axis, Gs(z) defines axial slices. Similarly, when Gs is applied along the y-axis, Gs(y) defines coronal slices, or when applied along the x-axis, Gs(x) defines sagittal slices. After slice selection (for example, axial, Fig. 1-10, *A*) a matrix of pixels is set up within the slice by applying the phase-encoding gradient along the y-axis, Gp(y), to define rows by $\phi = \omega_o t$ (Fig. 1-10, *B*). The frequency-encoding gradient is applied along the x-axis, Gf(x), to define the columns by $\Delta\omega_o$ (Fig. 1-10, *C*). The phase- (ϕ) and frequency- (ω) encoding gradient steps ($\Delta\phi$ and $\Delta\omega_o$, respectively) determine the matrix size (for example, 128 × 256, 192 × 256, 256 × 256, and so forth) and the field of view (FOV), the area of the region of interest displayed (for example, 32 cm FOV, 24 cm FOV, 16 cm FOV, and so on), and thus the pixel position (ϕ_y, ω_x) and size (FOV ÷ matrix). For example, a 25 cm FOV and 256 × 256 matrix provides a 1 mm × 1 mm pixel size, whereas a 25 cm FOV and 256 × 128 matrix gives a 1 mm × 2 mm pixel size. Voxel size (mm³) and position (slice Z and pixel ϕ_y, ω_x) are thus defined, again recalling that each voxel contains hydrogen (H1) proton microvectors "coherently" acting as a single, free-precessing macroscopic magnetic vector (formed by the 90°- and 180°-RF pulses) having magnitude, or intensity (I_v), spin frequency (ω_v), flip angle (θ_v), and spin phase (ϕ_v).

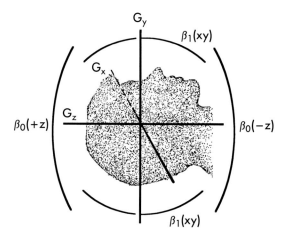

Fig. 1-8 The gradients. The gradient fields (G_x, G_y, G_z) superimposed on the static main field (β_o) and synchronized with the RF pulses [β_1(xy)] define voxels of a matrix within each slice (see Fig. 1-2).

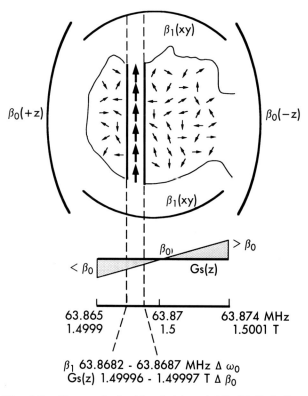

Fig. 1-9 The gradients. The Gs(z) and 90° RF [β_1(xy)] are simultaneously applied with the entire coil receiving RF energy, but only the *micro*vectors at the selected axial slice (1.49996-1.49997 T $\Delta \beta_o$) resonate at a frequency bandwidth (63.8682-63.8687 MHz $\Delta \omega_o$) according to $\Delta \omega_o = \gamma \Delta \beta_o$ and form *macro*vectors, which are diverted 90° into the xy plane.

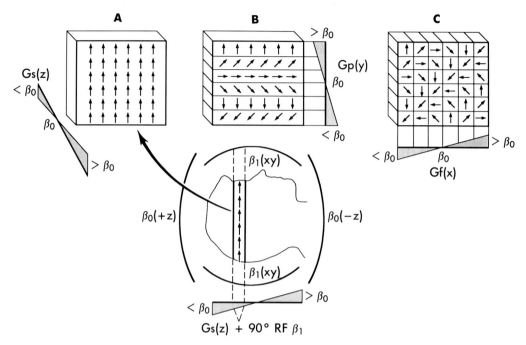

Fig. 1-10   The gradients. The simultaneous application of Gs(z) and 90° RF [β_1(xy)] defines a specific slice **(A)** containing *macro*vectors diverted 90° into the xy plane. The phase-encoding gradient [Gp(y)] is then applied (for example, $\Delta \beta_0$ at 0.1mT/cm), and each row of *macro*vectors in the matrix **(B)** precesses at slightly different rates compared with adjacent rows according to $\Delta \omega_0 = \gamma \Delta \beta_0$. When the Gp(y) is discontinued after a preset time interval (t), all *macro*vectors return to precessing at the same ω_0 but at different ϕs according to their row locations along the y-axis and $\phi = \omega_0 t$. The frequency-encoding gradient [Gf(x)] is then activated **(C)** and each column of *macro*vectors precesses at different ω_0s from adjacent columns, again according to $\Delta \omega_0 = \gamma \Delta \beta_0$. The *macro*vectors are thus encoded by different ω_0s according to their column locations along the x-axis. The voxels of the matrix (6 × 6 in this example) are now defined (ω_x, ϕ_y) within the slice, each with an encoded *macro*vector distinct from its neighbor along each row and column.

SPIN ECHO IMAGING
Basic extrinsic parameters—TR and TE

The spin echo (SE) is the primary pulse-sequencing technique used for brain and spine MRI, especially for providing stationary tissue parameters. Other important but adjunctive techniques include inversion recovery (IR), gradient echo (GE), and chemical shift (CS). The pulse sequence describes the type and timing of the RF and gradient pulses necessary to generate and encode the voxel MR signals. In the SE technique (Fig. 1-11) the initial RF pulse type is the 90° transmitter RF excitation pulse at the Larmor frequency that converts M_z (precessing H1-proton microvectors aligned $+z > -z$ at the same frequency but at random phases) to M_{xy} (saturated, focused, and coherently precessing microvectors of the same phase to form a free-precessing macrovector diverted 90° into the xy plane of the RF coil). The first 90°-RF pulse may convert M_o (equilibrium state, the maximum level of longitudinal magnetization, M_z) to maximum transverse magnetization, M_{xy} (the excitation state), whereas subsequent 90°-RF pulses may convert M_z ($\leq M_o$) to $\leq M_{xy}$, depending on the time spacing of the 90°-RF excitation pulses. This operator-adjustable time spacing, known as the repetition time (TR),[5,12] is the major determinant of the degree of T1 recovery (M_z toward M_o) after each 90°-RF excitation pulse, whether the recovery is incomplete ($M_z < M_o$), the partial saturation state, or complete (M_o), the saturation recovery state (Fig. 1-12).

The second RF pulse type used in the SE sequence is one or more 180°-receiver RF refocusing pulses (Fig. 1-11). This converts the FID (the original 90° focused and diverted free-precessing macrovector, M_{xy}, which decays due to proton microvector dephasing by extrinsic T2* factors) to one or more subsequent echoes (Fig. 1-13) by rephasing the microvectors and reestablishing a coherent, free-precessing macrovector, M_{xy}, which induces RF receiver coil voltage. The MR signal generated reflects the true, intrinsic T2. The degree of decay, or loss of M_{xy}, for a given tissue is determined by the operator-adjustable time spacing of the first and subsequent echoes from the immediately preceding 90°-RF pulse and is referred to as the echo time (TE).[5,12] By varying the TR and TE, the operator may emphasize a certain tissue parameter (T1, p, T2) as the dominant (weighted) determinant of voxel signal brightness and intervoxel contrast (Figs. 1-14 and 1-15).

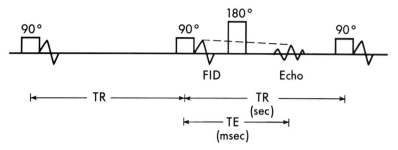

Fig. 1-11   The basic spin echo. The time interval between successive 90° RF pulses is known as the repetition time (TR); the interval between the preceding 90° RF pulse and the subsequent 180° RF-generated echo is the echo time (TE). Notice that the SE sequence begins with a solitary 90° RF excitation pulse to start the T1-recovery process with the TR determining the degree or extent of recovery for either T1, proton density, or T2 imaging. Notice also that the amplitude of the echo is less than that of the original FID (dashed line). Also see Figs. 1-6, 1-7, 1-12, and 1-13.

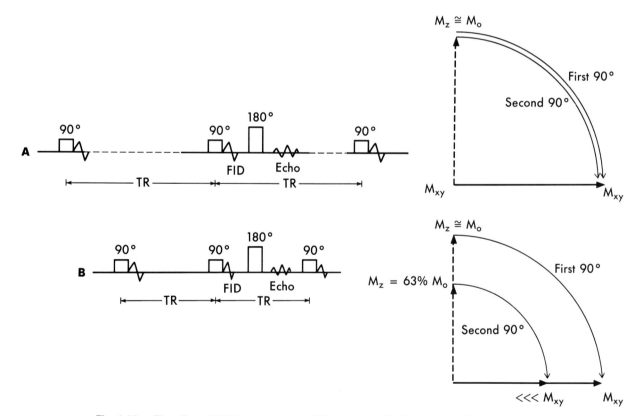

Fig. 1-12   The effect of TR in the spin echo. With very long TR (for example, TR 4000 msec/TE 20 msec) more complete proton realignment (saturation recovery) is allowed after the initial 90° pulse (A) so that subsequent 90° and 180° echo tandems produce maximum signal intensity (M_{xy}) and proton density contrast (short TE) or T2 contrast (long TE). With shorter TR (for example, TR 600 msec/TE 20 msec) proton realignment is incomplete after the initial 90° pulse (partial saturation), and subsequent 90° and 180° echo tandems (B) result in reduced overall signal ($<<< M_{xy}$) but T1 contrast (also see Figs. 1-6 and 1-7).

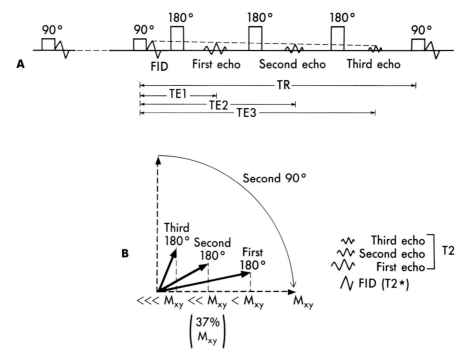

Fig. 1-13   Multiple spin echo imaging. Following the second 90° RF-generated FID (excitation), a series of 180° RF refocusing pulses **(A)** generate subsequent echoes (TE1, TE2, TE3) of progressively declining amplitude and signal intensity but increasing T2 contrast—the rate of amplitude decay *(dashed line)* being related to the true T2 relaxation time. The declining amplitude of each echo (T2) beyond the 90° RF FID (T2*) correlates with sequential 180° RF refocusing of the dephasing *micro*vectors to re-form free-precessing *macro*vectors during relaxation **(B)**, each *macro*vector composed of decreasing net transverse magnetization (M_{xy}) but increasing net longitudinal magnetization (M_z). Also see Fig. 1-7.

Fig. 1-14   CNS tissue contrast curves (T1, p,T2). The T1 relaxation curves for each tissue displayed represent recovery (spin realignment) of longitudinal magnetization along the first vertical axis (M_z) and are derived "indirectly" through the SE technique with echo intensity measurements for each tissue using fixed short TE and varying the TR (see Fig. 1-12). The T2 relaxation curves represent decay (spin dephasing) of transverse magnetization along the second vertical axis (M_{xy}) and are derived "directly" by measuring echo intensities for each tissue using the SE technique with fixed long TR and varying TE (see Fig. 1-13). The TR and T1 scales are in units of seconds, whereas the TE and T2 scales are in milliseconds. The third vertical axis represents the intensity gray scale from dark (low end) to bright (higher end). Along the horizontal axis 90° RF excitation and 180° RF refocusing pulses are displayed along with their respective echoes (vertical dashed lines intersecting the T2 decay curves). Also see Figs. 1-15 and 1-21. **A,** Short TR (0.6 sec) and short TE (20 msec) provide T1-dominant contrast with the following intensity scale: Fat *(F)* > white matter *(W)* > gray matter *(G)* > CSF *(C)*. Notice that short TR and long TE produce poor signal (low end of intensity scale) and poor contrast (convergence of intensity curves). See Figs. 1-15, *A,* and 1-21, *A.* **B,** Intermediate to long TR (2 sec) and short TE (30 msec) provide p-dominant contrast with the following intensity scale: F > G > W > C; with long TE (80 to 120 msec) T2-dominant contrast is provided with the following intensity scale: C > G > W > F. See Figs. 1-15, *B* and *C* and 1-21, *B* and *C.* **C,** Very long TR (4 to 6 sec) and short TE (for example, 30 msec) results in stronger signal and purer p weighting but relatively poor contrast, whereas with long TE (80 to 120 msec) there is purer T2 weighting with excellent contrast but longer imaging times unless the number of signals averaged (NSA) is decreased; also the p echo at this TR may not readily separate flowing $-OH_2$ (CSF) from nonflowing $-OH_2$ (lesion).

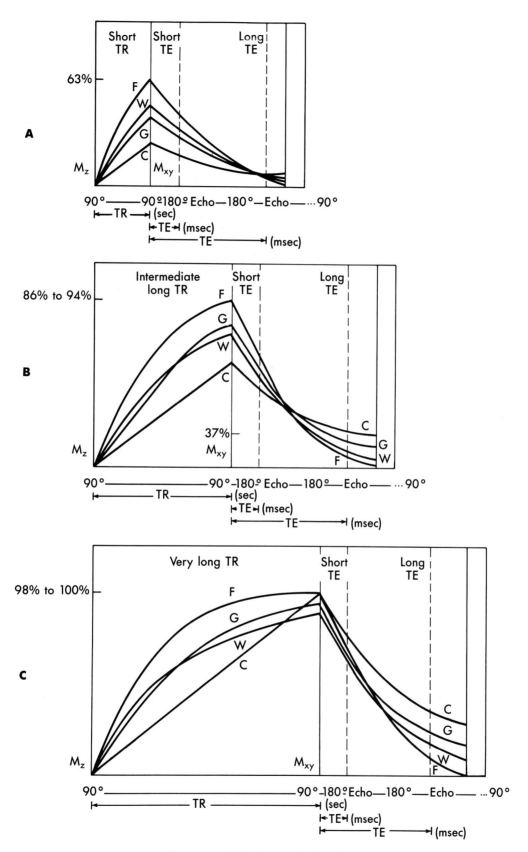

Fig. 1-14 For legend see opposite page.

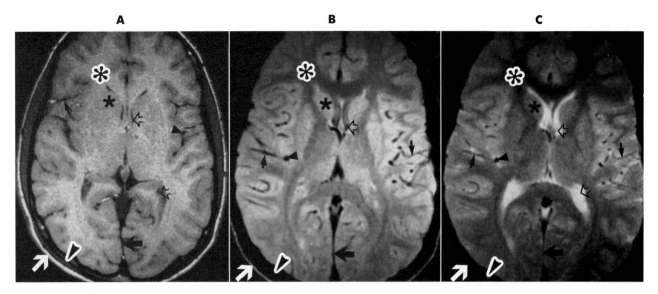

Fig. 1-15   A 15-year-old boy with normal brain MRI including axial T1-dominant image **(A)** (TR 600 msec/TE 20 msec), p-dominant image **(B)** (TR 2000 msec/TE 30 msec), and T2-dominant image **(C)** (TR 2000 msec/TE 80 msec) demonstrating normal intensity pattern for fat *(white arrow)*, white matter *(large asterisk)*, gray matter *(small asterisk)*, ventricular CSF *(open arrow)*, cortical bone *(arrowhead)*, and vascular structures with in-plane flow *(small arrow)* and through-plane flow *(triangle)* and dura *(large arrow)* at the junction of falx and tentorium. See also Fig. 1-14 and box on p. 19.

CNS tissue contrast

Depending on field strength (as previously stated, T1 relaxation times are longer at higher field) relatively short TR (for example, < 800 msec) and short TE (for example, < 30 msec) render T1-dominant images (Figs. 1-14, *A*, and 1-15, *A*), whereas longer TR (for example, > 2000 msec) sequences (Fig. 1-14, *B*) with shorter TE (for example, < 30 msec) give proton density–dominant images (Fig. 1-15, *B*) and with longer TE (for example, > 80 msec), as a second echo, gives T2-dominant images[5,8,12] (Fig. 1-15, *C*). With as short a TE as possible, varying the TR determines T1 (short TR) and proton-density (long TR) weighting. Short TR with long TE provides poor signal and poor contrast. With relatively short TR (between successive 90°-RF excitation pulses), and thus partial proton realignment (partial saturation) with incomplete recovery ($M_z < M_o$), T1 contrast between tissues is emphasized. In fact, the optimum T1 contrast[12] is usually achieved when the selected TR ≤ 1T1 (63% recovery toward M_o) for the voxel tissues studied (Figs. 1-14, *A*, and 1-15, *A*).

With longer TR (> 3T1 to 4T1 and 94% to 98% recovery of M_o) there is more complete proton realignment, with recovery nearing the equilibrium value ($M_z \cong M_o$) and T1 contrast is lost. At this level, contrast is now primarily proton-density determined (Figs. 1-14, *B*, and 1-15, *B*). If the TR is sufficiently prolonged (> 4T1) so that all voxel tissues have fully recovered to M_o, then their intensity differences (Fig. 1-14, *C*) are purely related to their proton density differences (different levels of M_o). However, such very long TR (4 to 6 seconds) may make imaging times

impractical. Furthermore contrast is lost between H1 tissues of different chemical composition but similar proton density (for example, water $-OH_2$ and lipid $-CH_2$), rendering the tissues indistinguishable (isointense). Moreover, the extremely long TR often overcomes flow differences, making flowing $-OH_2$ (for example, CSF) inseparable from nonflowing $-OH_2$ (for example, edema, tumor, and so forth), again, because of their similar proton densities. Therefore intermediate to long TR (2T1 to 3T1) is preferred (Figs. 1-14, *C*, and 1-15, *B*). The short TE minimizes spin dephasing and loss of M_{xy} and therefore minimizes T2 contrast when TE < 1T2 (loss of 63% M_{xy}) for the voxel tissues studied. This is important, therefore, for T1 (short TR/short TE) and proton-density (long TR/short TE) imaging. The optimum T2 contrast[12] (long TR/long TE) is achieved at TE > 1T2 of the voxel tissues examined (Figs. 1-14, *B*, and 1-15, *C*). Since the MR signal can be generated only in the xy plane (by M_{xy}) of the RF coil, T1 contrast is not directly observed, but rather is indirectly generated through the T2 decay process. However, the TR does determine the starting intensity for the T2 decay process (Fig. 1-14), that is, lower overall image intensity for T1 (short TR) images compared with higher overall image brightness for proton-density (long TR) images.

RF/gradient synchronization

As alluded to previously the gradient (G) pulses are applied in sequence (slice-, phase-, and frequency-encoding) and synchronized with the excitation (90°) and refocusing (180°) RF pulses as follows (Fig. 1-16): slice selection (Gs) + 90°-RF pulse at same $\Delta\omega_o$, then phase-

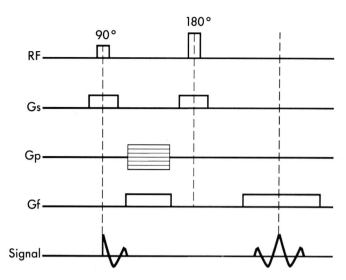

Fig. 1-16   2DFT spin echo RF and gradient pulse sequence profile (see pp. 14 and 15).

are also available for volume acquisitions and three-dimensional display[12] for example, in MR angiography. With the 2DFT method multiple slices may be efficiently acquired through the application of RF/gradient pulses with echo recording for a second set of alternate slices during the relaxation interval following RF/gradient application for the first slice set (multislice acquisition).[12]

REFERENCES
NMR and MRI

1. Axel L: *Glossary of MR terms,* ed 2, Reston, Va, 1986, American College of Radiology.
2. Balter S: An introduction to the physics of magnetic resonance imaging, *Radiographics* 7:371, 1987.
3. Boesch C, Martin E: Combined application of MR imaging and spectroscopy in neonates and children: installation and operation of a 2.35-T system in a clinical setting, *Radiology* 168:481, 1988.
4. Bottomley PA: Human in vivo NMR spectroscopy in diagnostic medicine: clinical tool or research probe? *Radiology* 170:1, 1989.
5. Fullerton GD: Magnetic resonance imaging signal concepts, *Radiographics* 7:579, 1987.
6. Hart HR, Bottomley PA, Edelstein WA, et al: Nuclear magnetic resonance imaging: contrast-to-noise ratio as a function of strength of magnetic field, *AJR* 141:1195, 1983.
7. Kjos BO, Ehman RL, Brant-Zawadzki M, et al: Reproducibility of relaxation times and spin density calculated from routine MR imaging sequences: clinical study of the CNS, *AJNR* 6:271, 1985.
8. Merritt CRB: Magnetic resonance imaging—a clinical perspective: image quality, safety and risk management, *Radiographics* 7:1001, 1987.
9. Pavlicek W: MR instrumentation and image formation, *Radiographics* 7:809, 1987.
10. Sprawls P: Spatial characteristics of the MR image. In Stark DD, Bradley WG, editors: *Magnetic resonance imaging,* St Louis, 1988, Mosby–Year Book.
11. Villafana T: Fundamental physics of magnetic resonance imaging, *Radiol Clin North Am* 26:701, 1988.
12. Wehrli FW, MacFall JR, and Newton TH: Parameters determining the appearance of NMR images. In Newton TH, Potts DG, editors: *Advanced imaging techniques,* San Anselmo, Calif, 1984, Clavadel.

encoding gradient (Gp), and frequency-encoding gradient (Gf), followed by reapplication of the Gs with the 180°-RF pulse (same $\Delta\omega_o$), then finally reapplication of the frequency-encoding (readout) gradient (Gf) with echo generation.[2,12] This entire RF/gradient cycle (of only a few milliseconds) must be repeated with varying amplitude for each phase-encoding gradient application (128, 256, and so on). Furthermore, to improve signal intensity, each entire "set" of RF/gradient cycles may be repeated and two or more excitations or measurements of each voxel signal (echo) averaged (number of signals averaged, or NSA). The total acquisition time (T)[9] may then be calculated by [TR] $\times$ [ϕ—matrix] $\times$ [NSA]. For example, for double-echo p T2 SE (2000/30, 80) with TR 2000 msec (and echoes of 30 msec and 80 msec), matrix of 128 (ϕ) $\times$ 256 (ω), and NSA of 2, T = (2000 msec), $\times$ (128) $\times$ (2) $\div$ 60 sec/min = 8 min 32 sec; or for T1 SE (600/20) with TR 600 msec (TE 20 msec), matrix 256 (ϕ) $\times$ 512 (ω), and NSA = 4, T = (600 msec) $\times$ (256) $\times$ (4) $\div$ 60 sec/min = 10 min 15 sec.

The Fourier transform

The voltage (analog signal) induced in the RF receiver by the echo, consisting of amplitude versus time, is converted by the two-dimensional Fourier transform (2DFT) as intensity versus frequency (digital signal) for display. The Fourier transform[2,12] is the acquisition and reconstruction computer algorithm that analyzes and records the MR signal intensities according to phase (ϕ) and frequency (ω), much like a prism separates white light into component colors of the rainbow (by frequency differences) for the human eye, or similar to the cochlear mechanism of the ear with its own 2DFT to distinguish individual voices of a choir or instruments of an orchestra by pitch (ω), tempo (ϕ), and loudness (intensity). Three-dimensional (3DFT) algorithms

Biomechanisms

STATIONARY TISSUES
Basic elements

Biological formulation of spin echo–MR signal patterns requires separate consideration for stationary tissues (fat, gray and white matter, bone, tumor, edema, and so forth) and flowing tissues (CSF, vascular, cyst, collections, and so on),[31,59,76,94,95] both normal and abnormal (see box on p. 16 and Fig. 1-17). For stationary tissues the intensities are determined by molecular and magnetic proton interactions (T1, p, T2) within the voxel (intravoxel). For flowing tissues the signals are primarily or additionally influenced by tissue movement (proton flow) through slices (transvoxel) and across voxels (intervoxel), as discussed in the next section. Furthermore, normal and abnormal stationary tissue states are usually composed of one or a combination of basic tissue elements[13,31,59] including fat ($-CH_2$), water ($-OH_2$), macromolecular matrix (for example, protein, $-NH_2$), or mineralization (for example, calcium and iron). Water is the dominant component in most instances and probably exists in primarily one of two biological forms—

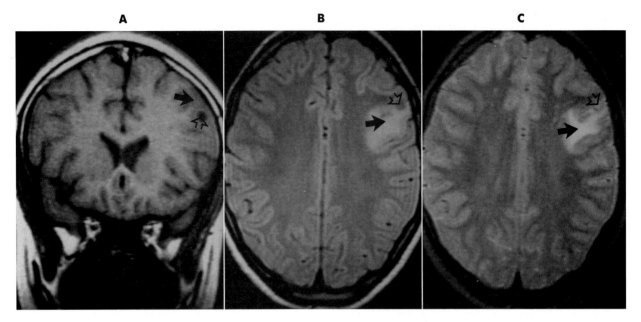

Fig. 1-17   An 8-year-old boy with focal seizure and left frontal cerebral infarction. MRI demonstration *(black arrow)* of nonflowing intracellular and extracellular free $-OH_2$ (infarction with edema) as low intensity on coronal T1 **(A)** and high intensity on axial p **(B)** and T2 **(C)** images. Flowing, extracellular free $-OH_2$ is demonstrated *(open arrow)* within an atrophic defect as low intensity on T1 **(A)** and p **(B)** images, and high intensity on T2 **(C)** images similar to ventricular and subarachnoid CSF. See also Fig. 1-18 and box on p. 16.

BIOLOGICAL BASIS OF PROTON RELAXATION

I. STATIONARY TISSUE ELEMENTS (*I*, INTENSITY)

A. Free $-OH_2$: T1, low I; T2, high I
  1. Extracellular (EC free $-OH_2$): stagnant blood, disk space, edema (vasogenic, interstitial), epidermoid (aqueous form of cholesterol)
  2. Intracellular (IC free $-OH_2$): gray matter, edema (cytotoxic), neoplasm, infarction, demyelination
B. Bound $-OH_2$ (Hydrous matrix: matrix $-OH_2$)
  1. Extracellular (EC matrix $-OH_2$): T1 shortening dominates (T1, iso-high I; T2, high I): abscess, empyema, hygroma, colloid cyst, Rathke's cyst, neurenteric cyst, craniopharyngioma, cystic or necrotic glioma, mucinous metastasis
  2. Intracellular (IC matrix): T2 shortening dominates (T1, variable I; T2, low I): white matter, hypercellular neoplasm (for example, lymphoma)
C. Anhydrous or anisotopic hydrous matrix: T1 and T2, low I: muscle, collagen, fibrin, keratin, mucin, colloid, ligament, dura, fibrocartilage

D. Fat: T1, high I; T2, low I: subcutaneous, epidural, marrow, lipoma, hamartoma, dermoid, teratoma, pantopaque (exception: the aqueous form of cholesterol in epidermoid and cholesterol cyst, renders T1, low I; T2, high I)
E. Mineralization and hemorrhage (proton relaxation enhancement)

II. FLOWING TISSUE ELEMENTS (EXTRACELLULAR FREE $-OH_2$)*

A. Blood
  1. Arterial
    a. Systole
    b. Diastole
  2. Venous
B. Cerebrospinal fluid (CSF)
  1. Bulk flow (CSF production/absorption)
  2. Pulsatile flow (transmitted arterial/venous pulsations)

*Intensity patterns depend on flow factors.

---

free or bound.[31,59,75,94] The molecular and magnetic character of free water (free $-OH_2$) is relatively unrestricted (for example, CSF and edema) in the absence of other tissue elements (Fig. 1-17). Macromolecular binding or structuring of water (hydration or bound $-OH_2$) alters the proton relaxation (T1,T2) of the bound $-OH_2$ whether it is intracellular (for example, the protein matrix of a neoplasm) or extracellular (for example, a proteinaceous collection). Often the different forms of water are in a state of continual exchange or equilibrium.

Spin-lattice (T1) relaxation

T1 (spin-lattice) relaxation (recovery of M_z) involves the exchange of energy between the relaxing, realigning protons (H1 spins) and their intravoxel molecular environment (lattice: water $-OH_2$, lipid $-CH_2$, protein $-NH_2$, and so forth) as related to molecular size, structure, motion, and collision[31,59,94] (Fig. 1-18). The closer the motional frequency (rotational, translational) or tumbling rate of the molecules to the Larmor frequency of H1 at a given field strength, the more efficient the energy exchange (spin-to-

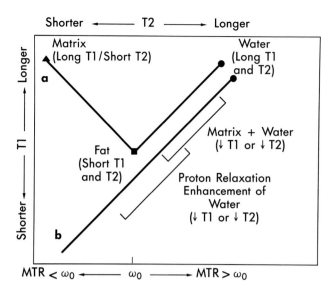

Fig. 1-18 Molecular basis for proton relaxation (intravoxel). The T1 and T2 relaxation times of the major tissue elements (fat [*square*], matrix, for example, protein [*triangle*], water [*circle*], and matrix + water) are depicted (*line a*) according to their molecular behavior (molecular tumbling rates, *MTR*) relative to the Larmor frequency for H1 (ω_o). Notice that the closer the MTR to ω_o the shorter the T1 (for example, fat), and the more remote the MTR relative to ω_o the longer the T1 (for example, matrix [MTR $< \omega_o$] and water [MTR $> \omega_o$]). The T2 of the elements relative to MTR is also shown. Also notice (*line b*) that the combination of matrix + water (see text) may shorten the T1 and T2 of the water component. A similar profound effect may also be observed (*line b*) with proton relaxation enhancement (PRE) by paramagnetic and magnetically susceptible substances.

lattice) and the faster and higher the M_z recovery toward M_o (fat, CH2). This is reflected by a shorter T1 relaxation time producing a stronger voxel MR signal (higher intensity, hyperintense, or increased brightness) relative to tissues of longer T1 on short TR/TE sequences. The higher the motional frequency (free $-OH_2$: CSF and edema) or lower the motional frequency (solid macromolecules or macromolecular matrix: protein and carbohydrate) relative to the ω_o of H1, the less efficient the energy exchange and the slower and less complete the M_z toward M_o. This is represented by a longer T1 and the production of a relatively weaker signal (lower intensity, hypointense, decreased brightness) on short TR/TE sequences.

Spin-spin (T2) relaxation

T2 (spin-spin) relaxation (decay of M_{xy}) represents the magnetic interaction among spins (processing H1 protons) as influenced by natural fluctuations (variations, inhomogeneities, nonuniformities) in local (intravoxel) tissue magnetic fields[31,59,95] (Fig. 1-18) and does not involve the exchange of energy per se. Such variations in local fields ($\Delta\beta_v$) produce changing proton precessional frequencies ($\Delta\omega_v$) and thus proton phase changes ($\Delta\phi_v$) with resultant spin dephasing and loss of coherence, including breakdown of the macrovector within the xy plane and loss of the MR signal. The more flexible or mobile molecular structures

(free $-OH_2$) with weaker and more homogeneous magnetic fields result in slower proton dephasing (longer maintained precessional coherence) and slower M_{xy} decay. This is reflected as longer T2 with stronger and longer sustained macrovector, echo, and signal (higher intensity, hyperintense, increased brightness) on long TR/TE sequences as opposed to tissues with shorter T2. The more rigid or fixed molecular structures (macromolecular matrix) with stronger, fixed magnetic fields and greater field variation (inhomogeneities), or structures associated with anisotropic[31,59] motion of water (discordant motion between $-OH_2$ and matrix), produce faster and more complete spin dephasing and faster M_{xy} decay. This is represented by a shorter T2 relaxation time with more rapid loss of coherent signal (lower intensity, hypointense, decreased brightness, or signal void) on long TR/long TE sequences. Fatty tissues, in general, have intermediate to short (relatively efficient) T2 relaxation.

Proton density

Proton density, or spin density (p), affects MR signal intensity so that tissues of higher p (higher voxel concentration of resonating H1 spins) are associated with a higher maximum level of tissue magnetization (M_o) and stronger signal (fat, nonflowing free $-OH_2$) than tissues of lower p (protein matrix and calcium) on long TR/short TE sequences.

Combined elements

Frequently, combining tissue components results in molecular and magnetic alterations that produce shortening of the T1 and T2 relaxation times[31,59,94] (Fig. 1-18). This is observed with macromolecular (protein, carbohydrate, mucoprotein, glycoprotein, and so forth) binding or structuring of water, forming a hydrous macromolecular matrix (matrix $-OH_2$). "Paradoxical" shortening of the T1 of the bound $-OH_2$ may result (decreased T1, therefore increased signal intensity relative to CSF) along with shortening of the T2 (decreased T2, therefore decreased intensity relative to CSF). With intracellular matrix $-OH_2$ (for example, cellular neoplasm) the T2 shortening may predominate.[59] The lesion core, therefore, may be of variable (iso-, low, or high) intensity on T1 (short TR/TE) images but of relatively low intensity on T2 (long TR/TE) images (Fig. 1-19) as contrasted especially with the higher intensity (long T2) of associated intracellular or extracellular free $-OH_2$ (for example, edema). Often, however, with extracellular matrix $-OH_2$ the T1-shortening effect dominates over the T2-shortening effect and produces higher starting intensity from which T2 decay proceeds, thus resulting in net signal increase.[59] This is observed with neoplastic, inflammatory, and other types of proteinaceous fluid collections or cysts (Fig. 1-20), as well as with some paramagnetic substances (gadolinium (Gd)-DTPA). In general, the greater the matrix component (for example, protein) in the matrix OH2, the more dominant the T2 shortening effect (lower intensity on T2 or on both T1 and T2 images). With lesser matrix concentrations, the more dominating the T1-shortening

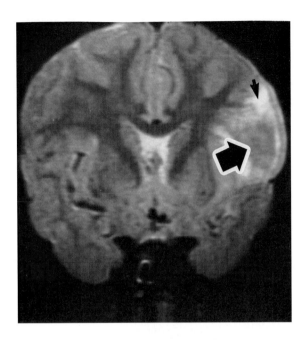

Fig. 1-19 A 4-year-old girl with focal seizures and left frontal cerebral primitive neuroectodermal tumor (PNET). T2 coronal MRI shows central low intensity tumor "core" *(large arrow)* with surrounding high intensity tumor plus edema *(small arrow)*. Also see Fig. 1-18 and box on p. 16.

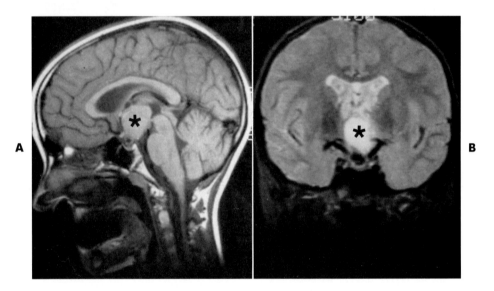

Fig. 1-20 An 8-year-old girl with short stature, visual difficulties, and headache with proteinaceous cystic craniopharyngioma. MRI shows isointense to hyperintense suprasellar mass *(asterisk)* on sagittal T1 image **(A)** with marked hyperintensity *(asterisk)* on coronal T2 image **(B)**. Also see Fig. 1-18 and box on p. 16.

effect (higher intensity on T1 and T2 images).

In summary, stationary (nonflowing) tissues of shorter T1 with faster proton realignment and M_z recovery toward M_o (fat, white matter, and proteinaceous collection) are of higher intensity than those of longer T1 with slower realignment and recovery (CSF, edema, gray matter, muscle, and collagen) on short TR/TE sequences (Figs. 1-15, *A*, 1-20, and 1-21, *A*). Tissue elements with higher p and higher level of M_o (fat, gray matter, edema, and so on) are of higher signal intensity than those of lower p with lower level of M_o (white matter, calcium, keratin, ligament, and dura) on long TR/short TE images (Figs. 1-15, *B*, and 1-21, *B*). Substances of longer T2 (slower spin dephasing and longer coherent M_{xy} macrovector) are of higher intensity (CSF, edema, gray matter, and proteinaceous collection) on long TR/TE sequences (Figs. 1-15, *C*, 1-19, 1-20, and 1-21, *C*) than those of shorter T2 (faster spin dephasing, shorter macrovector) with relative signal decrease or signal loss (fat, white matter, and hypercellular neoplasm).

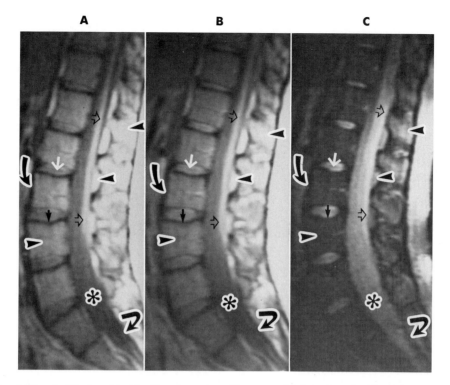

Fig. 1-21   A 16-year-old girl with urinary incontinence and tethered cord with thickened filum demonstrated by MRI including normal intensity patterns on **(A)** sagittal T1-dominant image (TR 600 msec/TE 20 msec), **(B)** p-dominant image (TR 2000 msec/TE 30 msec), and **(C)** T2-dominant image (TR 2000 msec/TE 80 msec) for subcutaneous, epidural, and marrow fat *(arrowhead)*, spinal cord *(open arrow)*, disk space *(white arrow)*, CSF *(asterisk)*, dura *(elbow arrow)*, ligament *(curved arrow)*, and cortical bone *(small arrow)*. Also see box below.

FLOWING TISSUES: PROTON FLOW

Different TR/TE settings afford correspondingly different tissue contrast scales for the brain and spine based on T1 (short TR/TE), p (long TR/short TE), or T2 (long TR/TE) as the dominant SE-contrast parameters for ordering of tissues along a signal-intensity continuum (see box at right). This ordering is relatively constant for the stationary tissues but varies for the flowing tissues (vascular, CSF, and so on) because of complex flow influences* (tissue movement through and across voxels).

Lower intensity flow signal

Flowing tissues (see box on p. 20) tend to be of low intensity[7,8,10] or signal void relative to stationary tissues within the slice when (1) flow is high velocity, turbulent (spin dephasing), or saturated (RF excitation), (2) when flow direction is either perpendicular or oblique through the slice plane, and (3) particularly when flow is parallel or oblique *within* the slice plane. Flowing spins directed perpendicularly or obliquely through the slice at flow rates exceeding the time interval between exposure to the 90°- and 180°-RF pulses at $\omega_o = \gamma\beta_o$ specific for the slice (slice-selection gradient) appear low intensity or without

---

*References 7, 8, 10, 16, 57, 83.

CNS TISSUE SCALES—SPIN ECHO*

T1: TR < 800 msec / TE < 30 msec (short TR/TE)
Fat > WM > GM > Disk > Muscle > CSF† > Calcium ‡ > Vascular †
p: TR > 2000 msec / TE < 30 msec (long TR/short TE)
Fat > GM > Disk > WM > Muscle > CSF† > Calcium ‡ > Vascular †
T2: TR > 2000 msec / TE > 80 msec (long TR/TE)
Disk > CSF† > GM > WM > Fat > Muscle > Calcium‡ > Vascular †

WM, White matter; *GM,* gray matter.
*See Figs. 1-14, 1-15, and 1-21; cord GM/WM may differ from brain GM/WM.
†Intensity depends on flow factors.
‡Includes cortical bone, ligament, and dura.

signal (signal void). This is known as time-of-flight signal loss and is seen with systolic arterial flow (Fig. 1-15) and vascular-pulsatile CSF flow. Also, because of the orderly changing phase- and frequency-encoding gradients (Figs. 1-15 and 1-21), proton flow, either vascular (arterial or venous), or CSF (pulsatile or bulk), within the slice volume is of low intensity because of the continual spin dephasing (phase loss) of the protons flowing from voxel to voxel

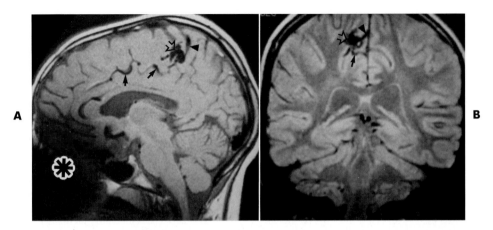

Fig. 1-22   A 12-year-old girl with asymptomatic cerebral arteriovenous malformation shown by MRI with high velocity, turbulent flow producing signal void on sagittal T1 **(A)** and coronal p **(B)** images including arterial feeder *(black arrows)*, nidus *(open arrow)*, and venous drainer *(triangle)*. Also notice ferromagnetic signal loss from dental braces *(asterisk)* in **A**. See box below.

PROTON FLOW (f)—SPIN ECHO

I. LOW INTENSITY OR SIGNAL VOID (T1, p, or T2)

  A. Flow variants
    1. In-plane arterial, venous, and bulk CSF (except T2) flow
    2. Through-plane high velocity, turbulent, saturated, or presaturated arterial, venous, or CSF flow
    3. Perivascular CSF
  B. Flow abnormalities
    1. Arteriovenous malformation (high flow, for example, arteriovenous shunt)
    2. Aneurysm, dissection
    3. Accentuated pulsatile CSF
      a. Hydrocephalus
      b. Hydrosyringomyelia
    4. Vascular occlusive disease
      a. Stenotic turbulence
      b. Collaterals
      c. Fibrin clot (for example, arterial)
      d. Deoxyhemoglobin clot (for example, venous or arterial aneurysm or dissection)

II. ISOINTENSITY TO HIGH INTENSITY (T1, p, or T2)

  A. Flow variants
    1. Venous or CSF entry slice enhancement
    2. Even echo rephasing
    3. Diastolic gating
    4. Pseudodiastole
    5. Gradient moment nulling
  B. Flow deficit
    1. Arterial occlusive
      a. Intraluminal (for example, stenosis [absent signal void] or aneurysm [methemoglobin clot])
      b. Extraluminal (for example, dissection [methemoglobin clot])
    2. Venous occlusive (methemoglobin clot)

---

across rows and columns of the matrix. Only on T2 (long TR/TE) sequences will the longer T2 of bulk CSF overcome its flow character (low intensity on T1 and p images) to produce higher signal intensity (Figs. 1-15, *C*, and 1-21, *C*).

Nonlaminar or turbulent flow[8] (arterial, venous, CSF, and so on) also promotes spin dephasing with signal loss. This is observed with arterial bifurcations, arteriovenous malformation (AVM) (Fig. 1-22), aneurysm,[8,52,86] and pulsatile CSF in hydrocephalus or hydrosyringomyelia.[10,16,32,82,84] Spins having received the 90°-RF excitation pulse and having incompletely recovered during relaxation are referred to as saturated or partially saturated. When flowing through (entering or leaving) the slice these spins are also of low intensity or signal void relative to the stationary tissues within the slice. This occurs for flow between slices during a multislice acquisition. Presaturation is the application of 90°-RF pulses to tissues immediately outside the specifically defined slice of interest (or multislice set) in the direction of flow (arterial, venous, or both) to saturate the flowing spins and render them without signal (signal void) as the spins flow through the slice. This flow-compensation technique helps eliminate entry slice flow-enhancement artifact and reduce pulsatile flow artifacts and flow-induced phase-shift artifacts along the phase-encoding gradient,[48,49,78] alone or combined with other methods such as gradient moment nulling.

Pulsatile CSF flow through narrow passages (aqueduct, foramina of Monro, fourth ventricular outlet foramina, and so forth), especially accentuated in obstructive hydrocephalus[10,32,84] (Fig. 1-23), often appears void of signal, even on long TR/TE sequences, as compared with other areas of ventricular or cisternal CSF bulk flow (related to CSF production/absorption dynamics). This pulsatile CSF flow void is caused by accentuated to-and-fro acceleration of CSF through narrow channels from transmitted systolic cerebral and choroid arterial pulsations. Such flow voids may produce phase-shift artifacts (Fig. 1-24). Pulsatile

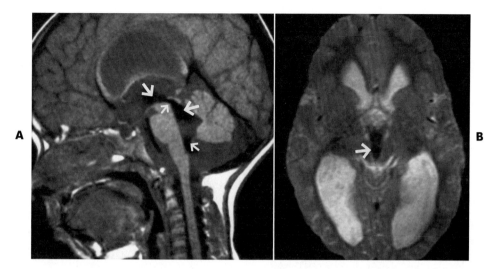

Fig. 1-23   4-year-old girl with increasing head circumference and nonspecific ventriculomegaly shown by CT. MRI shows fourth, third, and lateral ventricular dilation with accentuated pulsatile CSF flow signal voids *(arrows)* at the outlet foramina of the fourth ventricle, the aqueduct, the rostral fourth ventricle, and the posterior third ventricle on sagittal T1 **(A)** and axial T2 **(B)** images, all consistent with obstructive hydrocephalus. Notice the clarity of low intensity basilar artery **(A)** contrasted with the gray-appearing CSF using presaturation. Also notice the paucity of phase-shift artifacts **(B)** from the pulsatile third ventricle CSF flow void using gradient moment nulling. See box on p. 20.

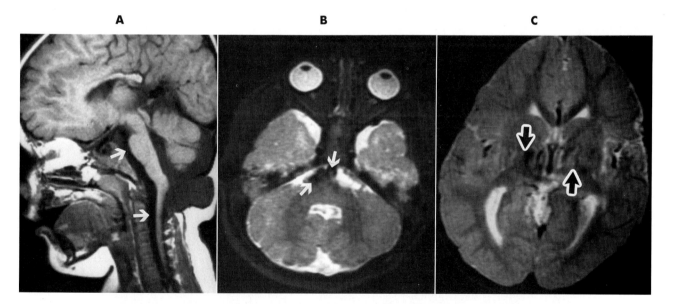

Fig. 1-24   A 2-year-old boy with macrocephaly and cervicooccipital meningocele. MRI shows accentuated CSF signal void *(white arrows)* ventral to brain stem and anterior to cervical cord along the course of the obscured vertebral, basilar, and anterior spinal arteries on sagittal T1 **(A)** and axial T2 **(B)** images. **C,** Axial T2 image shows accentuated third ventricular pulsatile CSF void *(black arrows)* with phase-shift artifacts (along the phase-encoding gradient). The T1 sagittal image was acquired without presaturation, whereas the axial T2 image was acquired without gradient moment nulling. See box on p. 20.

A   **B**

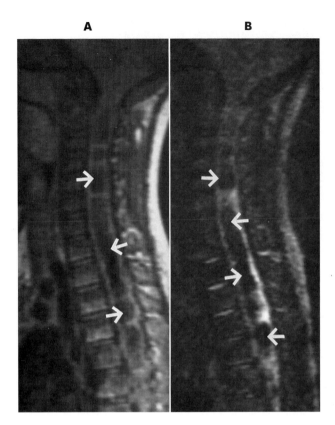

Fig. 1-25   A 3-year-old boy with paraparesis and hydrosyringomy-elia associated with lower cord astrocytoma. Sagittal p **(A)** and T2 **(B)** MRI show cervical cord expansion with saccular hydrosyringo-myelia exhibiting low intensity **(A)** and signal void **(B)** pulsatile intramedullary CSF flow *(arrows)*. See box on p. 20.

turbulent flow voids are often also seen, particularly with obstructive hydrocephalus, in ventricular and cisternal areas at and just beyond the entry or exit sites (Fig. 1-23) of the narrow passages (for example, posterior third ventricle preaqueductal, rostral fourth ventricle postaqueductal, and the like). Furthermore CSF protons in the subarachnoid spaces contiguous to arterial structures often undergo systolic, pulsatile dephasing that produces perivascular CSF signal loss and may exaggerate arterial dimensions (pseu-doectasia or pseudoaneurysm effect) especially along the basilar artery ventral to the brain stem and spinal arteries about the cord (Fig. 1-24). Transmitted accentuated arterial or venous pulsations may often produce a similar CSF signal void effect in the spinal canal,[10,16,69,70,85] especially in obstructive hydrosyringomyelia[28,82] (Fig. 1-25). Some of these effects may be partially or completely reversed with the use of flow-compensation techniques, which often provide sharper vascular and neural contours and a more homogeneous (grayer) appearance of the CSF (compare Fig. 1-23, *A* with Fig. 1-24, *A*).

Higher intensity flow signal

Normal laminar slow flow (usually venous and occasion-ally CSF) may be of relative high intensity (flow-related enhancement)[8,51] when the flow is directed perpendicularly or obliquely when entering a single slice or when entering the first or last slice (entry slice effect) of a multislice sequence. The resulting high intensity may have variable penetration into interior slices, depending on whether flow direction is the same or opposite to that of slice acquisition (Figs. 1-26 and 1-27). The high intensity intraluminal signal is the result of nonturbulent flow of fully magnetized

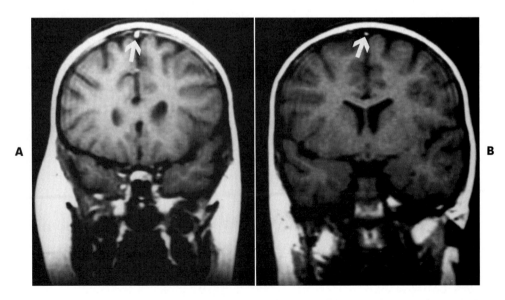

Fig. 1-26   A 4-year-old boy with normal T1 coronal MRI (**A** and **B**) of a multislice set demonstrating superior sagittal venous sinus entry slice enhancement *(arrows)* as high intensity across the entire vessel on the first slice **(A)** with central luminal high intensity seen on a deeper slice **(B)**, all as related to laminar flow with higher velocity and deeper penetration centrally. See box on p. 20.

protons (nonsaturated) originating outside of and flowing into the partially saturated slice at a rate (time of flight) that allows exposure to both the 90°- and 180°-RF pulses, resulting in an echo from fully recovered (M_o) protons (proton-density effect). This effect is most often seen with T1 (short TR/TE) images (occasionally with p and T2 sequences, especially for CSF flow enhancement) in which the stationary tissues within the slice are already partially saturated and of relatively lower intensity compared with the inflowing high intensity unsaturated protons. Again, this may be partially or completely eliminated (along with phase-shift artifacts) if the presaturation technique is applied along the direction of vascular or CSF flow, for example, above the axial slice to saturate venous flow (dural sinus, caval, jugular) and below to saturate arterial flow (aortic, carotid).

Relatively high signal intensity[8] of normal flowing tissues may occasionally be observed on p and T2 images related to incidental (physiological) or intentional (programmed) application of RF/gradient pulses. This includes even-echo rephasing, diastolic or pseudodiastolic gating, and gradient moment nulling. Flowing spins dephased and of low intensity through the initial 180° RF–generated echo (odd-echo dephasing) of a spin echo sequence may be rephased and made into high intensity spins by a subsequent echo applied as an even multiple of the first echo (TEs 20 and 40 msec, 30 and 60 msec, and so on). Also, timing of the TR to diastole either intentionally (cardiac gating) or coincidentally (pseudogating) may render the momentarily non- or slow-flowing spins (for example, stagnant arterial blood or stagnant CSF) as high intensity on p and T2 images (low intensity on T1 images).[25-27] Gradient moment nulling

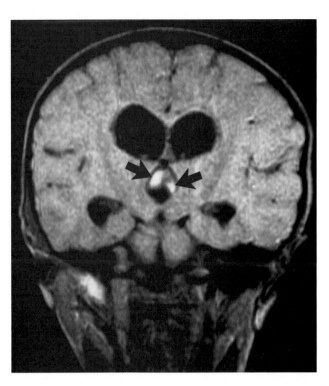

Fig. 1-27 A 4-year-old boy with posterior fossa tumor and obstructive hydrocephalus with accentuated third ventricular CSF flow and unusual entry slice enhancement *(arrows)* on the first slice of a T1 coronal multislice series. Similar phenomena may occasionally be seen as a normal flow variant in the aqueduct, ventricular foramina, or subarachnoid spaces (especially about the brain stem or cord). See box p. 20.

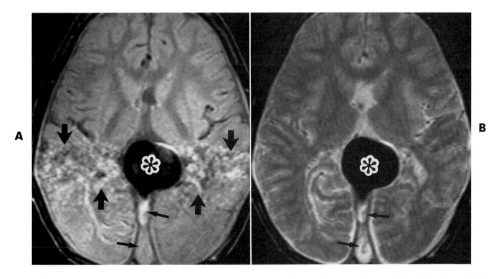

Fig. 1-28 A 6-year-old boy for follow-up of Galenic AVM and hydrocephalus after shunting. MRI demonstrates large turbulent vascular flow signal void *(asterisk)* within the vein of Galen aneurysm (or varix) and phase-shift artifacts *(large arrows)* on the axial p image **(A). B,** The artifacts are dramatically reduced on axial T2 image using gradient moment nulling. High intensity slow vascular flow and partial thrombosis are seen within the midline anomalous venous sinus posteriorly *(thin arrows)*. See box on p. 20.

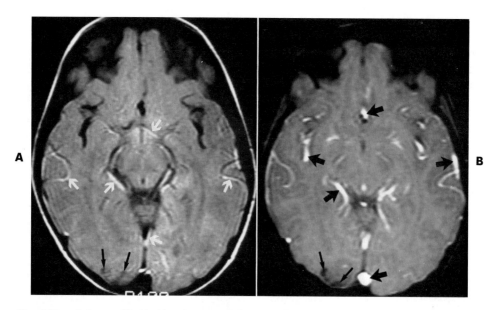

Fig. 1-29 A 4-year-old girl with seizures and abnormal right occipital cerebral high densities on CT. **A,** Axial p spin echo MRI demonstrates nonspecific right occipital low intensities *(black arrows)*. **B,** gradient echo sequence demonstrates magnetic susceptibility (T2*) signal loss consistent with calcification *(thin arrows)* ruling out vascular cause of the low intensities. Normal vascular highlighting is demonstrated elsewhere *(large arrows)*. Notice the vascular high-intensity edge effect due to gradient moment nulling (GMN) in **A** *(white arrows)*. See Tables 1-2 and 1-3 and Figs. 1-18 and 1-44.

(GMN) is a gradient form of flow compensation (presaturation is an RF form of flow compensation): an extra gradient pulse is applied in reverse direction to the original (usually slice-selection) gradient to rephase flowing spins dephased by the original gradient.[25,41,48,67,71] This results in relatively increased intensity and uniformity of signal (especially venous and CSF) while minimizing or eliminating flow-related, phase-shift artifacts (compare Fig. 1-23, *B* with 1-24, *C;* Fig. 1-28). Minor phase/frequency shift edge effect may be apparent, however, along vascular, especially venous, structures (Fig. 1-29).

Vascular occlusive phenomena

Flow deficit in occlusive vascular disease may produce a variety of intraluminal signal abnormalities depending on the sequence (T1,p,T2), the plane and direction of the section acquisition relative to flow direction and velocity, the vessel type (arterial versus venous), and the nature and timing of the occlusive process (stenosis, thrombosis, embolism, dissection, collaterals, and so forth). Slow or nonflowing blood (plasma plus cellular elements) alone may give signal abnormalities similar to nonflowing, extracellular $-OH_2$ (low intensity on T1 images, high intensity on p and T2 images) whether flow direction is through or within the slice and depending on flow rate (time of flight) relative to the slice acquisition time (Fig. 1-28). Slow arterial flow perpendicular or oblique to the slice plane may theoretically produce flow-related enhancement (high intensity entry-slice effect). Arterial stenosis or occlusion[46,49] may more

likely be identified as small caliber intraluminal low intensity (or signal void) or as the absence of normal arterial flow void (relative isointensity or hyperintensity) at the expected normal site (Fig. 1-30) with or without post-stenotic flow void due to turbulence.[46] Occasionally, arterial collaterals (for example, in moyamoya disease) may appear as pinpoint, linear, or curvilinear signal voids[30] (Fig. 1-31).

The presence, type (cellular or fibrinous), and timing (acute, subacute, or chronic) of the luminal clot (thrombus, embolus) within the slice also influence the signal pattern. Fibrinous arterial thrombosis or embolism may be of relatively low intensity throughout the sequences.[49] Venous thrombosis and arterial thrombosis associated with aneurysm (intraluminal clot) or dissection (extraluminal clot) are often of a cellular (RBC) nature[49,77,89] with intensity abnormalities determined by the age of the clot (breakdown products of hemoglobin). Acute to subacute thrombosis/dissection (deoxyhemoglobin) may be of isointensity to low intensity on T1 images and of lower intensity on p and T2 images. Subacute to chronic clot (methemoglobin) may be of high intensity on T1 images and of higher intensity on p and T2 images (Figs. 1-32 and 1-33). The signal patterns associated with the evolution of hemorrhage and clot formation are primarily determined by the mechanism of proton relaxation enhancement (PRE). Unpredictable variations in flow physiology and pathophysiology along with the application of MR system software, including RF and gradient flow compensation, make interpretation of vascular

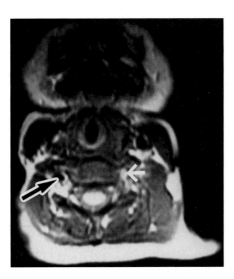

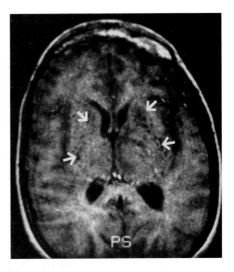

Fig. 1-30 An 8-year-old boy after therapy for cervicothoracic neuroblastoma with radiation-induced cervical spinal osteochondroma producing left vertebral artery occlusion. Axial proton density MRI shows normal right vertebral arterial flow void *(black arrow)* with absent flow void (isointensity to high intensity) on the left *(white arrow)* cephalad to the level of the osteochondroma. See box on p. 20.

Fig. 1-31 An 8-year-old girl with neurofibromatosis and optic glioma postradiation with moyamoya. Axial T1 MRI shows multiple basal ganglia and capsular pinpoint and linear signal voids representing telangiectatic collaterals *(arrows)*. See box on p. 20.

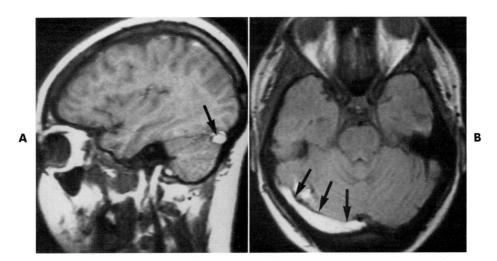

Fig. 1-32 An 18-year-old woman with seizures and pseudotumor cerebri syndrome. MRI shows right lateral dural venous sinus thrombosis as intraluminal high intensity *(arrows)* on sagittal T1 **(A)** and axial p **(B)** images consistent with extracellular methemoglobin content. See box on p. 20 and Table 1-2.

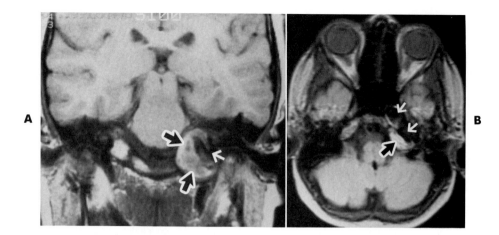

Fig. 1-33   An 8-year-old boy with acute left sensorineural hearing loss and facial palsy. Coronal T1 **(A)** and axial p **(B)** MRI demonstrate left petrous internal carotid arterial aneurysm and dissection with central luminal turbulent flow void *(white arrow)* and peripheral high intensity intraluminal and extraluminal thrombosis *(black arrow)* consistent with extracellular methemoglobin content. See box on p. 20 and Table 1-2.

intensity patterns problematic. Inconsistency of vascular signal findings from image to image, plane to plane, and sequence to sequence usually indicates a nonpathologic flow variant. Consistent findings throughout provide a higher level of certainty, especially for the diagnosis of occlusive vascular disease (Figs. 1-30 to 1-33). As an adjunct to SE sequencing, gradient echo techniques may assist in confirming vascular flow abnormalities.

PROTON RELAXATION ENHANCEMENT
Paramagnetic PRE

Certain intrinsic pathologies or extrinsically administered agents (Table 1-2) may facilitate (shorten) proton relaxation,[76] either T1, T2, or both. Paramagnetic substances, when placed within the main magnetic field, align with β_o (+z) and produce T1 PRE of $-OH_2$ protons (accelerated proton realignment and recovery of M_z toward M_o) with increased signal intensity on T1 (short TR/TE) images. This effect results from direct access and interaction of the paramagnetic substance in close proximity to the $-OH_2$ molecules, and is encountered with methemoglobin[35] in subacute-chronic hemorrhage or thrombosis[2] (Figs. 1-32 to 1-34), Gd-DTPA enhancement* (Fig. 1-35), melanin,[58] paramagnetic metals or alloys of tissue mineralization[19,92] (Fig. 1-36), and oxidative free radicals[43] (for example, abscess capsule). Depending on the paramagnetic concentration (relative to $-OH_2$), the T1-shortening effect with accelerated recovery of M_z toward M_o may carry over (higher starting intensity for T2 decay) into the longer TR sequences and dominate any T2-shortening effect. This results in continued high intensity on p and T2 images. Such a phenomenon has been observed with Gd-DTPA enhance-

*References 11, 33, 47, 65, 73, 88.

Table 1-2   Proton relaxation enhancement (PRE)

Element or agent	T1 image (short TR/TE)	T2 image (long TR/TE)
Gadolinium	High I	High I
Methemoglobin, extracellular	High I	High I
Methemoglobin, intracellular	High I	Low I
Melanin	High I	Low or high I
Deoxyhemoglobin	Iso-low I	Lower I
Hemosiderin	Iso-low I	Lowest I
Ferritin	Iso-low I	Lower I
Calcium	Iso-, low, or high I	Iso-low I

I, Intensity.

ment (Fig. 1-35) and extracellular methemoglobin (Figs. 1-32 to 1-34). Occasionally a paramagnetic substance in higher concentration may produce both effects, that is, T1 PRE with hyperintensity on short TR/TE images and T2 PRE with hypointensity on long TR/TE images (melanin, intracellular methemoglobin) (Fig. 1-37). With a very high concentration, or the anhydrous state, T2 PRE with low intensity may prevail throughout the sequences.

Magnetic susceptibility PRE

Substances containing iron (ferromagnetic) are of moderate to high magnetic susceptibility (measure of the ability of a substance to become magnetized within an external field) and induce local intrinsic tissue voxel magnetic field inhomogeneities (intravoxel gradients, $\Delta\beta_v$) that accelerate spin dephasing (T2* effect) of $-OH_2$ protons diffusing through the heterogeneous fields. As a result, there is signal

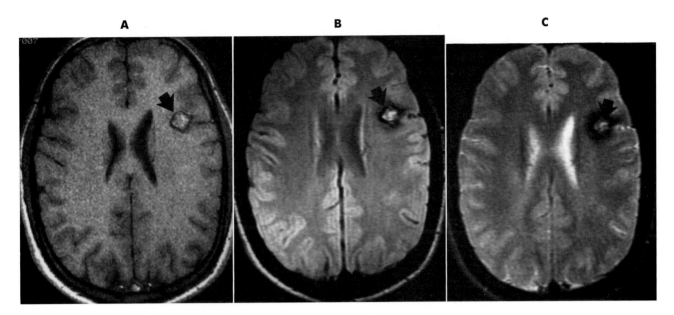

Fig. 1-34   A 14-year-old boy with focal seizures and nonspecific left frontal high density on CT. Axial T1 **(A)**, p **(B)**, and T2 **(C)** MRI show left frontal cavernous hemangioma *(arrows)* with central high intensity on all images consistent with extracellular methemoglobin content, plus peripheral low intensity exhibiting progressive signal loss and blurring from T1 **(A)** to p **(B)** to T2 **(C)** characteristic of hemosiderin ("iron effect"). See Table 1-2.

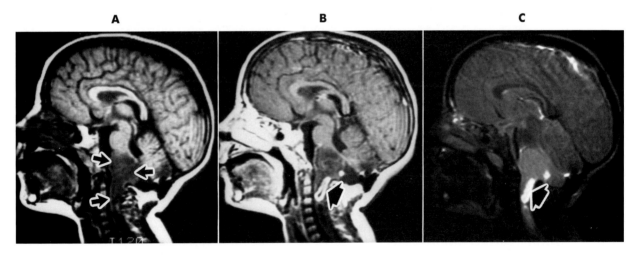

Fig. 1-35   A 9-year-old girl with residual postoperative cervicomedullary astrocytoma. **A,** Sagittal T1 MRI shows residual low intensity medullary and upper cervical cord expansion *(arrows)*. After intravenous Gd-DTPA injection sagittal T1 **(B)** and T2 **(C)** images demonstrate high-intensity enhancement *(arrows)*. See Table 1-2.

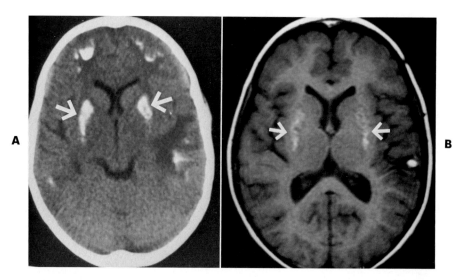

Fig. 1-36 A 10-year-old girl after chemotherapy and cranial irradiation for acute lymphoblastic leukemia. **A,** CT shows high density basal ganglia and cerebral calcifications *(arrows)*. **B,** Axial T1 MRI demonstrates bilateral putaminal high intensities *(arrows)* but no intensity abnormalities at other sites of CT calcification. The left temporal CT and MRI abnormalities represent previous hemorrhage. See Table 1-2.

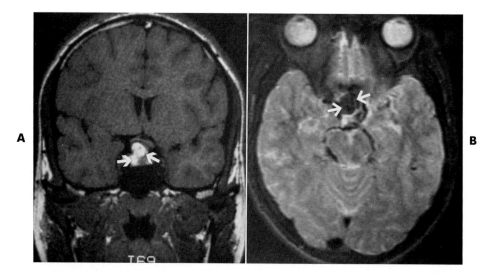

Fig. 1-37 A 19-year-old man with hemorrhagic prolactinoma. **A,** T1 coronal MRI shows high intensity intrasellar-suprasellar mass *(arrows)* compressing the chiasm. **B,** Lower intensity *(arrows)* on T2 axial image is consistent with intracellular methemoglobin content. See Table 1-2.

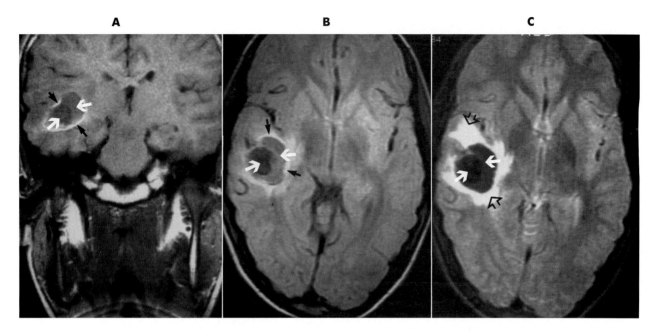

Fig. 1-38   A 17-year-old boy with minor head trauma and subsequent seizures. Coronal T1 **(A)**, axial p **(B)** and T2 **(C)** MRI show right temporal cavernous hemangioma and intracerebral hemorrhage, acute to subacute, with central hypointensity *(white arrows)* consistent with deoxyhemoglobin content (progressive lower intensity from **A** through **C**) and peripheral hyperintensity *(black arrows)* consistent with methemoglobin. Also notice surrounding edema *(open arrows)* hypointense on T1 **(A)** and hyperintense on p **(B)** and T2 **(C)** images. See Table 1-2.

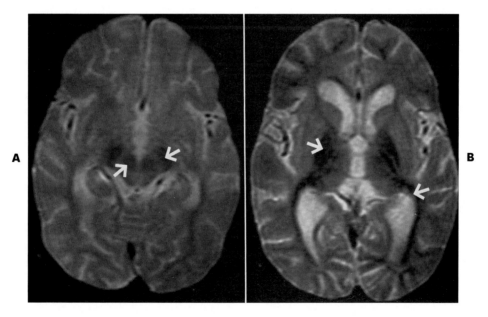

Fig. 1-39   A 6-year-old girl with perinatal brain injury and subsequent psychomotor retardation. **A** and **B**, Axial T2 MRI show bilateral marked hypointensity *(arrows)* of the red nuclei, substantia nigra, globus pallidus, and geniculocalcarine tracts consistent with excessive ferritin deposition probably caused by profound hypoxic-ischemic insult (notice cerebral atrophy). Basal ganglia and brain stem iron of lower intensity compared with adjacent white matter tracts is usually abnormal under 10 years of age. See Table 1-2.

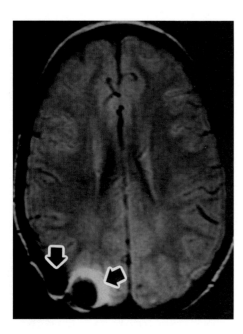

Fig. 1-40   A 9-year-old girl after surgery for parietal cortical glioma with scalp surgical staples in place. Axial p MRI shows ferromagnetic high and low intensity field distortion artifact *(arrows)* that obscures the operative tumor site.

decrease or loss on T2 (long TR/TE) images as seen with deoxyhemoglobin[35-37] in acute-subacute hemorrhage (Fig. 1-38), intracellular methemoglobin[35-37] in subacute-chronic hemorrhage (Fig. 1-37), ferritin[1,20] (Fig. 1-39) and hemosiderin[35,36] after hemorrhage (see Fig. 1-34). The signal loss is often apparent also on p (long TR/short TE) and T1 (short TR/TE) images when substances of higher magnetic susceptibility in greater concentration (iron as hemosiderin) produce such profound T2 shortening that the resultant voxel T2 is shorter than the user-selected TE. Furthermore the effect is often progressive (decreasing intensity and increasing blur with longer TR and TE) from T1 to p to T2 images (see Fig. 1-34), and is more pronounced at higher fields and with gradient echo techniques. With bulkier ferromagnetic or other metallic objects (dental braces, shunt apparatus, surgical clips and wires, scoliosis rods, and the like) gross field distortion with signal loss and high signal rimming is seen* (Figs. 1-22 and 1-40). Occasionally, substances of high magnetic susceptibility (iron) in low concentrations (for example, extracellular methemoglobin) or substances of low susceptibility (calcium), alone or in combination with other trace metals, produce paramagnetic high intensity[19] on short TR/TE sequences (see Fig. 1-36).

Hemorrhage and clotting

The T1 and T2 PRE mechanisms are particularly important as the basis for signal-intensity patterns in the evolution of hemorrhage and clotting.[35, 36, 39] The PRE-determined patterns parallel the appearance of red blood cell

(RBC) breakdown products associated with deoxygenation (deoxyhemoglobin) and reoxygenation (methemoglobin) of the oxyhemoglobin molecule, the deposition of dystrophic iron (ferritin, hemosiderin), as well as the involvement of these and other elements (platelets, thrombin, and fibrin) in the coagulation process. Fresh or hyperacute hemorrhage (less than 1 day) has been described as nonspecific and similar to that of nonflowing, free extracellular $-OH_2$ (stagnant blood, that is, plasma and cellular elements including oxyhemoglobin) with long T1 (low intensity on short TR/TE images), high p (high intensity on long TR/short TE images), and long T2 (high intensity on long TR/TE images). Acute-subacute hemorrhage (less than 10 to 14 days) has an appearance (Fig. 1-38) of isointensity to low intensity on short TR/TE images and of lower intensity on long TR (with short and long TE) images because of the magnetic susceptibility T2 PRE effects of deoxyhemoglobin (deoxygenation of oxyhemoglobin). In subacute-chronic hemorrhage (greater than 2 to 4 weeks), intracellular methemoglobin (reoxygenation of deoxyhemoglobin) provides high intensity (paramagnetic T1 PRE) starting at the periphery and advancing centrally over time on short TR/TE sequences (see Figs. 1-37 and 1-38) and low intensity (magnetic susceptibility T2 PRE) on long TR sequences, whereas extracellular (after RBC lysis) methemoglobin (see Figs. 1-32 to 1-34) gives T1 high intensity plus p and T2 high intensity (extracellular $-OH_2$ influx).

Difficulty in more precise matching of MR appearance with timing reflects the multifactorial complexity of the bleeding/clotting process, including the lack of accurate correlation between initiation, cessation, and continuation (or recurrence) of hemorrhage and the onset of, or change in, clinical symptoms and timing of the MR examination.[38,44,99] Furthermore, recent studies indicate that hyper-concentration of plasma and hemoglobin proteins during clot retraction may contribute significantly to these signal-intensity patterns.[45] Such consideration is logical, since the known T1- and T2- shortening effects of protein on water (matrix $-OH_2$), as discussed earlier, is equivalent to the PRE $-OH_2$ effect for paramagnetic and magnetically susceptible substances (see the box on p. 16 and Fig. 1-18). Fresh, acute, and subacute hemorrhages are usually accompanied by surrounding edema as low intensity on T1 images and high intensity on p and T2 images (see Fig. 1-38). Post-hemorrhage hemosiderin is primarily deposited at the periphery of the clot as a rim or a ring (chronic hemorrhage) and is of low intensity on the short TR/TE sequence and of even lower intensity on longer TR sequences, all as related to the strong and heterogeneous susceptibility T2 PRE effect of iron (Fig. 1-34). These signal patterns have been described primarily for intracerebral hemorrhage. With some variation, similar patterns have been observed for subdural and epidural hemorrhages[29] (Fig. 1-41). Because of the CSF flow and oxygenation dynamics of the compartment, subarachnoid hemorrhage does not often conform to these patterns (unless loculated) and may be more readily detected by CT in the acute or subacute stage.[15,44]

---

*References 6, 17, 42, 63, 80, 81, 91.

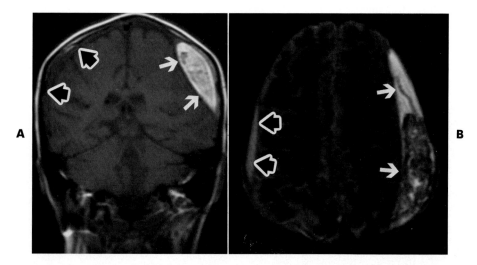

Fig. 1-41   A 16-year-old girl with hydrocephalus after shunting and nonspecific bilateral subdural collections shown by CT. Coronal T1 **(A)** and axial T2 **(B)** MRI show small right subdural collection *(black arrows)* of isointensity to low intensity on T1 images **(A)** and of higher intensity on T2 images **(B)** consistent with chronic subdural hematoma (or hygroma). Larger left high-intensity collection is present with low-intensity components *(white arrows)* consistent with recurrent subdural hematoma containing methemoglobin, fibrin, and ferritin or hemosiderin. Cortical venous landmarks are displaced with the brain surface, characteristic of the extraarachnoid location of the collections. "Chronic" extraarachnoid hematomas (especially subdural) usually do not contain methemoglobin or hemosiderin (absent blood-brain barrier) and should appear similar to the right-sided collection in this case. The presence of methemoglobin (high intensity) and hemosiderin or ferritin (low intensity) suggests rehemorrhage at this very chronic stage. See Table 1-2.

CHEMICAL SHIFT

Chemical shift (CS) refers to the measurable difference (shift) in Larmor frequency (ω_o) between different chemical or molecular states (electron shielding) of hydrogen.[66] This may allow, for example, separation of waterbound $(-OH_2)$ protons from lipidbound $(-CH_2)$ protons and is exaggerated at higher fields. CS artifacts may be encountered at water-fat interfaces (orbital fat/optic nerve, vertebral marrow/disk, and so forth), especially at higher fields along the frequency-encoding gradient (frequency shift) as alternating bright and dark lines[64,66,96] (Fig. 1-42). The CS effect may occasionally serve to distinguish fat from other tissue components exhibiting similar intensity patterns through the sequences (for example, intracellular methemoglobin).

ADJUNCTIVE IMAGING TECHNIQUES
Inversion recovery and chemical shift

Important adjunctive pulse-sequence techniques include inversion recovery (IR), chemical shift (CS), and gradient echo (GE). The spin echo (SE) is the standard for stationary tissue parameters (p, T1, T2), as well as for primary evaluation of proton flow, proton relaxation enhancement, and chemical shift.

IR is primarily a stationary tissue sequence providing the best T1 contrast,[94] although it provides a lower signal-to-noise ratio than SE for comparable acquisition time. A special modification of the IR is the STIR sequence (Fig.

1-43), which suppresses fatty high-intensity signal while providing additive water T1 and T2 effects as high intensity.[21] This is particularly effective for bone marrow imaging (neoplastic invasion) or orbit imaging (optic nerve abnormalities) so that water-containing lesions are not obscured by the dominant high intensity of normal marrow or orbital fat.[21,87,93] A similar result may be obtained by using fat-suppression CS imaging* to suppress the $-CH_2$ frequency peak of tissues and emphasize the $-OH_2$ peak, or using gradient echo imaging to promote tissues of long T2/T2* $(-OH_2)$ over those of short T2/T2* (fat).

CS imaging may be used for confirmation that an intensity pattern indeed represents fat, for suppression of fatty high intensity when using Gd-DTPA enhancement (orbit and marrow imaging), and for proton (H1) spectroscopy.[14,50,53]

Gradient echo imaging

Gradient echo (GE) techniques (GRE, GRASS, FLASH, FISP) employ lower flip-angle (10° to 50°) excitation RF pulses and gradient reversal or inversion, rather than 180°-RF refocusing, for echo generation[9,97] (Fig. 1-44 and Table 1-3). This technique is especially effective (combined with gradient moment nulling) for delineating flowing tissues. These flow-sensitive GE sequences highlight vas-

---

*References 12, 55, 68, 90, 97, 98.

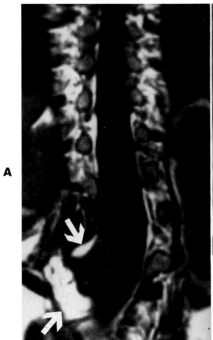

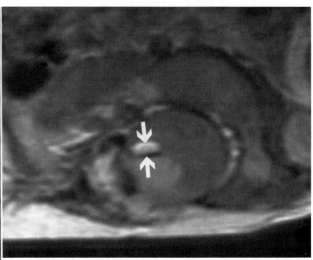

Fig. 1-42   A 2-year-old boy with lipomyelomeningocele. Coronal T1 **(A)** and axial p **(B)** MRI show terminal intradural tethering mass with T1 high intensity fatty components *(arrows)* interfacing water (CSF) and producing chemical shift artifacts as exaggerated high- and low-intensity bands *(arrows)* on the p image **(B).**

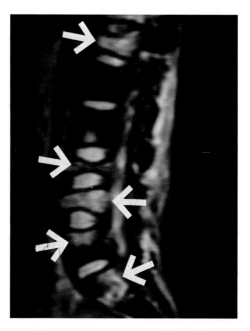

Fig. 1-43   A 7-year-old boy with metastatic rhabdomyosarcoma. Sagittal STIR (TR 2000, TE 35, TI 165) MRI demonstrates multilevel spinal metastases as high intensity, including vertebral collapse *(arrows).*

Table 1-3   Gradient echo sequences

	T1	p*	T2*†	T2/T1‡
TR(msec)	200-400	100-400	100-400	25-100
TE(msec)	12-15	12-15	30-60	12-15
θ(N°)	45-90	5-20	5-20	30-60

Best for CSF enhancement (myelogram effect) with minimal T2 artifact if as short a TE as possible is used.

†Best for magnetic susceptibility effect using longer TE.

‡Steady-state free precession is vascular flow-sensitive but provides poor stationary tissue contrast unless spoiler gradient and as short a TE as possible are used, thus giving T1-like contrast.

Multislice gradient echo acquisition is recommended for CSF enhancement* or magnetic susceptibility effect†; single slice gradient echo acquisition is recommended for vascular flow enhancement.‡

cular (MR angiography)* and CSF (MR myelography)[23,24] structures as hyperintense signals (Figs. 1-29 and 1-45) by gradient refocusing of spins originally dephased by flow-induced phase shifts. In addition to gradient-refocused echo generation and gradient moment nulling, GE techniques also use single-slice acquisitions (entry slice enhancement) to render normal vascular flow as high intensity. Shortcomings of this method may include difficulties in distinguishing GE high-intensity vascular flow from intraluminal subacute-chronic clot (methemoglobin) without T1 SE images, and GE low-intensity vascular flow deficit from intraluminal low intensity due to slow flow variant, turbulence, or acute-subacute thrombus (deoxyhemoglobin or intracellular methemoglobin). Unlike RF rephasing (SE technique), gradient reversal (GE) does not refocus proton dephasing (phase differences) caused by extrinsic magnetic field inhomogeneities ($\Delta\beta_o/T2^\star$) or intrinsic heterogeneous magnetic susceptibility ($\Delta\beta_v/T2^\star$), nor that caused by

---

*References 4, 22, 40, 54, 61, 72.

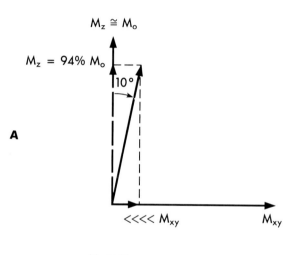

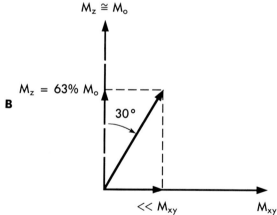

Fig. 1-44   Reduced flip angle gradient echo technique. With short flip angle (θ = 10°), proton density (short TE as possible) and T2* (longer TE) contrast (M_z = 94% M_o) may be obtained **(A)**, but with overall reduced image signal ($\lll M_{xy}$) as compared with SE techniques (θ = 90°). With somewhat longer flip angle (θ = 30°), T1 (short TE as possible) contrast (M_z = 63% M_o) may be achieved **(B)** with some increase in image signal. The reduced flip angle allows shorter TR, whereas the gradient echo allows shorter TE as compared with SE techniques. See Table 1-3 and text.

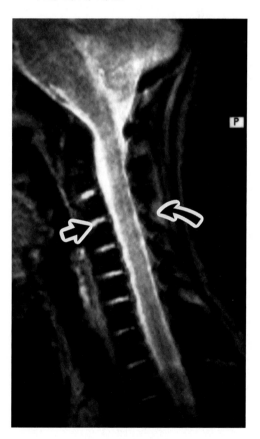

Fig. 1-45   An 8-year-old girl with persistent neck pain after head and neck trauma. Normal sagittal "proton density" gradient echo MRI (θ = 12°, TR 330 msec, TE 12 msec) demonstrates high-intensity "enhancement" of tissues with longer T2/T2*, including the water of disk space *(straight arrow)*, CSF, cord, and muscle *(curved arrow)* as contrasted against the lower-intensity, "suppressed" tissue intensities (shorter T2/T2*) of fat and bone. See Table 1-3 and Fig. 1-44.

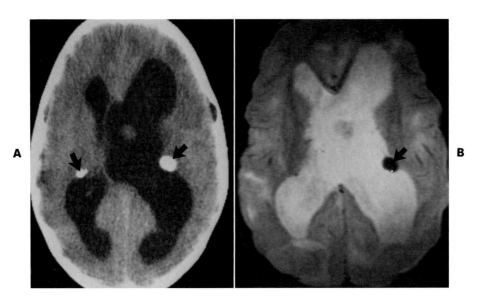

Fig. 1-46   A 6-year-old boy with tuberous sclerosis. **A,** CT shows two periventricular nodular high-density calcifications *(arrows)* and asymmetric hydrocephalus. **B,** Axial T2 MRI obviously shows the large left subependymal calcification as low intensity *(arrow).* See Table 1-2.

chemical shift. GE techniques therefore are extrasensitive to magnetic susceptibility sources (weak or strong) of T2* ($\Delta\beta_v$) including tissue mineralization[1,3] (calcium, ferritin, hemosiderin, and so on) and breakdown products (deoxy-hemoglobin, intracellular methemoglobin, hemosiderin) of red blood cells (hemoglobin) in hemorrhage and thrombosis.[5,79]

The GE techniques at high or low field are often more sensitive to the mineralization of weak magnetic susceptibility (calcification) than are SE techniques (see Fig. 1-29), in which the 180°-RF refocusing pulse eliminates or minimizes such effects (T2*) unless the calcification is concentrated (Fig. 1-46) and occupies a large portion of the voxel volume (low intensity due to low proton density). The stronger magnetic susceptibility effect of iron is directly and exponentially proportional to field strength, is usually not eliminated by SE 180° refocusing, and therefore, is almost always demonstrated (see Figs. 1-34, 1-38, and 1-39) with the SE technique at higher magnetic fields (1.0 to 1.5 T). Furthermore the iron effect (for example, hemosiderin) is characteristically exaggerated (progressive signal loss and blurring) with longer TR and TE. With bulkier ferromagnetic or other metallic objects gross field distortion is even more exaggerated on GE. At lower field strength, the SE technique may not readily detect iron in hemorrhage or thrombosis; therefore the GE technique may be more useful for hemorrhage detection especially at the lower field.[5,79]

With the proper selection of flip angle (θ), TR, and TE, the GE method may emphasize tissues (Fig. 1-45) of longer T2/T2* (free $-OH_2$: CSF, disk, muscle, hyaline cartilage, edema, tumor, and so forth) as contrasted with tissues of shorter T2/T2* (marrow fat, protein matrix, bone, calcifi-

cation, iron, and so forth).[9,23,24] However, T2* effects often produce artifacts at bone–soft tissue interfaces (cranial base, intraspinal) and air–soft tissue interfaces (sinuses, otomastoid). Furthermore, with the improper selection of GE parameters, stationary $-OH_2$ abnormalities may be obscured (see Table 1-3). In conclusion, the spin echo is the preferred primary pulse-sequencing technique for MRI of brain and spine abnormalities, particularly at the higher fields (β_o), not only for evaluation of stationary tissues but also for flowing tissues, PRE phenomena, and chemical shift. Gradient echo is considered secondary and adjunctive for evaluating and enhancing flowing tissues (vascular and CSF), calcium (at higher or lower β_o), iron (at lower β_o), and hemorrhage (especially at lower β_o).

SUMMATION: INTRINSIC PLUS EXTRINSIC MRI PARAMETERS

In summary, the voxel MR signal intensity (I_v) is directly and linearly proportional to proton density (p) and directly and exponentially proportional to transverse (spin-spin) relaxation time (T2), FID time (T2*), T1 proton relaxation enhancement (T1 PRE), repetition time (TR), and field strength (β_o). At the same time, I_v is inversely and exponentially proportional to longitudinal (spin-lattice) relaxation time (T1), T2 proton relaxation enhancement (T2 PRE), and echo time (TE), and more complexly influenced by proton flow (f), chemical shift (CS), and flip angle (θ). Using a modification of the Bloch equation*[94] for MR intensity (I_v) as related to intrinsic tissue parameters (p, T1, T2, T2*, PRE, f, CS) and extrinsic user-selected parame-

---

*$I \propto N(H)(1-e^{-TR/T1})e^{-TE/T2}$

ters, (TR, TE, θ, β_o) these relationships may be expressed as follows:

$$I_v \propto \frac{p, T2, T2^\star, T1 \, PRE, TR, \beta_o}{T1, T2 \, PRE, TE} \pm f \pm CS \pm \theta$$

From this expression one can readily see that diagnostic formulation of MR signal abnormalities is often complex. Pathologic elements may influence voxel intensity through more than one intrinsic parameter for a given set of extrinsic parameters. In addition, disease processes are often constituted by more than one pathological element. Image interpretation is further complicated when one element operating through a dominant parameter obscures the basic disease process expressed through another parameter. This may be encountered with hemorrhagic neoplasm in which the signal pattern is dominated by the PRE effects of hemoglobin breakdown. Therefore, as with any imaging modality, the proper interpretation of MR findings must always be guided by sound technological and clinical principles, as further discussed in the next section and subsequent chapters.

REFERENCES
Biomechanisms

1. Aoki S, Okada Y, Nishimura K, et al: Normal deposition of brain iron in childhood and adolescence: MR imaging at 1.5 T, *Radiology* 172:381, 1989.
2. Atlas SW, Grossman RI, Goldberg HI, et al: Partially thrombosed giant intracranial aneurysms: correlation of MR and pathologic findings, *Radiology* 162:111, 1987.
3. Atlas SW, Grossman RI, Hackney DB, et al: Calcified intracranial lesions: detection with gradient-echo-acquisition rapid MR imaging, *AJR* 150:1383, 1988.
4. Atlas, SW, Mark AS, Fram EK, et al: Vascular intracranial lesions: applications of gradient-echo MR imaging, *Radiology* 169:455, 1988.
5. Atlas SW, Mark AS, Grossman RI, et al: Intracranial hemorrhage: gradient-echo MR imaging at 1.5 T, *Radiology* 168:803, 1988.
6. Bellon EM, Haacke EM, Coleman PE, et al: MR artifacts: a review, *AJR* 147:1271, 1986.
7. Bradley WG: Flow phenomena in MR imaging. In Stark DD, Bradley WG, editors: *Magnetic resonance imaging,* St Louis, 1988, Mosby–Year Book.
8. Bradley WG: Flow phenomena in MR imaging, *AJR* 150:983, 1988.
9. Bradley WG: When should GRASS be used? *Radiology* 169:574, 1988.
10. Bradley WG, Kortman KE, Burgoyne B: Flowing cerebrospinal fluid in normal and hydrocephalic states: appearance on MR images, *Radiology* 159:611, 1986.
11. Brasch RC, Bennett HF: Considerations in the choice of contrast media for MR imaging, *Radiology* 166:897, 1988.
12. Brateman L: Chemical shift imaging: a review, *AJR* 146:971, 1986.
13. Braun IF, Malko JA, Davis PC: The behavior of pantopaque on MR: in vivo and in vitro analyses, *AJNR* 7:997, 1986.
14. Bruhn H, Frahm J, Gyngell ML, et al: Noninvasive differentiation of tumors with use of localized H-1 MR spectroscopy in vivo: initial experience in patients with cerebral tumors, *Radiology* 172:541, 1989.
15. Chakeres DW, Bryan RN: Acute subarachnoid hemorrhage: in vitro comparison of magnetic resonance and computed tomography, *AJNR* 7:223, 1986.
16. Citrin CM, Sherman JL, Gangarosa RE, et al: Physiology of the CSF flow-void sign: modification by cardiac gating, *AJR* 148:205, 1987.
17. Clark JA, Kelly WM: Common artifacts encountered in magnetic resonance imaging, *Radiol Clin North Am* 26:893, 1988.
18. Czervionke LF, Czervionke JM, Daniels DL, et al: Characteristic features of MR truncation artifacts, *AJNR* 9:815, 1988.
19. Dell LA, Brown MS, Orrison WW, et al: Physiologic intracranial calcification with hyperintensity on MR imaging: case report and experimental model, *AJNR* 9:1145, 1988.
20. Dietrich RB, Bradley WG: Iron accumulation in the basal ganglia following severe ischemic-anoxic insults in children, *Radiology* 168:203, 1988.
21. Dwyer AJ, Frank JA, Sank VJ, et al: Short T1 inversion-recovery pulse sequence: analysis and initial experience in cancer imaging, *Radiology* 168:827, 1988.
22. Edelman RR, Wentz KU, Mattle HP, et al: Intracerebral arteriovenous malformations: evaluation with selective MR angiography and venography, *Radiology* 173:831, 1989.
23. Enzmann DR, Rubin JB: Cervical spine: MR imaging with a partial flip angle, gradient-refocused pulse sequence. Part I. General considerations and disk disease, *Radiology* 166:467, 1988.
24. Enzmann DR, Rubin JB: Cervical spine: MR imaging with a partial flip angle, gradient-refocused pulse sequence. Part II. Spinal cord disease, *Radiology* 166:473, 1988.
25. Enzmann DR, Rubin JB, Wright A: Cervical spine MR imaging: generating high-signal CSF in sagittal and axial images, *Radiology* 163:233, 1987.
26. Enzmann DR, Rubin JB, Wright A: Use of cerebrospinal fluid gating to improve T2-weighted images. Part I. The spinal cord, *Radiology* 162:763, 1987.
27. Enzmann DR, Rubin JB, O'Donohue J, et al: Use of cerebrospinal fluid gating to improve T2-weighted images. Part II. Temporal lobes, basal ganglia, and brain stem, *Radiology* 162:768, 1987.
28. Enzmann DR, O'Donohue J, Rubin JB, et al: CSF pulsations within nonneoplastic spinal cord cysts, *AJR* 149:149, 1987.
29. Fobben ES, Grossman RI, Atlas SW, et al: MR characteristics of subdural hematomas and hygromas at 1.5 T, *AJR* 153:589, 1989.
30. Fujisawa I, Asato R, Nishimura K, et al: Moyamoya disease: MR imaging, *Radiology* 164:103, 1987.
31. Fullerton GD: Physiologic basis of magnetic relaxation. In Stark DD, Bradley WG, editors: *Magnetic resonance imaging,* St Louis, 1988, Mosby–Year Book.
32. Gammal TE, Allen MB, Brooks BS, et al: MR evaluation of hydrocephalus, *AJNR* 8:591, 1987.
33. Gibby WA: MR contrast agents: an overview. *Radiol Clin North Am* 26:1047, 1988.
34. Goldberg HI, Grossman RI, Gomori JM, et al: Cervical internal carotid artery dissecting hemorrhage: diagnosis using MR, *Radiology* 158:157, 1986.
35. Gomori JM, Grossman RI: Mechanisms responsible for the MR appearance and evolution of intracranial hemorrhage, *Radiographics* 8:427, 1988.
36. Gomori JM, Grossman RI, Goldberg HI, et al: Intracranial hematomas: imaging by high-field MR, *Radiology* 157:87, 1985.
37. Gomori JM, Grossman RI, Goldberg HI, et al: Occult cerebral vascular malformations: high-field MR imaging, *Radiology* 158:707, 1986.
38. Gomori JM, Grossman RI, Hackney DB, et al: Variable appearances of subacute intracranial hematomas on high-field spin-echo MR, *AJR* 150:171, 1988.
39. Grossman RI, Gomori JM, Goldberg HI, et al: MR imaging of hemorrhagic conditions of the head and neck, *Radiographics* 8:441, 1988.
40. Gullberg GT, Wehrli FW, Shimakawa A, et al: MR vascular imaging with a fast gradient refocusing pulse sequence and reformatted images from transaxial sections, *Radiology* 165:241, 1987.
41. Haake EM, Lenz GW: Improving MR image quality in the presence of motion by using rephasing gradients, *AJR* 148:1251, 1987.
42. Hahn FJ, Chu WK, Coleman PE, et al: Artifacts and diagnostic pitfalls of magnetic resonance imaging: a clinical review, *Radiol Clin North Am* 26:717, 1988.
43. Haimes AB, Zimmerman RD, Morgello S, et al: MR imaging of brain abscesses, *AJR* 152:1073, 1989.
44. Hayman LA, Pagani JJ, Kirkpatrick JB, et al: Pathophysiology of acute intracerebral and subarachnoid hemorrhage: applications to MR imaging, *AJR* 153:135, 1989.

45. Hayman LA, Taber KH, Ford JJ, et al: Effect of clot formation and retraction on spin-echo MR images of blood: an in vitro study, *AJNR* 10:1155, 1989.
46. Heinz ER, Yeates AE, Djang WT: Significant extracranial carotid stenosis: detection on routine cerebral MR images, *Radiology* 170:843, 1989.
47. Hesselink JR, Press GA: MR contrast enhancement of intracranial lesions with Gd-DTPA, *Radiol Clin North Am* 26:873, 1988.
48. Hinks RS, Quencer RM: Motion artifacts in brain and spine MR, *Radiol Clin North Am* 26:737, 1988.
49. Katz BH, Quencer RM, Kaplan JO, et al: MR imaging of intracranial carotid occlusion, *AJR* 152:1271, 1989.
50. Koschorek F, Gremmel H, Stelten J, et al: Characterization of CNS lesions by using high-resolution MR spectroscopy of CSF: preliminary results, *AJNR* 10:523, 1989.
51. Kucharczyk W, Kelly WM, Davis DO, et al: Intracranial lesions: flow-related enhancement on MR images using time-of-flight effects, *Radiology* 161:767, 1986.
52. Lee BCP, Herzberg L, Zimmerman RD, et al: MR imaging of cerebral vascular malformations, *AJNR* 6:863, 1985.
53. Luyten PR, den Hollander JA: Observation of metabolites in the human brain by MR spectroscopy, *Radiology* 161:795, 1986.
54. Masaryk TJ, Modic MT, Ross JS, et al: Intracranial circulation: preliminary clinical results with three-dimensional (volume) MR angiography, *Radiology* 171:793, 1989.
55. Matthaei D, Haase A, Frahm J, et al: Multiple chemical shift selective (CHESS) MR imaging using stimulated echoes, *Radiology* 160:791, 1986.
56. McMurdo SK, Brant-Zawadzki M, Bradley WG, et al: Dural sinus thrombosis: study using intermediate field strength MR imaging, *Radiology* 161:83, 1986.
57. Mills CM, Brant-Zawadzki M, Crooks LE, et al: Nuclear magnetic resonance: principles of blood flow imaging, *AJNR* 4:1161, 1983.
58. Mirowitz SA, Sartor K, and Gado M: High-intensity basal ganglia lesions on T1-weighted MR images in neurofibromatosis, *AJNR* 10:1159, 1989.
59. Mitchell DG, Burk DL, Vinitski S, et al: The biophysical basis of tissue contrast in extracranial MR imaging, *AJR* 149:831, 1987.
60. Mitchell MR, Tarr RW, Conturo TE, et al: Spin echo technique selection: basic principles for choosing MRI pulse sequence timing intervals, *Radiographics* 6:245, 1986.
61. Needell WM, Maravilla KR: MR flow imaging in vascular malformations using gradient-recalled acquisition, *AJNR* 9:637, 1988.
62. Oot RF, New PFJ, Pile-Spellman J, et al: The detection of intracranial calcifications by MR, *AJNR* 7:801, 1986.
63. Patton JA, Kulkarni MV, Craig JK, et al: Techniques, pitfalls and artifacts in magnetic resonance imaging, *Radiographics* 7:505, 1987.
64. Porter BA, Hastrup W, Richardson ML, et al: Classification and investigation of artifacts in magnetic resonance imaging, *Radiographics* 7:271, 1987.
65. Powers TA, Partain CL, Kessler RM, et al: Central nervous system lesions in pediatric patients: Gd-DTPA-enhanced MR imaging, *Radiology* 169:723, 1988.
66. Pusey E, Lufkin RB, Brown RKJ, et al: Magnetic resonance imaging artifacts: mechanism and clinical significance, *Radiographics* 6:891, 1986.
67. Quencer RM, Hinks RS, Pattany PH, et al: Improved MR imaging of the brain by using compensating gradients to suppress motion-induced artifacts, *Radiographics* 9:431, 1988.
68. Rosen BR, Fleming DM, Kushner DC, et al: Hematologic bone marrow disorders: quantitative chemical shift MR imaging, *Radiology* 169:799, 1988.
69. Rubin JB, Enzmann DR: Harmonic modulation of proton MR precessional phase by pulsatile motion: origin of spinal CSF flow phenomena, *Radiographics* 8:307, 1987.
70. Rubin JB, Enzmann DR: Imaging of spinal CSF pulsation by 2DFT MR: significance during clinical imaging, *AJNR* 8:297, 1987.
71. Rubin JB, Wright A, Enzmann DR: Lumbar spine: motion compensation for cerebrospinal fluid on MR imaging, *Radiology* 166:225, 1988.
72. Ruggieri PM, Laub GA, Masaryk TJ, et al: Intracranial circulation: pulse-sequence considerations in three-dimensional (volume) MR angiography, *Radiology* 171:785, 1989.
73. Runge VM, Schaible TF, Goldstein HA, et al: Gd-DTPA: clinical efficacy, *Radiographics* 8:147, 1988.
74. Runge VM, Wood ML, Kaufman DM, et al: The straight and narrow path to good head and spine MRI, *Radiographics* 8:507, 1988.
75. Sage MR: blood-brain barrier: phenomenon of increasing importance to the imaging clinician, *AJNR* 3:127, 1982.
76. Saini S, Frankel RB, Stark DD, et al: Magnetism: a primer and review, *AJR* 150:735, 1988.
77. Schick RM, Jolesz F, Barnes PD, et al: MR diagnosis of dural venous sinus thrombosis complicating L-Asparaginase therapy, *Comput Med Imaging Graph* 13:319, 1989.
78. Schultz CL, Alfidi RJ, Nelson AD, et al: The effect of motion on two-dimensional Fourier transformation magnetic resonance images, *Radiology* 152:117, 1984.
79. Seidenwurm D, Meng TK, Kowalski H: Intracranial hemorrhagic lesions: evaluation with spin-echo and gradient-refocused MR imaging at 0.5 and 1.5 T, *Radiology* 172:189, 1989.
80. Shellock FG: MR imaging of metallic implants and materials: a compilation of the literature, *AJR* 151:811, 1988.
81. Shellock FG, Crues JV: High field strength MR imaging and metallic biomedical implants: an ex vivo evaluation of deflection forces, *AJR* 151:389, 1988.
82. Sherman JL, Barkovich AJ, Citrin CM: The MR appearance of syringomyelia: new observations, *AJR* 148:381, 1987.
83. Sherman JL, Citrin CM: Magnetic resonance demonstration of normal CSF flow, *AJNR* 7:4, 1986.
84. Sherman JL, Citrin CM, Gangarosa RE, et al: The MR appearance of CSF flow in patients with ventriculomegaly, *AJNR* 7:1025, 1986.
85. Sherman JL, Citrin CM, Gangarosa RE, et al: The MR appearance of CSF pulsations in the spinal canal, *AJNR* 7:879, 1986.
86. Smith HJ, Strother CM, Kikuchi Y, et al: MR imaging in the management of supratentorial intracranial AVMs, *AJNR* 9:225, 1988.
87. Stimac GK, Porter BA, Olson DO, et al: Gadolinium-DTPA–enhanced MR imaging of spinal neoplasms: preliminary investigation and comparison with unenhanced spin-echo and STIR sequences, *AJR* 151:1185, 1988.
88. Sze G: Gadolinium-DTPA in spinal disease, *Radiol Clin North Am* 26:1009, 1988.
89. Sze G, Simmons B, Krol G, et al: Dural sinus thrombosis: verification with spin-echo techniques, *AJNR* 9:679, 1988.
90. Szumowski J, Plewes DB: Separation of lipid and water MR imaging signals by chopper averaging in the time domain, *Radiology* 165:247, 1987.
91. Teitelbaum GP, Bradley WG, Klein BD: MR imaging artifacts, ferromagnetism, and magnetic torque of intravascular filters, stents, and coils, *Radiology* 166:657, 1988.
92. Tsuruda JS, Bradley WG: MR detection of intracranial calcification: a phantom study, *AJNR* 8:1049, 1987.
93. Vogler JB, Murphy WA: Bone marrow imaging, *Radiology* 168:679, 1988.
94. Wehrli FW, MacFall JR, Newton TH: Parameters determining the appearance of NMR images. In Newton TH, Potts DG, editors: *Advanced imaging techniques,* San Anselmo, Calif, 1984, Clavadel.
95. Wehrli FW, MacFall JR, Shutts D, et al: Mechanisms of contrast in NMR imaging, *J Comput Assist Tomogr* 8:369, 1984.
96. Weinreb JC, Brateman L, Babcock EE, et al: Chemical shift artifact in clinical magnetic resonance images at 0.35 T, *AJR* 145:183, 1985.
97. Winkler ML, Ortendahl DA, Mills TC, et al: Characteristics of partial flip angle and gradient reversal MR imaging, *Radiology* 166:17, 1988.
98. Yeung HN, Kormos DW: Separation of true fat and water images by correcting magnetic field inhomogeneity in situ, *Radiology* 159:783, 1986.
99. Zimmerman RD, Heier LA, Snow RB, et al: Acute intracranial hemorrhage: intensity changes on sequential MR scans at 0.5 T, *AJNR* 9:47, 1988.

MRI examination and analysis of pediatric central nervous system disease

TECHNIQUES AND GUIDELINES

To accommodate the varying needs of the infant, child, and adolescent, a reliable, friendly, and versatile MR operation is required along with the proper immobilization, sedation, and monitoring capabilities. For pediatric CNS applications, we prefer the higher-field magnet (1.0 to 1.5 T) to provide an increased signal-to-noise ratio for more flexible use of operator-selectable parameters including thin sections with small fields of view (FOV) for a variety of RF coils to provide high spatial resolution of the cranial and spinal neuraxis at efficient scan times. Also, the higher field allows the potential for MR spectroscopy (proton, phosphorus, and so on). At the higher field, volume or surface RF coils closely applied to the region of interest (ROI) with reduced FOV (12 to 20 cm) allows lower-order phase encoding with higher-order frequency encoding (for example, 128×256 matrix) to provide smaller effective pixel size (FOV $\div$ matrix) for good spatial resolution at 3 to 5 mm slice thickness. Good contrast resolution is maintained at 1 to 2 NSA, thus preventing significant time penalty, especially for longer TR (p and T2 contrast) acquisitions. Also, higher-order phase and frequency encoding (for example, 256×256 matrix or 192×256 matrix) with thin slices (for example, 3 mm) may be used to achieve higher spatial detail for shorter TR/TE acquisitions with 1 to 4 NSA for T1 contrast.

Proper positioning of the ROI central to the RF coil at the common intersection of the gradient coordinates within the central bore of the magnet is critical for optimum image quality especially at smaller FOV. Nonaliasing software along the phase- and frequency-encoding gradients or the ability to switch phase- and frequency-gradient directions is also important to prevent or minimize image wraparound. Brain examinations may be conducted using the adult head coil for older children and adolescents, whereas smaller volume coils (for example, an extremity coil) may be used for neonates and infants. Spinal examinations of infants and small children may be conducted using the adult head coil (as a pediatric "body" coil) or using the smaller-volume coil for the neonate. Rectangular, elliptical, or circular surface coils within a "movable" coil holder, or as a multiple coil array, is preferred, however, since total spinal or craniospinal examination is often required. This is especially true for multilevel developmental malformations (for example, postrepair myelocele with Chiari II malformation, hydrosyringomyelia, or caudal retethering) or extensive craniospinal neuraxis involvement by neoplasm (for example, CSF/leptomeningeal seeding with medulloblastoma). The movable coil holder, or multicoil array, allows coil repositioning or electronic switching longitudinally along the entire extent of the craniospinal axis without disturbing the sedated or anesthetized patient and also

reduces total examination time. In children with ferromagnetic or other metallic implants (braces, clips, wires, shunts, rods, and the like) signal loss and distortion may be minimized by using as short TE (with short TR) as possible and selecting a scan plane that does not intersect the implant.

Sedation and immobilization are necessary to minimize motion, the most significant contributor to MR image degradation, especially in younger patients. Aggressive but safe sedation (or anesthesia, when necessary) is used along with firm application of head, arm, and body restraints for patient security and comfort. MRI-compatible vital monitoring and support (cardiac, respiratory, and pulse oximetry) are required to ensure the safety of the sedated patient. A nurse experienced in pediatrics and a crashcart with pediatric accessories are also important. Depending on the individual or institutional preference, sedation of infants may be achieved with chloral hydrate 50 to 75 mg/kg (maximum 1500 to 2000 mg), and of children 2 to 6 years of age with Demerol compound (meperidine 25 mg/ml, chloropromazine 6.25 mg/ml, and promethazine 6.25 mg/ml) administered intramuscularly (1 ml/10 to 15 kg, maximum 2 ml). Oral diazepam (0.3 mg/kg) may occasionally be helpful for an overanxious child or adolescent. The radiologist may prefer to consult with an anesthesiologist regarding intravenous sedation or anesthesia.

The child's urinary bladder should be empty before the examination. A firmly applied abdominal wrap may help decrease transmitted respiratory and bowel motion artifact. Flow-compensating and motion-suppression capabilities include RF presaturation, gradient moment nulling, respiratory compensation, cardiac or peripheral gating, and the ability to switch phase- and frequency-encoding gradient directions to divert phase-encoding motion artifact away from the ROI. These techniques are especially important for minimizing arterial or venous pulsation artifact near the skull base for temporal lobe, pituitary-hypothalamic, and posterior fossa imaging. These techniques are also critical to minimize arterial, venous, and CSF pulsatile flow artifacts in spine imaging. Guidelines[4,5] have been devised (Tables 1-4 and 1-5) that direct system hardware (gradient and RF electronics) and software (gradient and RF pulse sequencing) to produce the desired plane (axial, sagittal, coronal, oblique, and so forth), spatial resolution (slice thickness, FOV, and matrix), and contrast resolution (TR, TE, flip angle, and NSA) for imaging of a specified ROI within a desirable scan time (TR $\times$ phase-matrix $\times$ NSA), to emphasize certain intrinsic parameters (p, T1, T2, T2$\star$, flow, and so on), and to provide a gray-scale display that enhances certain tissue interfaces.

For brain imaging (Table 1-4), basic screening consists of a minimum of two planes and two acquisitions for T1, proton-density (p), and T2 information as follows: initial spin echo (SE) sagittal T1 (short TR/TE) acquisition followed by SE axial proton-density (long TR/short TE), and T2 (long TR/TE) acquisition. Presaturation (usually

Table 1-4   Brain imaging

Plane	Matrix(ϕ,ω)	TR(msec)	TE(msec)	NSA	Slice/gap(mm)	FOV(cm)	Parameters
Sagittal	128 or 192 × 256	600	20	1-2	5/1-2.5	20-24	T1
Axial	128 or 192 × 256	2000	15-30 and 80-120	1-2	5/2.5	20-24	p/T2

Then use the TR/TE that provides the best anatomical delineation or tissue characterization for additional planes.

Table 1-5   Spine imaging

Plane	Matrix(ϕ,ω)	TR(msec)	TE(msec)	NSA	Slice/gap(mm)	FOV(cm)	Parameters
Sagittal localizer	128 × 256	400	20	1	5/1	24-32	T1
Sagittal	128 or 192 × 256	400-600	20	2-4	3-4/0.5-1.0	20-24	T1
Sagittal	128 × 256	2000	15-30 and 80-120	1-2	4/1	20-24	p/T2

Then use the TR/TE that provides the best anatomical delineation or tissue characterization for additional planes.

with T1 SE) and gradient moment nulling (usually with p/T2 SE) may be used for flow compensation. The initial series provides a T1-weighted screen and a mid-sagittal slice to assist set-up for subsequent acquisitions. The second series gives long TR screening in the familiar axial plane, often important for CT correlation. After reviewing the screening sequences the operator may then select the TR and TE that provide the best anatomical delineation or tissue characterization for additional planes. If there are more specific clinical or imaging guides (US or CT), the initial screening MRI acquisitions may be tailored for the desired information. Additional axial T1 SE images may assist further in mapping myelination in the neonate and young infant. Thinner slices or smaller gaps between slices may be desired for closer examination of a specific ROI. Additional coronal p/T2 SE sections may be attained for seizure screening, especially for a temporal lobe focus. Multiple planes are often necessary, especially for surgical and radiotherapy planning and follow-up. In the posterior fossa, sagittal (T1) and axial (p/T2) planes are the minimum for defining cerebellar lesions relative to the brain stem, cord, cranial nerves, and vascular structures. Additional coronal planes may be important for cerebellopontine angle and cervicomedullary junction lesions. Additional sagittal p/T2 SE images may be important for intrinsic brain stem lesions regarding longitudinal extent. For lesions about the sella turcica and third ventricle (deep midline), sagittal, coronal, and axial slices are often needed to adequately delineate the relationship of lesions to the carotid-cavernous, deep venous, pituitary-hypothalamic, optic pathway, other cranial nerve, and the third ventricular landmarks. Coronal planes are also important for parasagittal and basal cerebral lesions. All three planes are frequently required for defining cerebral abnormalities relative to the major arterial, venous, lateral ventricular, motor pathway, language and memory, and visual radiation landmarks.

In general, T1 SE images have proven optimal for anatomical delineation, especially for gross developmental malformations (see Chapter 3). Proton-density and T2 spin-echo acquisitions usually provide the best sensitivity for water- ($-OH_2$) and iron- (Fe) containing lesions in subtle developmental or acquired lesions. All three parameters (T1, p, T2) are considered the minimum requirement for tissue characterization. Adjunctive brain imaging methods as outlined earlier include fat-suppression, gradient-echo, and Gd-DTPA enhancement techniques. The major indications for fat suppression include the need for clear delineation of water-containing lesions (with or without additional gadolinium enhancement) in areas where fat normally dominates and may obscure such abnormalities on T1 and proton-density images (for example, orbit and marrow), and to distinguish fat from other tissue elements that may have similar intensity patterns (for example, methemoglobin). The main indication for adjunctive gradient echo imaging (see Table 1-3) includes the delineation of vascular flow components or abnormalities (vascular occlusion, vascular malformation, and the like), the enhancement of CSF compartments or abnormalities (for example, myelogram, ventriculogram, or cisternogram effect and CSF dynamics), and the detection or confirmation of mineralization (for example, calcification and iron) or hemorrhage (for example, deoxyhemoglobin) through enhanced magnetic susceptibility. Although the indications for effective use of Gd-DTPA[6] as an imaging agent of the blood pool and blood-brain barrier have yet to be systematically worked out for pediatric CNS imaging, Gd-DTPA has primarily been helpful in the imaging of neoplastic processes. In general, preinjection sagittal T1 SE screening is conducted, followed by sagittal and axial or coronal T1 SE sections after intravenous Gd-DTPA injection (0.1 ml/kg, maximum 10ml). Axial p/T2 SE images are additionally important for nonenhancing tumor components and treatment effects (see Chapter 7).

Plain film findings are used as a guide to set up MR spine imaging (Table 1-5). A rapid T1 SE acquisition using a large FOV (24 to 32 cm) appropriate for patient size is done for surveying, positioning, and programming subsequent series. Total spine or craniospinal examination is facilitated by using the longest coil appropriately matched for patient weight within a movable coil holder or as part of a multicoil array, as previously described. After review of the initial series, the operator selects the TR/TE parameters that provide the best localization and characterization for additional planes. For most developmental abnormalities (for example, dysraphism), sagittal T1 SE longitudinal surveying (3- to 4- mm slice) is used, especially for craniocervical anomalies, conus terminations, hydrosyringomyelia, and diastematomyelia. Further coronal T1 SE longitudinal imaging is conducted to determine the extent of the hydrosyringomyelia or the diastematomyelia. Axial T1 SE sections (5/1-mm slice/gap and small FOV, 12 to 16 cm) are then recommended for screening of filar thickening (conus medullaris to filum terminus), for caudae equina nerve root anatomy, for dermal sinus tracts, and for lipomas. Axial p/T2 SE sections may be preferred for characterization of developmental masses other than lipoma (for example, cyst or dermoid), for diastematomyelic septation, and for canal dimensions. For most acquired conditions of the epidural space (for example, inflammatory or neoplastic processes), additional sagittal or axial p/T2 SE images may be desired. For intramedullary and intradural processes, additional sagittal, coronal, or axial T1 SE sections post-gadolinium may be necessary, especially for tumor mass, seeding, or hydrosyringomyelia (rule-out tumor). Sagittal p/T2 SE sections may be necessary to demonstrate intramedullary lesions producing minimal or no cord expansion (for example; infarction, demyelination, and myelitis) and for vascular malformations. Flow-compensation and motion-suppression techniques are critically important in MR spine imaging, especially for intradural lesions (seeding, and the like). As mentioned previously, fat suppression may be important (for example, STIR), especially for marrow imaging, whereas gradient echo techniques (see Table 1-3) may provide CSF enhancement (myelogram effect), vascular flow characterization, or magnetic susceptibility information.

DIAGNOSTIC SENSITIVITY AND SPECIFICITY

The superior contrast resolution of MRI provides unequaled sensitivity as compared with CT or US, especially for water- ($-OH_2$) containing lesions.[1-3] The sensitivity is more pronounced with proton-density (long TR/short TE) and T2 (long TR/TE) SE sequences than with T1 (short TR/TE) SE sequences (see Fig. 1-17). Abnormal voxel $-OH_2$ has higher proton density (greater concentration of resonating H1s) and much longer T2 (longer sustained proton macrovector coherence) with resultant higher intensity than adjacent normal stationary tissues (for example, gray and white matter). The T1 differences between abnormal and normal $-OH_2$ are usually not as great on SE sequences (lesions may be isointense to slightly hypointense). Inversion recovery (IR) sequences provide superior T1 contrast, particularly at lower field strength, but often with a poor signal-to-noise ratio relative to the longer acquisition time. Since many pathologies (neoplasm, edema, infarct, demyelination, cyst, and so forth) are associated with increased $-OH_2$ content, the sensitivity of MRI often does not translate into specificity, particularly if only T2 sequences are used. Specificity may be advanced, nonetheless, by identifying predominant or additional pathological components that are of higher intensity on T1 images or of lower intensity on T2 images (and also occasionally on p and T1 images).[7] Furthermore, the proton-density echo may often distinguish extracellular fluid (flowing) $-OH_2$ from extracellular nonfluid $-OH_2$ or intracellular free $-OH_2$.

Lesions, or lesional elements, which are either of short T1, produce T1 PRE (paramagnetic), or result in slow proton flow, appear higher intensity on T1 (short TR/TE) images. This includes fat ($-CH_2$), for example, in lipoma (see Fig. 1-42), hamartoma, dermoid, or teratoma. Also included is extracellular hydrous macromolecular matrix (EC matrix $-OH_2$) as with carbohydrate- or protein-containing developmental, neoplastic (see Fig. 1-20), or inflammatory lesions (colloid cyst, craniopharyngioma, cystic hygroma, mucinous metastases, abscess, and so on). Methemoglobin in subacute-chronic hemorrhage or thrombosis (see Figs. 1-32 to 1-34, 1-37, 1-38, and 1-41) is also of high intensity on T1 images, as is melanin (for example, in choroidal melanoma or the dysplastic foci of neurofibromatosis). T1 high intensity is seen with Gd-DTPA enhancement associated with absence or disruption of the blood-brain barrier and with blood-pool effects (see Fig. 1-35). Occasionally, paramagnetic alloys or metals and minerals in low concentration (calcium, iron) produce T1 hyperintensity (see Fig. 1-36). Relative high intensity (see Figs. 1-28, 1-30, and 1-32) may also be encountered with arterial occlusive disease (absence of normal flow void) or venous occlusive disease (methemoglobin thrombus).

Pathological components that are either of low proton density, short T2, produce T2 PRE (magnetic susceptibility), or result in rapid/turbulent proton flow, appear low intensity (or signal void) on T2 (long TR/TE) images. Occasionally the low intensity also may be apparent on proton-density and T1 images. Such low intensity may be seen with mineral deposition in high concentration including calcification (see Fig. 1-46), and iron as ferritin or hemosiderin (see Figs. 1-34, 1-39, and 1-41). Iron as deoxyhemoglobin in acute-subacute hemorrhage or thrombosis also appears low intensity (see Fig. 1-38). Anhydrous

Table 1-6   Tissue intensity (I) characteristics

Element	T1(Short TR/TE)	p(Long TR/Short TE)	T2(Long TR/TE)
Fat	High I	High I	Low I
EC matrix $-OH_2$ (proteinaceous collection or cyst)	Iso-high I	High I	High I
Nonfluid free $-OH_2$ (for example, edema)	Low I	High I	High I
Fluid free $-OH_2$ (CSF)	Low I	Low I	High I
IC matrix $-OH_2$ (for example, hypercellular tumor)	Variable I	Iso-high I	Low I
Anhydrous or anisotropic matrix (for example, collagen)	Low I	Low I	Low I
Methemoglobin (extracellular)	High I	High I	High I
Methemoglobin (intracellular)	High I	Variable-high I	Low I
Deoxyhemoglobin	Iso-low I	Low I	Lower I
Gadolinium-DTPA	High I	High I	High I
Melanin	High I	Variable I	Low or high I
Ferritin	Iso-low I	Low I	Lower I
Hemosiderin	Iso-low I	Lower I	Lowest I
Low concentration Fe	High I	Low I	Lower I
Calcification	Iso-, low, or high I	Iso-low I	Iso-low I
Vascular slow flow	Iso-, low, or high I	Iso-high I	Iso-high I
Vascular/CSF rapid flow	Low I	Low I	Low I

extracellular macromolecular matrix, bound hydrous intracellular matrix (IC matrix $-OH_2$), and anisotropic hydrous matrix include protein, carbohydrate, or combined complexes (for example, glycoprotein and mucoprotein) that are often hypointense (see Figs. 1-19 and 1-41). Examples are collagen, fibrin, keratin, colloid, mucin, and some hypercellular neoplasms (for example, medulloblastoma). High velocity or turbulent flow is of low intensity or signal void as with normal (for example, carotid and jugular) or abnormal (for example, AVM) vascular flow (see Figs. 1-22, 1-28, 1-31, and 1-33). Similar turbulent low intensity or signal void may be seen with accentuated pulsatile CSF flow in obstructive hydrocephalus or hydrosyringomyelia (see Figs. 1-23 and 1-25).

Fluid (flowing) and nonfluid $-OH_2$ may both appear hypointense on T1 images and hyperintense on T2 images. Proton-density echoes may easily distinguish them by demonstrating lower intensity for flowing extracellular free $-OH_2$ as with CSF-filled ventricles, cisterns, cysts, collections, clefts, or defects (see Fig. 1-17). Nonfluid extracellular free or bound $-OH_2$ and intracellular free $-OH_2$ appear as relatively high intensity on proton-density echoes (see Fig. 1-17) including neoplasm, infarction, demyelina-

tion, edema, and so forth. However, proteinaceous fluid collections or cysts (EC matrix $-OH_2$) may not be readily distinguished from solid (IC matrix $-OH_2$) masses (see Fig. 1-20). Combining the intensity (I) characteristics throughout the SE sequences for T1, p, and T2 weighting a pattern may emerge for a given abnormality that may further enhance specificity (Table 1-6).

REFERENCES
Techniques and guidelines

1. Barnes P: Magnetic resonance in pediatric and adolescent neuroimaging, *Neurol Clin North Am* 8:741, 1990.
2. Barnes P, Lester P, Yamanashi W, et al: MR imaging in childhood intracranial masses, *Magn Reson Imaging* 4:41, 1986.
3. Barnes P, Prince J, Galloway D, et al: Complementary roles of MR and CT in pediatric cranial and spinal imaging, *Pediatr Radiol* 17:345, 1987.
4. Bradley W, Kortman K, Crues J: Central nervous system high resolution MR imaging and effect of increasing spatial resolution on resolving power, *Radiology* 156:93, 1985.
5. Bradley W, Tsuruda J: MR sequence parameter optimization: an algorithmic approach, *AJR* 149:815, 1987
6. Elster A, Moody D, Ball M, et al: Is Gd-DTPA required for routine cranial MR imaging? *Radiology* 173:231, 1989.
7. Weinstein M: MRI versus CT: today's scoreboard, *Magnetic resonance imaging and CT update*, 1989, Harvard Medical School Postgraduate Course, Cambridge, Mass, October 27, 1989.

2 · Clinical Principles of Pediatric Neuroradiology

Patrick D. Barnes
David K. Urion
Jane C. Share

Ultrasonography, computed tomography, and magnetic resonance imaging

ULTRASONOGRAPHY

Ultrasonography (US) is noninvasive (nonionizing), inexpensive, portable, fast, real time, and multiplanar. It uses no contrast agents and infrequently requires patient sedation. US signals represent variations in acoustic reflectance of tissues and tissue interfaces so that echogenic structures (for example, choroid plexus, hemorrhage, solid tumor, edema, infarction, and cerebritis) and sonolucent structures (ventricular CSF, cysts, and so forth) may be separated from one another and from the more uniform brain substance. More complex disease processes (for example, ventriculitis) may exhibit more complex sonographic patterns. Although US provides moderately good soft tissue resolution, it is operator dependent and requires a window unimpeded by bone or air for cranial and spinal imaging. These drawbacks limit the range of use to the fetus (obstetrical US), infant (open fontanelle and sutures), immature or dysplastic cranium or spine (for example, dysraphism), and surgery (craniotomy and laminectomy). Cranial neurosonography is most effective for viewing echogenic supratentorial intraventricular, periventricular, and intracerebral lesions (for example, hemorrhage), as well as sonolucent CSF and other fluid-containing lesions (for example, hydrocephalus, cyst, and cleft).

US is considered the procedure of choice (see box at right) for prenatal and neonatal screening.* It is the first and

---

*References 2, 5, 6, 10, 18, 20, 21.

PRIMARY APPLICATIONS OF US

Fetal screen
Infant screen
Intraoperative
Doppler
Hemorrhage (intracerebral and intraventricular)
Gross malformation
Atrophy
Ventriculomegaly
Cysts
Dysraphism screen

---

usually definitive modality for neonatal hypoxic-ischemic encephalopathy (HIE), suspected developmental malformations, infection, and macrocephaly. Hemorrhagic manifestations of HIE readily detected by US (Figs. 2-1 and 2-2) include germinal matrix hemorrhage, intraventricular hemorrhage, and periventricular hemorrhagic infarction of prematurity, as well as hemorrhagic infarction in the term infant.[13,25-27] Computed tomography (CT) may more reliably detect extracerebral hemorrhage (subdural and subarachnoid) and posterior fossa collections (cerebellar or subdural). The nonhemorrhagic manifestations of HIE may be demonstrated by US as intraparenchymal echogenicities (IPE) representing ischemic edema or necrosis (infarction), including periventricular leukomalacia in the preterm infant.[25,26] This type of ischemic brain injury is the major determinant of neurological outcome. IPE may evolve into ventriculomegaly (atrophy), porencephaly, or cystic en-

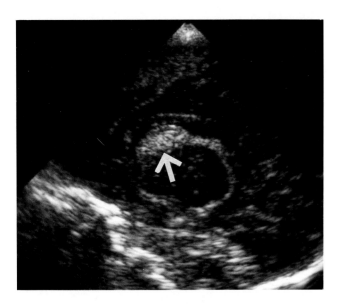

Fig. 2-1   Germinal matrix hemorrhage of prematurity shown by parasagittal US scan through the anterior fontanelle as an echogenic subependymal mass *(arrow)* at the caudothalamic notch anterior to the normally echogenic choroid plexus and beneath the sonolucent lateral ventricle.

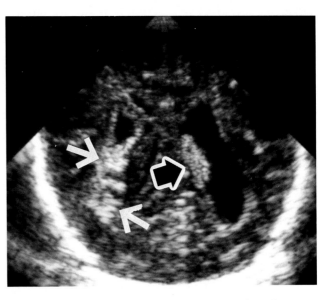

Fig. 2-3   Dandy-Walker cyst and hydrocephalus shown by posteriorly angled coronal US scan as a triangular infratentorial sonolucent cyst *(asterisk)* along with dilatation of the sonolucent lateral ventricles *(arrows).*

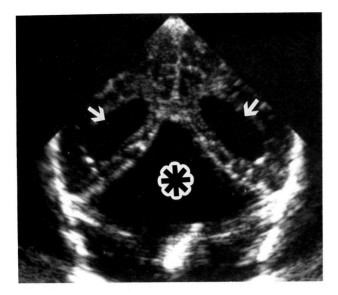

Fig. 2-2   Intraventricular hemorrhage and hydrocephalus of prematurity shown by posteriorly angled coronal US scan through the anterior fontanelle as an echogenic mass *(white arrows)* within the sonolucent right lateral ventricle. The normally echogenic choroid plexus is demonstrated *(black arrow)* within the sonolucent left lateral ventricle.

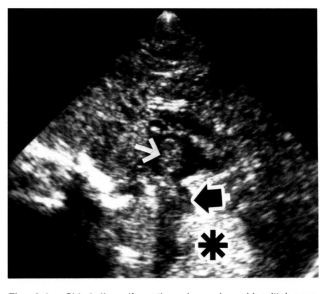

Fig. 2-4   Chiari II malformation shown by midsagittal scan, including large mass intermedia *(white arrow)*, bulbous tectum *(black arrow)*, and echogenic dysplastic cerebellum *(asterisk)* with poorly visualized fourth ventricle.

cephalomalacia. The more subtle ischemic periventricular lesions are occasionally better delineated by US than by CT, in which the low density of immature white matter often obscures the injury. US effectively images the evolution of ischemic IPE, as well as the progression or resolution of hemorrhage and its sequelae (for example, hydrocephalus). US also effectively delineates the potential hemorrhagic or

hypoxic-ischemic complications of extracorporeal membrane oxygenation (ECMO)[15,24] in asphyxic infants with meconium aspiration, diaphragmatic hernia, persistent fetal circulation, and so forth.

Developmental anomalies readily identified by US [1,9,14] are those involving the ventricular system or containing CSF (Fig. 2-3) and include congenital hydrocephalus,

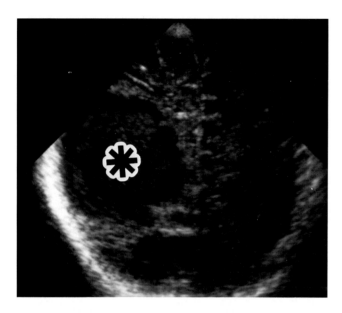

Fig. 2-5 Right parietal cerebral abscess *(asterisk)* shown by angled coronal US scan with echogenic central debris, liquified sonolucent periphery, and echogenic-surrounding edema. (Courtesy of Teele R, Share J: *Ultrasonography of infants and children,* Philadelphia, WB Saunders, in press.)

hydranencephaly, holoprosencephaly, absent septum pellucidum, agenesis of the corpus callosum, porencephaly (open schizencephaly), Dandy-Walker syndrome, arachnoid cyst, encephalocele, and so forth. Other anomalies often delineated by US include Chiari II malformation (Fig. 2-4), agyria-pachygyria, lissencephaly, and vascular malformations, especially aneurysm of the vein of Galen. US may not distinguish between hydranencephaly (absent cerebral mantle) and severe hydrocephalus (attenuated cerebral mantle). Other than for occasional identification of tubers (tuberous sclerosis), US is not considered the procedure for delineation of more subtle migrational, proliferative, or histogenetic malformations. Sonography is often used to delineate CNS infection[8,11] and the sequelae or complications (Fig. 2-5) that may accompany bacterial meningitis or TORCH infections (*t*oxoplasmosis, *o*ther viruses, *r*ubella, *c*ytomegalovirus, *h*erpes simplex viruses), such as ventriculitis, hydrocephalus, effusion, abscess, cystic encephalomalacia, edema, cerebritis, infarction, and calcification. CT with intravenous contrast enhancement may be preferred for the diagnosis and follow-up of suppurative collections, whereas US may serve as a guide for drainage. In the infant with macrocephaly[3,7,22,23] US provides an assessment of ventricular size for hydrocephalus, abnormal parenchymal echoes in dysplastic or degenerative megalencephaly, mass or collection (cyst, tumor, and subdural hematomas or hygromas), and large extracerebral spaces in external hydrocephalus.

Other special sonographic applications in pediatric CNS disease include spinal US, operative sonography, and Doppler neurosonography. Spinal US[4,16-18,28] is particularly effective for screening dysraphic myelodysplasia in the

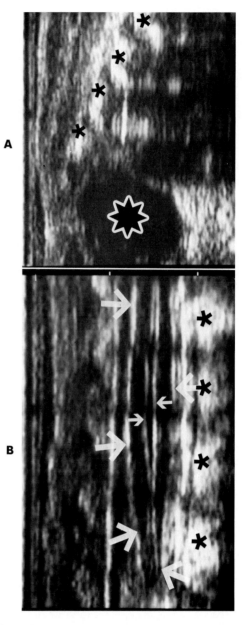

Fig. 2-6 Caudal presacral meningocele **(A)** and dilated central canal of the caudal spinal cord **(B)** shown by midsagittal US scans of the lower back. The sonolucent meningocele *(star)* lies anteroinferiorly to the tip of the sacrum. The echogenic cord outline is shown by the larger white arrows, and the echogenic outline of the large central canal is shown by the smaller white arrows. The black asterisks define the echogenic sacral and lumbar vertebral bodies.

first 3 to 6 months of life (Fig. 2-6), and can demonstrate conus level and cord pulsation through the cartilaginous posterior elements and interspinous gaps. US can delineate a variety of dysraphic abnormalities (Fig. 2-6) including meningocele, lipoma, hydromyelia, Chiari II malformation, diastematomyelia, lipomyelomeningocele, myelocystocele, and so forth. Spinal US is most effective for the screening of small infants with low-yield presentations (for example, sacral dimple only), and for clarifying ambiguous lum-

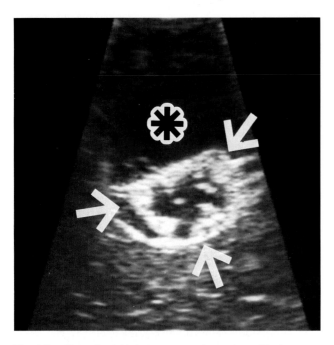

Fig. 2-7   Frontal cerebral astrocytoma demonstrated by intraoperative US, including the sonolucent cyst *(asterisk)* and echogenic solid tumor *(white arrows)* with central sonolucent necrosis.

bosacral spine films to rule out tethered cord and to evaluate anomalies of other systems (for example, hydronephrosis or solitary kidney). Occasionally sonography may be used for postoperative follow-up to detect cord retethering (lack of cord pulsation), although operative scarring often makes assessment difficult. Intraoperative sonography[16,18] has emerged as an important neurosurgical tool (Fig. 2-7) for safe and specific guidance in biopsy (separation of tumor core from edema), ventricular shunt placement, drainage of fluid collections, delineation of intraspinal traumatic bone fragments, monitoring of arteriovenous malformation (AVM) resection (Doppler), and localization of cord tumor or hydrosyringomyelia. Recently developed and refined Doppler techniques[7,15,19] have helped to identify specific intracranial vascular structures and to evaluate arterial patency, as well as flow direction and flow quantitation (resistive index). Specific applications include the evaluation of extracorporeal membrane oxygenation (ECMO) patients, assessment of brain death, delineation of vascular malformations, and discrimination of obstructive hydrocephalus from other causes of ventriculomegaly.

REFERENCES
Ultrasonography
1. Babcock D: Sonography of congenital malformations of the brain, *Neuroradiology* 28:428, 1986.
2. Babcock D, Han B: *Cranial ultrasonography of infants,* Baltimore, 1981, Williams & Wilkins.
3. Babcock D, Han B, Dine M: Sonographic findings in infants with macrocrania, *AJR* 150:1359, 1988.
4. Babyn P, Chuang S, Daneman A, et al: Sonography evaluation of spinal cord birth trauma with pathologic correlation, *AJNR* 9:765, 1988.
5. Benacerraf B: Fetal hydrocephalus, diagnosis, and significance, *Radiology* 169:858, 1988.
6. Filly R, Cordoza J, Goldstein R, et al: Detection of fetal CNS anomalies, *Radiology* 172:403, 1989.
7. Fischer A, Livingston J: Transcranial Doppler and real-time cranial sonography in neonatal hydrocephalus, *J Child Neurol* 4:64, 1989.
8. Frank J: Sonography of intracranial infection in infants and children, *Neuroradiology* 28:440, 1986.
9. Funk K, Siegel M: Sonography of congenital midline brain malformations, *Radiographics* 8:11, 1988.
10. Grant E, Tessler F, Perrella R: Infant cranial sonography, *Radiol Clin North Am* 26:1089, 1988.
11. Han B, Babcock D, Adams L: Bacterial meningitis in infants: sonographic findings, *Radiology* 154:645, 1985.
12. Han B, Babcock D, Oestreich A: Sonography of brain tumors in infants, *AJR* 143:31, 1984.
13. Kirks D, Bowie J: Cranial US of neonatal periventricular/intraventricular hemorrhage, *Pediatr Radiol* 16:114, 1986.
14. McGahan J, Ellis W, Lindfors K, et al: Congenital CSF-filled intracranial abnormalities: a sonographic classification, *JCU* 16:531, 1988.
15. Mitchell D, Merton D, Needleman L, et al: Neonatal brain, color Doppler imaging. Part I. Technique and vascular anatomy. Part II. Altered flow patterns from ECMO, *Radiology* 167:303-310, 1988.
16. Naidich T, Quencer R, editors: *Clinical neurosonography,* New York, 1987, Springer-Verlag.
17. Naidich T, Fernbach S, McLone D, et al: Sonography of the caudal spine and back: congenital anomalies in children, *AJR* 142:1229, 1984.
18. Rubin J, DiPietro M, Chandler W, et al: Spinal ultrasonography: intraoperative and pediatric applications, *Radiol Clin North Am* 26:1, 1988.
19. Rubin J, Hatfield M, Chandler W, et al: Intracerebral AVMs: intraoperative color Doppler flow imaging, *Radiology* 170:219, 1989.
20. Rumack C, Johnson M: *Perinatal and infant brain imaging: role of ultrasound and CT,* Chicago, 1984, Mosby–Year Book.
21. Sanders R, Blakemore K: Lethal fetal anomalies: sonographic demonstration, *Radiology* 172:1, 1989.
22. Shackelford G: Neurosonography of hydrocephalus in infants, *Neuroradiology* 28:452, 1986.
23. Strassburg H, Sauer M, Weber S, et al: Ultrasound diagnosis of brain tumors in infancy, *Pediatr Radiol* 14:284, 1984.
24. Taylor G, Fitz C, Miller M, et al: Intracranial abnormalities in infants treated with ECMO: imaging with US and CT, *Radiology* 165:675, 1987.
25. Volpe J: *Neurology of the newborn,* ed 2, Philadelphia, 1987, WB Saunders.
26. Volpe J: Current concepts of brain injury in the premature infant, *AJR* 153:243, 1989.
27. Volpe J: Intraventricular hemorrhage in the premature infant—current concepts. Part II. *Ann Neurol* 25:109, 1989.
28. Zieger M, D'orr U, Schulz R: Pediatric spinal sonography. Part II. Malformations and mass lesions, *Pediatr Radiol* 18:105, 1988.

COMPUTED TOMOGRAPHY

Computed tomography (CT) uses ionizing radiation with an image display of densities that are directly related to the attenuation coefficients (relative x-ray absorption) of tissues as a function of electron density (atomic number Z) of the component elements[5,15] (see box on p. 45). Tissue elements of higher atomic number are higher density and include calcium, iron, bone in mineralization, iodine in contrast-enhanced vascular structures, enhanced CSF spaces, or enhanced areas of absent or altered blood-brain barrier. Tissues of lower atomic number are lower density and include oxygen, nitrogen, or carbon in air, fat, CSF,

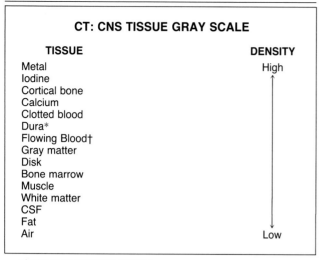

CT: CNS TISSUE GRAY SCALE

TISSUE	DENSITY
Metal	High
Iodine	
Cortical bone	
Calcium	
Clotted blood	
Dura*	
Flowing Blood†	
Gray matter	
Disk	
Bone marrow	
Muscle	
White matter	
CSF	
Fat	
Air	Low

*Includes ligament and cartilage.
†Depends on hematocrit and flow character.

PRIMARY APPLICATIONS OF CT

Acute trauma
Acute hemorrhage (extracerebral, posterior fossa)
Infarction screen
Gross malformation
Atrophy
Tuberous sclerosis (calcium)
Sturge-Weber syndrome (calcium)
Suppurative collection
Hydrocephalus (nontumor, postshunt)
Macrocephaly screen
Headache-only screen
Static encephalopathy
Acute seizure of known disease
Calcification/bone
Orbit, sinus, petrous bones
Localized spinal column abnormality
Stereotactic/three-dimensional
Postoperative state

muscle, white matter, gray matter, and water-containing lesions. CT is considered an excellent hard tissue imaging modality (for example, bone) with moderately good soft tissue resolution, especially at high-contrast interfaces such as air-water, bone-water, bone-fat, and fat-water in the orbits, sinuses, otomastoid, and so forth. CT artifact, however, often limits soft tissue resolution in areas where bone dominates (for example, skull base, intraspinal) or metallic objects are located (gunshot fragments, surgical clips, and the like). Although using ionizing radiation, current-generation scanners effectively restrict the exposure to the immediate volume of interest.

CT is fast and readily accessible for emergencies and for patients with other serious illnesses. Direct imaging is usually restricted to the axial or coronal plane. Reformatting in other planes (for example, sagittal) is associated with significant deterioration of spatial resolution unless high matrices (for example, 512 × 512), smaller fields of view, or thinner slices are used, all of which usually require higher radiation. CT often requires sedation in young children, occasionally needs intravenous contrast enhancement, and sometimes CSF contrast opacification. High resolution bone algorithms are important for fine bone anatomy (for example, temporal bone). Projection scout images may assist in lesion localization for surgery and radiotherapy planning. Three-dimensional reconstruction software is important for planning craniofacial reconstructive surgery[14] (see Fig. 2-42). Computer-assisted stereotactic CT techniques (see Chapter 7) provide guidance for neurosurgical biopsy or resection and for small-field radiotherapy (radiosurgery).[3] Real-time CT-guided needle biopsy procedures are also well established for spinal column and paraspinal lesions (see Chapter 10).

The role of CT has been redefined (see box above, right) in the context of accessible and reliable ultrasound (US) and magnetic resonance imaging (MRI).[1,2] In the neonate and young infant CT is often of secondary or adjunctive importance, but it serves a significant back-up role to US. When the US window is lost with age, CT becomes the primary screening and often definitive modality for brain imaging. In general, for most presentations nonenhanced CT is done as the initial or only screen. Intravenous contrast injection, preferably using low osmolar nonionic agents, is considered only after viewing the preinjection study. In a few well-defined situations contrast-enhanced CT is anticipated by design. Noncontrast examination is usually all that is required for CT screening of neonatal problems after US, nonvascular developmental anomalies[12] (Fig. 2-8), acute trauma,[7,9] acute hemorrhage[5] (Fig. 2-9), and suspected infarction,[4] especially that associated with known predisposing disease (for example, congenital heart disease). It is usually sufficient for displaying infection[4,5] (meningitis, encephalitis, TORCH), nonneoplastic hydrocephalus (posthemorrhage, postinfection, and congenital), and follow-up of hydrocephalus after shunting.[4,5] Noncontrast CT is often all that is required to evaluate macrocephaly, headache without neurological signs, and failure to thrive or developmental delay (psychomotor retardation) and in nonprogressive disease (atrophy, leukomalacia, mineralization) associated with static encephalopathies (Fig. 2-10). CT without contrast is often satisfactory for some neurocutaneous syndromes (for example, calcification in tuberous sclerosis) and for acute seizures related to known conditions (for example, trauma and infection).[4,5] CT without enhancement suffices in most instances for the orbits, sinuses, facial bones, temporal bones, and spinal column.[8,11,13]

Intravenous enhancement for blood-brain barrier disruption or blood pool effect is additionally recommended for CT evaluation of suspected or known vascular malformation, neoplasm, abscess, or empyema[5] (Fig. 2-11). Enhanced CT may help evaluate a mass or hemorrhage of

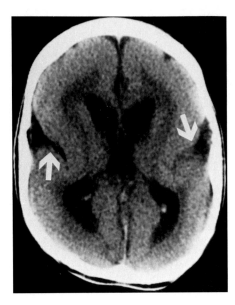

Fig. 2-8   Noncontrast CT demonstrates gross brain changes of lissencephaly including pachygyric-agyric cortex plus ventricular, Sylvian *(white arrows)*, and gray-white matter dysmorphia.

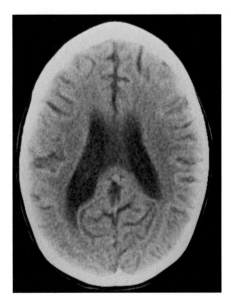

Fig. 2-10   Noncontrast CT showing cerebral atrophy after encephalitis with ventricular and sulcal dilatation plus loss of gray-white matter differentiation.

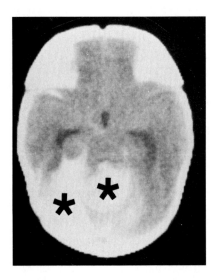

Fig. 2-9   Noncontrast CT showing high density tentorial and posterior fossa parturitional hemorrhage *(asterisks)* in a term newborn.

unknown etiology, unexplained focal seizures, and chronic subdural hematoma. It also may help differentiate infarction from neoplasm or abscess, serve as an indicator of disease activity, for example, in degenerative or inflammatory disease and vasculitis, or provide a high-yield guide for stereotactic or open biopsy (for example, tumor core). Follow-up or repeat CT studies may assist in distinguishing evolving infarction or focal inflammation from neoplasm (Fig. 2-12). Contrast-only CT may be employed for routine follow-up of neoplasm, vascular malformation, and suppurative collection, as well as for suspected metastasis or

seeding. CT study before and after contrast injection is recommended if an acute neurological change (suspected hemorrhage) is discovered at follow-up. Precontrast- and postcontrast-enhanced CT also is suggested in the immediate postoperative period to assess operative change versus residual disease (see Chapter 7). Additional coronal CT may be particularly important for complete assessment of the orbits, sinuses (to detect ostiomeatal complex disease), temporomandibular joints, or temporal bones.[8,13] Coronal planes may also be indicated for intrasellar, skull base, midline, and vertex intracranial lesions. Ventricular or subarachnoid CSF-contrast opacification may further assist in evaluating or confirming CSF compartment lesions or communication (for example, arachnoid cyst or ventricular encystment). As a rule, and except for suppurative infection, MRI should be the alternative to contrast-enhanced CT in the circumstances just enumerated.

As mentioned before, CNS tissues are displayed by CT according to density based on x-ray attenuation coefficients.[4,15] CT abnormalities are characterized as low density, isodensity, or high density relative to gray matter and by the degree and pattern of enhancement after iodinated contrast administration. Abnormal low density, or low attenuation, approaching that of CSF usually implies increased free water content but is nonspecific. A wide variety of lesions appear as low density (Fig. 2-12) including cyst, edema, necrosis, neoplasm, infarction, dysplasia, inflammation, degeneration, and so forth. Abnormalities of very low density, or negative attenuation coefficients, include those containing fat (for example, lipoma, dermoid, teratoma) or air (for example, pneumocephalus after trauma or surgery). Isodense abnormalities may be detected only if there is distortion of normal anatomy, if they are contrasted against lower or higher

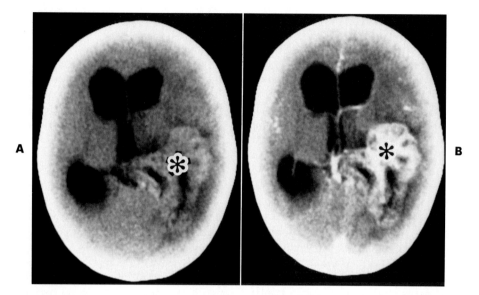

Fig. 2-11   Precontrast **(A)** and postcontrast **(B)** CT of choroid plexus papilloma *(asterisks)* showing high density **(A)** consistent with a combination of tumor hypercellularity, hypervascularity, and calcification. **B,** Abnormal enhancement correlates with blood-brain (or tumor) barrier breakdown and hypervascularity.

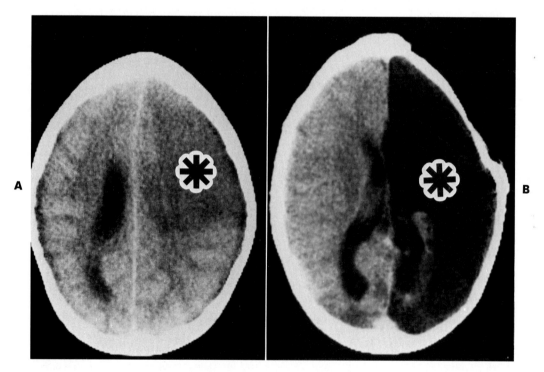

Fig. 2-12   Serial CT studies showing the evolution from acute cerebral infarction **(A)** with left frontal low density mass effect *(asterisk)* to hemispheric atrophy **(B)** with extensive low density, CSF-filled defect *(asterisk)* and ventricular dilatation.

density structures (for example, intraventricular tumor), or if there is contrast enhancement of the abnormality itself or of adjacent tissues (for example, isodense hematoma). As mentioned earlier, enhancement after intravenous administration of iodinated agents implies either absent or disrupted blood-brain barrier or blood pool effect. Enhancement is expected in a number of normal tissues including vascular and dural structures, as well as the pituitary, infundibulum, pineal gland, choroid plexus, and so forth. Abnormal enhancement is often nonspecific (see Fig. 2-11), since it appears with any of a variety of pathologies producing barrier breakdown (for example, neoplasm or infarction) or those associated with abnormal vascularity (for example, vascular malformation). Abnormalities of higher density (see Fig. 2-11) than gray matter (high attenuation) on nonenhanced CT include mineralization (ossification, calcification, iron), acute or subacute hemorrhage or thrombosis, abnormal blood pool effect such as vascular malformation (for example, vein of Galen aneurysm), hypervascular tumor (choroid plexus papilloma, and the like), and hypercellular neoplasm (high nuclear-to-cytoplasmic ratio) such as medulloblastoma, other primitive neuroectodermal tumors, germinoma, lymphoma, and so forth. Another important CT sign is loss of gray matter/white matter differentiation (see Figs. 2-10 and 2-26), though again nonspecific, and may be seen acutely (hypoxic-ischemic injury) or chronically (hypomyelination).

REFERENCES
Computed tomography

1. Barnes P: Magnetic resonance in pediatric and adolescent neuroimaging, *Neurologic Clinics of North America,* vol 8, Philadelphia, 1990, WB Saunders.
2. Barnes P, Lester P, Yamanashi W, et al: MR imaging in childhood intracranial masses, *Magn Reson Imaging* 4:41, 1986.
3. Davis D, Kelly P, Marsh W, et al: Computer-assisted stereotactic biopsy of intracranial lesions in pediatric patients, *Pediatr Neurosci* 14:31, 1988.
4. Diebler E, Dulac O: *Pediatric neurology and neuroradiology,* New York, 1987, Springer-Verlag.
5. Faerber E: *Cranial computed tomography in infants and children,* Philadelphia, 1986, JB Lippincott.
6. Fredericks B, Boldt D, Tress B, et al: Diseases of the spinal canal in children with noncontrast CT, *AJNR* 10:1233, 1989.
7. Gentry L, Godersky J, Thompson B, et al: Comparative study of MR and CT in closed head trauma, *AJR* 150:673, 1988.
8. Humphrey C, Strand R, Barnes P: Head and neck imaging in childhood. In Healy G, editor: *Common problems in pediatric otolaryngology,* Chicago, 1990, Mosby–Year Book.
9. Kleinman P: *Diagnostic imaging of child abuse,* Baltimore, 1987, Williams & Wilkins.
10. Legido A, Zimmerman R, Packer R, et al: Significance of basal ganglia calcification on CT in children, *Pediatr Neurosci* 14:2:64, 1988.
11. Petterson H, Harwood-Nash D: *CT and myelography of the spine and cord,* New York, 1982, Springer-Verlag.
12. Sarwar M: *CT of congenital brain malformations,* Boston, 1985, Martinus Nihoff.
13. Strand R, Humphrey C, Barnes P: Imaging of petrous temporal bone abnormalities in infancy and childhood. In Healy G, editor: *Common problems in pediatric otolaryngology,* Chicago, 1990, Mosby–Year Book.
14. Vannier M, Hildebolt C, Marsh J, et al: Craniosynostosis: three-dimensional CT reconstruction, *Radiology* 173:669, 1989.
15. Yamada N: *Pediatric cranial computed tomography,* New York, 1983, Igaku-Shoin.

MAGNETIC RESONANCE IMAGING

As one of the less invasive or relatively noninvasive neuroimaging technologies, magnetic resonance imaging (MRI) is neither ionizing, as are CT and isotope scanning, nor requires a pathway unobstructed by bone or air, as does US. Furthermore the MRI signal is exponentially derived from multiple parameters (T1, T2, PRE, and so on), whereas CT (x-ray attenuation) and US (acoustic impedance) signals are linear derivatives of single parameters. MRI provides multiplanar imaging with equivalent resolution in all planes without repositioning the patient or machine. Bone does not interfere with soft tissue resolution, although metallic objects often produce signal void or field distortion artifacts. Some ferromagnetic or electronic devices (for example, aneurysm clips and pacemakers) pose a hazard, and MRI is usually contraindicated in these cases. MRI is not as fast as US or CT, and patient sedation is required in most infants and younger children, since image quality is easily compromised by gross motion. MRI may not be as readily accessible to the pediatric patient as is US or CT and may not be feasible in emergencies or for intensive care cases unless magnet-compatible vital monitoring and support is available.

Although more expensive than US or non-contrast CT, MRI is less expensive than the more invasive modalities such as angiography, myelography, or even ventriculographic or cisternographic CT, all of which often require anesthesia. In general, MRI should be the primary alternative[2,3] for processes often known to be isodense by CT (for example, occult tumor in seizure disorder), for suspected soft tissue abnormalities near bone (for example, low posterior fossa lesions), for situations in which CT requires vascular, CSF, or blood-brain barrier enhancement (for example, AVM, cyst, neoplasm) and especially when the more invasive procedures are under consideration. In these circumstances MRI has made the greatest impact and has displaced or replaced less sensitive and more invasive neuroradiological procedures. In a number of important circumstances, MRI also may provide specificity by further characterizing nonspecific US or CT abnormalities.

MRI has demonstrated superior sensitivity in a number of circumstances (see box on p. 49). It is the only modality that can provide an accurate assessment of brain maturation, that is, myelination[1] (Fig. 2-13). MRI provides superior sensitivity and disease extent in demyelination, dysmyelination, and extrapyramidal degeneration[10] (Fig. 2-14) and effectively displays encephalitis (Fig. 2-14), vasculitis, gliosis, and small foci of leptomeningeal suppuration not revealed by CT. MRI is often better than CT in demonstrating traumatic injuries (Fig. 2-15), including axonal shear injury, cortical contusion, brain stem injury, and sequelae such as microcystic encephalomalacia and gliosis.[7] MRI can detect anomalies that elude CT, including malformations of neural and glial migration and proliferation (Fig. 2-16) such as heterotopias, fused schizencephaly, and the phacomatoses (for example, neurofibromatosis).[4,13] MRI has demonstrated minute seizure foci including hippocampal sclerosis and mesial temporal glioma, as well as small

PRIMARY APPLICATIONS OF MRI

Myelination
Neurodegenerative disease
Brain inflammation
Nonhemorrhagic trauma
Migrational anomalies
Neurofibromatosis
von Hippel–Lindau disease
Infarction (hemorrhagic, multiple, vasculitis)
Vascular malformation
Hemorrhage (subacute, chronic, atypical)
Venous occlusive disease
Unexplained focal seizure
Unexplained hydrocephalus
Neuroendocrine disorder
Nonspecific CT/US findings (calcification, enhancement, ventriculomegaly, extracerebral collection)
Surgical anatomy
Radiotherapy planning
Tumor response and treatment effects
Spinal neuraxis
Spinal marrow

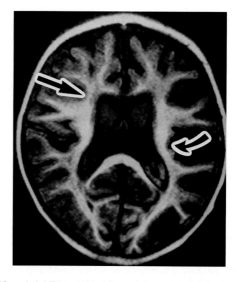

Fig. 2-13   Axial T1-weighted inversion recovery MRI demonstrating normal myelination *(black arrows)* as high intensity in this young infant.

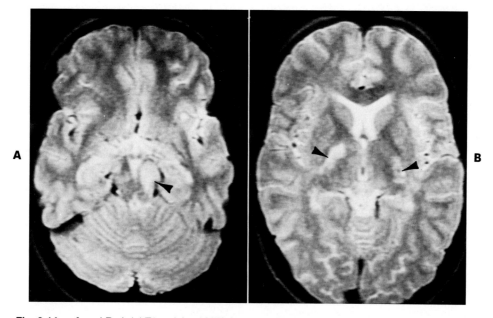

Fig. 2-14   **A** and **B,** Axial T2-weighted MRI demonstrating encephalitis with demyelination including high-intensity foci *(black arrowheads)* within the midbrain, basal ganglia, and deep capsular tracts.

tumors about the aqueduct, sella, or lower brain stem, despite negative or equivocal CT findings[2,3,9] (Figs. 2-17 to 2-19). MRI is the preferred procedure for neurological presentations beyond infancy, when tumor becomes the likely cause, and especially for increased pressure, unexplained focal epilepsy, and central neuroendocrine disorders.

MRI frequently offers greater diagnostic specificity than does CT or US for delineating vascular and hemorrhagic processes.[2,8,12] This includes the clear depiction of vascular structures and abnormalities based on proton flow parameters and software enhancements not requiring the injection of contrast agents. It also provides more specific identification and staging of hemorrhage and clot formation according to the evolution of hemoglobin breakdown (Fig. 2-20; see Figs. 1-38 and 1-41) and can often differentiate arterial from venous occlusive disease (see Fig. 1-32). MRI is the procedure of choice before or instead of angiography for evaluating unexplained hemorrhage shown by CT, especially for angiographically occult lesions (cavernous hemangioma), and distinguishing vascular malformation from neoplasm when CT shows nonspecific calcification or

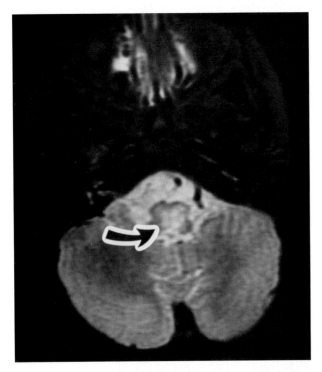

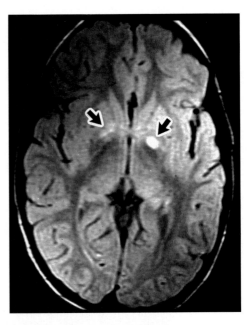

Fig. 2-15   Axial T2-weighted MRI showing high-intensity medullary lesion *(black arrow)* consistent with brain stem infarction with negative CT.

Fig. 2-16   Axial proton density MRI demonstrating bilateral high-intensity dysplastic foci *(black arrows)* in neurofibromatosis 1. (From Barnes P: *Neurol Clin North Am* 8:741,1990.)

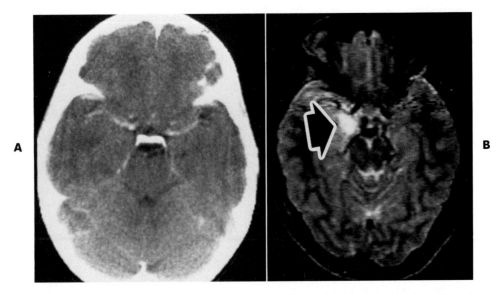

Fig. 2-17   Partial complex seizure disorder due to right mesial temporal astrocytoma *(arrow)* negative by CT **(A)** but shown as high-intensity abnormality by axial T2 MRI **(B).** (From Barnes P: *Neurol Clin North Am* 8:741, 1990.)

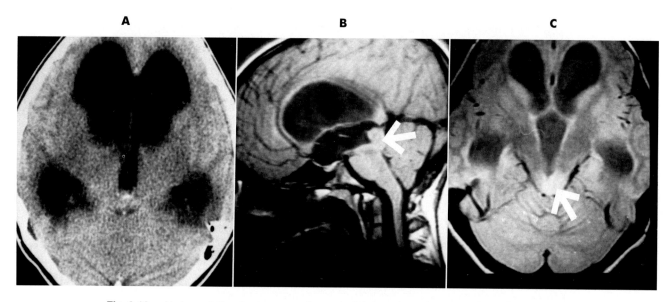

Fig. 2-18   Hydrocephalus due to apparent aqueductal stenosis as shown by CT **(A).** Sagittal T1 **(B)** and axial proton density **(C)** MRI demonstrate a tectal tumor *(white arrows).* (From Barnes P: *Neurol Clin North Am* 8:741, 1990.)

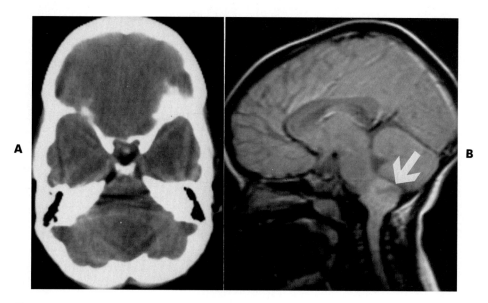

Fig. 2-19   Cervicomedullary astrocytoma with negative or equivocal CT **(A)** but abnormal sagittal proton density MRI **(B)** showing a high-intensity mass *(arrow).*

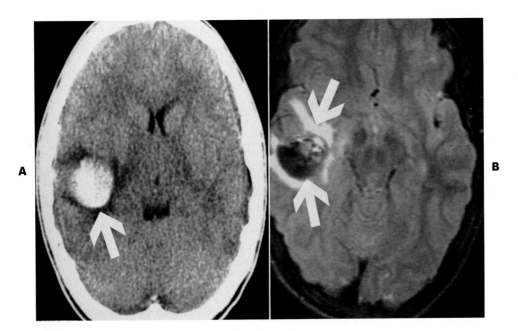

Fig. 2-20   Temporal cavernous angioma with hemorrhages of multiple age shown by CT **(A)** after trivial trauma as a high-density mass *(white arrow)* with surrounding low density, and by axial T2 MRI **(B)** as mixed high and low intensities *(white arrows)* consistent with both subacute and chronic hemorrhage.

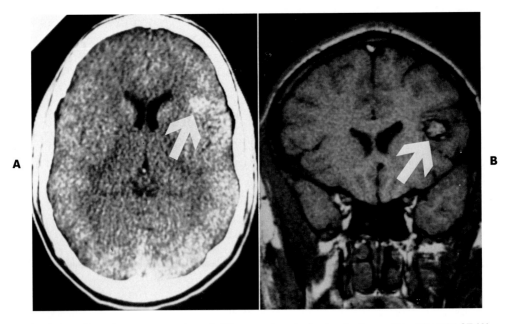

Fig. 2-21   Frontal cavernous angioma *(white arrows)* producing focal seizures shown by axial CT **(A)** as a nonspecific calcific high density and by coronal T1 MRI **(B)** as a central high intensity with peripheral low intensity characteristic of cavernous angioma. In childhood the differential diagnosis of a solitary cerebral calcification as shown by CT includes tumor (for example, glioma), hamartoma (for example, tuber), vascular malformation (for example, cavernous angioma), and infection (for example, cysticercosis).

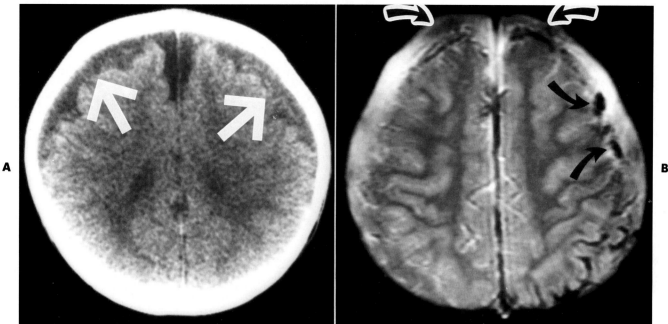

Fig. 2-22 Bilateral subdural hematomas shown by CT **(A)** as nonspecific, low-density extracerebral collections *(arrows)* and by axial gradient MRI **(B)** as high-intensity subdural collections with low-intensity areas *(arrows)* consistent with both chronic and acute hemorrhage.

enhancement (Fig. 2-21). It may further clarify nonspecific extracerebral collections first shown by CT or US (Fig. 2-22) by differentiating benign infantile collections (for example, external hydrocephalus) from subdural hematomas (for example, in child abuse). MRI readily confirms CSF-containing compartments and lesions (for example, arachnoid cysts) without requiring cisternography or ventriculography (Fig. 2-23). MRI may also offer supportive (physiological) or causative (anatomical) information regarding obstructive hydrocephalus[2,6] (see Fig. 1-23) when CT or US demonstrates nonspecific ventriculomegaly. This includes hydrocephalus due to occult tumor, for example, periaqueductal glioma or neoplastic seeding. The proton flow characteristics of CSF make CSF-contrast opacification unnecessary in these circumstances, although occasionally intravenous contrast administration is required (for example, gadolinium-enhanced seeding).

Although comparatively less sensitive and less specific than MRI in the instances just described, cranial CT and US still provide practical cost-effective screening (and often definitive evaluation) in the majority of cases. This is especially the case for "rule-out" indications or for confirmation in acute trauma, acute hemorrhage (especially neonatal), infection (for example, meningitis), gross developmental malformations (for example, Chiari II, agenesis of the corpus callosum), and atrophy associated with static encephalopathies (that is, cerebral palsy). CT or US often adequately assesses large masses (cyst, tumor), hydroceph-

alus in infancy, hydrocephalus after shunting, and the immediate postoperative state. In some of these cases MRI's precise delineation of anatomy (multiplanar) and disease extent (multiparameter) may serve as an adjunct to US or CT for complete evaluation regarding more specific treatment or prognosis,[2] including developmental conditions (Fig. 2-23). Furthermore, MRI has become the primary method in neuroncological imaging (Fig. 2-24) for surgery, radiotherapy, and chemotherapy planning, as well as for follow-up of tumor response and treatment effects, particularly with the more recent addition of intravenous Gd-DTPA[11] contrast enhancement for barrier breakdown imaging and the detection of leptomeningeal/CSF dissemination.

With regard to spinal imaging, the plain film, or US in the very young, remains the primary screening procedure along with the occasional use of isotope bone scanning for extradural reactive, inflammatory, or neoplastic processes. CT is usually chosen next, especially in acute trauma or for localized bony disease, for example, fracture-dislocation, spondylolysis, benign tumor, or bone anomaly. For the most part, MRI has replaced myelography and CSF-contrast CT as the definitive procedure for spinal neuraxis imaging (Fig. 2-25; see Fig. 1-42) including developmental conditions (for example, myelodysplasia) and acquired processes (for example, neoplasia).[2,5,13,14] MRI also is the procedure of choice for evaluating spinal marrow involvement in neoplastic diseases or hematopoietic disorders (see Fig.

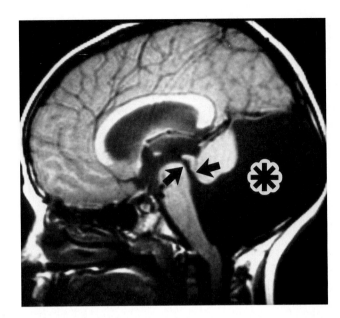

Fig. 2-23   Dandy-Walker cyst with hydrocephalus shown by sagittal T1 MRI as a large retrocerebellar CSF-intensity cyst *(asterisk)*. Accentuated CSF flow voids *(arrows)* are seen across the patent aqueduct.

A   B   C

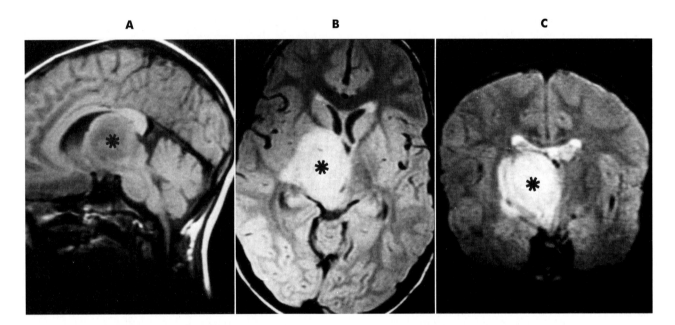

Fig. 2-24   Right thalamic glioma *(asterisk)* demonstrated by sagittal T1 **(A)**, axial proton density **(B)**, and coronal T2 **(C)** MRI for treatment planning.

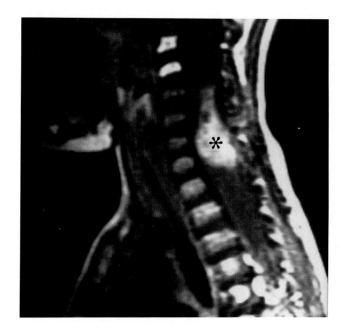

Fig. 2-25 Cervical cord ganglioglioma shown by sagittal T1 MRI as a gadolinium-enhancing intramedullary tumor *(asterisk)* with hydrosyringomyelia or cystic cord expansion above and below. (From Barnes P: *Neurol Clin North Am* 8:741, 1990.)

1-43). Water soluble, low osmolar, nonionic contrast CT or myelography is only rarely indicated for subarachnoid space lesions (for example, cysts) poorly identified by MRI or when artifact from metallic instrumentation (for example, Harrington rods) limits MRI use.

REFERENCES
Magnetic resonance imaging

1. Barkovich A, Kjos B, Jackson D, et al: Normal maturation of the neonatal and infant brain: MR imaging at 1.5 T, *Radiology* 166:173, 1988.
2. Barnes P: *Magnetic resonance in pediatric and adolescent neuroimaging, Neurologic Clinics of North America,* vol 8, Philadelphia, 1990, WB Saunders.
3. Barnes P, Lester P, Yamanaski W, et al: MR imaging in childhood intracranial masses, *Magn Reson Imaging* 4:41, 1986.
4. Braffman B, Bilaniuk L, Zimmerman R: CNS manifestations of the phakomatoses on MR, *Radiol Clin North Am* 26:773, 1988.
5. Davis P, Hoffman J, Ball T: Spinal abnormalities in pediatric patients: MR imaging, *Radiology* 166:679, 1988.
6. Gammal T, Allen M, Brooks B, et al: MR evaluation of hydrocephalus, *AJR* 149:807, 1987.
7. Gentry L, Godersky J, Thompson B, et al: MR and CT in closed head trauma, *AJR* 150:673, 1988.
8. Gomori J, Grossman R, Goldberg H, et al: Intracranial hematomas: high-field MR, *Radiology* 157:87, 1985.
9. Heinz E, Heinz T, Radtke R, et al: Efficacy of MR vs CT in epilepsy, *AJR* 152:347, 1989.
10. Newell M, Grossman R, Haskney D, et al: MR imaging of white matter disease in children, *AJNR* 9:503, 1988.
11. Powers T, Partain C, Kessler R, et al: CNS lesions in pediatric patients: Gd-DTPA-enhanced MR imaging, *Radiology* 169:723, 1988.
12. Smith H, Strother C, Kikuchi Y, et al: MR in the management of supratentorial AVMs, *AJR* 150:1143, 1988.
13. van der Knaap M, Valk J: Congenital abnormalities of the CNS, *AJNR* 9:315, 1988.
14. Vogler J, Murphy M: Bone marrow imaging, *Radiology* 168:679, 1988.

Symptoms and signs in pediatric CNS disease: a clinical guide to neuroimaging

DEVELOPMENTAL DELAY

Failure to thrive (FTT) broadly refers to failure of somatic growth and development (weight and height). Developmental delay, also known as psychomotor retardation, refers to failure of the infant or child to achieve the expected motor milestones (sitting, crawling, walking, hand-eye coordination) or cognitive milestones (speech, memory, learning) as part of normal growth and development.[3,15] Somatic as well as neurological delay may result from a variety of CNS diseases, systemic illnesses, or diseases of other organ systems. Psychomotor impairment may result from a previous brain insult no longer active (static encephalopathy), from an active, ongoing, progressive process (progressive encephalopathy), or from a recurring process (paroxysmal or episodic syndrome). Developmental delay may be manifest in the neonate or infant as hypotonia (flaccid motor impairment), the so-called "floppy infant syndrome." This is usually indicative of damage to the immature, premyelinated pyramidal white matter tracts (upper motor neuron involvement, that is, cerebral cortex to anterior horn cells of the spinal cord) or to lower motor neuron disease (anterior horn cell to muscle). In the older infant or child the expression may be that of hypertonia (spastic or rigid motor impairment) including paraparesis or diparesis (legs), hemiparesis (arm and leg), quadraparesis (legs and arms), or monoparesis (arm or leg). This is usually a reflection of damage to the myelinating or myelinated tracts. There may be associated or isolated involvement of gray matter manifested as seizures, mental retardation, language and speech delay, learning difficulties, or behavioral disorders (hyperactivity, autism, and the like).[2,11] Occasionally there is extrapyramidal (for example, basal ganglia) involvement with involuntary motor phenomena (choreoathetosis, and the like), brain stem involvement (cranial neuropathy), or a cerebellar component (for example, ataxia). There may be associated craniofacial dysmorphism, microcephaly, or macrocephaly.

Cerebral palsy is the nonspecific designation for static encephalopathy of prenatal or perinatal origin (perinatal encephalopathy).[3,4,8,13,15] This terminology implies fixed or static, nonprogressive deficit(s). The cause includes, but is not limited to, prenatal or perinatal asphyxia (also known as perinatal hypoxic-ischemic encephalopathy, HIE), whether hemorrhagic or nonhemorrhagic, in the preterm or term infant.[14] Other important causes are parturitional trauma, prenatal or perinatal infection (for example, TORCH infections, bacterial meningitis, and HIV), and primary brain malformations, whether confined to the CNS or associated with anomalies of other organ systems. Brain malformations are often part of genetic or chromosomal syndromes (neurofibromatosis, trisomy 21, and so forth).[5,6,12] If the causative insult occurs at the early embryological or fetal stages of the first or second trimester, the result is arrested or altered development of the forming brain, that is, malformation (for example, anencephaly, holoprosencephaly, lissencephaly, callosal agenesis, Chiari II, and so forth). Later insults in the third trimester, perinatal period, or postnatal period result in incomplete development or destruction (encephaloclasis) of the formed or near-formed brain (for example, cerebral hypoplasia, porencephaly, leukomalacia, encephalomalacia and the like).[6]

In the floppy infant, hypotonia may occasionally be related to a fixed deficit as the result of spinal cord injury (for example, transection) or myelodysplasia (for example, myelocele or myelomeningocele).[3,15] If the neurological disorder is a progressive encephalopathy or myelopathy, then the major consideration is a CNS mass or expansion versus a neurodegenerative disease. Intracranial or spinal processes in the former category include hemorrhage, hydrocephalus, inflammatory collection, cyst, neoplasm, hydrosyrinx, and or the tension/ischemia of dysraphic cord tethering. Often more specific signs are present to direct the neuroimaging. Neurodegenerative disorders comprise a variety of heredofamilial metabolic disorders, genetic and chromosomal malformative syndromes, as well as certain systemic diseases and connective tissue disorders.[9,10] Episodic or paroxysmal neurological syndromes are covered in subsequent sections.

In general, US is the imaging procedure of first choice for prenatal screening and postnatal examination for most of the considerations just discussed. CT is recommended when US is not applicable, for example, lack of a bone window, or is inconclusive regarding the clinical query. US is an effective modality especially for viewing the supratentorial intracranial compartment, gross malformations, intraventricular and intracerebral hemorrhage, cystic lesions, and hydrocephalus (see Fig. 2-1 to 2-3). CT is somewhat better for demonstrating posterior fossa lesions, edema, infarction, and extracerebral hemorrhage or other collection (see Fig. 2-9). MRI is reserved for exceptional cases in which US or CT does not provide the desired information and especially for progressive disease in either the mass/expansion or neurodegenerative category, and particularly for spinal neuraxis evaluation. [1]

REFERENCES
Developmental delay

1. Barkovich A: *Pediatric neuroimaging*, New York, 1990, Raven.
2. Barlow C: *Mental retardation and related disorders*, Philadelphia, 1987, FA Davis.
3. Dunn D, Epstein L: *Decision making in child neurology*, Philadelphia, 1987, BC Decker.
4. Fenichel G: *Clinical pediatric neurology*, Philadelphia, 1988, WB Saunders.
5. Jones K: *Smith's recognizable patterns of human malformation*, ed 4, Philadelphia, 1988, WB Saunders.
6. Lemire R, Loeser J, Leech R, et al: *Normal and abnormal development of the human nervous system*, New York, 1975, Harper & Row.
7. Menkes J: *Textbook of child neurology*, ed 3, Philadelphia, 1985, Lea & Febiger.
8. Nelson K: Cerebral palsy. In Swaiman K: *Pediatric neurology*, St Louis, 1989, Mosby–Year Book.

9. Rapin I: Cerebral degenerations of childhood: differential diagnosis. In Rowland LP, editor: *Merritt's textbook of neurology,* ed 7, Philadelphia, 1984, Lea & Febiger.
10. Swaiman K: Intellectual and motor deterioration. In Swaiman K: *Pediatric neurology,* St Louis, 1989, Mosby–Year Book.
11. Swaiman K: Mental retardation. In Swaiman K: *Pediatric neurology,* St Louis, 1989, Mosby–Year Book.
12. Taybi H: *Radiology of syndromes and metabolic disorders,* ed 2, Chicago, 1983, Mosby–Year Book.
13. Thompson G, Rubin I, Bilenker R: *Comprehensive management of cerebral palsy,* New York, 1983, Grune & Stratton.
14. Volpe J: *Neurology of the newborn,* ed 2, Philadelphia, 1987, WB Saunders.
15. Weiner H, Urion D, Levitt L: *Pediatric neurology for the house officer,* ed 3, Baltimore, 1988, Williams & Wilkins.

ENCEPHALOPATHY, COMA, AND BRAIN DEATH

Acute or progressive impairment of consciousness in the infant, child, or adolescent may present as encephalopathy (abnormal sensorium) or coma (loss of consciousness, LOC).[3-6,9,10] Other important symptoms or history include pain, headache, seizure, fever, paresis, movement disorder, or infection. More specific neurological findings of a focal or lateralizing nature or the presence of elevated intracranial pressure provide the indication for emergent versus elective imaging. Encephalopathy in the absence of lateralizing signs is likely of toxic or metabolic origin,[8] including asphyxia (for example, after cardiopulmonary arrest), poisoning (lead and the like), drug ingestion, or metabolic abnormalities such as hypoglycemia, hypocalcemia, hyponatremia, uremia, or hyperammonemia (for example, Reye's syndrome). CNS infection such as meningitis or encphalitis is another important consideration for emergent imaging. More specific signs such as hemiparesis, unilateral cranial nerve palsy, or elevated pressure indicate a destructive or expanding lesion and provide the requirement for immediate imaging, usually CT. Imaging is important also in the difficult to examine, uncooperative, or unresponsive patient and particularly when toxic encephalopathy is

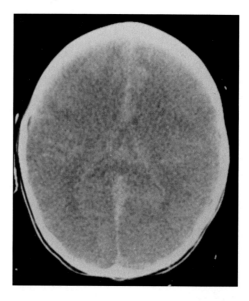

Fig. 2-26 A 3-year-old victim of a motor vehicle accident shows hypoxic-ischemic injury and brain death as demonstrated by CT as diffuse cerebral low densities with loss of ventricular and subarachnoid space landmarks, as well as loss of gray-white matter differentiation.

complicated by possible trauma, infection, or hemorrhage. In this situation, and particularly when there are signs of raised pressure, imaging may distinguish a focal mass from a diffuse process so that lumbar puncture for CSF analysis can be carried out with relative safety. Imaging may be important for uncovering not only the cause of neurological impairment, for example, hematoma as a result of AVM, but also the effect of insults on the CNS, for example, edema in asphyxia (Fig. 2-26). The initial imaging examination also serves as a baseline for follow-up to evaluate

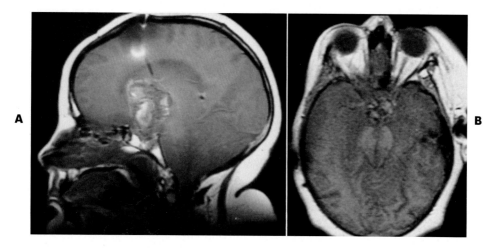

Fig. 2-27 Adolescent girl with progressive suprasellar tumor growth, extensive edema, tonsillar herniation, and brain death with sagittal T1 MRI **(A)** and axial gradient echo MRI **(B)** failing to demonstrate normal vascular intensities consistent with absent cerebral blood flow. (From: Jones K, Barnes P: *AJNR,* in press.)

disease progression, sequelae, treatment response, and treatment effects. Altered mental status also may be associated with seizure disorder (aura, postictal, status epilepticus, and so forth), as well as other paroxysmal or episodic disorders including syncope, migraine (aura), and acute schizophrenia (hallucinations, delusions). The definition of brain death is usually based on neurological and EEG evidence of total and irreversible cessation of brain function.[2,7] Imaging studies are rarely if ever indicated for determining brain death but have been employed to confirm absence of blood flow to the brain, including dynamic isotope scanning, contrast-enhanced CT, Doppler US,[1] and, rarely, angiography or MRI (Fig. 2-27).

REFERENCES
Encephalopathy, coma, and brain death

1. Bode H, Sauer M, Pringsheim W: Diagnosis of brain death by transcranial Doppler sonography, *Arch Dis Child* 63:1474, 1988.
2. Coulter D: Neurologic uncertainty in newborn intensive care, *N Engl J Med,* 316:840.
3. Dunn D, Epstein L: *Decision making in child neurology,* Philadelphia, 1987, BC Decker.
4. Fenichel G: *Clinical pediatric neurology,* Philadelphia, 1988, WB Saunders.
5. Lockman L: Impaired consciousness. In Swaiman K: *Pediatric neurology,* St Louis, 1989, Mosby–Year Book.
6. Menkes J: *Textbook of child neurology,* ed 3, Philadelphia, 1985, Lea & Febiger.
7. Schneider S, Ashwal S: Determination of brain death in childhood. In Swaiman K: *Pediatric neurology,* St Louis, 1989, Mosby–Year Book.
8. Schwartz J: Poisoning and drug-induced neurologic diseases. In Swaiman K: *Pediatric neurology,* St Louis, 1989, Mosby–Year Book.
9. Vannucci R, Young R: Diagnosis and management of coma in children. In Pellock J, Myer E, editors: *Neurologic emergencies in infancy and childhood,* Philadelphia, 1984, Harper & Row.
10. Weiner H, Urion D, Levitt L: *Pediatric neurology for the house officer,* ed 3, Baltimore, 1988, Williams & Wilkins.

PAROXYSMAL DISORDERS

Paroxysmal disorders involve recurring or episodic motor or sensory neurological impairment.[6,7,14,21,26] Epilepsy (convulsive or seizure disorder) composes the largest group referred for imaging, whereas migraine constitutes the most common of the nonepileptic paroxysmal conditions. Convulsive disorders in childhood fall into two major categories: generalized and partial seizures (see box above).[11,12,15] Clinical and EEG findings suggesting involvement of both cerebral hemispheres or the deep midline structures (brain stem, thalamus, and so forth) define a generalized seizure disorder, whereas findings indicating a seizure focus limited to part of one hemisphere define a partial seizure disorder. Generalized seizures may often occur in partial seizure disorders (partial seizures with secondary generalization). Epileptic syndromes in the generalized category include absence (petit mal), tonic-clonic (grand mal), infantile spasms, minor motor seizures (Lennox-Gastaut), and benign myoclonic epilepsy. The partial epilepsy category comprises simple and complex partial disorders including benign epilepsy of childhood with rolandic spikes (BECRS), benign occipital epilepsy, gelastic seizures, and epilepsia partialis continua syndrome.

CHILDHOOD EPILEPSY

GENERALIZED	PARTIAL
Absence	Simple
Tonic-clonic	Complex
Infantile spasms	BECRS
Minor motor	Benign occipital
Lennox-Gastaut syndrome	Gelastic
Benign myoclonic	Epilepsia partialis continua

The commonest cause of acute or episodic hemiparesis in childhood is a seizure disorder, that is, a postictal paralysis (Todd's paralysis).[26] It should be noted that a seizure is only a symptom of CNS dysfunction and, as with any neurological symptom, requires evaluation to discriminate among fixed nonprogressive disease states, progressive intracranial processes, and idiopathic disorders.

Seizures in the neonatal period, by distinction, may be focal or generalized (see box on p. 59). These are often the result of a metabolic derangement such as hypoglycemia, hypocalcemia, pyridoxine deficiency, or narcotic withdrawal.[5] Perinatal asphyxia (HIE) including intracranial hemorrhage is a major cause of neonatal seizures.[24] Other important causes include brain malformation, CNS infection (TORCH and the like), and the initial expression of an inborn error of metabolism (for example, maple syrup urine disease). Occasionally the seizures are idiopathic, benign, and transient (benign familial neonatal convulsion). Correctable metabolic derangement or electrolyte imbalance must also be ruled out in the older child with new onset of seizures, especially when associated with a systemic or gastrointestinal illness. Toxic exposure, drug ingestion, or hematologic disorder with anemia should also be excluded. Convulsions may also accompany trauma, hypoxia, or febrile infection. Focal seizures may be the initial indication of an otherwise occult focal brain lesion (see Figs. 2-17 and 2-21) such as a neoplasm, vascular malformation, hamartoma, or sclerosis.[12,23,26]

Typical febrile seizures are brief, often familial, and associated with a rising fever.[6] Again, correctable metabolic derangement must be excluded and infection investigated if necessary (for example, to rule out meningitis or encephalitis). It is essential to distinguish "typical" benign febrile seizures from fever-induced epilepsy of another cause. *Absence* seizures (petit mal) with characteristic EEG findings are rarely if ever the result of specific CNS disease.[11] Tonic-clonic seizures (grand mal) are the commonest form of idiopathic epilepsy in childhood. These may be primary generalized or partial with secondary generalization.[15] *Infantile spasms* are an age-specific convulsive syndrome indicating diffuse disease of the immature CNS, often with characteristic hypsarrhythmic EEG.[26] These may be idiopathic but are often related to known or identifiable disease including prenatal infection, malformation (for example, callosal dysgenesis, Aicardi's syndrome), peri-

---

NEONATAL SEIZURES

Benign familial
Metabolic
Narcotic withdrawal
Hypoxic-ischemic
Malformation
Infection
Inborn error of metabolism

---

natal asphyxia, trauma, phacomatosis (for example, tuberous sclerosis), meningitis, encephalitis, hemorrhage, chromosomal anomaly (for example, trisomy 21), or metabolic/neurodegenerative disorder (for example, aminoacidopathy). *Minor motor seizures* are generalized with akinetic, atonic, or myoclonic components and include Lennox-Gastaut syndrome (epilepsy with mental retardation).[15] The causes are many and similar to the list for infantile spasms. A benign form of myoclonic seizures first described by Janz also exists as part of the spectrum of *primary generalized epilepsy of adolescence.*

Partial epilepsies (simple and complex) are focal disorders and idiopathic in 30% to 50% of cases.[12,15] *Simple partial seizures* may be motor or sensory, depending on the location of the focus, and occur without impaired consciousness. *Focal seizures* may be encountered with a variety of CNS pathologies, as previously enumerated, to include neoplasm. Well-known benign forms are the benign focal epilepsies of childhood including sylvian or rolandic (BECRS) and occipital. *Complex partial seizures* (temporal lobe or psychomotor seizures) are distinguished from simple partial epilepsy by impaired consciousness and frequent complex behavioral aspects (aura).[12] Causes of complex seizures are similar to those of simple seizures. Rarely, major personality, behavioral, or psychiatric disorders may coexist with complex seizures. Other partial epilepsy syndromes include gelastic seizures (or laughing spells) associated with hypothalamic or mesial temporal lesions, and epilepsia partialis continua, a rare prolonged focal seizure without loss of consciousness and usually secondary to a focal encephalitis or a diffuse cortical/subcortical process.[15]

Intractable seizures are those that are refractory to anticonvulsant treatment, once inadequate drug choice and inadequate drug levels have been ruled out.[6,26] Diagnostic reassessment is often necessary along with consideration for surgery, for example, temporal lobectomy, corpus callosotomy, cortisectomy, or hemispherectomy. The evaluation often requires extensive electrophysiological assessment including long-term EEG monitoring and Wada testing, along with sophisticated imaging for surgical planning with MRI, single photon emission computed tomography (SPECT), or positron emission tomography (PET).[4,13,25] *Status epilepticus* denotes the state of recurring or continual seizures without recovery of consciousness for 30 minutes

or more.[23,26] Prolonged status may require clinical reevaluation and exclusion or correction of metabolic imbalances. Imaging may help demonstrate previously unrecognized CNS disease, especially if there are abnormal neurological signs (increased intracranial pressure, retinal hemorrhage, and so on), and particularly if the status was precipitated by trauma or infection.

In general, imaging is not routinely recommended for initial evaluation of the benign convulsive disorders, that is, the classic absence and typical febrile epilepsies, as well as the benign rolandic, occipital, and myoclonic seizure disorders.[11] Imaging is recommended for seizures associated with abnormal neurological signs, history of CNS abnormality, focal clinical or EEG features, or deterioration of school performance. Imaging is also indicated when there is a change in seizure or EEG pattern including worsening of otherwise adequately treated seizures or focal EEG slowing.[11,15,26] US (for the infant) or CT is recommended for the initial imaging of seizures (for example, neonatal seizures, infantile spasms, or Lennox-Gaustaut syndrome) with known or expected disease (for example, HIE, infection, trauma, or malformation). Focal epilepsy (simple or partial) without obvious cause demonstrated by clinical, US, or CT evaluation should be evaluated by MRI because of its proven superior sensitivity[3,10,18,22] (see Fig. 2-17). Even with negative initial imaging results, close follow-up is important and repeat study warranted for any change in neurological examination, seizure pattern, or EEG. Again, imaging assists in evaluating not only the cause of seizures but also the effects of chronic epilepsy and chronic anticonvulsant therapy including atrophy that may be diffuse or regional. The latter may be an indirect indication of seizure origin. Occasionally, transient focal or unilateral CT-density or MR-intensity abnormalities may be seen associated with focal prolonged or repeated convulsions (Fig. 2-28). This presumedly represents perifocal edema and commonly resolves after a period of seizure control as documented on follow-up imaging.

Seizures are to be distinguished from a variety of other common episodic but *nonepileptic disorders* (that is, those with normal EEG) including breathholding spells, syncope, migraine, pseudoseizures, cyclic vomiting, vertigo, ataxia, movement disorders, apnea, and sleep disorders.* Neuroimaging is not ordinarily required for evaluating many of these syndromes, especially breathholding spells, syncope, pseudoseizures, and sleep disorders, unless associated with abnormal neurological signs, abnormal EEG (seizure disorder), history of preexisting CNS disease, trauma, or a hypoxic episode. Cyclic vomiting may be epileptic, migrainous, metabolic, gastrointestinal, or psychogenic. Rarely a lower brain stem lesion, for example, medullary glioma may produce continual vomiting (see Fig. 2-19). Syncope implies impaired cerebral perfusion and is usually of cardiovascular or vasomotor origin. Sleep disorders of childhood (for example, somnambulism, night terrors, insomnia, or hypersomnia) rarely require further neurolog-

---

*References 1, 2, 6, 8, 9, 19, 26.

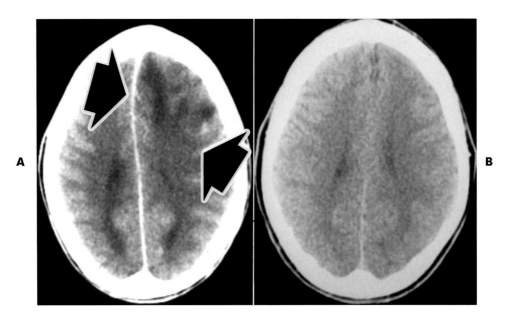

Fig. 2-28   **A** and **B,** Serial CT scans demonstrating left frontal low-density edema *(arrows)* associated with repeated focal seizures that resolves on follow-up **(B)** after a period of seizure control.

ical or imaging evaluation unless associated with a seizure disorder or for the reasons previously enumerated above.[1,8,9,19] Hypersomnia may occur after head trauma, encephalitis, cranial irradiation, systemic illness, or with narcolepsy, obstructive apnea, depression, or drug use. *Apnea* (absent respiratory effort) in the newborn may be a sign of CNS immaturity or related to a developmental malformation (for example, Chiari II), asphyxia, drugs, infection, metabolic imbalance, systemic disease, or seizures.[6,26] Occasionally it is a sign of progressive neuromuscular disease, for example, Landry-Guillain-Barré-Strohl syndrome. Prolonged apnea may be associated with the *sudden infant death syndrome* (SIDS) or near-SIDS. It also has been linked to gastroesophageal reflux. Obstructive sleep apnea is often associated with adenotonsillar enlargement, oropharyngeal anomalies, or neuromuscular disease. Migraine, vertigo, ataxia, and movement disorders are discussed in forthcoming sections.

REFERENCES
Paroxysmal disorders

1. Anders T, Keener M: Sleep/wake state development and disorders of sleep in infants, children, and adolescents. In Levine M, Carey W, Crocker A, Gross R, editors: *Developmental behavioral pediatrics,* Philadelphia, 1983, WB Saunders.
2. Barlow C: *Headaches and migraine in childhood,* Philadelphia, 1984, JB Lippincott.
3. Brooks B, King D, El Gammal, et al: MR imaging in patients with intractable complex partial epileptic seizures, *AJNR* 11:93, 1990.
4. Denays R, Rubinstein M, Ham H, et al: Single photon emission computed tomography in seizure disorders, *Arch Dis Child,* 63:1184, 1988.
5. Doberczak T, Shanser S, Senie R, et al: Neonatal neurologic and encephalographic effects of intrauterine cocaine exposure, *J Pediatr* 113:354, 1988.
6. Dunn D, Epstein L: *Decision making in child neurology,* Philadelphia, 1987, BC Decker.
7. Fenichel G: *Clinical pediatric neurology,* Philadelphia, 1988, WB Saunders.
8. Ferber R: Sleep, sleeplessness, and sleep disruptions in infants and young children, *Ann Clin Res* 234:227, 1985.
9. Guillemin C, editor: *Sleep and its disorders in children,* New York, 1987, Raven.
10. Heinz E, Heinz T, Radtke R, et al: Efficacy of MR vs CT in epilepsy, *AJNR* 9:1123, 1988.
11. Holmes GL: *Diagnosis and management of seizures in children,* Philadelphia, 1987, WB Saunders.
12. Holmes GL: EEG and neuroradiologic evaluation of children with epilepsy, *Pediatr Clin North Am* 36:395, 1989.
13. Jack C, Sharbrough F, Marsh W: Use of MR imaging for quantitative evaluation of resection for temporal lobe epilepsy, *Radiology* 169:463, 1988.
14. Menkes J: *Textbook of child neurology,* ed 3, Philadelphia, 1985, Lea & Febiger.
15. Mikati M, Brown T: Seizure disorders in children. In Dershewitz A, editor: *The practice of office-based pediatrics,* Philadelphia, 1988, JB Lippincott.
16. Mizroli E: Childhood epileptic syndromes, *Int Pediatr* 4:201, 1989.
17. Schorner W, Meencke H, Felix R: Temporal lobe epilepsy: CT and MR imaging, *AJNR* 8:773, 1987.
18. Smith A, Weinstein M, Quencer R, et al: Association of heterotopic gray matter with seizures: MR imaging, *Radiology* 168:195, 1988.
19. Smith S: Sleep disorders in children. In Swaiman K: *Pediatric neurology,* St Louis, 1989, Mosby–Year Book.
20. Soges L, Cacayorin E, Petro G, et al: Migraine: evaluation by MR, *AJNR* 9:425, 1988.
21. Swaiman K: *Pediatric neurology,* St Louis, 1989, Mosby–Year Book.
22. Triulzi F, Franceschi M, Fazio F, et al: Nonrefractary temporal lobe epilepsy: 1.5 T MR imaging, *Radiology* 166:181, 1988.
23. Urion D, Avery M, Sabry J, et al: Neurology. In Avery M, First L: *Pediatric medicine,* Baltimore, 1989, Williams & Wilkins.
24. Volpe J: *Neurology of the newborn,* ed 2, Philadelphia, 1987, WB Saunders.
25. Vries J, Crumrino P, Dasheiff R: Epilepsy surgery in childhood. In McLaurin R, Schut L, Venes J, Epstein F, editors: *Pediatric neurosurgery,* ed 2, Philadelphia, 1989, WB Saunders.
26. Weiner H, Urion D, Levitt L: *Pediatric neurology for the house officer,* ed 3, Baltimore, 1988, Williams & Wilkins.

HEADACHE AND OTHER PAIN SYNDROMES

Acute headache in a child often occurs with a febrile illness, especially with head and neck infections, for example, eye, sinus, or otomastoid.[1,3,8] It may be a main or early presenting symptom of meningitis or encephalitis. Headache commonly accompanies head trauma and is a major symptom of subarachnoid hemorrhage, whether traumatic or spontaneous (for example, vascular malformation). However, other, more revealing signs are often present. Neoplasm is a rare cause of acute-onset headache unless the tumor is hemorrhagic (for example, primitive neuroectodermal tumor, high grade glioma, or malignant germ cell tumor) or involves the leptomeninges (for example, leukemia, medulloblastoma seeding, gliomatosis, and so forth).[1] Hydrocephalus is an infrequent source of acute pain except in instances of shunt malfunction. Other causes of acute headache include hypertension (for example, pheochromocytoma), drug abuse, and the initial episode of migraine or muscle tension headache syndromes.

More *chronic persistent, recurring,* or *progressive headache* may be a sign of an expanding intracranial lesion.[1,3,4,6,8] The headache may precede the onset of other neurological symptoms or signs by weeks or months. Persistent pain may also occur with chronic meningitis, pseudotumor cerebri, or be of migraine or muscle tension origins. Recurring episodes are more characteristic of migraine but also occur with sinus, dental, temporomandibular joint, or ocular muscle causes. Rarely, recurring headache is part of the symptom complex of an heredofamilial neurodegenerative disorder. Trigeminal neuralgia is rare in childhood but requires investigation including imaging. *Migraine* is a common source of nonepileptic paroxysmal neurological impairment, especially headache. The family history is positive in 90% of cases. The syndrome is of a vascular or vasomotor mechanism and manifested as classic (with visual aura or other prodrome), common (without prodrome), or complicated (with accompanying hemiplegia, ophthalmoplegia, aphasia, vertigo, and the like).[1,6,8] Psychogenic causes of headache are more frequent into adolescence.

Barlow[1] has emphasized certain clinical indications for neuroimaging in children with subacute or chronic headache as follows:

1. Abnormal neurological signs, unexplained reduction in visual acuity, or enlarged head circumference
2. Associated constitutional symptoms such as recent school failure, behavioral change (for example, anorexia or apathy), and somatic growth retardation
3. Frequent nocturnal or morning headache, especially of increasing frequency and severity
4. Periodic headache with seizures especially in the same episode (especially focal seizures), or as a complex syndrome
5. Cluster headaches (migrainous neuralgia) in a child, or headache in any child under 6 years of age
6. Focal neurological signs during the headache (complicated migraine)
7. Focal neurological signs during the aura with fixed laterality or persisting beyond the aura
8. Visual gray-out at the peak of headache
9. Brief cough headache

Neuroimaging is recommended to search for intracranial tumor, vascular malformation, or ischemic changes (migraine). CT may suffice for screening of tumor or vascular malformation. MRI is often more sensitive or specific in demonstrating vascular lesions including the ischemic edema or infarction associated with complicated migraine[7] (Fig. 2-29).

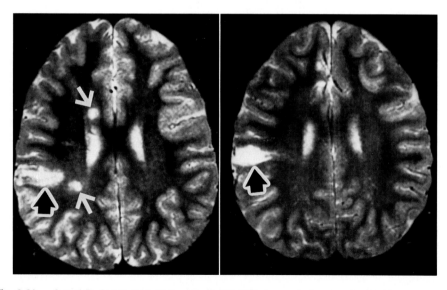

Fig. 2-29 **A** and **B,** Serial axial proton density/T2 MRI demonstrating transient *(white arrows)* and more permanent *(black arrow)* intensity abnormalities associated with complicated migraine in a young girl.

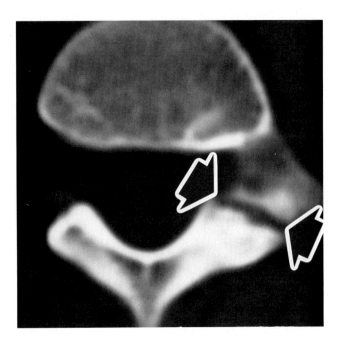

Fig. 2-30   Axial CT demonstrating spondylolysis *(arrows)* with left neural arch defect and adjacent sclerotic reaction.

Neck or back pain of spinal or paraspinal origin is usually related to musculoskeletal strain, overuse, postural factors, or trauma. Pain associated with scoliosis, torticollis, tenderness, positive straight leg raising, fever, or neurological signs warrants investigation.[3,5,9] Occult traumatic or dysplastic bony defects (spondylolysis) are frequent causes of such pain, whereas facet arthropathy and disc protrusion (traumatic) are unusual causes (Fig. 2-30). Muscle or bone pain may be a presenting symptom of leukemia or sickle cell anemia. Spinal column infection or neoplasm may produce pain, percussion tenderness, or a palpable mass. Intraspinal neoplasms of cord or nerve root origin may cause pain. Extremity pain, especially when associated with a limp or an abnormal gait, may also reflect muscle, bone, or joint disease, but occasionally such pain may be related to spinal column or spinal neuraxis disease,[2] or to a reflex sympathetic dystrophy. The neuroimaging work-up should initially include plain films of the spine. An isotope bone scan should follow if film results are negative. CT is recommended if a benign bony lesion is expected (for example, spondylolysis or osteoid osteoma), whereas MRI is preferred for an anticipated invasive bone, soft tissue, or marrow process, especially when neurological signs are present (see Chapter 10).

Paresthesias (pain, numbness, and tingling) alone or with other symptoms and signs may be associated with lesions at a variety of levels from the cerebral cortex to muscle.[3,8] The sensory symptoms or deficit may originate at the cerebral hemispheric, thalamic, or brain stem level (for example, infarction, demyelination, neoplasm, or inflammation). Segmental or longitudinal intramedullary cord lesions (for example, ischemia, myelitis, syrinx, or tumor)

or extramedullary lesions (for example, tumor) with Brown-Séquard's syndrome may be responsible for the sensory impairment. Nerve root compression or irritation by infection, tumor, or disc protrusion, and neuropathy (traumatic, neurofibromatosis, inflammatory, vasculitis, and so forth) are other causes of paresthesias. Episodic sensory symptomatology may be observed with migraine, seizure disorder, hyperventilation, drugs, neuromuscular disease, or systemic illness. MRI (cranial or spinal) is probably the best choice for evaluating convincing symptoms and signs in this category (see Chapter 4).

REFERENCES
Headache and other pain syndromes

1. Barlow C: *Headaches and migraine in childhood,* Philadelphia, 1984, JB Lippincott.
2. Bowyer S, Hollister J: Limb pain in childhood, *Pediatr Clin North Am,* 31:1053, 1984.
3. Dunn D, Epstein L: *Decision making in child neurology,* Philadelphia, 1987, BC Decker.
4. Fenichel G: *Clinical pediatric neurology,* Philadelphia, 1988, WB Saunders.
5. Hensinger R: Back pain in children. In Bradford D, Hensinger R: *The pediatric spine,* New York, 1985, Thieme.
6. Rothner A: Headache. In Swaiman K: *Pediatric neurology,* St Louis, 1989, Mosby–Year Book.
7. Sageo L, Cacayorin E, Petro G, et al: Migraine: evaluation by MR, *AJNR* 9:425, 1988.
8. Weiner H, Urion D, Levitt L: *Pediatric neurology for the house officer,* ed 3, Baltimore, 1988, Williams & Wilkins.
9. Winter R: Spinal problems in pediatric orthopedics. In Morrissy R, editor: *Lovell & Winter's pediatric orthopedics,* ed 3, Philadelphia, 1990, JB Lippincott.

TORTICOLLIS AND SCOLIOSIS

Torticollis, which includes wry neck or head tilt, may be painful or nonpainful, of developmental or acquired origin, and isolated or associated with other neurological findings [3,6] (see box on p. 63). Developmental causes include craniocervical junction and cervical spinal anomalies (for example, occipitalization of the atlas, Klippel-Feil spectrum, and so forth), skeletal dysplasias with odontoid hypoplasia and atlantoaxial or atlantooccipital subluxation (for example, isolated, Down's syndrome, spondyloepiphyseal dysplasia, or Morquio's syndrome). Developmental tumors or cysts of the neck (hemangioma, cystic hygroma, and so forth) are rarely associated with torticollis unless very large. Acquired causes include congenital muscular torticollis, trauma (for example, rotary C1-2 fixation or subluxation), childhood arthritis, head and neck inflammatory processes (adenopathy, cellulitis, or abscess), cervical spinal or paraspinal bone or soft tissue tumor (for example, histiocytosis or sarcoma), and idiopathic torticollis.

Congenital muscular torticollis, or congenital wry neck, is the commonest cause of torticollis in infancy and childhood. The wry neck deformity results from a contracture of the sternocleidomastoid muscle. Intrauterine or obstetrical injury may produce venous outflow interruption with edema and subsequent myodegeneration and fibrosis. Initially a neck mass appears and then subsides. Secondary craniofacial deformity (that is, plagiocephaly) is frequently

---

TORTICOLLIS (HEAD TILT)

Idiopathic torticollis
Transient torticollis
Congenital muscular torticollis
Craniocervical anomaly
Klippel-Feil spectrum
Chiari malformation
Skeletal dysplasia
Developmental neck tumor
Trauma
Head and neck inflammation
Childhood arthritis
Strabismus/ophthalmoplegia
Dystonia
Spinal column tumor
Posterior fossa or cervical cord tumor

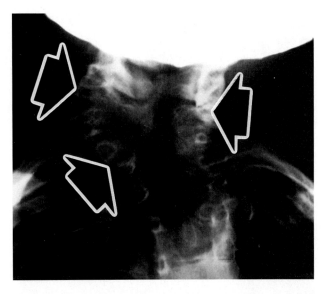

Fig. 2-31 Frontal plain film in torticollis demonstrating congenital cervicothoracic scoliosis in Klippel-Feil syndrome including multiple formation-segmentation bony anomalies *(arrows)*.

present. Torticollis may also be caused by isolated dystonia. Abnormal neurological signs usually accompany wry neck or head tilt due to strabismus, IV or VI cranial neuropathy, posterior fossa tumor, cervical cord tumor, or dystonia associated with neurodegenerative disease. Transient torticollis may be isolated and benign or part of Sandifer's syndrome, spasmus nutans, or drug-induced dystonia.

Initial evaluation of the patient with torticollis should include frontal and lateral plain films of the craniocervical junction and cervical spine (Fig. 2-31). CT may suffice to further delineate traumatic, developmental, or inflammatory processes.[9] Neuroanatomical evaluation requires MRI (see Chapters 9 and 10) especially when neurological signs are present, malignant extradural neoplasm is expected, myelodysplasia is anticipated (for example, Klippel-Feil syndrome with Chiari I malformation, diastematomyelia, or hydrosyringomyelia), or neuraxis tumor is suspected.[1,2,8,10] Craniocervical or cervical spinal instability is evaluated with flexion and extension plain films or fluoroscopy. Tomography may occasionally be helpful for bony delineation in planes not easily accessible by CT (coronal and sagittal). Flexion and extension cervical spinal MR examination may be carried out only with careful positioning and close monitoring.

Abnormal spinal curvatures include scoliosis, kyphosis, lordosis, kyphoscoliosis, and straightening or contour reversal.[4,5,11] A curvature abnormality may be the initial or major presenting feature in a child with disease of the spinal column or neuraxis. A complete classification is presented in Chapter 9. A simplified scheme is presented in the box on the right. The great majority of childhood scolioses fall into the *idiopathic* category, commonly a rightward thoracic or double thoracolumbar curve in an otherwise healthy preadolescent or adolescent girl (female-to-male ratio, 10:1). Lordosis may be a prominent feature, especially in patients with severe spinal curves. Orthopedic management is usually nonoperative unless the scoliosis progresses. Further imaging before surgical correction or stabilization is usually not necessary unless atypical signs or symptoms

occur (pain, numbness, weakness, left curve, or neurological deficit), which may indicate an otherwise occult tumor or syrinx, a consequence of increasing curvature with disc protrusion, nerve impingement, or cord attenuation. In these rare circumstances, MRI is the imaging procedure of choice[2,4,8,11] (Fig. 2-32).

COMMON SPINAL CURVATURE ABNORMALITIES OF CHILDHOOD

Idiopathic scoliosis
Congenital/dysraphic
Skeletal dysplasias
Neurofibromatosis
Painful
Neuropathic

Congenital scoliosis results from formation or segmentation anomalies of the bony column, such as a hemivertebra or a pedicle bar.[5,11] There tends to be curvature progression with growth, occasional underlying myelodysplasia in the neurenteric spectrum (for example, diastematomyelia or neurenteric cyst), associated dysraphism, or anomalies of other systems (for example, solitary kidney). Klippel-Feil anomaly is included in this category. MRI is recommended for neuroanatomical delineation (see Chapter 9) before orthopedic intervention.[1,2,8] CT or tomography is a useful adjunct to plain films for better definition of the bony anomalies. The radiographic hallmark of *dysraphism* is a spinolaminal defect (spina bifida) often with characteristic

A   B

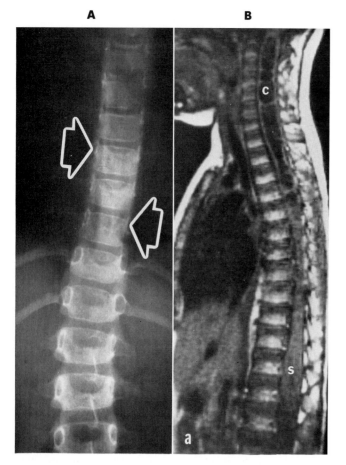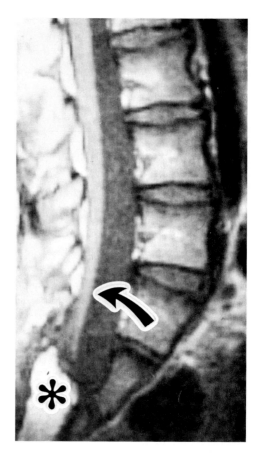

Fig. 2-32   **A,** Atypical idiopathic scoliosis due to cord tumor with thoracic pedicle thinning *(arrows)* on frontal plain film. **B,** Sagittal T1 MRI shows cervicothoracic cystic cord expansion *(C)* and lower thoracic solid intramedullary tumor *(S); a,* Astrocytoma.

Fig. 2-33   Sagittal T1 MRI showing lipomyelomeningocele with low placement of the cord *(arrow)* and caudal lipoma *(asterisk).*

dorsal cutaneous stigmata clinically (lipoma, dimple, hairy-patch), lower limb deformity (for example, cavus foot), neurogenic bladder or bowel dysfunction, or associated imperforate anus complex.[9] The scoliosis may be progressive and congenital (formation-segmentation anomaly) or neuropathic (for example, ischemic cord tethering or hydrosyringomyelia). MRI is the procedure of choice (Fig. 2-33) for definitive neuroanatomical evaluation.[1,8]

Skeletal dysplasias commonly associated with spinal deformities include neurofibromatosis, Down's syndrome, achondroplasia, spondyloepiphyseal dysplasia, and the mucopolysaccharidoses.[9] In *neurofibromatosis* there may be an underlying mesodermal dysplasia (dural ectasia or meningocele) or neoplasia (neurofibroma). Mechanical neural compression is the primary concern in the other skeletal dysplasias and is usually related to canal stenosis, kyphoscoliosis, or atlantoaxial subluxation. After initial radiographs, flexion-extension filming may be important along with CT or tomography, as discussed previously. MRI is the preferred imaging modality to evaluate neuroanatomical involvement (see Chapter 9), particularly in neurofibromatosis patients with scoliosis, a paraspinal

mass, or both.[1,2]

Painful curvatures may be traumatic, inflammatory, or neoplastic, as discussed previously. Another "red-flag" curvature abnormality is the unexplained, chronic or progressive, and often nonpainful, *neuropathic curve.* The curve is often S-shape and may be associated with canal expansion. The condition may be readily explained with an established clinical diagnosis of neurodegenerative or neuromuscular disease (for example, cerebral palsy or muscular dystrophy). However, the child with unexplained scoliosis or a diagnosis of "idiopathic" scoliosis inappropriate for age or gender should be evaluated further for intraspinal (or intracranial) pathology, including intramedullary neoplasm (astrocytoma or ependymoma) or hydrosyringomyelia.[8] Other entities to consider in cases of spinal canal expansion may include dural ectasia, arachnoid cyst, extramedullary tumor, or connective tissue disorder (for example, Marfan's syndrome). Definitive evaluation is carried out by MRI (see Figs. 2-25 and 2-32), often with Gd-DTPA enhancement, especially to detect neoplasia when the hydrosyringomyelia is not obviously of a developmental cause (for example, Chiari I malformation).

REFERENCES
Torticollis and scoliosis

1. Barkovich A: *Pediatric neuroimaging,* New York, 1990, Raven.
2. Davis P, Hoffman J, Ball T, et al: Spine abnormalities in pediatric patients: MR imaging, *Radiology* 166:679, 1988.
3. Dunn D, Epstein L: *Decision making in child neurology,* Philadelphia, 1987, BC Decker.
4. Gillespie R: Juvenile and adolescent idiopathic scoliosis. In Bradford D, Hensinger R: *The pediatric spine,* New York, 1985, Thieme.
5. Hall J: Congenital scoliosis. In Bradford D, Hensinger R: *The pediatric spine,* New York, 1985, Thieme.
6. Hensinger R, Fielding J: The cervical spine. In Morrissy R, editor: *Lovell & Winter's pediatric orthopedics,* ed 3, Philadelphia, 1990, JB Lippincott.
7. Naidich T, Quencer R, editors: *Clinical neurosonography,* New York, 1987, Springer-Verlag.
8. Nokes S, Murtagh F, Jones J, et al: Childhood scoliosis: MR imaging, *Radiology* 164:791, 1987.
9. Petterson H, Harwood-Nash D: *CT and myelography of the pediatric spine and cord,* New York, 1982, Springer-Verlag.
10. Walker H, Dietrich R, Flannigan B, et al: MR imaging of the pediatric spine, *Radiographics* 7:1129, 1987.
11. Winter R: Spinal problems in pediatric orthopedics. In Morrissy R, editor: *Lovell & Winter's pediatric orthopedics,* ed 3, Philadelphia, 1990, JB Lippincott.

MOTOR DISTURBANCES
Voluntary motor disorders

Voluntary motor weakness *(-paresis)* or paralysis *(-plegia)* requires further neurological characterization to discriminate upper motor neuron origin (pyramidal tract: cerebral cortex to anterior horn cells of the spinal cord) from lower motor neuron origin (neuromuscular pathway: anterior horn cells to muscle)[4,7,15] and whether the lesion is acute, static, episodic, or progressive (see box above). The distribution of weakness, that is, proximal or distal limb, upper or lower extremity, ocular, facial, bulbar, and unilateral or bilateral, further localizes the level(s) of nervous system involvement. Assessment of muscle tone and reflexes usually provides differentiation of upper motor neuron involvement (hypertonia, hyperreflexia, and Babinski's sign) from lower motor unit involvement (normal tone to hypotonia and normal to depressed reflexes).[7,9,14,15] Often, however, with acute upper motor neuron insults, areflexia or hyporeflexia with hypotonia may be present initially with subsequent evolution to hyperreflexia and hypertonia. The distribution identifies the specific level or levels of involvement along the craniospinal neuraxis for upper motor disease or along the neuromuscular pathway for lower motor disease.

Acute hemiparesis or *hemiplegia* (including central facial palsy) in a previously healthy child, and without trauma, usually indicates cerebrovascular disease or a convulsive disorder.[2,8,10,15] Vascular causes include acute spontaneous hemorrhage (for example, vascular malformation) and acute vascular occlusion, whether arterial or venous (for example, congenital heart disease, moyamoya, or sickle cell disease).[7,9,11,12] Other unusual causes of acute hemiplegia include viral necrotizing encephalitis that is initially focal (for example, herpes), purulent or granulomatous infection (for example, meningitis with arteritis or thrombophlebitis),

acute hemorrhagic leukoencephalitis (hemolytic-uremic syndrome, Henoch-Schönlein purpura), acute multiple sclerosis, and postinfection demyelination (acute disseminated encephalomyelitis).[2,7,15] Neoplasm is a rare cause of acute hemiplegia when associated with acute hemorrhage, severe edema, or vessel occlusion with ischemia. CT (or US) is the imaging procedure of choice initially (Fig. 2-12). MRI may provide clarification when the results of the screening examination are negative or inconclusive (see Chapter 6).

Quadriparesis (or *-plegia*) of upper motor origin usually indicates brain stem or cervical cord level involvement (and rarely bilateral cerebral involvement). *Paraparesis* (or *-plegia*) of upper motor origin implies thoracic or lumbar spinal cord involvement (the conus medullaris usually terminates above L2-3) or rarely a parasagittal high convexity intracranial lesion. Paraparesis of lower motor origin may indicate lumbar or sacral intraspinal disease (caudae equina). *Brown-Séquard's syndrome* denotes hemicord involvement with ipsilateral motor loss and contralateral pain and thermal deficit.[4,7,15] Acute or progressive spinal level quadriparesis or paraparesis indicates a destructive, expansile, compressive, or tension lesion. Other characteristic neurological findings include a sensory deficit level along dermatomes, and bladder or bowel dysfunction. These findings require emergent spinal imaging including plain films followed by CT or MRI, depending on the cause suspected after evaluating the clinical and plain film findings (see Figs. 2-25, 2-32, and 2-33). Acute onset of spinal neuraxis deficit(s) may be related to obvious trauma. Acute neurological impairment out of proportion with the traumatic incident (minor trauma) may indicate a preexisting condition such as an unstable craniocervical anomaly, Chiari malformation, tethered cord, tumor, or a pathological fracture. Other causes of acute deficit include myelitis (for example, viral), hemorrhage or ischemia (for example, vascular malformation), or abscess. Tumor (neoplasm, cyst, and the like) usually has a more insidious course,[5] as does myelodysplasia (for example, diastematomyelia or lipomyelomeningocele) with cord compression or tethering and ischemia. In these instances the patient may not seek medical attention until the impairment becomes acutely disabling. In the straightforward trauma case plain films and CT scans probably suffice. In more complicated trauma or nontraumatic presentations plain films and MRI are preferred (see Chapter 10).

Acute or progressive lower motor neuron paraparesis

(unilateral or bilateral) may require lumbosacral spinal imaging (plain film, CT, or MRI) to exclude a compressive or tension lesion (see Fig. 2-33) involving the caudae equina nerve roots (for example, tumor, dysraphic tethering, or abscess). Other causes include the acute neuromuscular diseases of anterior horn cell origin (for example, viral, poliomyelitis), peripheral nerve origin (for example, after infection, Landry-Guillain-Barré-Strohl syndrome), neuromuscular junction origin (for example, toxicity, botulism, myasthenia gravis), or myopathy (myositis, viral).[3,6] Landry-Guillain-Barré-Strohl syndrome (postinfection polyneuritis) is the most common of this group encountered in childhood.[1]

Chronic upper motor weakness due to intracranial or spinal level disease is unusual without previous history or neurological signs. Static upper motor deficits of childhood (cerebral palsy) were discussed in "Developmental Delay." Also, as mentioned earlier, progressive encephalopathy or progressive myelopathy with *"paresis"* or *"plegia"* requires further investigation including imaging for an expanding or compressive lesion or a neurodegenerative process. Chronic paresis of lower motor origin not related to an intraspinal process usually indicates disease in the neuromuscular spectrum (anterior horn cell, peripheral nerve, neuromuscular junction, or muscle).[3,6,13] Motor neuron (anterior horn cell) disorders include spinomuscular atrophies (for example, Werdnig-Hoffmann disease) organic acidopathies, glycogen storage diseases, and congenital or infantile neuroaxonal dystrophy. A chronic degenerative peripheral neuropathy (classically with distal limb weakness) may be axonal (for example, heredofamilial metabolic disorder or sensorimotor neuropathy) or demyelinating (chronic inflammatory or diabetes mellitus). Mixed central and peripheral nervous system involvement occurs in a number of neurodegenerative disorders including metachromatic leukodystrophy and Krabbe's disease. Neuromuscular junction disorders (myasthenic syndromes) include congenital and juvenile forms of myasthenia gravis and drug-induced disorders (for example, aminoglycosides). Chronic myopathies classically produce proximal limb weakness. Myopathies may be congenital, dystrophic (muscular dystrophies), metabolic (for example, mitochondrial disorders or lipid or glycogen storage diseases), or endocrine (thyroid, parathyroid, or adrenal disease). Chronic inflammatory diseases may also be responsible for a longstanding myopathy including polymyositis, collagen vascular disease, tuberculosis, or trichinosis. MRI is probably the definitive modality for imaging neurodegenerative processes of brain and cord (see Chapter 4). It may also serve an adjunctive role in the evaluation of peripheral nervous system and muscular diseases.

REFERENCES
Voluntary motor disorders

1. Asbury A: Diagnostic considerations in Guillain-Barré syndrome, *Ann Neurol* 9:1, 1981.
2. Barlow C: *Headaches and migraine in childhood,* Philadelphia, 1984, JB Lippincott.
3. Brooke MH: *A clinician's view of neuromuscular diseases,* ed 2, Baltimore, 1986, Williams & Wilkins.
4. Carpenter G: *Core text of neuroanatomy,* ed 3, Baltimore, 1985, Williams & Wilkins.
5. Cohen M, Duffner P: Tumors of the brain and spinal cord including leukemic involvement. In Swaiman KF: *Pediatric neurology,* St Louis, 1989, Mosby–Year Book.
6. Dubowitz V: *Muscle disorders in childhood,* Philadelphia, 1978, WB Saunders.
7. Dunn D, Epstein L: *Decision making in child neurology,* Philadelphia, 1987, BC Decker.
8. Edwards M, Hoffman H: *Cerebrovascular disease in children and adolescents: current neurosurgical practice,* Baltimore, 1988, Williams & Wilkins.
9. Fenichel G: *Clinical pediatric neurology,* Philadelphia, 1988, WB Saunders.
10. Golden G: Stroke syndromes in childhood, *Neurol Clin North Am* 3:59, 1985.
11. Golden G: Cerebrovascular disease. In Swaiman KF: *Pediatric neurology,* St Louis, 1989, Mosby–Year Book.
12. Menkes J: *Textbook of child neurology,* ed 3, Philadelphia, 1985, Lea & Febiger.
13. Rapin I: Cerebral degenerations of childhood: differential diagnosis. In Rowland LP, editor: *Merritt's textbook of neurology,* ed 7, Philadelphia, 1984, Lea & Febiger.
14. Swaiman K: *Pediatric neurology,* St Louis, 1989, Mosby–Year Book.
15. Weiner H, Urion D, Levitt L: *Pediatric neurology for the house officer,* ed 3, Baltimore, 1988, Williams & Wilkins.

Disorders of movement and coordination

The extrapyramidal system mediates motor activity and includes the basal ganglia and their interconnections with the pyramidal system.[1] Disorders involving this system in childhood may result in abnormal involuntary movements (dyskinesias) and abnormal muscle tone (see box on p. 67). The manifestations include chorea, athetosis, tics, myoclonus, tremor, and dystonia.[3,4,7,8] Although motor coordination involves input and output at many levels of the nervous system (visual, vestibular, proprioceptive, and so on), disorders of coordination in childhood are usually of cerebellar origin and manifest as ataxia.[3,8]

Chorea refers to rapid, irregular, dancelike movements and is often accompanied by *athetosis* (slow writhing movements).[3,8] Acute chorea or choreoathetosis is often caused by intoxication or toxic exposure (carbon monoxide), trauma (for example, burns, electrical), and hypothermic arrest for cardiac surgery. Subacute chorea may be associated with streptococcal infection (Sydenham's disease), metabolic disorder (hypocalcemia, adrenal insufficiency, and the like), or vascular disease (Henoch-Schönlein purpura, lupus, or infarction). Chorea due to basal ganglia involvement by neoplasm, inflammation (encephalitis), or infarction is usually accompanied by other neurological symptoms and signs. A chronic isolated and benign form also exists. Static chorea or choreoathetosis may be a major feature of cerebral palsy. Progressive chorea is seen with a variety of genetic, metabolic, and neurodegenerative diseases, most frequently ataxia telangiectasia, Huntington's disease, and phenylketonuria.

Myoclonus denotes sudden muscle jerks that occasionally are physiological (for example, hiccups).[3,8] Myoclonus may be the main feature of epilepsy (for example, infantile

---

DISORDERS OF MOVEMENT AND COORDINATION

Chorea
Athetosis
Myoclonus
Tics
Tremors
Dystonia
Ataxia

ATAXIA OF CHILDHOOD

ACUTE	EPISODIC	STATIC	PROGRESSIVE
Infection	Epilepsy	Cerebral	Hydrocephalus
Postinfection	Migraine	palsy	"Mass"
Posttrauma	Metabolic	Posttoxicity	Posterior
Intoxication	Familial	Metabolic	fossa tumor
Opsoclonus-		Postinfec-	Degenerative
myoclonus		tion	disorder
		Posttrauma	
		Idiopathic	

---

spasms), as previously discussed. Myoclonic encephalopathy (polymyoclonus, ataxia, and opsoclonus) occurs after viral infections or is associated with occult neuroblastoma. Muscle jerks may accompany toxic or metabolic encephalopathy (renal or hepatic failure, hypoglycemia, and so forth) and trauma with anoxia. Myoclonus may occur acutely or chronically with infections such as subacute sclerosing panencephalitis or HIV encephalitis (AIDS). Myoclonic paroxysms are occasionally a feature of a progressive, metabolic neurodegenerative disease (for example, Tay-Sachs, lipofuscinosis, or Gaucher).

Tics are brief movements, usually of the head and face, that may be accompanied by vocalizations. Tics may be isolated and transient on an emotional basis, or multiple as with Gilles de la Tourette's syndrome.[8] *Tremors* are subclassified as static, intention, postural, or head tremor.[3] Static tremors are classically associated with Parkinson's disease, juvenile Huntington's chorea, Hallervorden-Spatz disease, and Wilson's disease. Postural tremors are usually physiological or familial, but may be exaggerated with CNS stimulants. They also may accompany peroneal muscular atrophy. An intention tremor is characteristic of cerebellar dysfunction, with causes similar to those associated with ataxia. Forms of head tremor include spasmus nutans (head nodding, head tilt, and monocular nystagmus) that may be idiopathic or associated with optic glioma, and the bobble-head doll syndrome accompanying third ventricular lesions (for example, colloid cyst).

Dystonia denotes abnormal posturing that may involve the head and neck, trunk, or an extremity.[3] Acute dystonia is usually drug induced (for example, phenothiazines) but may result from toxic exposure (for example, strychnine) or tetanus. Chronic dystonia that is isolated and persistent may be drug related, posthemiplegic, associated with Wilson's disease, or inherited. Episodic heredofamilial forms also exist. Dystonia may occur as a component of a neurodegenerative disease, including Huntington's disease, Hallervorden-Spatz disease, Niemmann-Pick disease, or the lipidoses.[5]

Ataxia, or incoordination, in childhood is most often manifested as a gait abnormality[8] (see box above, right). Acute ataxia is usually related to infection (viral cerebellitis or meningitis) or occurs after viral infection (for example,

varicella). Occasionally it is an accompanying feature of a more widespread postinfectious or parainfectious encephalopathy. Other important causes of acute ataxia are postconcussion syndrome, in which a posterior fossa hematoma must be excluded, and intoxication with drugs or alcohol. Acute cerebellar ataxia is a major feature of opsoclonus-myoclonus syndrome associated with occult neuroblastoma. Chronic persistent ataxia as a static process may exist with cerebral palsy or following hypoglycemia, meningitis, trauma, or lead poisoning. The "clumsy child" syndrome is an idiopathic form of persistent ataxia, often associated with hypotonia. Episodic or intermittent ataxia may accompany epileptic disorders, migraine, or certain metabolic errors. A benign familial form also exists. Progressive ataxia is the hallmark of an intracranial expansion or mass, including hydrocephalus and especially posterior fossa tumors. Progressive ataxia is often a major feature of some degenerative disorders, particularly metachromatic leukodystrophy, ataxia telangiectasia, Friedrich's ataxia, and juvenile Refsum's syndrome.

Imaging of movement disorders or impaired coordination is important in instances of acute unexplained presentations to establish cause or, when the cause is known, to document effects or degree of involvement for purposes of establishing prognosis and planning treatment. Progressive unexplained forms obviously require imaging to potentially uncover a destructive process or a mass lesion.[2] Tics alone usually do not require imaging. Progression of known disease may require imaging to detect or document sequelae or complications of a process that may require more specific management, such as edema, hemorrhage, or hydrocephalus, and to rule out causes of the symptoms or signs other than disease progression or sequelae. Although US (in the infant) or CT may suffice for screening in these situations, MRI is more sensitive, especially regarding disease extent and distribution in neurodegenerative diseases.[5,6]

REFERENCES
Disorders of movement and coordination

1. Carpenter M: *Core text of neuroanatomy,* ed 3, Baltimore, 1985, Williams & Wilkins.
2. Cohen M, Duffner P: Tumors of the brain and spinal cord including leukemic involvement. In Swaiman KF: *Pediatric neurology,* St Louis, 1989, Mosby–Year Book.

3. Dunn D, Epstein L: *Decision making in child neurology,* Philadelphia, 1987, BC Decker.
4. Fenichel G: *Clinical pediatric neurology,* Philadelphia, 1988, WB Saunders.
5. Rapin I: Cerebral degenerations of childhood: differential diagnosis. In Rowland LP, editor: *Merritt's textbook of neurology,* ed 7, Philadelphia, 1984, Lea & Febiger.
6. Rutledge J, Hilal S, Silver A, et al: Study of movement disorders and brain iron by MR, *AJNR* 8:397, 1987.
7. Swaiman K: *Pediatric neurology,* St Louis, 1989, Mosby–Year Book.
8. Weiner H, Urion D, Levitt L: *Pediatric neurology for the house officer,* ed 3, Baltimore, 1988, Williams & Wilkins.

EYE SYMPTOMS AND SIGNS

Important eye symptoms and signs in child neurology are listed in the box above. Episodic impairment of *visual acuity* may be psychogenic, drug related, toxic, epileptic, migrainous, or related to increased intracranial pressure.[4,12,14] Persistent or progressive visual loss may occur with ocular, orbital, optic nerve (cranial nerve II), or intracranial abnormalities.[1,2,6-8] *Ocular causes* of visual impairment include chorioretinitis (for example, toxoplasmosis), hemorrhage (for example, persistent hyperplastic primary vitreous), or tumor (for example, retinoblastoma). *Orbital lesions* may also produce proptosis or abnormal ocular movements and include trauma, cellulitis or abscess, pseudotumor, developmental malformations (for example, sphenoorbital dysplasia, or encephalocele), neoplasm (for example, leukemia, lymphoma, rhabdomyosarcoma, neuroblastoma, or primitive neuroectodermal tumor), or vascular anomalies (for example, hemangioma). *Optic nerve lesions* include dysplasia or hypoplasia, glioma, leukemia, meningeal seeding, neuroma or meningioma (rarely), neuritis, or demyelination. Bilateral *optic atrophy* denotes chronicity and may occur with optic nerve hypoplasia syndromes (for example, absent septum pellucidum, holoprosencephaly, or callosal dysgenesis) and other midline developmental malformations (for example, sphenoidal encephalocele, arachnoid cyst, and so forth). Optic atrophy also may occur following neuritis, in neurodegenerative disorders, with chiasmatic tumor involvement (for example, glioma or craniopharyngioma), or from chronically elevated intracranial pressure. *Papilledema* is usually a sign of increased intracranial pressure but also may occur with idiopathic or parainfectious neuritis and inflammatory or neoplastic meningeal infiltration.[4,14] *Visual field defects* may localize optic pathway involvement as chiasmatic (bitemporal hemianopsia) or optic tract/optic radiation (homonymous hemianopsia), as with tumor, inflammation, infarction, demyelination, and so forth.

Double vision (diplopia) or *blurred vision* may indicate extraocular muscle imbalance, malalignment, or ophthalmoplegia.[4,12] The imbalance is often transient in the newborn up to 4 months of age. Unilateral involvement is usually ophthalmoplegic. Bilateral impairment (strabismus) may be static and nonophthalmoplegic (supranuclear), as with cerebral palsy. Persistent or progressive impairment may be the result of orbit disease (trauma, infection, tumor, myositis), myasthenia gravis (with associated ptosis), isolated cranial nerve III (oculomotor) palsy, isolated

---

IMPORTANT EYE SYMPTOMS AND SIGNS

Visual acuity loss
Visual field defects
Optic atrophy
Papilledema
Diplopia
Ophthalmoplegia
Horner's syndrome
Parinaud's syndrome
Nystagmus

---

cranial nerve IV (trochlear) palsy, or isolated cranial nerve VI (abducens) palsy. *Oculomotor palsy* may be partial (ophthalmoplegia) or complete (ophthalmoplegia plus pupillary dilation) and congenital, traumatic, inflammatory, neoplastic, or resulting from aneurysm, herniation, or complicated migraine. *Trochlear palsy* alone may be congenital, posttraumatic, or associated with encephalitis. Unilateral or bilateral *abducens palsy* may be a nonlocalizing manifestation of raised intracranial pressure, especially hydrocephalus, or related to trauma, an inflammatory process, neoplasm, benign postviral or postvaccinal effects, or Duane's syndrome. Ophthalmoplegia due to multiple or bilateral cranial nerve involvement may arise with demyelination, vascular occlusive disease, Möbius sequence, myasthenia gravis, Landry-Guillain-Barré-Strohl syndrome, botulism, or brain stem glioma. Traumatic, neoplastic, or inflammatory involvement of the cavernous sinus or superior orbital fissure may produce unilateral total ophthalmoplegia.

Horner's syndrome is unilateral ptosis, miosis, and facial anhydrosis.[4,11] It may occur with first order neuron involvement (hypothalamus to C8-T1), as seen with brain stem glioma or spinal cord tumor. Second order neuron involvement (C8-T1 paravertebral sympathetic chain) may arise with brachial plexus lesions, neoplasms (for example, neuroblastoma or ganglioneuroma) or cervical lymphadenopathy. Although third order neuron disease (superior cervical ganglion to the iris dilator muscle) is usually idiopathic in children, Horner's syndrome may coincide with internal carotid thrombosis, aneurysm, or trauma, and with nasopharyngeal or otomastoid disease (for example, tumor or infection). *Parinaud's syndrome* refers to upward gaze paralysis and often accompanies midbrain involvement, especially by tumor (for example, pineal region neoplasms).

Nystagmus is rhythmic involuntary oscillations of the eyes and may be of ocular, optic nerve, brain stem, cerebellar, or vestibular origin.[3,4,14] Pendular nystagmus may be congenital (isolated), associated with ophthalmic disease, or part of the spasmus nutans complex in which optic glioma must be excluded. Conjugate jerk nystagmus may be congenital, drug induced, due to myasthenia gravis, or related to cerebellar abnormalities. Although disassociate jerk nystagmus is an unusual finding in children, it occurs

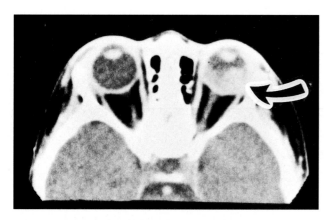

Fig. 2-34   Contrast-enhanced axial CT of retinoblastoma showing left calcified and enhancing intraocular tumor *(arrow)*.

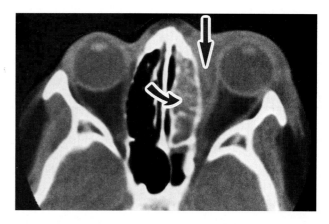

Fig. 2-36   Axial CT of left preseptal periorbital cellulitis with ethomoid sinusitis *(curved arrow)* and medial orbital cellulitis *(straight arrow)*.

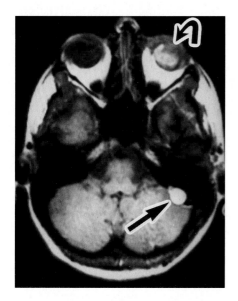

Fig. 2-35   Axial T1 MRI in von Hippel–Lindau syndrome showing high-intensity hemorrhage associated with the left ocular *(curved arrow)* and left posterior fossa *(straight arrow)* hemangioblastomas.

ocular bobbing (pontine lesion), and ocular dysmetria (cerebellar abnormality). Opsoclonus was discussed earlier.

If the process producing abnormal eye findings is primarily or exclusively intraocular, then ophthalmic assessment and ultrasonography may suffice, except for evaluation of neoplasm (for example, retinoblastoma). CT may then be indicated (Fig. 2-34) for assistance with diagnosis, disease extent, and treatment planning (for example, radiotherapy). CT or MRI may be indicated for ocular findings implying CNS disease (Fig. 2-35), for

with posterior fossa lesions, large suprasellar masses involving the midbrain, and pineal region tumors. Vestibular nystagmus (horizontal jerk) is usually associated with vertigo and may be of central origin, as with brain stem glioma or acoustic neuroma involving cranial nerve VIII. Vestibular nystagmus of peripheral origin (inner ear) is usually caused by infection (for example, viral labyrinthitis). Long-standing jerk nystagmus in the primary position is usually congenital. Vertical nystagmus is also rare in childhood, but occurs with lesions at the level of the foramen magnum (for example, Chiari I malformation or tumor) or with midline cerebellar or medullary lesions. Other syndromes with abnormal eye movements include oculomotor apraxia (which may be related to third ventricular lesions, cerebellar degeneration, or may be idiopathic),

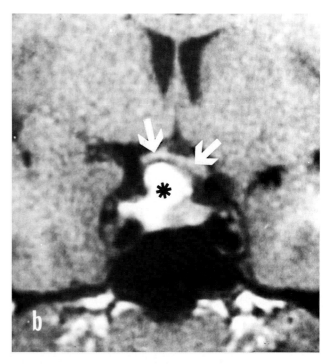

Fig. 2-37   Coronal T1 MRI demonstrating high-intensity hemorrhagic pituitary adenoma *(asterisk)* elevating and deforming the optic chiasm *(arrows)*.

example, chorioretinitis with toxoplasmosis or retinal hemangioblastoma with von Hippel-Lindau syndrome. Extraocular orbital lesions are usually best evaluated first with high resolution axial or coronal CT.[9,10,15] CT often provides definitive evaluation, especially in trauma, infection, and pseudotumor (Fig. 2-36). CT also may suffice for detecting acute intracranial trauma, inflammation, and vascular or developmental causes of abnormal eye signs, as well as for hydrocephalus. MRI is the preferred procedure for delineating processes extending beyond the orbit intracranially and for discriminating neoplastic and other progressive or destructive processes involving the optic pathways and cranial nerves along the skull base (Fig. 2-37). Disease processes and abnormalities confined to the temporal bone are usually best evaluated with high resolution axial and coronal CT.[13]

REFERENCES
Eye symptoms and signs

1. Avery M, Robb R: Ophthalmology. In Avery M, First L: *Pediatric medicine,* Baltimore, 1989, Williams & Wilkins.
2. Burde R, Savino P, Trobe J: *Clinical decisions in neurophthalmology,* St Louis, 1985, Mosby–Year Book.
3. Carpenter M: *Core text of neuroanatomy,* ed 3, Baltimore, 1985, Williams & Wilkins.
4. Dunn D, Epstein L: *Decision making in child neurology,* Philadelphia, 1987, BC Decker.
5. Fenichel G: *Clinical pediatric neurology,* Philadelphia, 1988, WB Saunders.
6. Harley R: *Pediatric ophthalmology,* ed 2, Philadelphia, 1983, WB Saunders.
7. Mortyn L: Pediatric neurophthalmology. In Harley R: *Pediatric ophthalmology,* ed 2, 1983, WB Saunders.
8. Nelson L: *Pediatric ophthalmology,* Philadelphia, 1984, WB Saunders.
9. Peyster R, Hoover E: *CT in orbital disease and neurophthalmology,* Chicago, 1984, Mosby–Year Book.
10. Roden D, Savino P, Zimmerman R: MR imaging in orbital diagnosis, *Radiol Clin North Am,* 26:535, 1988.
11. Sauer C, Levinsohn N: Horner's syndrome in childhood, *Neurology* 26:116, 1976.
12. Sher P: Visual loss associated with neurologic disease in childhood. In Swaiman K: *Pediatric neurology,* St Louis, 1989, Mosby–Year Book.
13. Strand R, Humphrey C, Barnes P: Imaging of petrous temporal bone abnormalities in infancy and childhood. In Healy G, editor: *Common problems in pediatric otolaryngology,* Chicago, 1990, Mosby–Year Book.
14. Weiner H, Urion D, Levitt L: *Pediatric neurology for the house officer,* ed 3, Baltimore, 1988, Williams & Wilkins.
15. Wells R, Sty J, Gonnering R: Imaging of the pediatric eye and orbit, *Radiographics* 9:1023, 1989.
16. Yousem D, Atlas S, Grossman R, et al: MR imaging of Tolosa-Hunt syndrome, *AJNR* 10:1181, 1989.

FACIAL PALSY

Facial weakness (cranial nerve VII palsy) may occur in the newborn with parturitional trauma or posterior fossa hemorrhage.[6,10,16] Absence or hypoplasia of the depressor anguli oris muscle may mimic facial palsy. Bilateral seventh nerve palsy in the newborn may be part of the Möbius sequence or caused by hypoxic-ischemic encephalopathy or neuromuscular disease. Beyond the neonatal period unilateral facial palsy is usually idiopathic (Bell's palsy) but may be related to diabetes mellitus, trauma (basilar skull fracture), otomastoid disease (infection,

tumor), meningeal infection or neoplasm (for example, leukemia), brain stem glioma, cerebellopontine angle tumor, acoustic neuroma, histiocytosis, or, rarely, sarcoidosis.[1,6,8,9,11] Bilateral impairment is rare in Bell's palsy but may occur with Landry-Guillain-Barré-Strohl syndrome, hypertension, botulism, myasthenia gravis, myotonic dystrophy, or brain stem glioma. CT is preferable to US for screening (Fig. 2-38), especially for skull base and temporal bone abnormalities.[5,13-15] Neuroanatomical evaluation is best provided by MRI[14] (Fig. 2-39).

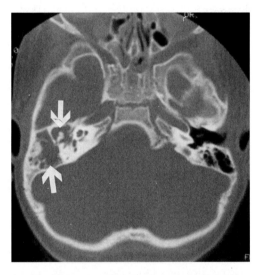

Fig. 2-38   Axial CT in an infant with right congenital cholesteatoma *(arrows).* There is a middle ear and mastoid opacification with compartment expansion and bony destruction. (From: Strand R, et al: Imaging of petrous temporal bone abnormalities in infancy and childhood. In Healy G, editor *Common problems in pediatric otorhinolaryngology,* Chicago, 1990, Mosby–Year Book.)

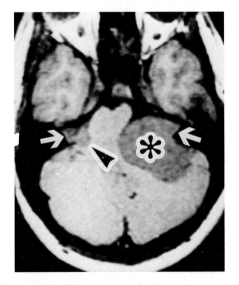

Fig. 2-39   Axial T1 MRI showing neurofibromatosis 2 with bilateral acoustic neuromas. Larger *(asterisk)* and smaller *(arrowhead)* cerebellopontine angle masses are demonstrated with bilateral internal auditory canal widening *(white arrows).*

VERTIGO

Acute vertigo may occur with viral labyrinthitis, encephalitis, meningitis, or drug intoxication.[6,7,16] Vertigo also may be a feature of otomastoid infection, trauma, or tumor (for example, cholesteatoma or rhabdomyosarcoma).[1-3,9,11] Chronic recurrent vertigo may be associated with epilepsy, migraine, the postmeningitic or posttraumatic state, or rarely with posterior fossa tumor (cranial nerve VIII involvement).[6,16] A benign form of paroxysmal vertigo also occurs in childhood. Again, CT is the choice for imaging temporal bone disease, whereas MRI is better for neuroanatomical assessment, especially for neoplastic processes[14,15] (Fig. 2-39).

HEARING LOSS

Conductive hearing loss is most commonly associated with acute or chronic otomastoid infection including cholesteatoma, but may be developmental (otomastoid dysplasia/hypoplasia) and manifested initially as microtia.[1-3,9,11,12] Other causes include trauma (ossicular disruption) and neoplasm with pain or mass (for example, histiocytosis, rhabdomyosarcoma, primary cholesteatoma, and primitive neuroectodermal tumor).[3] *Sensorineural hearing loss* may arise at the cochlear (inner ear) or retrocochlear (cranial nerve VIII) level. It may be related to cochlear dysplasia (Mondini spectrum), the postinfectious state (meningitis), cerebral palsy, or associated with genetic or chromosomal syndromes or craniofacial complexes (for example, Treacher Collins syndrome or hemifacial microsomia). Sensorineural hearing loss also may be isolated and idiopathic or heredofamilial, or, rarely, due to a neoplasm (for example, brain stem glioma or acoustic neuroma in neurofibromatosis).[1,9,11,12] High-resolution CT is the choice for imaging otomastoid disease and assessing cochlear sensorineural hearing loss, whereas MRI is better for detecting intracranial extension of temporal bone disease and evaluating retrocochlear sensorineural hearing loss when tumor is suspected[14,15] (Figs. 2-39 and 2-40).

OTHER CRANIAL NERVE PALSIES

Isolated palsies of cranial nerves V (trigeminal), IX (glossopharyngeal), X (vagus), XI (accessory), and XII (hypoglossal) are rare in childhood.[6,16] When these cranial nerves are involved, there are usually multiple cranial neuropathies, as with brain stem glioma, encephalitis, demyelination, hypoxic-ischemic encephalopathy, malformation (Chiari II), Möbius sequence, or a neurodegenerative disorder. The anatomical location, that is, medulla, and disease processes under consideration may make MRI preferable to CT for imaging evaluation (see Fig. 2-19).

REFERENCES
Facial palsy, vertigo, hearing loss, and other cranial nerve palsies
1. Avery M, Healy G: Otolaryngology. In Avery M, First L: *Pediatric medicine,* Baltimore, 1989, Williams & Wilkins.
2. Balkany T, Pashley N: *Clinical pediatric otolaryngology,* St Louis, 1986, Mosby–Year Book.
3. Bluestone C, Stool S: *Pediatric otolaryngology,* ed 2, Philadelphia, 1990, WB Saunders.

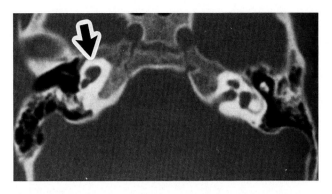

Fig. 2-40 Axial CT in Mondini's anomaly with sensorineural hearing loss. Cochlear dysplasia is demonstrated as a cavity or lack of normal cochlear turns *(arrow).* (From Strand R, et al: Imaging of petrous temporal bone abnormalities in infancy and childhood. In Healy G, editor: *Common problems in pediatric otorhinolaryngology,* Chicago, 1990, Mosby–Year Book.)

4. Carpenter M: *Core text of neuroanatomy,* ed 3, Baltimore, 1985, Williams & Wilkins.
5. Curtin H: Modern imaging in ear, nose, and throat problems, *Pediatr Infect Dis J* 7:S174, 1988.
6. Dunn D, Epstein L: *Decision making in child neurology,* Philadelphia, 1987, BC Decker.
7. Eviator L, Eviator A: Vertigo in children, *Pediatrics* 59:833, 1977.
8. Fenichel G: *Clinical pediatric neurology,* Philadelphia, 1988, WB Saunders.
9. Healy G, editor: *Common problems in pediatric otolaryngology,* Chicago, 1990, Mosby–Year Book.
10. Manning J, Adour K: Facial paralysis in children, *Pediatrics* 49:102, 1972.
11. Myer C, Cotton R: *A practical approach to pediatric otolaryngology,* Chicago, 1988, Mosby–Year Book.
12. Rapin I: Hearing and cranial nerve VIII. In Swaiman K: *Pediatric neurology,* St Louis, 1989, Mosby–Year Book.
13. Schwaber M, Zealear D, et al: MR imaging and high-resolution CT in facial paralysis, *Otolaryngol Head Neck Surg* 101:449, 1989.
14. Strand R, Humphrey C, Barnes P: Imaging of petrous temporal bone abnormalities in infancy and childhood. In Healy G, editor: *Common problems in pediatric otolaryngology,* Chicago, 1990, Mosby–Year Book.
15. Valvassori G, Buckingham R, Carter B, et al: *Head and neck imaging,* New York, 1988, Thieme.
16. Weiner H, Urion D, Levitt L: *Pediatric neurology for the house officer,* ed 3, Baltimore, 1988, Williams & Wilkins.

CRANIOFACIAL DYSMORPHIA

Microcephaly, macrocephaly, hypertelorism, hypotelorism, and midface, orbital, and cranial anomalies are dysmorphias that may be isolated, indicators of intracranial abnormality, or associated with anomalies of other systems including genetic or chromosomal syndromes and the amniotic band–disruption complex* (see box on p. 72). A normal increase in head circumference appropriate for somatic growth and development reflects a normally growing brain. *Microcephaly* refers to a head circumference of more than two standard deviations below normal relative to body size.[5,19] The small brain may result from a malformation or an encephaloclastic process. Microcephaly at birth

*References 5, 6, 11, 14, 17, 19.

CRANIOFACIAL DYSMORPHIA

Microcephaly
Macrocephaly
Hypertelorism
Hypotelorism
Midface anomalies
Cranioceles
Craniosynostosis
Neurocutaneous syndromes
Head and neck anomalies

---

may be related to an extensive brain malformation (for example, holoprosencephaly, lissencephaly, or large encephalocele), a genetic defect (for example, Cockayne's syndrome, or Menkes' kinky-hair disease), a chromosomal aberration (for example, Down's syndrome, trisomy 13, and so forth), intrauterine growth retardation, TORCH infection, hypoxia-ischemia, or may be heredofamilial (micrencephaly). Postnatal microcephaly may be postmeningitic or postencephalitic, neurodegenerative, postirradiation, or postanoxic. A small, nongrowing brain may result in secondary craniosynostosis.

Macrocephaly refers to a head circumference of more than two standard deviations above normal. Evaluation of head growth rate (serial head circumference measurements) is important along with assessment of developmental milestones, perinatal history, and signs of raised intracranial pressure.[3-5,19] Macrocephaly with normal growth rate and normal neurological examination is characteristic of megalencephaly and is usually familial. Dysplastic megalencephaly is often associated with developmental delay, seizures, neurocutaneous syndrome (for example, neurofibromatosis), genetic syndromes (for example, Soto's syndrome—cerebral gigantism), or elevated central venous pressure (for example, achondroplasia). Macrocephaly related to "rebound" or "catch-up" brain growth occurs in the thriving infant after prematurity or after a period of deprivation or serious illness. Familial, dysplastic, and rebound types may manifest mild to moderate degrees of ventricular or subarachnoid space dilatation. Macrocephaly and accelerated head growth in infancy without elevated pressure may occur as nonprogressive ventricular or subarachnoid space dilatation. This is known as benign communicating or external hydrocephalus and probably results from immaturity of the arachnoid villi. There may be associated so-called "benign subdural collections of infancy."[5,7,13,19] This form of macrocephaly usually stabilizes as a form of megalencephaly in later infancy (Fig. 2-41). Progressive hydrocephalus is usually associated with signs of increased pressure (and often declining milestones) except in the infant or child with preexisting brain injury, for example, hydrocephalus after intraventricular hemorrhage in a premature infant with coexistent periventricular leukomalacia. This and other sources of raised intracranial pressure are discussed in upcoming sections. Other causes

of macrocephaly with megalencephaly, hydrocephaly, or craniomegaly include lipid storage diseases, leukodystrophies such as Canavan's disease and Alexander's disease (see Chapter 4), cranial dysplasias (for example, craniometaphyseal dysplasia), and marrow hyperplasia (chronic hemolytic anemia, for example, thalassemia).

Hypertelorism (wide interorbital distance) may be isolated or associated with median cleft syndrome, nasofrontal or basal encephalocele (see Chapter 3), or other dysmorphic syndromes including Crouzon's syndrome, Apert's syndrome, cleidocranial dysostosis, osteogenesis imperfecta, or mucopolysaccharidoses.[2,16] The median cleft syndrome (cleft lip/palate) with hypertelorism may be associated with agenesis or dysgenesis of the corpus callosum, callosal lipoma, or, rarely, with holoprosencephaly.[15,16] *Hypotelorism* (narrowed interorbital distance) reflects ethmoid hypoplasia and is seen with holoprosencephaly complexes, Down's syndrome, and trigonocephaly of premature metopic synostosis.[2,15,16] Other midface anomalies (aplasia or hypoplasia of the midfacial skeleton) associated with holoprosencephaly include cebocephaly, ethmocephaly, cyclopia, median cleft lip, and intermaxillary rudiment. Type I lissencephaly is associated not only with microcephaly but also with dysmorphic facies and is seen in heredofamilial syndromes such as Miller-Dieker syndrome.[2]

Other cranial or craniofacial dysmorphias often associated with brain malformations include overt *cranioceles* (encephalocele or meningocele) such as occipital, cervicooccipital (Chiari III malformation), and frontal cranioceles. The more occult basal cranioceles (for example, frontonasal, frontoethmoidal, or midline sphenoidal) may be associated with hypertelorism or other midline intracranial anomalies such as optic and pituitary-hypothalamic hypoplasia or callosal dysgenesis.[2,16] Sphenoid wing or alar craniocele may occasionally occur as an isolated malformation with proptosis, but may also represent the sphenoorbital dysplasia of neurofibromatosis (pulsating exophthalmos). A *facial cutaneous malformation* may be the main feature of a neurocutaneous syndrome, including the orbitofacial port-wine stain of encephalotrigeminal angiomatosis in Sturge-Weber syndrome, or the palpebral plexiform neurofibroma with underlying buphthalmos and sphenoorbital dysplasia in neurofibromatosis.

Also included in the group of craniofacial dysmorphias are the premature *craniosynostoses*, whether primary and isolated, primary and associated with congenital syndromes, or secondary.[8,10,12] The primary isolated subcategory includes unilateral coronal or lambdoidal synostosis (plagiocephaly), sagittal synostosis (scaphocephaly or dolichocephaly), bilateral coronal or lambdoidal synostosis (brachycephaly), metopic synostosis (trigonocephaly), combined coronal and sagittal synostosis (turricephaly or oxycephaly), and combined coronal, lambdoidal, and sagittal synostosis (cloverleaf skull). Congenital craniofacial complexes associated with craniosynostosis include heredofamilial genetic and chromosomal syndromes.[11,17]

A   B   C

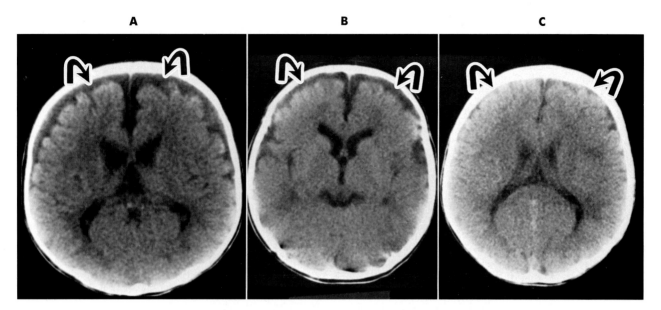

Fig. 2-41   Serial axial CT scans covering 18 months demonstrate progressive resolution of the low-density extracerebral collections *(curved arrows)* and ventriculomegaly characteristic of "benign" subdural collections and external hydrocephalus of infancy.

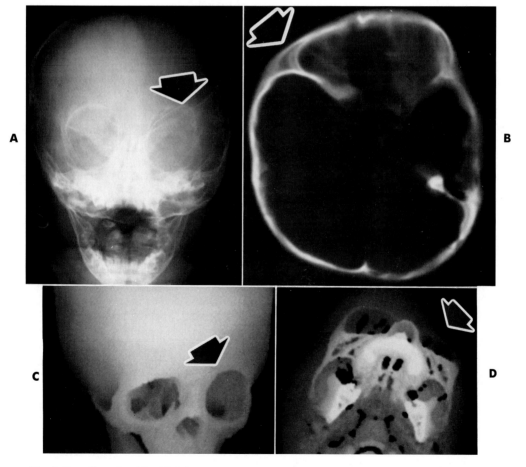

Fig. 2-42   Plain film **(A),** CT **(B),** and three-dimensional CT reconstructions (**C** and **D**) of coronal synostosis with orbital and cranial deformites *(black arrows).*

These consist of multiple synostoses, often with midface hypoplasia, orbital deformity, or digit anomalies (syndactyly, polydactyly, and so on), and include the syndromes of Apert, Crouzon, Pfeiffer, Carpenter, and so forth. Secondary suture closure may occur with bone dysplasias (for example, treated rickets), arrested hydrocephalus, trauma, or failure of brain growth (micrencephaly). Brain malformations or hydrocephalus may occasionally be associated with primary craniosynostosis. Multisuture or universal craniosynostosis may manifest increased intracranial pressure related to brain growth against an unyielding skull. *Head and neck dysmorphias*[9] indicative of underlying temporal bone or other anomalies include microtia, anomalies of the first branchial arch (cyst, sinus, and so on), Treacher Collins syndrome, hemifacial microsomia, and so forth.

Imaging of craniofacial dysmorphia (Fig. 2-42) may involve initial screening with skull films, US, or CT followed occasionally by more definitive MRI for delineation of intracranial and intraorbital malformations.[1,2,16] Often, high-resolution CT with three-dimensional reconstruction (Fig. 2-42) is needed for orbit, facial, sinus, skull base, and temporal bone anatomy for craniofacial reconstructive planning, especially when surgery is indicated to prevent progressive neurological impairment (visual, intellectual, and so forth).[10,18]

REFERENCES
Craniofacial dysmorphia

1. Babcock D, Han B, Dine M: Sonographic findings in infants with macrocrania, *AJR* 150:1359, 1988.
2. Byrd S, Naidich T: *Common congenital brain anomalies,* Philadelphia, 1988, WB Saunders.
3. DeMyer W: Megalencephaly in children: clinical syndromes, genetic patterns, and differential diagnosis from hydrocephalus, *Neurology* 22:634, 1972.
4. DeMyer W: Megalencephaly: types and differential diagnosis. In Swaiman K: *Pediatric neurology,* St Louis, 1989, Mosby–Year Book.
5. Dunn D, Epstein L: *Decision making in child neurology,* Philadelphia, 1987, BC Decker.
6. Fenichel G: *Clinical pediatric neurology,* Philadelphia, 1988, WB Saunders.
7. Hamza M, Bodensteiner J, Noorani P, et al: Benign extracerebral fluid collections: a cause of macrocrania in infancy, *Pediatr Neurol* 3:218, 1987.
8. Harwood-Nash D, Fitz C: *Neuroradiology in infants and children,* St Louis, 1976, Mosby–Year Book.
9. Healy G, editor: *Common problems in pediatric otolaryngology,* Chicago, 1990, Mosby–Year Book.
10. Hoffman H, Raffel C: Craniofacial surgery. In McLaurin R, Schut L, Venes J, Epstein F, editors: *Pediatric neurosurgery,* ed 2, Philadelphia, 1989, WB Saunders.
11. Jones K: *Smith's recognizable patterns of human malformation,* ed 4, Philadelphia, 1988, WB Saunders.
12. Laurent J, Cheek W: Craniosynostosis. In McLaurin R, Schut L, Venes J, Epstein F, editors: *Pediatric neurosurgery,* ed 2, Philadelphia, 1989, WB Saunders.
13. Maytal J, Alvarez L, Elkin C, et al: External hydrocephalus: radiologic spectrum, *AJNR* 8:271, 1987.
14. Menkes J: *Textbook of child neurology,* ed 3, Philadelphia, 1985, Lea & Febiger.
15. Naidich T, Osborn R, Bauer B: Median cleft face syndrome, CT and MR, *J Comput Assist Tomogr* 12:57, 1988.
16. Sarwar M: *CT of congenital brain malformations,* Boston, 1985, Martinus Nihoff.
17. Taybi H: *Radiology of syndromes and metabolic disorders,* ed 2, Chicago, 1983, Mosby–Year Book.
18. Vannier M, Hildebolt, et al: Craniosynostosis: diagnostic value of three-dimensional CT reconstruction, *Radiology* 173:669, 1989.
19. Weiner H, Urion D, Levitt L: *Pediatric neurology for the house officer,* ed 3, Baltimore, 1988, Williams & Wilkins.

INCREASED INTRACRANIAL PRESSURE

Symptoms and signs of elevated intracranial pressure include macrocephaly, accelerating head circumference, full or bulging fontanelle, split sutures, headache, vomiting, visual impairment, irritability, poor feeding, lethargy, stupor, encephalopathy, Parinaud's syndrome, bilateral or unilateral sixth nerve palsy, lower extremity hyperreflexia/hypertonia, and papilledema.[4,5,11,16,18] Causes include trauma, hemorrhage, acute hypoxic-ischemic insult, infection, parainfectious sequelae, metabolic derangement, hydrocephalus, tumors, pseudotumor cerebri, and universal craniosynostosis.[12-16] Neuroimaging is necessary to define a mass, fluid collection, edema, or hydrocephalus.[1,8,9,18] The mass may be a cyst, neoplasm, abscess, or hematoma. The abnormal fluid collection may be subdural or epidural, whether a hematoma, empyema, effusion, or hygroma. Edema may be traumatic, hypoxic-ischemic, toxic (for example, lead poisoning), metabolic (for example, ketoacidosis), infectious (meningitis or encephalitis), parainfectious inflammatory (postviral or postvaccinial) or parainfectious noninflammatory (for example, Reye's syndrome), or due to pseudotumor cerebri. Hydrocephalus is discussed in more detail in the next section.

HYDROCEPHALUS

Hydrocephalus is the state of excessive CSF accumulation with progressive dilatation of the ventricles, subarachnoid spaces, or both. Hydrocephalus is caused by an imbalance between CSF production and absorption or by a blockage of CSF flow.[9,14] Hydrocephalus due to CSF overproduction is rare but may occur with choroid plexus papilloma or villous hypertrophy. Obstructive hydrocephalus (CSF flow block or absorptive block) may be described as communicating with the obstructive lesion occurring outside the ventricular system (usually within the cisterns or at the parasagittal arachnoid villi), or noncommunicating and due to an intraventricular block (at or proximal to the fourth ventricular outlets). The vast majority of childhood hydrocephalus occurs in infancy (see box on p. 75), with the commonest cause being acquired adhesive ependymitis or arachnoiditis after hemorrhage or infection. Hydrocephalus is a well-known sequela of neonatal intracranial hemorrhage, especially in premature infants (germinal matrix–intraventricular hemorrhage).[17] Prenatal infection (for example, TORCH) or postnatal infection (for example, meningitis) may also lead to hydrocephalus. By far the commonest developmental source of hydrocephalus is Chiari II malformation associated with myelocele or myelomeningocele, which often develops after repair of the spinal defect. Other common developmental causes are aqueductal anomalies (forking, stenosis, septum, gliosis)

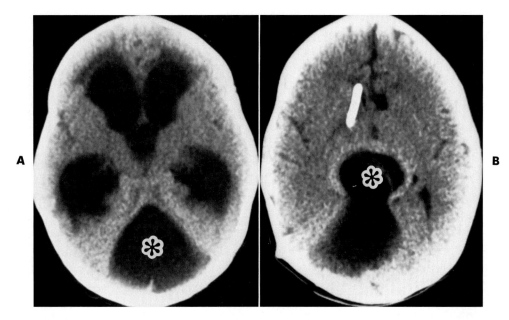

Fig. 2-43   Dandy-Walker cyst demonstrated by CT before **(A)** and after **(B)** ventricular shunting with upward herniation of the nondecompressed Dandy-Walker cyst through the tentorial hiatus *(asterisk)*.

CHILDHOOD HYDROCEPHALUS

DEVELOPMENTAL	ACQUIRED
Chiari II malformation	Posthemorrhage
Aqueductal anomalies	Postinfection
Congenital cysts	Posterior fossa tumors
Encephalocele	Tumors about the
Hydranencephaly	third ventricle
Craniosynostosis	Cerebral hemispheric tumors
Skull base anomalies	
Foraminal atresia	
Immature arachnoid villi	
Vein of Galen aneurysm	

---

and Dandy-Walker syndrome. Less common or rare causes of hydrocephalus include atresia of the foramen of Monro, skull base anomaly (achondroplasia), benign intracranial cyst, craniosynostosis, encephalocele, holoprosencephaly, hydranencephaly, and lissencephaly.

Neoplasm as an expanding mass or an obstructive lesion is a rare cause of elevated pressure or hydrocephalus in infancy.[3,9] Most masses of infancy are cystic or cystlike, including the Dandy-Walker spectrum, arachnoid or glioependymal cysts (retrocerebellar, suprasellar, intraventricular, quadrigeminal plate cistern, and so forth), porencephaly, encephalocele, and vein of Galen aneurysm as a blood-filled cyst. The rare neoplasms occuring in the first 2 years are astrocytomas, choroid plexus tumors (papilloma, carcinoma), germ cell tumors (for example, teratoma), and primitive neuroectodermal tumors (PNET). Beyond infancy neoplasm becomes the major cause of increased pressure and hydrocephalus.[2-4,18] Tumors in children have a predi-

lection for the midline along the ventricular and interventricular CSF pathways, including the posterior fossa along the fourth ventricle and aqueduct and the supratentorial compartment about the third ventricle (perisellar, foramina of Monro, pineal region, and so forth). Deep cerebral tumors (for example, thalamic or basal ganglia origin) and cerebral hemispheric tumors may produce increased pressure by mass effect and intracranial shift or cause seizures, hemiparesis, or other focal neurological deficits (see Chapter 7).

Increased pressure and hydrocephalus in the fetus and infant, especially when of developmental or acquired nonneoplastic origin, is first displayed with ultrasound and then CT before shunting.[1] MRI may be indicated to further delineate hydrocephalus (see Fig. 2-23) when surgery is more specifically directed beyond that of simple shunting (for example, cyst or other causative mass and encysted or complex ventricular system).[6] Further delineation may be important in Dandy-Walker syndrome (patency of the aqueduct), isolation of the fourth ventricle, porencephaly, or postventriculitis encystment. Proper placement of catheters for balanced shunting of the Dandy-Walker cyst and the lateral ventricles prevents upward or downward herniation due to unbalanced decompression of one compartment relative to the other (Fig. 2-43). Although CT may be a practical screening examination after infancy, MRI is preferred because neoplasm becomes the leading consideration. The multiplanar and multiparametric capability of MRI makes it the procedure of choice for delineation of anatomy and tumor extent for surgery, radiotherapy, and chemotherapy planning, as well as for follow-up of tumor response and treatment effects (see Chapter 7).

MRI may offer more supportive or causative information

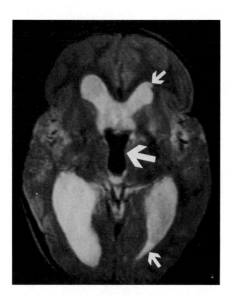

Fig. 2-44   Axial T2 MRI in obstructive hydrocephalus showing accentuated CSF flow voids in the third ventricle *(large white arrow)* and foramina of Monro. The high-intensity periventricular edema *(small white arrows)* is poorly separated from the high-intensity CSF within the dilated ventricles.

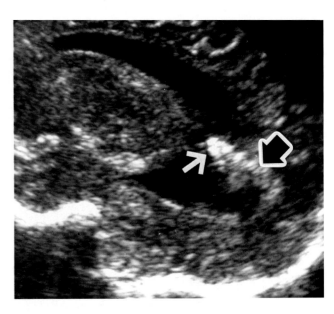

Fig. 2-45   Parasagittal US scan in hydrocephalus with shunt malfunction showing the echogenic ventricular catheter *(black arrow)* imbedded in the echogenic choroid plexus of the trigone *(white arrow)*, all as contrasted against the sonolucent dilated lateral ventricle.

when CT or US demonstrates nonspecific ventriculomegaly.[6] Supportive information that may indicate obstructive hydrocephalus includes MRI demonstration of accentuated aqueductal, foraminal, or ventricular CSF flow voids or periventricular edema (Fig. 2-44). Unexplained obstructive hydrocephalus after infancy requires thorough investigation for an occult inflammatory (infection) or neoplastic process (see Fig. 2-18). MRI may demonstrate periaqueductal tumor in presumed aqueductal stenosis, or leptomeningeal enhancement (Gd-DTPA) in inflammatory or neoplastic infiltration (for example, granulomatous infection, sarcoidosis, leukemia, seeding, and so on).

Treatment of hydrocephalus involves the resection or decompression of the causative mass, ventricular diversion, or both.[9,10,14] Prognosis depends on the origin of the hydrocephalus and on timing of the treatment. The prognosis for hydrocephalus associated with extensive brain malformation or injury is generally poor. The secondary pathological effects of hydrocephalus on the malformed, injured, or developing (myelinating) brain may be devastating. Progressive hydrocephalus unchecked produces interstitial edema, ependymal disruption, spontaneous ventriculostomy, possible herniation, and, ultimately, subependymal gliosis, demyelination, cystic leukomalacia, neuronal injury, and atrophy.[9] The goal of shunting is to reduce pressure to safe levels and to protect brain tissue volume.[10,14] Successful shunting is demonstrated on follow-up imaging as a proportionate decrease in ventricular size and as reestablishment of brain mantle thickness. Follow-up imaging of shunted, nonneoplastic hydrocephalus may be adequately done with US or CT (Figs. 2-45 and

2-46). Its portability and multiplanar capability makes US an ideal guide for shunt placement intraoperatively and shunt position evaluation on follow-up. After loss of the acoustic window in older infants and children, CT becomes the modality of choice for routine follow-up and for evaluating shunt complications including malfunction and subdural fluid collections. MRI may provide multiplanar anatomical and multiparametric delineation, including CSF flow dynamics, especially for complex, compartmentalized, or encysted hydrocephalus (Fig. 2-47).

Shunt malfunction (for example, infection, shunt obstruction, and so forth) is suspected when there are symptoms and signs of acute pressure, seizures, or fever. Imaging evaluation of shunt complications includes assessment of catheter position, ventricular size and configuration, and any change thereof.[10,14] Shunt malfunction may occur as a result of catheter obstruction, disconnection, migration, or inadequate length for growth of the child. The ventricular end of the catheter may be obstructed by choroid plexus or glial tissue if the catheter tip is not situated above and anterior to the foramen of Monro within the anterior body or frontal horn of the lateral ventricle (Figs. 2-45 and 2-46). Catheter obstruction by ependymal or neural tissue may also occur with an extraventricular position or ventricular collapse (embedded catheter). Shunt infection is a major cause of shunt malfunction. Shunt complications due to overdrainage include subdural hematomas or effusions, slit ventricle syndrome, craniosynostosis, and seizures. Distal ventriculovascular (for example, ventriculoatrial) shunt problems may include catheter or large vessel thrombosis, endocarditis, embolism, arrhythmia, perfora-

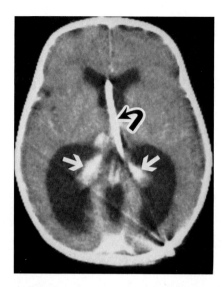

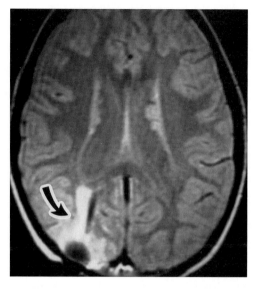

Fig. 2-46   Axial CT of shunted hydrocephalus in an unusual case of CSF overproduction due to choroid plexus villous hypertrophy. The ventricular catheter *(curved arrow)* is positioned into the frontal horn of the right lateral ventricle near the midline. There is marked enhancement of the prominent choroid plexus *(white arrows).*

Fig. 2-47   Axial proton density MRI in hydrocephalus with shunt malfunction due to disseminated medulloblastoma. There is high intensity CSF tracking along the shunt catheter *(arrow).*

tion, or detached tubing. Ventriculoperitoneal distal shunt complications (Fig. 2-48) include hernia, hydrocele, ascites, cyst formation, intestinal volvulus and obstruction, viscus or peritoneal perforation, and neoplastic or infectious seeding.

Along with CT imaging and comparison with previous CT studies, evaluation often includes shunt series radiographs (usually anteroposterior and lateral filming of the head and neck, thorax, abdomen, and pelvis), or ultrasonography, for ventriculoperitoneal shunt system discontinuity and abdominal complications[7] (Fig. 2-48). Ventricular shunt tap is usually essential, whereas contrast shuntogram is rarely needed. Occasionally CT with CSF contrast enhancement may be necessary to evaluate the complex, encysted, or compartmentalized system to assist in proper drainage or shunt catheter placement. Isolation of the fourth ventricle may occur after lateral ventricular shunting and secondary aqueductal closure in the presence of a preexisting outlet fourth ventricular obstruction. Expansion of the fourth ventricle results from continued choroid plexus CSF production, and there may be progressive compression of the brain stem. Isolation of the fourth ventricle is most commonly encountered after shunting of hydrocephalus for Chiari II malformation or for outlet foraminal adhesive occlusion from infection or hemorrhage. Again, multiplanar MRI or CSF–contrast enhanced CT may assist in preoperative planning along with stereotactic techniques or intraoperative US guidance to facilitate catheter placement.

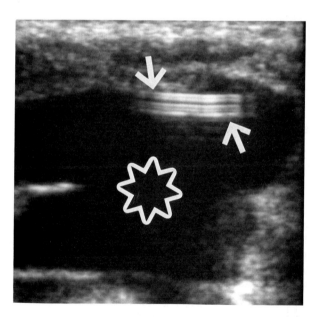

Fig. 2-48   Abdominal US scan in hydrocephalus with shunt malfunction showing the echogenic distal end *(white arrows)* of the ventriculoperitoneal shunt catheter within a loculated sonolucent intraperitoneal CSF collection *(star).*

REFERENCES
Increased intracranial pressure and hydrocephalus

1. Babcock D, Han B, Dine M: Sonographic findings in infants with macrocrania, *AJR* 150:1359, 1988.

2. Barlow C: *Headaches and migraine in childhood,* Philadelphia, 1984, JB Lippincott.
3. Cohen M, Duffner P: Tumors of the brain and spinal cord including leukemic involvement. In Swaiman KF: *Pediatric neurology,* St Louis, 1989, Mosby–Year Book.
4. Dunn D, Epstein L: *Decision making in child neurology,* Philadelphia, 1987, BC Decker.
5. Fenichel G: *Clinical pediatric neurology,* Philadelphia, 1988, WB Saunders.
6. Gammal T, Allen M, Brooks B, et al: MR evaluation of hydrocephalus, *AJR* 149:807, 1987.
7. Grunebaum M, Ziv N, Komreich L, et al: Sonographic signs of peritoneal pseudocyst obstructing ventriculoperitoneal shunts in children, *Neuroradiology* 30:433, 1988.
8. Maytal J, Alvarez L, Elkin C, et al: External hydrocephalus: radiologic spectrum, *AJNR* 8:271, 1987.
9. McCullough D: Hydrocephalus: etiology, pathologic effects, diagnosis, and natural history. In McLaurin R, Schut L, Venes J, Epstein F, editors: *Pediatric neurosurgery,* ed 2, Philadelphia, 1989, WB Saunders.
10. McLaurin R: Ventricular shunts: complications and results. In McLaurin R, Schut L, Venes J, Epstein F, editors: *Pediatric neurosurgery,* ed 2, Philadelphia, 1989, WB Saunders.
11. Menkes J: *Textbook of child neurology,* ed 3, Philadelphia, 1985, Lea & Febiger.
12. Michell J, Ward J: Evaluation and treatment of intracranial hypertension. In Pellock H, Myer E, editors: *Neurologic emergencies in infancy and childhood,* Philadelphia, 1984, Harper & Row.
13. Moser F, Hilal S, Abrams G, et al: MR imaging of pseudotumor cerebri, *AJR* 150:903, 1988.
14. Rekate H: Treatment of hydrocephalus. In McLaurin R, Schut L, Venes J, Epstein F, editors: *Pediatric neurosurgery,* ed 2, Philadelphia, 1989, WB Saunders.
15. Rockoff MA, Kennedy SK: Physiology and clinical aspects of raised intracranial pressure. In Repper A, Kennedy S, Zervas N, editors: *Neurological and neurosurgical intensive care,* ed 2, Rockville, Md, 1988, Aspen.
16. Trauner D: Increased intracranial pressure. In Swaiman K: *Pediatric neurology,* St Louis, 1989, Mosby–Year Book.
17. Volpe J: *Neurology of the newborn,* ed 2, Philadelphia, 1987, WB Saunders.
18. Weiner H, Urion D, Levitt L: *Pediatric neurology for the house officer,* ed 3, Baltimore, 1988, Williams & Wilkins.

NEUROENDOCRINE DISORDERS

Neuroendocrine, that is, pituitary-hypothalamic, disorders often encountered in childhood and adolescence (see box above) include hypopituitarism with growth failure (short stature), hyperpituitarism with growth excess (tall stature), precocious puberty, and delayed sexual development.[1-4] Other central endocrine syndromes occurring in childhood are diencephalic syndrome, diabetes insipidus, and the syndrome of inappropriate ADH secretion. Although there are many causes for *growth failure* (see Developmental Delay and Failure to Thrive), growth hormone deficiency is the major neuroendocrine cause, whether isolated and idiopathic (50%) or associated with other hormone deficiency (hypopituitarism). *Hypopituitarism* may be congenital and manifested as pituitary aplasia or hypoplasia (isolated or associated with anencephaly), holoprosencephaly, septooptic dysplasia, midface anomalies, empty sella, basal encephalocele, and genetic or chromosomal syndromes (for example, familial endocrinopathies, or Turner's syndrome). Acquired causes of hypopituitarism (Fig. 2-49) include trauma, hemorrhage, anoxia (perinatal asphyxia), toxoplasmosis, tuberculosis, histiocytosis, sarcoidosis, irradiation, autoimmune hypophysitis, infarction,

---

CHILDHOOD NEUROENDOCRINE DISORDERS

Hypopituitarism
  Growth failure
  Delayed puberty
Hyperpituitarism
Precocious puberty
Diabetes insipidus
Inappropriate ADH syndrome
Diencephalic syndrome

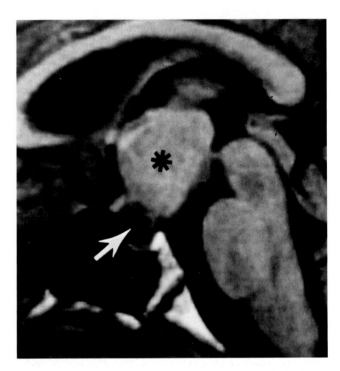

Fig. 2-49   Sagittal T1 MRI in craniopharyngioma producing hypopituitarism with short stature (growth hormone deficiency). There is a large suprasellar tumor *(asterisk)* with intrasellar calcification *(white arrow)* but intact posterior pituitary bright spot.

surgery, and neoplasm. Common neoplasms of childhood producing growth failure or hypopituitarism include craniopharyngioma, optic or hypothalamic glioma, germinoma, and pituitary adenoma.

Hyperpituitarism may be primary (pituitary hypersecretion from tumor) or secondary (target organ failure). Pituitary gigantism or juvenile acromegaly from pituitary adenoma with growth hormone excess is a rare cause of tall stature. Other causes of tall stature include constitutional, cerebral gigantism (Soto's syndrome), other genetic or chromosomal syndromes, Marfan's syndrome, and homocystinuria. Cushing's syndrome (ACTH hypersecretion due to pituitary adenoma) is also very rare in childhood. Prolactin-secreting adenoma is the most common type of

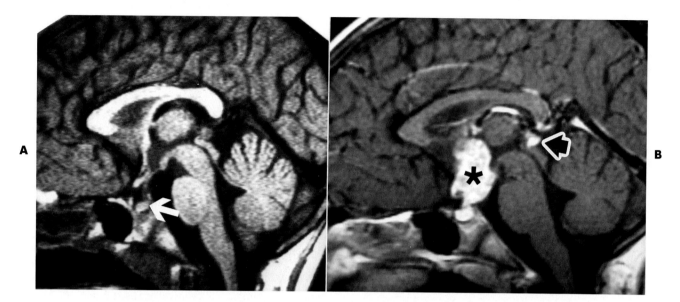

Fig. 2-50   Young girl with "idiopathic" diabetes insipidus. **A,** Initial sagittal T1 MRI reveals absence of the posterior pituitary bright spot *(arrow)*. **B,** Follow-up sagittal T1 MRI with gadolinium-DTPA over 1 year later shows a large enhancing suprasellar mass *(asterisk)* along with other enhancing foci *(arrow)*, again with absence of the posterior pituitary bright spot, all consistent with germinoma. (Courtesy of D. O'Leary, Brigham and Women's Hospital, Boston.)

pituitary adenoma in childhood and adolescence. Hyperprolactinemia results from macroadenomas more often than from microadenomas and manifests headache, growth retardation, delayed puberty, primary or secondary amenorrhea, galactorrhea, or advanced puberty.

Disorders of sexual development usually fall into one of two categories, *delayed puberty* or *precocious puberty.* Normal development relies on proper hypothalamic and anterior pituitary gonadotropic control of gonadal hormone activity. *Delayed sexual maturation* may be constitutional, related to pituitary gonadotropin failure, either isolated or associated with other deficiencies (hypopituitarism), or due to primary gonadal dysfunction. Causes include chromosomal aberrations (for example, Klinefelter's syndrome), genetic defects (for example, Noonan's syndrome), or familial. Developmental and acquired pituitary-hypothalamic causes of delayed sexual development are similar to those for growth failure or hypopituitarism as enumerated above and also include meningoencephalitis and pineal region tumors.

Advanced sexual development or *precocity* is more often isosexual than heterosexual and frequently idiopathic, especially in girls. However, a central lesion may often be implicated, particularly in boys. CNS causes include developmental anomaly (for example, suprasellar arachnoid cyst or hydrocephalus), encephalitis or meningitis, trauma, neurocutaneous syndrome (for example, neurofibromatosis), McCune-Albright syndrome, and tumor. The tumor may be primarily hypothalamic (hamartoma, glioma, germ cell tumor), arise in the pineal region (teratoma, pinealoma, and so on), or involve both the pineal and hypothalamic regions (for example germinoma). Non-CNS causes include

gonadal tumors (testicular or ovarian), ectopic gonadotropin tumors (mediastinal, hepatoblastoma, and so forth), hypothyroidism, exogenous sources, and adrenal disease (congenital adrenal hyperplasia or adrenal neoplasm).

Diabetes insipidus (DI) of central origin is caused by the neurohypophyseal deficiency of antidiuretic hormone (ADH, or vasopressin) and classically presents with polyuria and polydipsia. Central DI is to be distinguished clinically from nephrogenic and psychogenic causes. CNS causes include heredofamilial, idiopathic, meningoencephalitis, intraventricular hemorrhage, trauma or surgery with stalk injury, leukemia, histiocytosis, sarcoidosis and the pituitary-hypothalamic anomalies enumerated above, plus empty sella and neoplasm. Common neoplastic processes associated with DI are germinoma (hypothalamic, pineal region, or both) glioma and, rarely, craniopharyngioma. MRI may demonstrate absence of the normal posterior pituitary bright spot (Fig. 2-50) in addition to other findings such as tumor (see Chapters 3 and 7). Although DI is idiopathic in approximately 20% of cases, it may precede other neurological symptoms and signs of CNS tumor by months or even years (Fig. 2-50).

Inappropriate ADH secretion results in fluid and electrolyte imbalance and often encephalopathy. The syndrome may be associated with a variety of CNS and non-CNS diseases including meningitis or encephalitis, tumor, abscess, subarachnoid hemorrhage, Guillain-Barré syndrome, trauma, pneumonia, tuberculosis, cystic fibrosis, asphyxia, and neoplasms of other systems, or may be drug-induced (for example, vincristine) or follow surgery for a pituitary tumor. *Diencephalic syndrome* is an important anterior hypothalamic disorder classically seen in infancy as emaciation, hyperkinesis, increased or normal appetite, euphoria, overalertness, and hypoglycemia. The syndrome is usually associated with a hypothalamic neoplasm, most commonly astrocytoma (see Chapter 7).

Imaging evaluation of neuroendocrine disorders may not be necessary when the origin is confirmed by clinical and laboratory means and progressive CNS disease is not suspected. US or CT may be adequate for screening when the cause is known or expected, for instance, meningitis, trauma, or congenital causes. For unexplained disorders and suspected tumor, MRI is preferred over contrast-enhanced CT.

REFERENCES
Neuroendocrine disorders

1. Behrman R, Vaughan V, editors: *Nelson's textbook of pediatrics*, ed 13, Philadelphia, WB Saunders.
2. Brook C: *Clinical paediatric endocrinology*, ed 2, Boston, 1989, Blackwell.
3. Jacobson R, Abrams G: Disorders of the hypothalamus and pituitary gland in adolescence and childhood. In Swaiman K: *Pediatric neurology*, St Louis, 1989, Mosby–Year Book.
4. Villee D: Endocrinology. In Avery M, First L: *Pediatric medicine*, Baltimore, 1989, Williams & Wilkins.

DERMATOLOGICAL MANIFESTATIONS

Cutaneous or subcutaneous abnormalities that may indicate an underlying CNS abnormality[1-4] often fall into one of two major categories: neurocutaneous syndromes (phacomatoses) and dysraphism (neural tube closure malformations). The common *phacomatoses* of childhood include neurofibromatosis types 1 and 2 (cafe-au-lait spots, cutaneous neurofibromata, and axillary freckling), tuberous sclerosis (adenoma sebaceum, ungual fibroma, hypopigmented macule, and shagreen patch), and Sturge-Weber syndrome (orbitofacial port-wine stain). Less common or rare syndromes include von Hippel–Lindau syndrome, Klippel-Trenaunay-Weber syndrome, ataxia telangiectasia, hereditary hemorrhagic telangiectasia, Bannayan's syndrome, epidermal nevus syndrome, linear sebaceous nevus syndrome, hypomelanosis of Ito, and incontinentia pigmenti. *Dysraphic conditions* include overt or open defects with exposed neural tissue (for example, anencephaly, myelocele, and so forth) and the more occult or skin-covered defects (for example, lipomyelomingocele, low conus–tight filum, cephalocele, or dermoid). The latter group may be suspected in the presence of a cutaneous or subcutaneous lump (for example, lipoma or cyst), hairy patch, hemangioma or telangiectasia, dimple, sinus tract, skin tag, scoliosis, hypertelorism, or nasopharyngeal mass. Although CT may be recommended as the initial brain screen for neurocutaneous syndromes (see Chapter 7) with a high incidence of calcification (for example, tuberous sclerosis and Sturge-Weber syndrome) MRI clearly provides greater sensitivity for soft tissue dysplastic and neoplastic components (for example, tuberous sclerosis and neurofibromatosis), as well as vascular components (for example, Sturge-Weber syndrome and so on). US may be the preferred screening modality for dysraphic cranial and spinal conditions in the young infant, whereas CT is recommended for brain screening in older children (see Chapter 3). Plain films and MRI are recommended as the definitive combination for demonstrating spinal dysraphism (see Chapter 9).

REFERENCES
Dermatological manifestations

1. Berg B: Neurocutaneous syndromes. In Swaiman K: *Pediatric neurology*, St Louis, 1989, Mosby–Year Book.
2. Hurwitz S: *The skin and systemic disease in children*, Chicago, 1985, Mosby–Year Book.
3. Weiner H, Urion D, Levitt L: *Pediatric neurology for the house officer*, ed 3, Baltimore, 1988, Williams & Wilkins.
4. Weston W: *Practical pediatric dermatology*, ed 2, Boston, 1985, Little Brown.

PART TWO

Brain Imaging

3 · Congenital and Developmental Abnormalities of the Brain

Richard L. Klucznik
Samuel M. Wolpert
Mary L. Anderson

Recent advances in neuroimaging have brought the identification and classification of congenital brain anomalies to the forefront of pediatric neuroradiology. In utero, ultrasonography (US) is an invaluable tool for detecting severe intracranial abnormalities, assisting in determining prognosis and possible intervention. CT and US can readily diagnose most malformations occurring after birth. MRI provides the most elaborate display of malformations when more complete delineation is necessary for therapy, prognosis, or genetic counseling. The multiplanar capabilities and superior tissue contrast resolution of MRI allow more precise identification of absent, malformed, or displaced brain structures. The disorders of organogenesis, on which this chapter concentrates, can be adequately evaluated with short TR/short TE spin echo images (T1-weighted) in most cases. Structural abnormalities are best depicted in the sagittal and coronal planes, but each case must be individualized. Axial images may be helpful as well, especially when comparison to CT examination is required. Long TR spin echo images (proton-density and T2-weighted) are most helpful in the evaluation of lesions associated with disorders of histiogenesis, for example, neurocutaneous syndromes (Chapter 8), and the disorders of neuronal migration. Currently, MRI contrast enhancement with gadolinium-DTPA has little role in the evaluation of congenital malformations.

Once anatomical delineation of a structural abnormality is obtained, the lesion can then be classified. However, classification has been a difficult task and a topic of controversy among anatomists and pathologists. Etiologically, intrauterine environmental factors and chromosomal mutations each account for 10% of the congenital CNS abnormalities, whereas inheritance accounts for approximately 20%.[7] No definite cause has yet been elucidated for the remaining percentage. Furthermore specific insults may not lead to predictable abnormalities. An understanding of embryology and of various factors affecting development at different embryologic milestones may help explain many of the morphologic abnormalities. Brain abnormalities have been classified according to cellular (histogenesis) or anatomical (organogenesis) derangement.[5] Recently van der Knaap and Valk[12] modified Volpe's classification,

VAN DER KNAAP AND VALK CLASSIFICATION OF CONGENITAL, CEREBRAL, CEREBELLAR, AND SPINAL MALFORMATIONS

	GESTATIONAL TIME OF ONSET
DISORDERS OF DORSAL INDUCTION	
Primary neurulation	3 to 4 weeks
Cranioschisis (anencephaly, cephalocele)	
Rachischisis (myelocele, myelomeningocele, Chiari malformation, hydromyelia)	
Secondary neurulation	4 weeks to postnatal
Myelocystocele	
Diastematomyelia	
Diplomyelia	
Meningocele	
Lipomeningocele	
Lipoma	
Dermal sinus	
Tight filum terminale	
Neurenteric anomalies	
Caudal regression syndrome	
DISORDERS OF VENTRAL INDUCTION	5 to 10 weeks
Holoprosencephaly	
Septooptic dysplasia	
Agenesis of septum pellucidum	
Cerebral hemiatrophy/hemihypoplasia	
Hypoplasia/aplasia of cerebellar hemispheres	
Hypoplasia/aplasia of cerebellar vermis	
Dandy-Walker syndrome	
Craniosynostosis	
Diencephalic cyst	
DISORDERS OF NEURONAL PROLIFERATION DIFFERENTIATION AND HISTIOGENESIS	2 to 6 months
Micrencephaly	
Megalencephaly	
Unilateral megalencephaly	
Aqueductal anomalies	
Colpocephaly	
Porencephaly	
Multicystic encephalopathy	
Hydranencephaly	
Disorders of histiogenesis	
Neurocutaneous syndromes	
Tuberous sclerosis	
Sturge-Weber syndrome	
Von Hippel–Lindau disease	
Neurofibromatoses	
Vascular malformations	
Malformative tumors	
DISORDERS OF SULCATION AND MIGRATION	2 to 5 months
Agyria/pachygyria	
Lissencephaly	
Polymicrogyria	
Schizencephaly	
Neuronal heterotopias	
Hypoplasia/aplasia of corpus callosum	
MYELINATION DISORDERS	7 months to 2 years
Hypomyelination, retarded myelination	
SECONDARILY ACQUIRED INJURY OF NORMALLY FORMED STRUCTURES	
Encephaloclastic hydranencephaly	
Encephaloclastic porencephaly	
Encephaloclastic schizencephaly	
Encephaloclastic multicystic encephalopathy	
Hydrocephalus secondary to aqueductal stenosis	
Hemorrhage and infarction	
UNCLASSIFIED	
Arachnoid cysts	

Adapted and modified from van der Knaap MS, Valk J: *AJNR* 9:315, 1988.

which had arranged congenital disorders to reflect the onset of disturbance to the developing neural tissue. In Volpe's classification, the reason for the disturbance is not as important as the embryologic timing. Insults early in gestation can have more devastating effects on the developing neural structures than those later in gestation.

This chapter initially discusses normal myelination and then, using the van der Knaap and Valk system as a framework (see box on p. 84), provides MRI characteristics of the more commonly encountered congenital brain abnormalities. Emphasis remains on disorders of organogenesis. Vascular malformations, malformative tumors, and neurocutaneous syndromes (phacomatoses) are discussed in Chapters 6, 7, and 8 respectively. Malformations of the spinal cord, and encephaloclastic and degenerative disorders are presented in Chapters 4 and 9.

NORMAL MYELINATION

Ever since imaging modalities became available, the process of myelination of the brain has been investigated.[9,11] Early work with baboons and humans quantified myelination by the change from lower to relatively higher attenuation values of white matter on CT scans caused by a decrease in water content.[11] MRI is now considered the best imaging modality for evaluating myelination.

Myelination is a complex process that is still not completely understood. As myelination proceeds the water content of the white matter decreases from 88% at birth to 85% at 6 months[4,13]; simultaneously, surface membrane glycolipids, proteins, and cholesterol increases.[4,10] These structural alterations form the basis for the evolution of MRI signal patterns, with the changing water content of the brain being the major determinant. With the progressive loss of water content of the white matter the relaxation times of adjacent lipoprotein-bound water protons are affected.[1,8] Increase in the lipid content has a minor contribution to the changing signal. At birth there is relatively poor differentiation between white matter and gray matter especially on T1- and proton-density weighted images. As myelination proceeds, protein, cholesterol, or glycolipids cause shortening of the T1 relaxation time of water, which produces higher signal intensity on T1-weighted images.[1] The lower signal intensity on proton-density and T2-weighted images primarily results from a decrease in water content of the brain.[8] During the myelination process the gray matter retains more water than does white matter, and proton-density and T2-weighted images can then be used to differentiate the white matter as maturation proceeds. Recent investigators[1,3,6] have recommended using T1-weighted images primarily in the first 6 postnatal months of infancy for evaluating myelination and T2-weighted images for subsequent evaluations.

The development of myelination coincides with the establishment of neurological function. Structures necessary for information integration are myelinated first. The median longitudinal fasciculus, inferior and superior cerebellar peduncles, and thalamus are myelinated at birth[14]; this is manifested by hyperintensity on T1-weighted images[1] and hypo-

intensity on T2-weighted images. The posterior limb of the internal capsule and thalamus may also be myelinated.[14] Myelination then proceeds superiorly and peripherally. By 3 months the cerebellar white matter has increased signal intensity on T1 images[1,3] and hypointensity on T2 images. Myelination of the anterior limb of the internal capsule commences at 2 to 3 months and is completed by 11 months. Myelination of the deep or periventricular white matter begins in the occipital region by about 9 months, and continues anteriorly to the parietal and frontal regions. The centrum semiovale is completed by 7 to 11 months. First order arborization of the U fibers occurs by 1.5 years and second order branching by 3 years.[1,2,13]

The splenium of the corpus callosum begins to myelinate at 4 to 6 months, with low signal intensity on T2-weighted images spreading anteriorly to the rostrum by about 8 months of age; simultaneously the corpus callosum thickens to a nearly adult pattern by 1 year. The entire brain should have an adult pattern by 18 to 24 months of age. There may be persistent areas of increased signal intensity on T2-weighted images in the peritrigonal white matter or occasionally in the frontal periventricular white matter.[1] These areas may not myelinate until the fourth decade and are known to be normal areas of delayed myelination or hypomyelination called terminal zones.[14]

The following illustrations depict the normal pattern of myelination (Figs. 3-1 to 3-8).   *Text continued on p. 91.*

REFERENCES
Introduction and normal myelination

1. Barkovich AJ, Kjos BO, et al: Normal maturation of the neonatal and infant brain: MR imaging at 1.5 T, *Radiology* 166:173, 1988.
2. Bignami A, Palladini G, Zappella M: Unilateral megalencephaly with nerve cell hypertrophy: an anatomical and quantitative histochemical study, *Brain Res* 9:103, 1968.
3. Bird CR, Hedberg M, Drayer BP, et al: MR assessment of myelination in infants and children: usefulness of marker sites, *AJNR* 10:731, 1989.
4. Braun PE: Molecular organization of myelin. Morell P, editor: *Myelin*, ed 22, New York, 1984, Plenum.
5. DeMyer M: Classification of cerebral malformations: Original Article Series, *Birth Defects* 7:78, 1971.
6. Dietrich RB, Bradley WG, Zaragoza EJ, et al: MR evaluation of early demyelination patterns in normal and developmentally delayed infants, *AJNR* 9:69, 1988.
7. Faerber EN: Congenital disorders. In Faerber EN, editor: *Cranial computed tomography in infants and children*, Philadelphia, 1986, JB Lippincott.
8. Holland BA, Haas DK, Norman D: MRI of normal brain maturation, *AJNR* 7:201, 1986.
9. Johnson MA, Pennock JM, Bydder GM, et al: Clinical NMR imaging of the brain in children: normal and neurologic disease, *AJNR* 4:1013, 1983.
10. Norton WT: Formation, structure, and biochemistry of myelin. In Siegel GJ, Albers R, Arganoff BU, Katzman R, editors: *Basic neurochemistry*, Boston, 1981, Little, Brown.
11. Quencer RM: Maturation of normal primate white matter: computed tomographic correlation, *AJNR* 3:365, 1982.
12. Van der Knaap MS, Valk J: Classification of congenital abnormalities of the CNS, *AJNR* 9:315, 1988.
13. Yakovlev PI, Lecirirs AR: The myelogenetic cycles of regional maturation of the brain. In Narkovshe A, editor: *Regional development of the brain in early life*, Philadelphia, 1967, Davis.
14. Yakovlev PI, Wadsworth RC: Schizencephalies: A study of the congenital clefts in the cerebral mantle. II. Clefts with hydrocephalus and lips separated, *J Neuropathol Exp Neurol* 5:169, 1946.

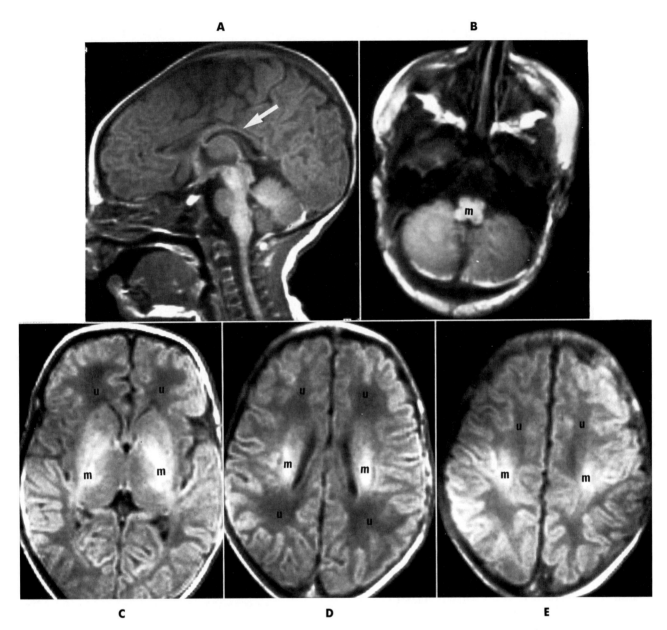

Fig. 3-1   Normal myelination at 4 days. **A,** Short TR/short TE images (650/20 msec). Sagittal images reveal high signal intensity of the medulla, mesencephalon, and cerebellar peduncle white matter indicating myelination. Note that the corpus callosum is thin and isointense to gray matter *(arrow)*. **B,** Axial images (650/20 msec) at the level of the medulla demonstrate the myelinated white matter tracts of the brain stem *(m)* compared with the cerebellum on the same level. **C,** On short TR/short TE images at the level of the basal ganglia the posterior limb of the internal capsule is of high signal intensity *(m)*, whereas the frontal *(u)* and occipital white matter is of low intensity (reversal of the normal adult pattern). **D** and **E,** The myelinated fibers of the corona radiata extend superiorly *(m)* and the unmyelinated white matter is of low intensity *(u)*.

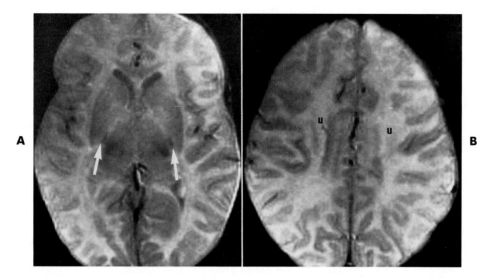

Fig. 3-2   Normal myelination at 21 days. **A** and **B,** Axial long TR/long TE images (3000/70 msec) demonstrate the unmyelinated white matter *(u)* as increased signal intensity because of its increased water content. Notice areas of low signal intensity in the posterior limb of the internal capsule indicating commencing myelination *(arrows).*

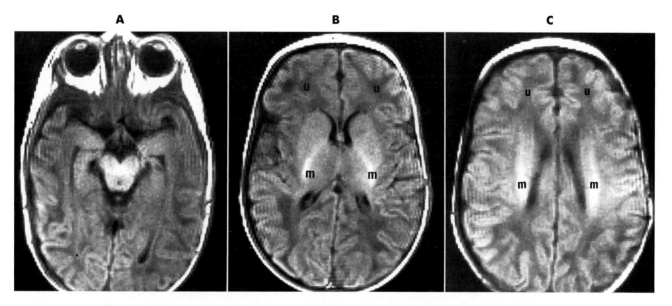

Fig. 3-3   Normal myelination at 1 month. **A** to **C,** Axial short TR/short TE images (650/19 msec) demonstrate myelinated white matter tracts of the pons, posterior limb of internal capsule (*m* in **B**), and proximal coronal radiata (*m* in **C**). Myelination *(u)* has not arborized in the U fibers.

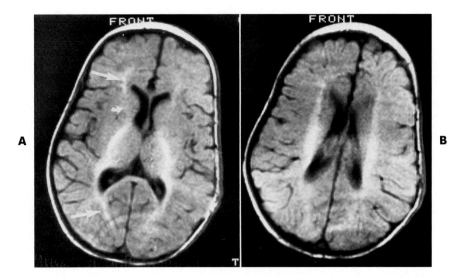

Fig. 3-4   Normal myelination at 3 months. As myelination proceeds superiorly the anterior limb of the internal capsule develops increased signal *(curved arrow)* on short TR/short TE images (650/20 msec). There is commencing myelination in the frontal and occipital white matter as well (**A,** *arrows*). Note also the myelination of the corona radiata (**B).**

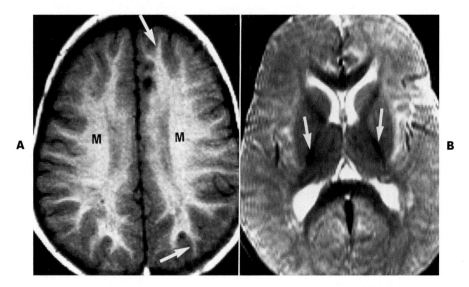

Fig. 3-5   Normal myelination at 9 months. Axial short TR/TE (600/17 msec) images. **A,** The centrum semiovale is myelinated *(M),* and there is arborization of the U fibers *(arrows).* The white matter has a higher signal than the gray matter, as in the adult. **B,** The long TR/long TE image (4000/100 msec) now shows myelination of the corpus callosum and the internal capsule (dark signal) *(arrows).*

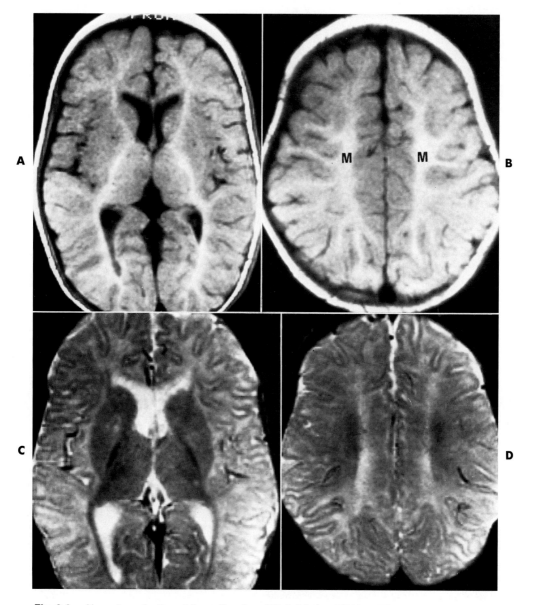

Fig. 3-6   Normal myelination at 5 months. **A** and **B,** Axial short TR/short TE images (650/20 msec). **C** and **D,** Axial long TR/long TE images (3000/90 msec). On T1-weighted images the internal capsule has completely myelinated. Myelination has also proceeded superiorly to the corona radiata *(M)*. On T2-weighted images the dark signal of the internal capsule indicates loss of water as myelination proceeds. However, in the centrum semiovale there is no corresponding dark signal. The T2-weighted images are not as sensitive as the T1-weighted images, which demonstrate the myelination as increased signal in the first 6 months.

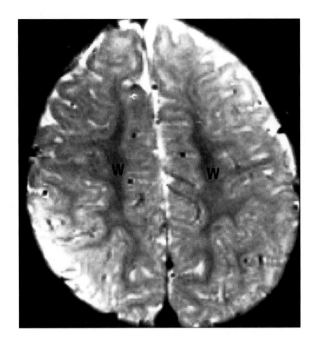

Fig. 3-7   Normal myelination at 1 year. The long TR/long TE image demonstrates the normal low signal of the white matter *(W)* with arborization and myelination of the U fibers.

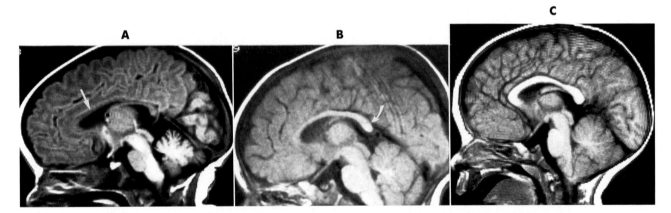

Fig. 3-8   Development of the corpus callosum. Sagittal short TR/short TE (650/20 msec) images at 21 days **(A),** 4 months **(B),** and 9 months **(C). A,** Within the first month the corpus callosum is not myelinated and remains isointense to gray matter and is relatively thin *(arrow).* **B,** As myelination proceeds there is increased signal intensity evident particularly in the splenium, which has begun to thicken *(curved arrow).* By 9 months the corpus callosum has thickened to a more normal adult configuration with increased signal indicating that the myelination is complete. Notice also the bright signal of the pituitary gland at 21 days, which is a normal finding at this age. Note the normal bright signal in the brain stem but not in the belly of the pons **(A).** This is a normal finding at 21 days.

DISORDERS OF MYELINATION

Children can develop white matter disorders as a result of demyelination, dysmyelination, and developmental delay, as well as idiopathically.[1] Demyelinating disorders may be divided into primary disorders, such as multiple sclerosis (see Chapter 4) and acute disseminated encephalomyelitis (see Chapter 5), and secondary disorders due to toxic or anoxic syndromes (see Chapter 6) or viral disorders (see Chapter 5). The dysmyelinating lesions such as metachromatic leukodystrophy, Krabbe's disease, Canavan's disease, Alexander's disease, and Pelizaeus-Merzbacher disease are discussed in Chapter 4.

White matter abnormalities may also be caused by delayed myelination on a developmental basis. For this diagnosis to be made, a careful comparison between the patient's scan and the expected onset of myelination pathways as seen on normal MRI scans will identify areas of delayed myelination.

Congenital muscular dystrophy

Delayed myelination is found in congenital muscular dystrophy of the Fukuyuma type, a disease with a particularly high frequency in Japan. Afflicted children are usually born floppy and severely mentally retarded. CT scans show a variety of abnormalities including white matter lucencies.[2] As the children grow older the lucencies disappear in a caudorostral progression. Marked morphological changes also occur in the brain, including agyria, pachygyria, microgyria, brain stem heterotopias, ventricular dilatation, enlarged sulci, and aqueductal stenosis. Pachygyria and delayed myelination have been found on MRI scans.[3]

REFERENCES
Disorders of myelination

1. Nowell MA, Grossman RI, Hackney DB, et al: MR imaging of white matter disease in children, *AJNR* 9:503, 1988.
2. Yoshioka M, Sawai S: Congenital muscular dystrophy (Fukuyuma type)—changes in the white matter low density on CT, *Brain Dev* 10:41, 1988.
3. Yoshioka M, Sawai S, Kuroki S, et al: MR imaging of the brain in Fukuyuma type congenital muscular dystrophy, *AJNR* 12:63, 1991.

DISORDERS OF DORSAL INDUCTION

The major categories of cranial and intracranial malformations include anomalies of dorsal induction, anomalies of ventral induction, and disorders of migration and neuronal proliferation. Although a review of embryology is beyond the scope of this text, some basic embryologic principles are described to make these abnormalities more understandable. The pathogenesis of these entities is best understood through basic embryologic principles.

During the first month of gestation one germ layer has the potential of inducing a change in another (induction). Dorsal induction refers to the process in which the midline notochord (derived from mesoderm) induces a thickening of the adjacent ectoderm to form the neural plate. Neural folds develop from the plate on each side and join in the midline to form a tubular structure, the primitive neural tube. The process is called primary neurulation. Disorders of dorsal induction as they pertain to cranial and brain development are discussed here (see box on p. 84); those pertaining to spinal development are discussed in Chapter 9.

Cranioschisis

Cranioschisis refers to abnormal formation of the cranium where the intracranial contents either do not develop or lie outside the cranial vault. The abnormalities range from complete absence of the cranium (anencephaly) to herniation of the contents (cephaloceles). In anencephaly, because the neural tube fails to close at the cranial end at 24 days' gestation, the cranial vault above the level of the orbits is completely absent. The intracranial contents are absent above the brain stem. There is no telencephalon (cerebrum), and the facies are dysmorphic. The prognosis is universally fatal. Ultrasonographically these lesions can be detected in utero in the first trimester, when a therapeutic abortion can be performed. The diagnosis is confirmed by examination of the amniotic fluid for elevated alpha-fetoprotein.

Cephaloceles

Cephaloceles occur with a frequency of 1/4000 to 1/5000 live births, three times more frequently than agenesis of the corpus callosum.[4] The defect occurs early in neurulation at approximately 28 to 45 days and is caused by partial failure of rostral neural tube closure. Isolated defects can occur later in development where progressive ossification of the chondrocranium can trap intracranial contents. The ossification centers may fail to unite, sometimes associated with increased intracranial pressure, and the calvarium may thin.[4] Associated anomalies have been reported, including *h*ydrocephalus, *a*gyria, *r*etinal *d*ysplasia, *e*ncephalocele (HARD + E syndrome)[4] and agenesis of corpus callosum with midline facial clefts.[6]

Cephaloceles are classified by location and their intracranial contents. A meningocele contains meninges and CSF, an encephalocele contains cerebral tissue, and an encephalocystomeningocele contains brain, meninges, and ventricles.[3,4] The cerebral tissue is usually extremely dysplastic without recognized architecture.[5]

OCCIPITAL. In North America occipital cephaloceles are the most common cephaloceles (71%), followed by parietal, frontal, and sphenoidal cephaloceles.[3] Encephaloceles are four times more common than meningoceles.[4] Infratentorial occipital cephaloceles are associated with Chiari malformations in half of the cases, including Chiari III malformation, which is herniation of the cerebellum into a cervical-occipital encephalocele (Fig. 3-9). Occipital cephaloceles, some of which may exceed the infant's head in size, have also been associated with Dandy-Walker malformations or other cystic lesions of the posterior fossa. There is also an association with amniotic bands in utero.[3]

MRI has two important roles in the evaluation of occipital cephaloceles: it helps to diagnose the contents of the defect

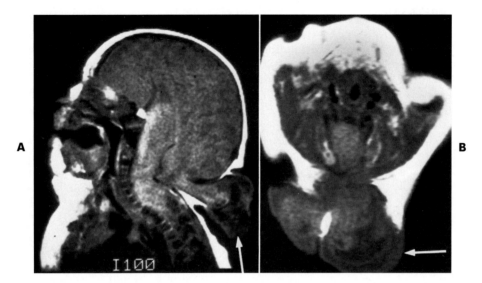

Fig. 3-9   Chiari III malformation. A cervicooccipital encephalomeningocele is evident. **A** and **B,** There is herniation of brain and meninges through a defect in the superior cervical region *(arrows).* There is severe hindbrain dysgenesis, with inferior displacement and herniation of the cerebellum through a posterior defect. No fourth ventricle or aqueduct is evident. The brain stem is misshapen in this severe deformity.

(Fig. 3-10) and to identify the vascular changes, particularly with the venous sinuses, that may occur.[9] Absence of brain tissue is the single most favorable prognostic feature for survival.[7] On MRI examination the straight sinus may be absent. The identification of the position of dural venous sinuses, especially the superior sagittal sinus, is critical for surgical management. If only a small meningocele is present, surgery may not be necessary, as the defect may close spontaneously. On occasion an occipital meningocele may be associated with other midline anomalies such as Dandy-Walker malformation (Fig. 3-10, *D* and *E*).

Hydrocephalus is associated in half of the patients with occipital encephaloceles and one fifth of the patients with meningoceles. It is important to identify the presence of hydrocephalus, since adequate shunting may have prognostic importance before surgical intervention can be attempted.

SPHENOIDAL. Sphenoidal cephaloceles are usually clinically occult. The herniation occurs through the floor of the sella turcica in the midline. The lesions may be purely sphenoidal or sphenoethmoidal,[3] but they are rarely sphenopharyngeal.[2] Callosal agenesis may be associated with the latter. Since the infundibulum and third ventricle may herniate through the defect, associated endocrine dysfunction may occur[2,8] (Fig. 3-11). Hypertelorism and facial malformations with labial or palatine fissures may occur. Two thirds of patients may have true midline clefts of the nose, upper lip, or both.[4] Approximately 40% have unilateral coloboma or hypoplasia of the eye. The cephaloceles may present in the nose as a pulsatile mass covered by nasal mucosa. Spontaneous fistula and meningitis are rare.

When a nasopharyngeal mass is present in an infant, a cephalocele must be considered in the differential diagnosis.

FRONTOETHMOIDAL. Frontoethmoidal lesions are uncommon in Europe and North America but are among the most common type seen in Southeast Asia.[4] They can be grouped according to location of the osseous defect, as described in the literature: nasoethmoidal, nasofrontal, nasoorbital, and interfrontal. Nasoethmoidal cephaloceles protrude through the lamina cribrosa and may present as a nasal mass, or polyp, rather than a facial or cerebral malformation. Nasal polyps are unusual in children, except in those with cystic fibrosis or allergies, and on their discovery a possible encephalocele should be suspected. If the intracranial connection of such an encephalocele is obliterated, the nasal mass has been incorrectly called a *nasal glioma.* Ectopic gliomas, however, may also occur prenasally at the bridge of the nose and are also called nasal gliomas.[10] These lesions are benign congenital neuroectodermal heterotopias rather than true gliomas and are not premalignant. They need to be distinguished from nasal or prenasal dermoids (see Chapter 7).

Nasofrontal cephaloceles occur through the bregma and may split the crista galli. There is associated hypertelorism, and the patients may have a glabellar mass. Larger lesions may contain part of the olfactory tracts and frontal lobes. Associated malformations include agenesis of the corpus callosum, holoprosencephaly, agyria, and hydrocephalus.[4] In nasoorbital cephaloceles the defect occurs between the ethmoid and frontal process of the maxilla and may pass into the orbits, appearing as medial orbital masses. Com-

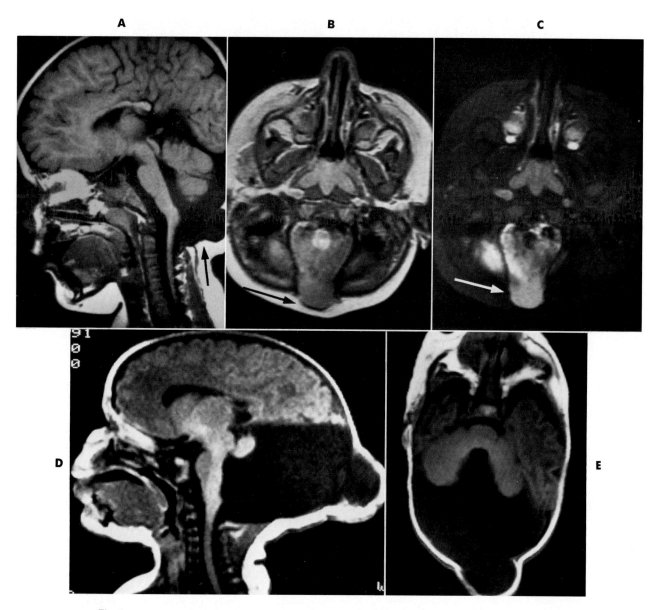

Fig. 3-10 **A** and **B,** Occipital meningocele. T1-weighted images demonstrate a defect in the occipital bone at the cervicomedullary junction, with herniation of the meninges only *(arrows)*. **C,** Similar changes are seen on the long TR/TE image *(arrow)*. The cerebellum remains in a normal position. **D** and **E,** Occipital meningocele associated with the Dandy-Walker syndrome in a newborn infant. Sagittal **(D)** and axial **(E)** (650/20 msec) images demonstrate a meningocele extending through the calvarium in association with absence of most of the vermis and a huge fourth ventricle.

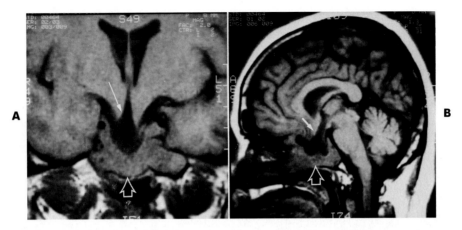

Fig. 3-11   Sphenoidal encephalocele. Coronal **(A)** and sagittal **(B)** T1-weighted images (600/25 msec). There is no sella turcica. The meninges, inferior frontal lobe, infundibulum, hypothalamus, and third ventricle *(arrow)* have herniated through a large defect in the sphenoid sinus. The encephalocele extends into the posterior nasopharynx *(open arrows)*.

plex deformities may occur, including hypertelorism, hypoplasia of the lacrimal ducts, dysgenesis of the corpus callosum, and frontal lobe hypoplasia.[6] Interfrontal cephaloceles occur along the metopic suture.

PARIETAL. Parietal cephaloceles are rare. They usually occur within 1 or 2 cm of the lambda. They have been associated with amniotic bands,[3] dysgenesis of the corpus callosum,[1] large interhemispheric cysts, and anomalous venous development.

REFERENCES
Disorders of dorsal induction

1. Barkovich AJ, Norman D: Anomalies of the corpus callosum: correlation with further anomalies of the brain, *AJNR* 9:493, 1988.
2. Boulanger T, Mathurin P, Dooms G, et al: Sphenopharyngeal meningoencephalocele: unusual clinical and radiologic features, *AJNR* 10:S80, 1989.
3. Byrd SE, Naidich TP: Common congenital brain anomalies. In Lee HS, Zimmerman RA, editors: *The radiologic clinics of North America,* Philadelphia, 1988, WB Saunders.
4. Diebler C, Dulac O: Cephaloceles: clinical and neurological appearance—associated cerebral malformations, *Neuroradiology* 25:199, 1983.
5. Karch SB, Urich H: Occipital encephalocele: a morphological study, *J Neurol Sci* 15:89, 1972.
6. Levy RA, Wald SL, Aitken PA, et al: Bilateral intraorbital meningoencephaloceles and associated midline craniofacial anomalies: MR and three-dimensional CT imaging, *AJNR* 10:1272, 1989.
7. Lorber J: The prognosis of occipital encephalocele, *Dev Med Child Neurol Suppl* 13:75, 1967.
8. Rice JF, Eggers DM: Basal transsphenoidal encephalocele: MR findings, *AJNR* 10:S79, 1989.
9. Wolpert SM: Vascular studies of congenital anomalies. In Newton TH, Potts DC, editors: *Radiology of the skull and brain,* St Louis, 1974, Mosby–Year Book.
10. Younus M, Coode PE: Nasal glioma and encephalocele: two separate entities. Report of two cases, *J Neurosurg* 64:516, 1986.

Chiari malformation

In 1891 Hans von Chiari described a series of patients with malformations of the posterior fossa in which inferior extension of the cerebellar tonsils through a large foramen magnum was the primary abnormality.[2] The term *Arnold-Chiari malformation* was coined in 1907 by Schwalbe and Gredig, pupils of Arnold, based on a case reported by Arnold in 1894 without an associated myelomeningocele. Following appropriate current convention, the anomaly will be called the Chiari malformation. The malformation is readily diagnosed with CT in virtually all cases, but MRI now affords more detailed delineation, and thin section sagittal, axial, and coronal T1-weighted images can provide precise anatomical delineation. Associated hydrocephalus and hydrosyringomyelia of the spinal cord can also be precisely defined by MRI.

Four anomalies of the hindbrain were classified by Chiari. Chiari IV malformation is severe cerebellar hypoplasia and has been placed in a separate category in the van der Knaap and Valk classification. Chiari III malformation is a cervicooccipital encephalocele with cerebellar herniation (see Fig. 3-9). Chiari I and Chiari II malformations are discussed in detail in the following pages.

Chiari I malformation

Chiari I malformation, which occurs less commonly in children than in adults, is defined as an extension of the cerebellar tonsils below the foramen magnum. Tonsils extending less than 3 mm below the foramen may not be clinically significant. In two thirds of the cases the tonsils extend to C1 (Fig. 3-12). In 25%, there may be extension as far as C3. Chiari I malformation differs from Chiari II malformation in that no associated myelomeningocele is present and supratentorial anomalies are lacking. It is an abnormality of hindbrain development, and there may be associated findings. The cisterna magna is small. Hydrocephalus is present in 25% of patients and has been postulated as the cause of tonsilar herniation due to a pressure effect.[4]

Clinical presentations include headaches, neck pain, and nystagmus. Craniocervical dysgenesis with atlantooccipital

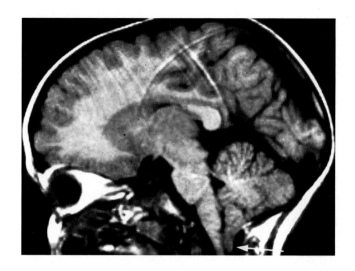

Fig. 3-12   Chiari I malformation. There is inferior herniation of the cerebellar tonsils to the level of C2 posterior to the cervical spinal cord *(arrow)*. There is no brain stem compression. No other anomalies were noted. This was an incidental finding on the sagittal T1 image (650/20 msec). (Note: the curvilinear "structures" seen above the corpus callosum are artifacts due to wrap-around.)

assimilation, associated Klippel-Feil syndrome,[14] spina bifida occulta, and lower cranial nerve palsies may occur. In another subgroup of patients basilar invagination (25% of patients) and syringohydromyelia (60% of patients)[14] may occur.

Chiari II malformation

The Chiari II malformation is a complex anomaly involving the entire neuroaxis. It is classified as a disorder of dorsal induction, since almost all patients have an associated myelomeningocele, usually in the lumbar region. Several theories concerning its pathogenesis have been postulated. The traction theory proposes that the primary cause is the myelomeningocele. The cord is tethered, pulling the brain stem and cerebellum into the upper cervical canal. The hydrodynamic theory suggests that hydrocephalus is the primary cause, with forced reopening of the closed neural tube producing the myelomeningocele with downward herniation of the hindbrain. The overgrowth theory proposes that an overgrowth of neural tissue prevents closure of the vertebral arches and a large supratentorium forces the hindbrain inferiorly.[5] Teratological theories stem from animal models in which varying teratogens have simulated the deformity. An alternative theory postulates lack of distention of the embryonic ventricular system secondary to the leaking myelomeningocele as the cause of the malformation.[8] Clinically there is a spectrum of severity ranging from asymptomatic to brain stem dysfunction including apnea.

Chiari II malformations are characterized by an elongated small cerebellum and brain stem with caudal displacement through an enlarged foramen magnum. There is often associated subependymal heterotopias, aqueductal stenosis, beaked collicular plate, diastematomyelia, diplomyelia, and syringomyelia (see Chapter 9).[9,15] The abnormality may be analyzed by considering the malformations occurring in different parts of the brain.

SUPRATENTORIAL. Abnormalities of the corpus callosum are common and may occur in up to 80% of patients with Chiari II malformation.[1] Complete agenesis occurs in 33% of patients[15] (Fig. 3-13). There may be associated absence of the cingulate gyrus. Although anteroinferior pointing of the anterior horns of the lateral ventricles is a nonspecific finding seen in other congenital anomalies, it is a near-constant feature of Chiari II malformation.[11] The supratentorial CSF spaces, most notably the quadrigeminal plate cistern, interhemispheric fissure, and cistern of the velum interpositum may be wide, especially after shunting[11] (Figs. 3-13 and 3-14). Colpocephaly, a disproportionate enlargement of the occipital horns,[6,11] may also be present. Stenogyria, multiple small gyri in which the cytologic architecture is normal, may be seen (Fig. 3-13). Usually the latter abnormality is located in the medial aspect of the occipital lobes and may be the result of dysplasia of the hemispheres medial to the atria. The falx can be thinned anteriorly, allowing visualization of interdigitations of the medial surfaces of the two cerebral hemispheres on axial or coronal examination (Figs. 3-13 and 3-14). The tentorium is low, inserting sometimes close to the foramen magnum, and can have a sickle shape.

A characteristic diencephalic appearance is that of a large massa intermedia, which can give the third ventricle a biconcave appearance on a coronal scan. The hypothalamus can be stretched and elevated. The heads of the caudate nuclei are enlarged, indenting the lateral horns of the ventricles.

INFRATENTORIAL. Mesencephalic abnormalities involving the aqueduct and colliculi are often present.[11] The aqueduct is dysfunctional and can be shortened, stretched, or dilated (Figs. 3-13 and 3-16) but not necessarily occluded.[9] Pressure from the occipital lobes at the level of the tentorial hiatus can cause compression of the midbrain.[7] One constant feature of Chiari II malformation is an abnormal appearance of the colliculi (see Fig. 3-13). The tectum may have a variable appearance ranging from bulbous to beaked. Although the fusion of the colliculi may be intrinsic to the malformation, hydrocephalus itself may cause this appearance.

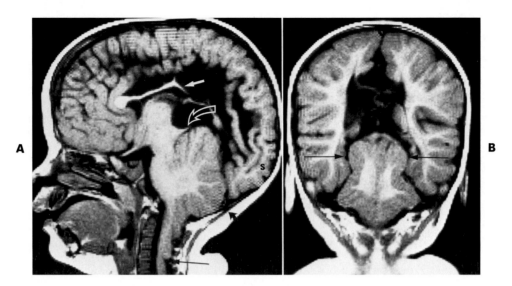

Fig. 3-13   Chiari II malformation. **A,** Sagittal (650/20 msec) image demonstrates a compendium of findings seen in Chiari II malformation. Partial agenesis of the posterior corpus callosum is present *(white closed arrows)* with wide interhemispheric CSF-containing spaces. The tectum is beaked *(open arrow).* The posterior fossa is small with a low insertion of the torcula *(short black arrow).* There is inferior extension of the nodulus and possibly uvula and a cervicomedullary kink at C4 *(long arrow).* Multiple small, shallow, convoluted gyri are present in the posterior parietal and occipital regions referred to as stenogyria *(S).* The aqueduct and fourth ventricle are not visualized. **B,** The appearance of a towering cerebellum is demonstrated with low insertion of the tentorium and small posterior fossa; the cerebellum extends superiorly *(long arrows).*

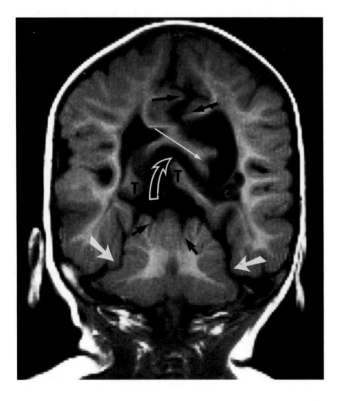

Fig. 3-14   Chiari II malformation (coronal scan). Absence of the falx allows interdigitation of the medial interhemispheric gyri *(upper black arrows).* The curved open arrow indicates a large supracerebellar cistern communicating with a wide interhemispheric fissure. The posteromedial temporal lobes indent the cistern *(T).* Note also indentation of the medial occipital gyrus into interhemispheric fissure *(long white arrow).* The cerebellum herniates superiorly *(white arrows).* The lower arrows indicate sagittally oriented sulci on the superior surface of the cerebellum. (From Wolpert SM, Anderson ML, Scott RM, et al: *AJR* 149:1033, 1987.)

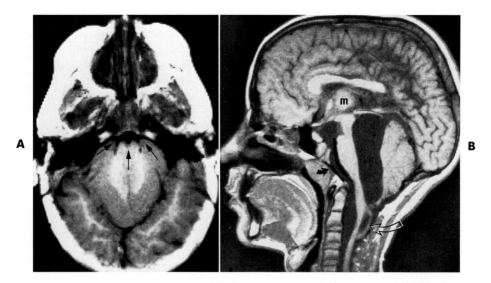

Fig. 3-15   Chiari II malformation. Other features of Chiari II malformation are demonstrated here. **A,** As the cerebellum sweeps around the brain stem "a triple-peak appearance" is formed *(arrows).* **B,** In another patient the fourth ventricle is trapped and enlarged. The foramen magnum is enlarged. A small syrinx is evident at C3 *(curved arrow).* The tectum is markedly stretched as the fourth ventricle expands. The massa intermedia is enlarged *(m).* The upper cervical cord is atrophic, and the subarachnoid space anterior to the upper cord is wide. The clivus is concave *(arrow).* (From Wolpert SM, Anderson ML, Scott RM, et al: *AJR* 149:1033, 1987.)

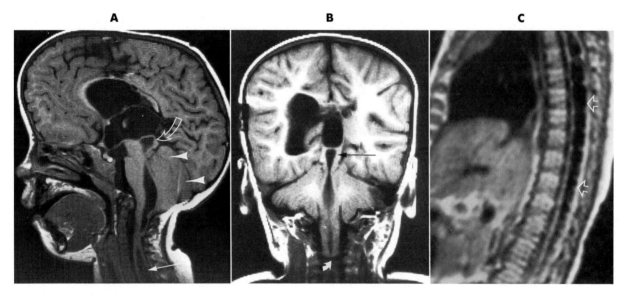

Fig. 3-16   Chiari II malformation. **A,** A syringohydromyelia extends inferiorly to the level of C5 *(long arrow).* No folia are identified over the surface of the vermis *(arrowheads).* A diverticulum of the aqueduct *(open arrow)* does not communicate with the third ventricle. The fourth ventricle is slightly deformed as it extends through the foramen magnum. **B,** The coronal view shows the aqueductal dilatation *(black arrow).* A medullary kink is indicated by the white arrow. **C,** A sagittal image of the spine reveals the extent of syringohydromyelia. Note the typical stack-of-coins *(open arrows)* appearance. (From Wolpert SM, Anderson ML, Scott RM, et al: *AJR* 149:1033, 1987.)

The rhombencephalon contains most of the characteristic features of infratentorial Chiari II malformation. Some form of cerebellar dysplasia is not uncommon. In contrast to the normal coronal orientation, there may be dorsal angulation of the cerebellar sulci, with consequent nonvisualization of the folia on the sagittal view (Fig. 3-16). The cerebellum and brain stem is inferiorly displaced through a wide foramen magnum. Owing to this impaction, the pyramis, uvula, and nodulus may be compressed and necrosis may occur. Prepontine migration of the cerebellum at the level of the middle cerebellar peduncle gives the brain stem a "triple peak" or "angel wing" appearance on axial views (see Fig. 3-15). Due to the low-lying, sickle-shaped tentorium, upward bulging of the cerebellum appears on coronal scans, the so-called towering cerebellum (see Figs. 3-13 and 3-14).

Inferior vermian pegs posterior to the medulla and fourth ventricle are a constant feature.[15] The dentate ligaments hold the upper cervical cord in position, and as the medulla and cerebellum impact downward on the upper cervical canal, tethering occurs. If the medulla is displaced below these ligaments, a cervicomedullary kink is formed, which is seen in 70% of patients[9,15] (see Figs. 3-13 and 3-15).

The cervicomedullary deformities are classified according to shape and contents.[9] Three types of cervicomedullary deformities can occur. In the first there is an inferior vermian peg alone. In the second the fourth ventricle is elongated and descends anterior to the vermian peg. In the third the medulla is buckled below the cervical cord, forming the cervicomedullary kink, which does not usually extend below C4. The fourth ventricle is either collapsed or dilated, particularly if it is trapped (see Fig. 3-15). As a result of herniation the exiting cranial nerve nuclei may at times make an upward turn to reach their skull base foramina. The most important complications are hydrocephalus (often after myelomeningocele closure) and isolation of the fourth ventricle following ventricular shunting.

Controversy exists over treatment for neurological symptoms referable to brain stem compression at the foramen magnum. In patients with a cervicomedullary kink to C4 or lower the majority were symptomatic,[3] and surgical decompression has been recommended. Others, however, found no correlation between the degree of hindbrain herniation and the symptomatology.[16] Aplasia or hypoplasia of cranial nerve nuclei, including the basal pontine nuclei, olivary nuclei, and disorganization of the brain stem nuclei, has been found in autopsy specimens and may be intrinsic to the anomaly.[5] Disorganization of brain stem nuclei may be the basis for neurological symptoms; if so, posterior decompression may not be beneficial.[16]

Syringohydromyelia of the upper cervical cord, extending inferiorly, is seen in 70% to 80% of cases[9] (see Fig. 3-16) (see Chapter 9).

MESODERMAL. Lückenshädl, or craniofenestria, a condition characterized by marked thinning of the occipital or parietal bones, is identified in 85% of Chiari malformations examined before 6 months, after which time it becomes unrecognizable.[9,10] Clival and petrous bone scalloping is identified in a majority of patients, secondary to pressure from the cerebellum. The petrous scalloping is above the jugular tubercles and internal auditory canals. Gyral indentations in the skull, particularly in the occipital bone posterior to the foramen magnum, are seen frequently on plain films and CT, but are difficult to identify on MR examinations.

Chiari III malformation

See occipital cephelocele (p. 91).

REFERENCES
Chiari malformation

1. Barkovich AJ: Congenital malformations of the brain. In Barkovich AJ, editor: *Pediatric neuroimaging*, New York, 1990, Raven.
2. Chiari H: Ueber Veränderungen des Kleinhirns Infolge von Hydrocephalie des Grosshirns, *Deutsche Medicinische Wochenschrift* 17:1172, 1891.
3. Curnes JT, Oakes WJ, Boyko OB: MR imaging at hindbrain deformity in Chiari II patients with and without symptoms of brainstem compression, *AJNR* 10:293, 1989.
4. De La Paz RL, Brody TJ, Buonanno FS, et al: Nuclear magnetic resonance imaging of Arnold-Chiari type I malformation with hydromyelia, *J Comput Assist Tomogr* 7:126, 1983.
5. Gilbert JN, Jones KL, Rorke LB, et al: Central nervous system anomalies associated with meningomyelocele, hydrocephalus, and the Arnold-Chiari malformation: reappraisal of theories regarding the pathogenesis of posterior neural tube closure defects, *Neurosurgery* 18:559, 1986.
6. Herskowitz J, Rosman NP, Wheeler CB: Colpocephaly: clinical, radiologic, and pathogenetic aspects, *Neurology* 35:1594, 1985.
7. Masters CL: The pathogenesis of the Arnold-Chiari malformation: the significance of hydrocephalus and aqueduct stenoses, *J Neuropathol Exp Neurol* 37:56, 1978.
8. McClone DG, Knepper PA: The cause of the Chiari II malformation: a unified theory, *Pediatr Neurosci* 15:1, 1989.
9. Naidich TP, McLone DG, Fulling KH: The Chiari II malformation: Part IV. The hindbrain deformity, *Neuroradiology* 25:179, 1983.
10. Naidich TP, Pudlowski RM, Naidich JB, et al: Computed tomographic signs of the Chiari II malformation. I. Skull and dural partitions, *Radiology* 134:65, 1980.
11. Naidich TP, Pudlowski RM, Naidich JB: Computed tomographic signs of the Chiari II malformation. III. Ventricles and cisterns, *Radiology* 134:657, 1980.
12. Naidich TP, Zimmerman RA: Common congenital malformations of the brain. In Brandt-Zawadski M, Norman D, editors: *Magnetic resonance imaging of the central nervous system*, New York, 1987, Raven.
13. Noorani PA, Bodensteiner JB, Barnes PD: Colpocephaly: frequency and associated findings, *J Child Neurol* 3:100, 1988.
14. Spinos E, Laster DW, Moody DM, et al: MR evaluation of Chiari I malformations at 0.15 T, *AJNR* 6:203, 1985.
15. Wolpert SM, Anderson ML, Scott RM, et al: Chiari II malformation: MR imaging evaluation. *AJR* 149:1033, 1987.
16. Wolpert SM, Scott RM, Platenberg RC, et al: The clinical significance of hindbrain herniation and deformity as shown on MR images of patients with Chiari malformation, *AJNR* 9:1075, 1988.

DISORDERS OF VENTRAL INDUCTION

Ventral induction is the process whereby the basic segments of the cranial neural tube are formed and separated from the notochord and overlying mesoderm. The developing notochord expands at its superior extent to form the primitive brain. This process is intimately intertwined with the development of the face, as the mesoderm of the

A   B   C

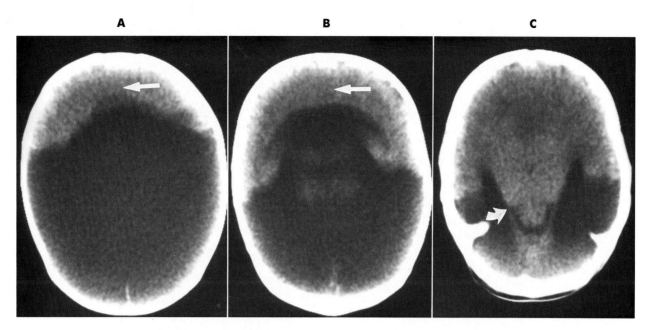

Fig. 3-17   Alobar holoprosencephaly. **A** and **B,** CT examination shows fusion of the frontal hemispheres anteriorly *(arrows)* and a large monoventricle. Posteriorly the single monoventricle replaces the cerebral hemispheres. No differentiation into separate hemispheres or ventricles is discernible. **C,** Inferiorly the thalami and corpus striatum form one fused mass *(arrow).*

notochord also induces the overlying ectoderm to form the facial structures. Overgrowth of the lamina terminalis occurs (marking the end of the primitive notochord), with expansion and diverticulation. With this overgrowth, there is the formation of the prosencephalon (forebrain), mesencephalon (midbrain), and rhombencephalon (hindbrain). The forebrain divides into two telencephalic vesicles, which become the cerebral hemispheres, and the diencephalon, which becomes the thalami and hypothalamus. The induction process also influences the development of the optic vesicles, which form as outpouchings of the diencephalon at about 4 weeks. Any abnormality affecting the ventral induction process from 4 to 7 weeks can affect the brain and facial structures. Disorders included in this category include holoprosencephalies, septooptic dysplasia, and agenesis of the septum pellucidum.

Holoprosencephaly

Holoprosencephaly is a disorder of diverticulation resulting in complete or partial absence of cleavage of the prosencephalon. The condition is associated with maternal diabetes, first trimester bleeding, and dizygotic twinning and has been induced experimentally with irradiation.[16,26] A number of chromosomal aberrations are associated with holoprosencephaly, including trisomy D (13 to 15), trisomy E (16 to 18 or 17 and 18), 13q syndrome, short arm deletion of 18, Meckel's syndrome, and Kallmann's syndrome. Although the overall incidence is 1/16,000 live births, if the child has the chromosomal aberration of trisomy 13, the incidence can be as high as 1/2,000.[16]

Holoprosencephaly is preferred over the terms *arhinencephaly* or *holotelencephaly,* which have been used previ-

ously. Arhinencephaly (olfactory agenesis) almost always accompanies all but the mildest form of holoprosencephaly. Callosal agenesis is also a uniform feature except in the mildest forms. The association of multiple heterotopias and poorly laminated cortical gray matter indicates that although holoprosencephaly can be dated to about 33 days' gestation at onset, the pathological process extends throughout most of fetal life.[32]

The primary abnormality is a failure of cleavage and diverticulation of the prosencephalon, particularly the frontal region. If the induction of the nasal ridges and premaxilla is also interfered with there will also be lack of induction of the frontonasal prominence and the facial structures may be hypoplastic. In the severe forms it has been stated that the "face predicts the brain."[14] This condition needs to be contrasted with the median cleft face syndrome characterized by various combinations of upper lip and/or nose clefting, hypertelorism, and midline brain anomalies such as callosal dysgenesis and lipomas.[28] The spectrum of cerebral abnormalities that may occur with holoprosencephaly can range from a near normal brain to a monoventricle to a cyclops.

Other clinical manifestations include macrocephaly or microcephaly and severe developmental delay. DeMeyer[14] and others have classified the spectrum of disorders into alobar, semilobar, and lobar types. Needless to say, the prognosis for the more severe alobar and semilobar types can be dismal.

Alobar.   Alobar holoprosencephaly is the most severe form of holoprosencephaly—no diverticulation occurs. The brain is small with a unilobed cerebrum and a single horseshoe-shaped monoventricle (Fig. 3-17). The corpus

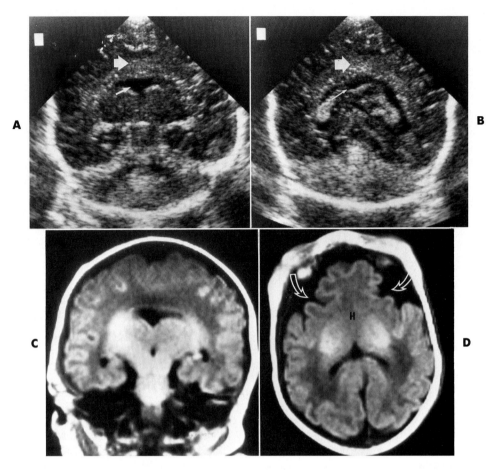

Fig. 3-18 Semilobar holoprosencephaly. **A** and **B,** Ultrasound demonstrates a single ventricle *(small arrow)* and fused cerebral hemispheres *(large arrow)* characteristic of holoprosencephaly. **C** and **D,** The coronal and axial MRI identify attempted differentiation of the cerebral hemispheres, especially the temporal lobes *(curved arrows).* The posterior interhemispheric fissure is formed. There is also an attempted differentiation of the anterior horns of the lateral ventricles. The frontal hemispheres *(H)* are fused into a single structure best delineated on axial images **(D).** (Ultrasound images courtesy Dr. Deborah ter Meulen, New England Medical Center Hospitals.)

callosum, interhemispheric fissure, falx, olfactory bulbs, and olfactory nerves are absent. The membranous roof of the third ventricle may balloon into a dorsal sac or cyst. [14,26] A number of facial deformities have been described. In mythology the cyclops monster represents an example of holoprosencephaly.

1. Cyclopia—one orbit with a proboscis and absent nose
2. Ethmocephaly—median proboscis between two orbits
3. Cebocephaly—rudimentary nose with one aperture and orbital hypotelorism
4. Median cleft lip with hypertelorism[13,14]
5. Hypotelorism

The thalamus and basal ganglia are fused (Fig. 3-17). On angiography the anterior cerebral artery is single (azygous), and the internal cerebral veins, superior sagittal sinus, and straight sinus are absent. The superior sagittal sinus may be replaced by a network of large abnormal veins that resembles the early embryonic pattern of venous drainage. The differential diagnoses may include hydranencephaly, which can be ruled out by both absence of the falx and fusion of the thalami (see Hydranencephaly) and congenital hydrocephalus.

SEMILOBAR. Semilobar holoprosencephaly is a less severe form of the entity. The brain is small. Again a single ventricular cavity is present, but some attempt at brain sulcation has occurred and there may be rudimentary occipital lobes and temporal lobes (Fig. 3-18). The falx may be present, and an interhemispheric fissure may be visible, at least posteriorly. The corpus callosum may be absent or incomplete. The olfactory bulbs and tracts are lacking. As in the more severe type the thalamus and basal ganglia are fused. Severe facial anomalies are not a constant feature, although a median cleft lip or hypotelorism can be associated.

LOBAR. The least severe form of holoprosencephaly is

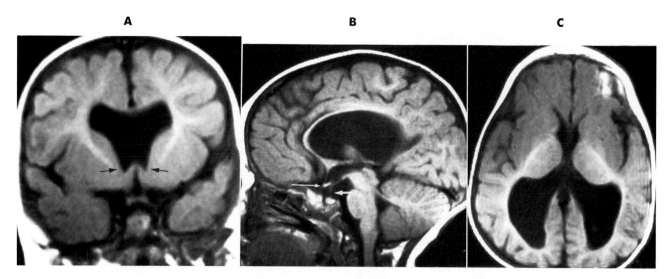

Fig. 3-19   Septooptic dysplasia. **A,** Coronal image (650/20 msec) demonstrates absence of the septum pellucidum and inferior pointing of the lateral ventricles *(arrows).* **B,** Sagittal image shows a thin optic chiasm and optic nerve *(long thin arrow).* The infundibulum is also small *(arrow).* **C,** Axial image (650/20 msec) displays normal anterior horns with enlarged occipital horns and atria, a condition called colpocephaly.

the lobar type. The brain is normal is size. The ventricles now begin to assume a more normal appearance, as the occipital and temporal horns are well individualized and the indusium griseum and cingulate gyri are fused from side to side. The lack of cleavage is usually frontal. The septum pellucidum is absent, and the corpus callosum also may be absent or dysplastic. Facial deformities are usually absent.

Septooptic dysplasia and absence of the septum pellucidum

Septooptic dysplasia (De Morsier syndrome) is also a disorder of ventral induction and has been considered a mild form of holoprosencephaly. It is a disorder of abnormal induction of the midline mesoderm occurring at the same time as the development of the optic vesicles. Failure of differentiation of the mesoderm into the optic stalk results in aplasia of the stalk.[18] Septooptic dysplasia is a heterogeneous group of abnormalities in which associated anomalies include pituitary hypothalamic insufficiency[27] and abnormalities of the corpus callosum and fornix. One half of these patients have schizencephaly.[10] These patients usually have hypotonia in the first days of life. Blindness is inferred by wandering nystagmus.[18,27] Associated pituitary hypothalamic abnormalities seen in two thirds of these patients range from panhypopituitarism to isolated GH, ACTH, or ADH insufficiency (diabetes insipidus).[27] Hypothalamic hamartomas, gliosis, and absence of some hypothalamic nuclei may be associated with a histologically normal pituitary.[31] The syndrome affects the firstborn child of healthy mothers, but environmental factors implicated include maternal diabetes, ingestion of quinidine, anticonvulsants, alcohol and drug abuse, as well as cytomegalovirus.[27]

On MR imaging, there is partial or complete absence of the septum pellucidum (one or both leaflets), best identified on coronal imaging (Fig. 3-19). Similar changes are seen on ultrasound imaging (Fig. 3-20). The frontal horns are flattened with nonspecific inferior pointing on coronal scans; they occur in Chiari II malformation as well (Figs. 3-19 and 3-20). The suprasellar and chiasmatic cisterns may be dilated with diverticular expansion of the optic recess. The optic chiasm is small. Hypoplasia of the optic nerves can be identified but is best visualized by ophthalmoscopy when the discs are small and atrophic. Other associated abnormalities include absence of the fornix and callosal dysgenesis.[25] There may be two subsets of patients with septal dysplasia/aplasia: those with schizencephaly and normal optic pathways, and those without schizencephaly but with hypoplasia of the optic nerves and hypothalamic-pituitary dysfunction.[2] Patients with posterior pituitary deficiency are likely to be without the typical normal hyperintense posterior pituitary gland on T1 images.[24]

Although a constant feature of septooptic dysplasia, complete or partial absence of the septum pellucidum occurs in other anomalies. It is rarely an isolated finding and has been associated with holoprosencephaly, dysgenesis of the corpus callosum, Chiari II malformation, schizencephaly,[11,21,30] hydranencephaly, and severe hydrocephalus as seen in aqueductal stenosis.[5] Absence of the septum should prompt a search for these associated anomalies.[1] Both the corpus callosum and septum pellucidum are derived from the commissural plate. Therefore absence of the septum may be associated with callosal dysgenesis. In Chiari malformations and aqueductal stenosis, the absence is probably the result of septal necrosis from long-standing hydrocephalus.[5]

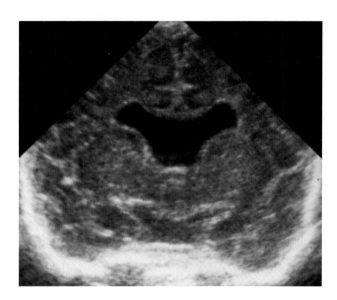

Fig. 3-20 Septooptic dysplasia. Coronal ultrasound image in a 7-day-old infant demonstrates absence of the midline septum pellucidum. (Courtesy Dr. Deborah ter Meulen, New England Medical Center Hospitals.)

Cerebral hemiatrophy

Cerebral hemiatrophy was initially described by Dyke et al.,[15] who recorded the plain radiographic findings and pneumoencephalographic findings in patients with hemiparesis, seizures, facial asymmetry, and mental retardation. Cerebral hemiatrophy is a small cerebral hemisphere with an ipsilateral dilated lateral ventricle (Fig. 3-21). The calvarium is thickened on the affected side, and the frontal, ethmoidal, and mastoid air cells are enlarged. The underdevelopment of the hemisphere is probably the result of in utero unilateral ischemia or infarction after infection or trauma.[9,15]

Posterior fossa cystic malformations

The cerebellum has the longest period of embryological development of any major structure of the brain.[33] Neuroblastic proliferation in the cerebellar plates is recognized at 32 days, but neuronal migration from the external granular layer is not complete until 1 year postnatally. As a result of this extended ontogenesis, the cerebellum is vulnerable to teratogenic insult for longer than most parts of the central nervous system.[32]

Dandy and Blackfan[12] were the first to describe a malformation of the posterior fossa in which the inferior vermis was absent and the fourth ventricle ballooned to form a cystic lesion posterior to the cerebellum. There was no communication between the cyst and the perimedullary cistern. They postulated atresia or postnatal obstruction of the foramen of Magendie as the cause of the abnormality. Taggart and Walker[35] also postulated that the cause was in utero atresia of the foramen of Magendie. Benda[8] coined the term *Dandy-Walker malformation* and commented that the foramen may be patent in the malformation. Since these initial investigations many descriptions and postulates concerning pathology have appeared in the literature.*

*References 3, 8, 17, 20, 29, 34.

Probably the best single unifying concept is that of impaired permeability of the fourth ventricle membranous roof together with vermian dysgenesis.

Although the pathogenesis is still uncertain, it is clear that the primary defect in posterior fossa cystic malformations is not obstruction of the foramen of Magendie alone. More recent reviews[3] classifying posterior fossa cystic lesions have considered that there is a spectrum of diseases involving the fourth ventricle and cerebellum, including the Dandy-Walker malformation, the so-called Dandy-Walker variant, and the retrocerebellar cyst. Currently, maldevelopment of the anterior and posterior membranous areas around the fifth week of gestation is considered the probable cause of the lesion.[3] The anterior membranous area is incorporated into the developing cerebellum, and the posterior membranous area forms the foramen of Magendie.[3,20,29] If the anterior membranous area fails to incorporate into the cerebellum and the posterior membranous area is malformed, the foramen of Magendie will balloon outward to form the posterior fossa cystic malformation.

The most common sign is macrocephaly with hydrocephalus and cerebellar dysfunction. The patients may have nystagmus, truncal ataxia, and cranial nerve palsies. Associated anomalies have been described, including complete or partial agenesis of the corpus callosum (25% of patients), polymicrogyria, cortical heterotopias, occipital encephalocele, and holoprosencephaly (minority of patients). Systemic anomalies include polydactylism, syndactylism, Klippel-Feil syndrome, and Cornelia de Lange's syndrome.[3,20]

The malformation is characterized by hypoplasia of the cerebellar hemispheres, hypoplasia or absence of the inferior cerebellar vermis, and marked dilatation of the fourth ventricle so that it balloons posterior to the remainder of the cerebellum, which is anterolaterally displaced (Fig. 3-22, *B*). The posterior fossa is enlarged, and the tentorial

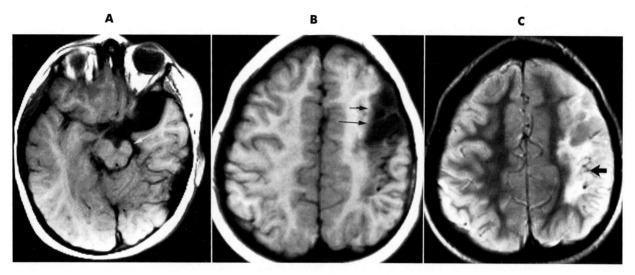

Fig. 3-21   Dyke-Davidoff-Masson syndrome. **A** and **B,** Axial short TR/short TE images demonstrate left cerebral hemiatrophy. Wallerian degeneration of the left cerebral peduncle is evident *(white arrow).* Encephalomalacic changes are seen in the distribution of the middle cerebral artery *(black arrows).* **C,** The long TR/long TE image (3000/90 msec) demonstrates increased signal intensity of the white matter caused by gliosis.

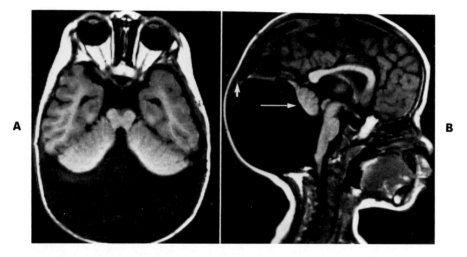

Fig. 3-22   Dandy-Walker malformation. A large posterior fossa cystic lesion is identified in continuity with the fourth ventricle on both sagittal and axial images. **A** and **B,** On the sagittal image only the superior vermis is present *(long arrow).* The torcula is elevated *(short arrow).* The remaining cerebellar tissue is displaced superiorly and anteriorly by the posterior fossa cyst. (From Robertson SJ, Wolpert SM: Brain: congenital. In Runge VM, editor: *Clinical magnetic resonance imaging,* Philadelphia, 1990, JB Lippincott.)

insertion and confluence of dural venous sinuses is elevated above the lambda, accounting for "torcular-lambdoid inversion," often with a wide, vertically oriented incisura (Fig. 3-22). The falx cerebelli is absent. Hydrocephalus is variable and may not be present at birth.[22] There is no correlation between the size of the posterior fossa expansion, vermian hypoplasia, and the degree of hydrocephalus.[20]

Harwood-Nash and Fitz[21] first coined the term *Dandy-Walker variant* to encompass those entities not satisfying all

the criteria for the true Dandy-Walker malformation. In this entity there is posterior evagination of the tela choroidea of the fourth ventricle with partial vermian agenesis without torcular elevation.[21,29] If a lesion does not satisfy the criteria for a true Dandy-Walker malformation and cannot be ascribed either to a retrocerebellar cyst or mega cisterna magna, it is probably best described anatomically without placement in a single category.

Absence of all or part of the inferior vermis may occur as an isolated anomaly or in association with Down's syn-

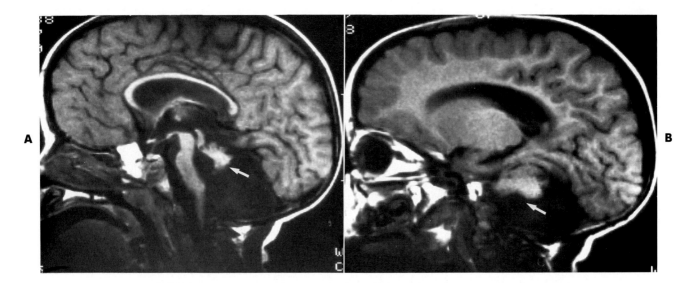

Fig. 3-23   Inferior vermian hypoplasia. The posterior fossa is small. The fourth ventricle opens into a posterior fossa CSF collection. However, the torcula is low, unlike that seen in Dandy-Walker malformation. The inferior vermis (**A,** *arrows*) and cerebellar hemisphere (**B,** *arrows*) are hypoplastic (short TR/short TE [650/20 msec] images). (From Robertson SJ, Wolpert SM: Brain: congenital. In Runge VM, editor: *Clinical magnetic resonance imaging,* Philadelphia, 1990, JB Lippincott.)

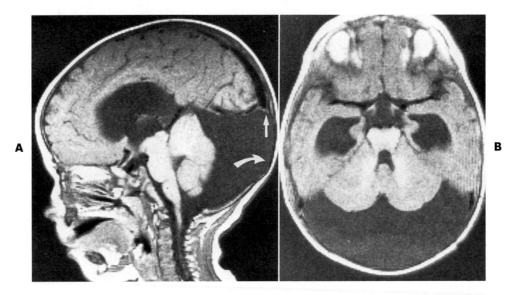

Fig. 3-24   Retrocerebellar arachnoid cyst. Sagittal **(A)** and axlal **(B)** short TR/short TE images (650/20 msec) show an intact cerebellar hemisphere and vermis. The fourth ventricle appears normal. Posterior to the cerebellum is a large cerebrospinal fluid collection displacing the cerebellum anteriorly. The torcula is also elevated *(arrow).* Thinning of the inner table of the posterior calvarium is noted *(curved arrow).*

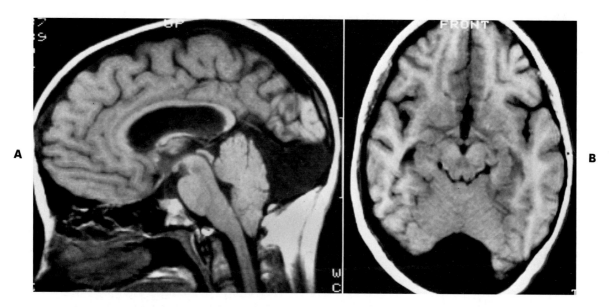

Fig. 3-25   Retrocerebellar arachnoid cyst. All images are short TR/short TE (650/20 msec). **A,** On the sagittal image a localized collection of cerebrospinal fluid is present posterior to the cerebellum, which is displaced anteriorly. The tonsils are extending inferiorly below the foramen magnum, probably because of the mass effect of the cyst. The occipital calvarium is thinned. The fourth ventricle is normal in size. The cerebellar vermis is intact. **B,** The cyst is well defined on the axial image, displacing an intact cerebellum anteriorly.

drome. This results from failure of development of the cerebellar midline primordia. Many of the cases ascribed to the Dandy-Walker variant may represent vermian or cerebellar hypoplasia (Fig. 3-23). Usually the inferior lobules are hypoplastic. The cerebellar peduncles, pons, and brain stem may be small. The fourth ventricle, basal cisterns, vallecula, and cisterna magna are prominent.[10] If accompanied by clinical signs of cerebellar and brain stem dysfunction, the appearances are probably the result of Joubert's syndrome.

The retrocerebellar arachnoid cyst, sometimes called Blake's pouch cyst because of its similarity to the embryonic appearance of the posterior fossa, is the posterior evagination of the tela choroidea, but without cerebellar agenesis. There is mass effect on the cerebellum, which may be displaced anteriorly (Figs. 3-24 and 3-25). The torcular may or may not be elevated, although the tentorium may bulge (Fig. 3-24). The cyst may extend through the tentorium.[19]

The mega cisterna magna is defined as a prominent CSF space posterior to the cerebellum without significant mass effect or cerebellar vermial agenesis. The architecture of the fourth ventricle is normal. The torcular is normal in position, and the posterior fossa is normal in size. Minor positional asymmetry of the dural venous sinuses may be present along with minor tentorial, falx, or inner table deformities.

Joubert's syndrome is characterized by absence of the cerebellar vermis, dysplasia of the cerebellar nuclei and brain stem, and anomalies of the inferior olives and spinal tracts. Patients with Joubert's syndrome have abnormal eye movements, ataxia, and episodic hyperpnea. They are usually mentally retarded.[23] Selective agenesis of the cerebellar hemispheres is much less common than vermial agenesis. Global cerebellar hypoplasia can be seen in patients with Tay-Sachs disease, Menkes' kinky-hair disease, and spinal muscular atrophy.[33] In all these cases the subarachnoid spaces surrounding the cerebellum are prominent, resemble cystic malformations, and must be distinguished from other posterior fossa cysticlike lesions, including encysted fourth ventricle (see Fig. 3-15) and cystic tumors.

Multiplanar imaging is indicated to distinguish among the entities, particularly if symptoms and signs of pressure are present (that is, hydrocephalus). This is critical for surgical planning directed at the cystic lesion or hydrocephalus. Patency of the aqueduct is the critical factor in deciding whether to shunt only the cyst or to shunt both the cyst and the ventricles to prevent upward or downward herniation when only one compartment is shunted.

Craniosynostosis

Whereas long and broad heads may be familial or molded during infancy according to ethnic or tribal customs, such shapes may also be caused by sutural synostoses, that is, premature closure (bony fusion) of the cranial sutures.[21] The synostoses may be primary and isolated (sagittal, coronal, metopic, lambdoidal) or associated with congenital syndromes (Apert's syndrome, Carpenter's syndrome, and Crouzon's disease). Sagittal synostosis results in scaphocephaly (dolichocephaly), unilateral coronal or lambdoidal synostosis in plagiocephaly, bilateral coronal or lambdoidal synostosis in brachycephaly, metopic synostosis in trigonocephaly, coronal and sagittal synostosis in oxycephaly (turricephaly), and a combination of coronal, lambdoidal, and sagittal synostoses in a cloverleaf skull. For further discussion of the plain film appearances of the skull in these conditions, the reader is referred to neuroradiology texts such as that by Harwood-Nash and Fitz.[21]

Hydrocephalus occurs in some cases of sutural synostosis and is then recognized on the CT or MR scan (see Chapter 2). In cases of Crouzon's disease, because of a small posterior fossa, the cerebellum is crowded and secondary tonsillar herniation may be present.

REFERENCES
Disorders of ventral induction

1. Aicardi J, Goutieres F: The syndrome of absence of the septum pellucidum with porencephalies and other developmental defects, *Neuropediatrics* 12:319, 1981.
2. Barkovich AJ, Fram EK, Norman D: Septooptic dysplasia: MR imaging, *Radiology* 171:189, 1989.
3. Barkovich AJ, Kjos BO, Norman D, et al: Revised classification of posterior fossa cysts and cystlike malformations based on the results of multiplanar MR imaging, *AJNR* 10:977, 1989.
4. Barkovich AJ, Newton TH: MR of aqueductal stenosis: evidence of a broad spectrum of tectal distortion, *AJNR* 10:471, 1989.
5. Barkovich AJ, Norman D: Absent septum pellucidum: a useful sign in the diagnosis of congenital brain malformations, *AJNR* 9:1107, 1988.
6. Barkovich AJ, Norman D: Anomalies of the corpus callosum: correlation with further anomalies of the brain, *AJNR* 9:493, 1988.
7. Becker H: Uber Hirngefassausschaltungen. Part 2. Interkranielle Gefassverschlusse: Uber Experimentelle Hydranencephalie (Blasenhirn), *Dtsch Z Nervenheilk* 161:446, 1949.
8. Benda CE: The Dandy-Walker syndrome, or the so-called atresia of the foramen Magendie, *J Neuropathol Exp Neurol* 13:14, 1954.
9. Brennan RE, Stratt BJ, Lee KF: Computed tomographic findings in cerebral hemiatrophy, *Neuroradiology* 17:17, 1978.
10. Byrd SE, Naidich TP: Common congenital brain anomalies. In Lee HS, Zimmerman RA, editors: *The radiologic clinics of North America*, Philadelphia, 1988, WB Saunders.
11. Chuang SH, Fitz CR, Chilton SJ, et al: Schizencephaly: spectrum of CT findings in association with septooptic dysplasia. Presented at the 70th Scientific Assembly and Annual Meeting of the Radiologic Society of North America, Washington, DC, November 1984.
12. Dandy WE, Blackfan KD: Internal hydrocephalus: an experimental, clinical, and pathologic study, *Am J Dis Child* 8:406, 1914.
13. DeMorsier G: Etudes sur les dysgraphies cranioencephaliques. III. Agenesie due septum lucidum avec malformation du tractus optique: la dysplasie septooptique, *Schiveig Arch Neurol Neurochir Psychiatr* 77:267, 1956.
14. DeMyer M, Zeman W, Palmer CG: The face predicts the brain: diagnostic significance of median facial anomalies for holoprosencephaly (arhinencephaly), *Pediatrics* 34:256, 1964.
15. Dyke CG, Davidoff LM, Masson CG: Cerebral hemiatrophy with homolateral hypertrophy of the skull and sinuses, *Surg Gynecol Obstet* 57:588, 1933.
16. Fitz CR: Holoprosencephaly and related entities, *Neuroradiology* 25:225, 1983.
17. Gardner E, O'Rahilly R, Prolo D: The Dandy-Walker and Arnold-Chiari malformations: clinical, developmental, and teratological considerations, *Arch Neurol* 32:393, 1975.
18. Hale BR, Rice P: Case reports—septooptic dysplasia: clinical and embryological aspects, *Develop Med Child Neurol* 16:812, 1974.
19. Haller JS, Wolpert SM, Rabe EF, et al: Cystic lesions of posterior fossa in infants: a comparison of clinical, radiological, and pathological findings in the Dandy-Walker syndrome and extraaxial cyst, *Neurology* 21:494, 1971.
20. Hart MN, Malamud N, Ellis WG: The Dandy-Walker syndrome: a clinicopathological study based on 28 cases, *Neurology* 22:771, 1972.
21. Harwood-Nash D, Fitz CR: *Neuroradiology in infants and children*, St Louis 1976, Mosby–Year Book.
22. Hirsch JF, Pierre-Kahn A, Renier D, et al: The Dandy-Walker malformation, a review of 40 cases, *J Neurosurg* 61:515. 1984.
23. Joubert N, Eisenring JJ, Robb JP, et al: Familial agenesis of the cerebellar vermis: a syndrome of episodic hyperapnea, abnormal eye movements, ataxia, and retardation, *Neurology* 19:813, 1969.
24. Kelly WM, Kucharczyk W, Kucharczyk J, et al: Posterior pituitary ectopia: an MR feature of pituitary dwarfism, *AJNR* 9:453, 1988.
25. Manelfe C, Rochiccioli P: CT of septooptic dysplasia, *AJR* 133:1157, 1979.
26. Manelfe C, Sevely A: Etude neuroradiologique des holoprosencephalies, *J Neuroradiol* 9:15, 1982.
27. Morishima A, Aranoff GS: Syndrome of septooptic-pituitary dysplasia: the clinical spectrum, *Brain Dev* 8:233, 1986.
28. Naidich TP, Osborn RE, Bauer B, et al: Median cleft face syndrome: MR and CT data from 11 children, *J Comput Assist Tomogr* 12:57, 1988.
29. Raybaud C: Cystic malformations of the posterior fossa, *J Neuroradiol* 9:103, 1982.
30. Reeves DL: Congenital absence of the septum-pellucidum, *Bull Johns Hopkins Hosp* 69:61, 1941.
31. Roessman V, Valesco ME, Small EJ, et al: Neuropathology or septooptic dysplasia (de Morsier syndrome) with immunohistochemical studies of hypothalamus and pituitary gland, *J Neuropathol Exp Neurol* 46:597, 1987.
32. Sarnat HB: Developmental disorders of the nervous system. In Bradley WG, Danoff RB, Fenichel GM, et al, editors: *Neurology in clinical practice*, vol 2, Boston, 1990, Butterworth Heinemann.
33. Sarnat HB, Alcala H: Human cerebellar hypoplasia: a syndrome of diverse causes, *Arch Neurol* 37:300, 1980.
34. Sawaya R, McLaurin RL: Dandy-Walker syndrome: clinical analysis of 23 cases, *J Neurosurg* 55:89, 1981.
35. Taggart JK, Walker AE: Congenital atresia of the foramens of Luschka and Magendie, *Arch Neurol Psychiatr* 48:583, 1942.

DISORDERS OF NEURONAL PROLIFERATION AND DIFFERENTIATION
Micrencephaly

The term *micrencephaly* refers to an abnormally small brain. In the context of congenital malformations (for example, lissencephaly and holoprosencephaly) it often reflects an early intrauterine insult usually of ischemic or infectious origin (TORCH group) (see Chapter 5), but it is also seen in some patients with metabolic disorders such as phenylketonuria (see Chapter 4). The cerebral hemispheres are usually symmetrical in appearance and anatomically intact in heredofamilial forms (see Chapter 2). Atrophy may be present in encephaloclastic forms, with prominence of the sulci and ventricles. Other findings include calvarial thickening, diffuse encephalomalacia, or focal porencephaly. Commonly these patients additionally manifest developmental delay, without focal neurological deficit.

Megalencephaly—generalized

Megalencephaly, or enlargement of the brain, may be caused by metabolic disorders or may be anatomical.[6] The abnormality can be unilateral or bilateral. Metabolic causes include Canavan's disease, Alexander's disease, metachromatic leukodystrophy, and mucopolysaccharidoses (see Chapter 4). Anatomical megalencephaly is seen in cases of pituitary gigantism and in neurocutaneous syndromes. The most common type is familial megalencephaly, in which the

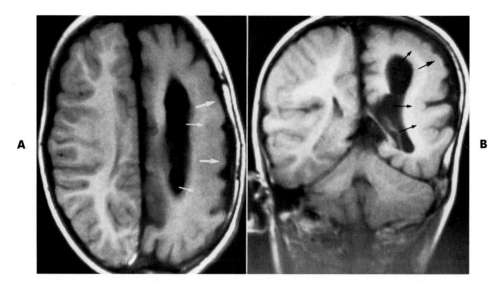

Fig. 3-26   Hemimegalencephaly with unilateral lissencephaly. **A** and **B,** The right hemisphere is normal in comparison with the larger left hemisphere, which contains a few shallow gyri (pachygyria) *(large arrows).* The cortex is also thickened *(small arrows),* and the ventricle is dilated.

cerebrum is larger than expected for the patient's age without specific parenchymal abnormalities.[6] On MRI the cerebrum may be unremarkable except for increased size for age, which can be overlooked if attention is not paid to the degree of magnification of the image (see Chapter 2).

Megalencephaly—unilateral

Unilateral megalencephaly is characterized by unilateral enlargement of one of the cerebral hemispheres. It can be focal, involving part of the hemisphere, or diffuse, involving the whole hemisphere. Microscopically the cortical neurons are enlarged, have an unusual morphology with a threefold increase in nuclear volume and sixfold increase in nucleolar volume.[5,13] Polymicrogyria, heterotopic gray matter, and lissencephaly (Fig. 3-26) are associated disorders.[1,2] Hemihypertrophy has been associated with diploid-triploid mosaicism.[8] The condition also shares features with granular cell hypertrophy of the cerebellum (Lhermitte-Duclos disease),[18] also called *gangliocytoma dysplasticum,* in which the hemispheric folia are enlarged and abnormal enlarged ganglion cells may be present (see Chapter 7).[16]

Patients have intractable seizures, hemiplegia, and developmental delay.[2,18] If the overgrowth is focal, involving the occipital and temporal lobes, MRI can aid in surgical resection of these lobes, which may be necessary to treat intractable seizures.

Unilateral megalencephaly on MRI appears as homolateral hemigigantism with a distorted thickened cortex and ventricular dilatation[1,2,18] (Fig. 3-26). The hemisphere can be so anomalous as to appear hamartomatous.[1] Recently MRI studies have indicated that decreased myelination as evidenced by increased water content of the centrum semiovale may occur in patients with unilateral megalencephaly.[1,2]

Colpocephaly

Colpocephaly is a nonspecific abnormality in which the occipital horns and atria are disproportionately enlarged in comparison to the remainder of the ventricular system[11,14] (Fig. 3-27). Colpocephaly represents a persistence of fetal ventricular morphology.[14] A similar pattern may be seen, however, with perinatal- or postnatal-acquired inflammatory insults (TORCH) or hypoxic-ischemic injury (for example, periventricular leukomalacia). It may also be associated with other congenital anomalies such as Chiari II malformation and agenesis or dysgenesis of the corpus callosum. As an isolated deformity, chromosomal abnormalities (such as trisomy 8), toxic agents (alcohol, diethylpropion, and hydrochloride), and intrauterine malnutrition have been implicated.[11] The patients may present with mental retardation, motor deficit, seizures, and spasticity.[14]

Hydranencephaly

By combining the words *hydrocephalus* and *anencephaly,* Spielmeyer[17] introduced the term *hydranencephaly.* Initially believed to be caused by primary agenesis of the neural wall,[19,20] the abnormality is now believed to be caused by occlusion of the supraclinoid internal carotid arteries[10] in the third to sixth months of gestation. By this time normal ventral induction and diverticulation has occurred, which accounts for the presence of the falx and some remaining normal cortex. Experimentally the lesion has been produced by the injection of paraffin into the supraclinoid carotid artery in developing embryos.[4] The cortical plate as well as the subjacent white matter is destroyed and resorbed, implying an encephaloclastic process.[15] The cerebral hemispheres are replaced by a membranous sac consisting of leptomeninges overlying a glial layer that is the remnant of the cortex and white matter.

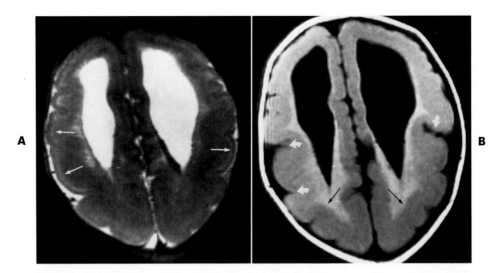

Fig. 3-27   Colpocephaly and lissencephaly. **A,** Axial short TR/TE images (650/20 msec). Selective dilatation of the atria and occipital horn is evident (colpocephaly). The brain has a smooth contour with a few areas of broad gryi *(white arrows)*. The gray matter of the cortex is thickened *(black arrows)*. The white matter is thin. **B,** On the long TR/long TE images (3000/90 msec) a circumferential band of increased signal intensity is present immediately below the surface of the hemisphere *(arrows)* indicating the cell-sparse zone of laminar necrosis. (From Robertson SJ, Wolpert SM: Brain: congenital. In Runge VM, editor: *Clinical magnetic resonance imaging,* Philadelphia, 1990, JB Lippincott.)

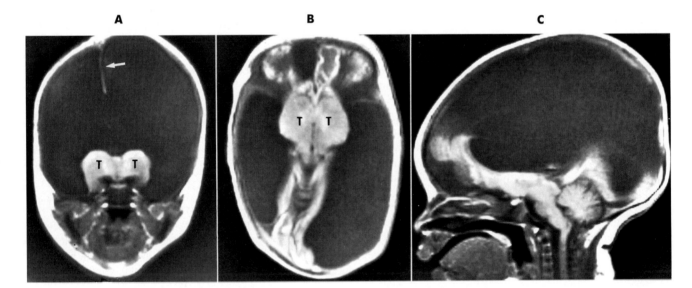

Fig. 3-28   Hydranencephaly. The cerebral hemispheres are largely replaced by two membranous fluid-filled sacs, best demonstrated on the coronal image **(A),** where the thalami *(T)* are surrounded by the fluid-filled hemispheres **(A** and **B).** The falx is present and can be seen in the coronal planes *(arrow).* Remaining residual frontal and occipital cortex is present. The posterior fossa is small, as is the brain stem **(C).**

In humans, causative agents include maternal syphilis, cytomegalovirus, toxoplasmosis, herpes infection, radiation, and abdominal trauma.[10,15]

On MRI most of the cerebral hemispheres is replaced by a membranous cerebrospinal fluid intensity sac in the distribution of the middle cerebral arteries (Fig. 3-28). The occipital lobes, inferior temporal lobes, and portions of the frontal cortex may remain. The vertebral arteries are intact, so there is preservation of the cerebellum, pons, and midbrain.[7] However, the posterior fossa may be small (Fig. 3-28), and coexistent cerebellar and brain stem anomalies may occur. The corticospinal tracts may be small. The olivary nuclei may be hypoplastic, and therefore the brain stem may appear atrophic.[10] The falx is intact, can remain in the midline, or be deviated to one side. The thalami are not fused and are usually surrounded by the membranous sac,[7] giving them a rounded appearance (Fig. 3-28).

Alobar holoprosencephaly is differentiated from hydranencephaly by the presence of the falx and the nonfusion of the thalami of the diencephalon. The findings of hydranencephaly can be mimicked by massive hydrocephalus (thinned cortical mantle present), porencephaly (usually more focal), and multiple cystic encephalomalacia.[7,9,10]

Neurocutaneous disorders

See Chapter 8.

Aqueductal anomalies

Narrowing of the aqueduct of Sylvius may be caused by a wide variety of conditions such as postinflammatory, neoplastic (periaqueductal tumors), and congenital causes. Pathologically there are four types of intrinsic congenital narrowings of the aqueduct: septum or membrane formation, forking, gliosis, and stenosis.[12] Membrane formation is the rarest of the four types and may result from intrauterine infection with a granular ependymitis, or from a developmentally acquired glial overgrowth. Forking of the aqueduct is commonly seen in association with spina bifida. Aqueductal gliosis often results from infection; stenosis represents narrowing without evidence of gliosis.

MRI, particularly when obtained in the sagittal plane, is an excellent modality to define the patency of the aqueduct. Usually short TR/short TE images are adequate for demonstration of the dimension, configuration, and patency of the aqueduct. In cases of aqueductal deformity due to periaqueductal masses, gadolinium-DTPA administration or follow-up MRI studies may be necessary to differentiate a glioma[3] from benign lesions such as aqueductal stenosis with tectal dysplasia, hamartoma, or gliosis (Fig. 2-18).

REFERENCES
Disorders of neuronal proliferation

1. Barkovich AJ, Chuang SH: Unilateral megalencephaly: correlation of MR imaging and pathologic characteristics, *AJNR* 11:523, 1990.
2. Barkovich AJ, Chuang SH, Norman D: MR of neuronal migration anomalies, *AJR* 150:179, 1988.
3. Barkovich AJ, Newton TH: MR of aqueductal stenosis: evidence of a broad spectrum of tectal distortion, *AJNR* 10:471, 1989.
4. Becker H: Uber Hirngefassausschaltungen, Part 2. Interkranielle Gefassverschlusse: Uber experimentelle hydranencephalie (Blasenhirn), *Dtsch Z Nervenheilk* 161:446, 1949.
5. Bignami A, Palladini G, Zappella M: Unilateral megalencephaly with nerve cell hypertrophy: an anatomical and quantitative histochemical study, *Brain Res* 9:103, 1968.
6. DeMyer W: Megalencephaly in children: clinical syndromes, genetic patterns, and differential diagnosis from other causes of megalocephaly, *Neurology* 22:634, 1972.
7. Dublin AB, French BN: Diagnostic image evaluation of hydranencephaly and pictorially similar entities, with emphasis on computed tomography, *Radiology* 137:81, 1980.
8. Ferrier P, Ferrier S, Stalder G, et al: Congenital asymmetry associated with diploid-triploid mosaicism and large satellites, *Lancet* 1:80, 1964.
9. Fowler M, Dow R, White TA, et al: Congenital hydrocephalus-hydrencephaly in five siblings, with autopsy studies: a new disease, *Develop Med Child Neurol* 14:173, 1972.
10. Halsey JH, Allen N, Chamberlin HR: The morphogenesis of hydranencephaly, *J Neurol Sci* 12:187, 1971.
11. Herskowitz J, Rosman NP, Wheeler CB: Colpocephaly: clinical, radiologic, and pathogenic aspects, *Neurology* 35:1594, 1985.
12. James HE: Narrowing of the aqueduct of Sylvius. In Hoffman HJ, Epstein F, editors: *Disorders of the developing nervous system: diagnosis and treatment*, Boston, 1986, Blackwell.
13. Manz HJ, Phillips TM, Rowden G, et al: Unilateral megalencephaly, cerebral cortical dysplasia, neuronal hypertrophy, and heterotopia: cytomorphometric, fluorometric, cytochemical, and biochemical analyses, *Acta Neuropathol* 45:97, 1979.
14. Noorani PA, Bodensteiner JB, Barnes PD: Colpocephaly: frequency and associated findings, *J Child Neurol* 3:100, 1988.
15. Raybaud C: Destructive lesions of the brain, *Neuroradiology* 25:265, 1983.
16. Smith RR, Grossman RI, Goldberg HI, et al: MR imaging of Lhermitte-Duclos disease: a case report, *AJNR* 10:187, 1989.
17. Spielmeyer W: Ein Hydranencephales Zwillingspaar, *Arch Psychiat Nervenkr* 39:807, 1904.
18. Townsend JJ, Nielsen SL, Malamud N: Unilateral megalencephaly: hamartoma or neoplasm? *Neurology* 25:448, 1975.
19. Yakovlev PI, Wadsworth RC: Schizencephalies: a study of the congenital clefts in the cerebral mantle. I. Clefts with fused lips, *J Neuropathol Exp Neurol* 5:116, 1946.
20. Yakovlev PI, Wadsworth RC: Schizencephalies: a study of the congenital clefts in the cerebral mantle. II. Clefts with hydrocephalus and lips separated, *J Neuropathol Exp Neurol* 5:169, 1946.

DISORDERS OF SULCATION AND MIGRATION

It is an axiom in the developing nervous system that neurons are generated in a site remote from where they will ultimately reside. Neuroblasts that lie in the subependymal zones at about the second gestational month lose their mitotic capabilities and begin migrating centrifugally along radially aligned glial cells to their destination in the cerebral cortex.[16] In the cerebral cortex immature nerve cells reach the pial surface, then reverse their direction as more recent arrivals displace the earlier migrated cells into deeper layers. Waves of migrating cells continue until the sixteenth week of gestation, with smaller waves continuing until the twenty-fifth week.[4] Cells generated later in gestation therefore lie in the cortex more superficial than those generated earlier, which lie in the deeper cortex.[2,4] The laminated arrangement of the mammalian cortex requires a large cortical surface to accommodate increasing numbers of migrating neurons. Convolutions provide this large surface area without incurring a concomitant increase in cerebral volume. Gyri and sulci are thus a direct result of neuronal migration. The pattern of gyral formation is so predictable that at autopsy the gestational age of an infant may be determined within a 2-week period from the convolutional pattern of the brain.[7] Once migration is complete the neurons integrate and interconnect to form functional units. Any insult to the developing brain in the migration period may result in a migration anomaly. The anomalies included in this category are agyria (lissencephaly), pachygyria, schizencephaly, and gray matter heterotopias.[13]

Lissencephaly

The normal human cortex is six layered. If an insult occurs to the early developing brain, the cortex may develop a four-layered appearance: a molecular layer, an outer cellular layer, a cell-sparse zone, and an inner cellular layer of disorganized neurons.[2,6] The cell-sparse zone contains a region of gliosis with an abnormally high water content. Neuronal migration beyond this region is impaired, and the neurons that develop later cannot follow their radial glial fibers. Because of the interruption to migrating neurons, the brain will have a smooth appearance, lacking gyral and sulcal definition as well as normal gray-white interdigitations. The term *agyria* applies to a brain with a smooth surface. *Pachygyria* refers to broad, flat gyri. Commonly the two coexist in the same brain often with frontal pachygyria and parietooccipital agyria. The term *lissencephaly* encompasses the agyria-pachygyria complex.

With severe forms of lissencephaly the prognoses is uniformly poor. The children are severely mentally retarded, usually presenting with seizures, hypotonia, and craniofacial dysmorphism. Three clinical syndromes have been described. Type I is associated with microcephaly. Constituting this group are the Miller-Dieker, Norman-Roberts, and Neau-Laxova syndromes. In the Miller-Dieker syndrome, there is lissencephaly, colpocephaly, and agenesis of the corpus callosum. The dysmorphic features include microcephaly, anteverted nares, epicanthal folds, and micrognathia. It is associated with a deletion of the short arm of chromosome 17 (band 17 p 13.3).[10,12] Norman-Roberts syndrome is not associated with chromosomal abnormalities. These patients are severely retarded, microcephalic with a prominent occiput, and usually have micrognathia and a prominent nasal bridge.[10]

Type II lissencephaly syndromes include Walker-Warburg syndrome and cerebroocularmuscular syndrome. These patients are macrocephalic with hydrocephalus. Walker-Warburg syndrome is characterized by lissencephaly, obstructive hydrocephalus, retinal dysplasia, and hypoplasia of the vermis with or without Dandy-Walker syndrome.[11] If the above findings are present along with congenital muscular dystrophy, the term applied is *cerebroocularmuscular syndrome* (COMS). The HARD + E syndrome encompasses *h*ydrocephalus, *a*gyria, *r*etinal *d*ysplasia, and *e*ncephalocele.[11] Type III encompasses isolated lissencephaly with cerebrocerebellar lissencephaly.

The MRI findings are characteristic. The overall appearance of the brain is smooth (see Fig. 3-26). There is underopercularization of the sylvian fissures with an exposed insula, which on axial images causes the brain to adopt a "figure of eight" appearance.[6,9,13] The cortex is thickened and contains a band of high signal intensity on T2-weighted images corresponding to the cell-sparse zone[2] (see Fig. 3-27). The claustrum and extreme capsule may be absent. Colpocephaly is present, and the corpus callosum may be dysplastic or absent. Associated gray matter heterotopias are common. Since neurons have degenerated, the brain stem is hypoplastic with smaller corticospinal tracts.

Polymicrogyria

Once the later migrating neurons arrive at the superficial cortex but do not distribute normally, numerous small gyri may form. The cortex is excessively convoluted and thickened. There is an abnormal histological pattern with a zone of laminar necrosis that is not as severe as that seen in the agyria-pachygyria complex, and no corresponding signal change is seen on T2-weighted images as is seen in lissencephaly. Polymicrogyria may be diffuse or focal, and commonly occurs in the insular region (Fig. 3-29). It is usually associated with other anomalies; for example it lines the cleft (pial-ependymal seam) in schizencephaly.[2,19] Also, polymicrogyria is the dominant histopathology in cortical dysplasias. The dysplasia may be focal, as an area of cortical infolding, or more diffuse; it has an irregular inner gray-white margin.

Polymicrogyria may not be "directly" demonstrated by MRI. It also may not be apparent on CT examination because of the overlying bone artifact. In many cases MRI reveals multiple, small, shallow convolutions that can be so complex that the superficial cortex may appear smooth. The underlying white matter may appear diminished, and the cortex itself is thickened.[2] In pachygyria, polymicrogyria, and schizencephaly, enlarged anomalous cortical venous drainage is present as the normal arborization of cortical veins fails to develop.[1] Polymicrogyria has been reported in Zellweger's cerebrohepatorenal syndrome, maternal carbon dioxide poisoning, congenital cytomegalic viral disease, and focal epilepsy associated with cortical dysplasias.[19]

Schizencephaly

Yakovlev and Wadsworth[17,18] initially described lesions with bilateral holohemispheric clefts of the parietal lobes and coined the term *schizencephaly*. Their initial description, however, also included cases of hydranencephaly and porencephaly. The term *schizencephaly* refers to full-thickness clefts of the cerebral hemispheres that are lined with gray matter and most commonly involve the parasylvian regions bilaterally and symmetrically.[2,18] The gray matter lining the cleft may be polymicrogyric. The cells of the ventricular ependyma meet the pial cells of the cortex, forming the so-called pial-ependymal seam.[14,18] Gray matter heterotopias may also be found in close association with the cleft. The malformation is probably caused by an insult (for example, ischemia) early in the migration process, causing focal destruction in the germinal matrix.[2] Schizencephaly and septooptic dysplasia frequently coexist (absence of the septum pellucidum).[2,8,19]

Two types of schizencephaly have been described depending on the size of the area involved and the separation

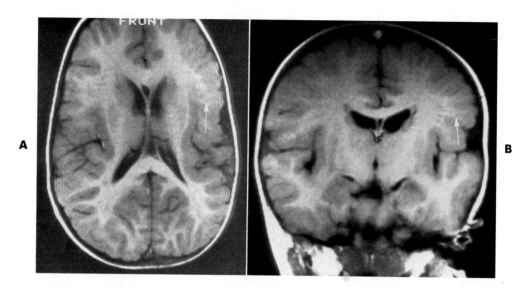

Fig. 3-29   Polymicrogyria. A few shallow convoluted gyri *(arrows)* are seen in the perisylvian region. The white matter interdigitations follow the convolutions. **A,** Axial scan. **B,** Coronal scan.

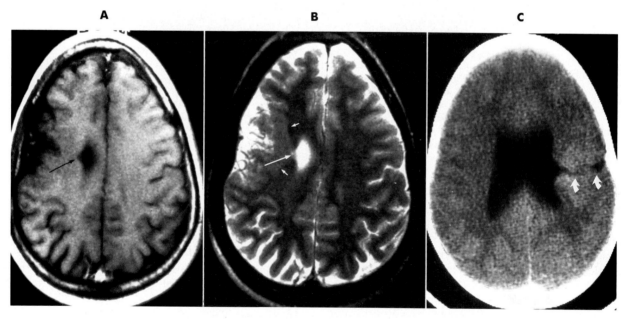

Fig. 3-30   Schizencephaly type I. A dimple is seen on the lateral wall of the lateral ventricle *(arrow)* on both short TR/short TE (650/20 msec) **(A)** and long TR/long TE (3000/90 msec) images **(B).** Gray matter is seen extending from the cortex toward the ventricle *(small arrows),* lining an almost indiscernible cleft. **C,** Axial CT examination of another patient demonstrates a small cleft extending from the cortex to the ventricle, representing the pial-ependymal seam *(arrows).*

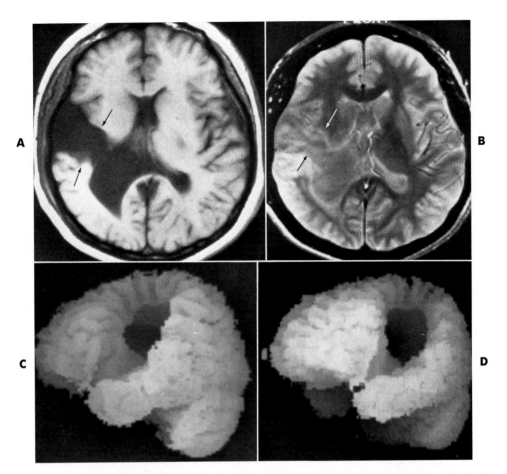

Fig. 3-31   Type II schizencephaly. A widely spaced cleft is present in the right parietal lobe. **A,** Short TR/short TE image demonstrates communication between the ventricle and the subarachnoid space through the pial-ependymal seam *(arrows).* **B,** This cleft is lined by gray matter *(arrows),* best seen on the long TR/long TE image. The gray matter lining distinguishes this case from that of porencephaly, which is lined by gliosis or white matter. **C** and **D,** Three-dimensional reconstructed images from a three-dimensional FLASH series demonstrate the cleft and gyri lining the cleft. With computer manipulatations the image can be rotated about its axis, offering different projections of the abnormality. (From Robertson SJ, Wolpert SM: Brain: congenital. In Runge VM, editor: *Clinical magnetic resonance imaging,* Philadelphia, 1990, JB Lippincott.)

of the clefts. Type I schizencephaly consists of a fused cleft[5] (Fig. 3-30). This fused pial-ependymal seam, forming a furrow in the developing brain, is lined by polymicrogyric gray matter that may be difficult to identify. The lesion can be unilateral or bilateral and is usually situated at or near the precentral or postcentral sulcus.[2,5] In Type II schizencephaly there is a large defect, a true holohemispheric cleft in the cerebral cortex filled with CSF and lined by polymicrogyria gray matter. The cleft is lined by a membrane consisting of two layers, an inner layer of ependyma and an outer layer of pia forming the pial-ependymal seam. Large portions of the cerebral hemispheres may be absent (Fig. 3-31). The clinical manifestations depend on the severity of the lesion. Patients with type I are often normal but may have seizures and spasticity. In the Type II abnormality usually there is severe mental retardation, seizures, hypotonia, spasticity,

inability to walk or speak, and blindness.[2,14]

MR imaging is excellent for identifying both type I and type II schizencephaly. Axial images demonstrate the small ventricular dimple and infolding of the cortical gray matter in type I. If short TR/short TE images do not provide high contrast between gray and white matter, it may be difficult to demonstrate the gray matter lining of the seam. Long TR/long TE images may then be needed. Imaging in two planes can help identify the pial-ependymal seam in type II, usually as a fan-shaped perisylvian cleft lined with polymicrogyria. The septum pellucidum may be absent, and the corpus callosum may be hypoplastic. We have seen a case of type II schizencephaly that increased in size concomitant with a developing hydrocephalus. When the hydrocephalus was shunted, the ventricles and schizencephalic clefts decreased in size.

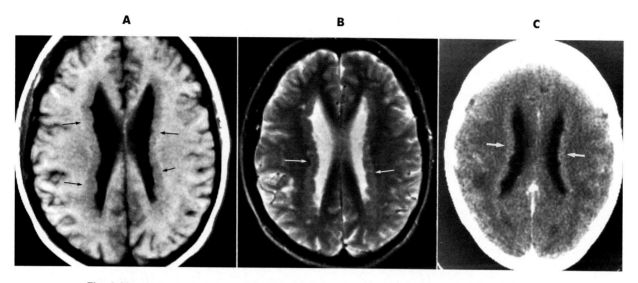

Fig. 3-32 Heterotopic gray matter. A subependymal region isointense with gray matter on both T1-weighted **(A)** and T2-weighted **(B)** images *(arrows)* is seen lining the ventricles on either side. The cortex is thin because the gray matter has not migrated from the subependymal region. **C,** CT scan demonstrates similar findings with gray matter lining the ventricles *(arrows).*

Heterotopic gray matter

Neuronal heterotopia may be an isolated anomaly or associated with other abnormalities such as schizencephaly or agenesis of the corpus callosum. Heterotopic gray matter consists of neurons in abnormal locations due to arrest in their radial migration to the pial surface of the brain. The abnormality may manifest as single, multiple, unilateral, or bilateral nodular masses of varying sizes appearing anywhere from the subependymal zone to the cortex.[2,19] Heterotopic gray matter may also be seen as diffuse nodular masses that line the ventricles and extend into adjacent white matter (Fig. 3-32). It may be difficult to exclude tuberous sclerosis on the basis of MRI signal characteristics alone. Heterotopias are not enhanced after intravenous contrast administration and rarely, if ever, calcify. Recently, band heterotopias have been described in patients with heterotopic gray matter in which a continuous band of heterotopic neurons is evident in the white matter between the lateral ventricles and cerebral cortex.[3] In these cases intervening white matter is seen between the ventricle and the band of gray matter, as well as between the heterotopic gray matter and the cortex[3] (Fig. 3-33).

Clinically, heterotopias may be foci of seizure activity. MRI can easily detect heterotopias as their signal intensity on all imaging sequences follows that of normal gray matter.

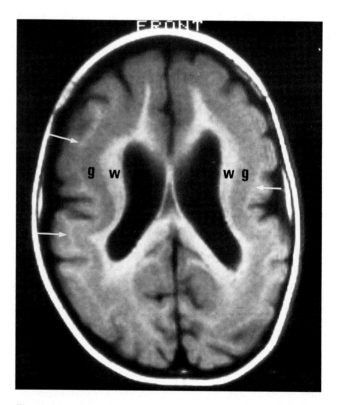

Fig. 3-33 Band heterotopia. Axial short TR/short TE (650/20 msec) images. The cortex consists of a few broad, shallow gyri (pachygyria). From the ventricle outward is a region of white matter *(w),* isointense gray matter *(g),* another thin layer of increased signal indicating white matter *(thin arrows),* and then cortex. The band of gray matter in the middle is the heterotopic gray matter.

REFERENCES
Disorders of sulcation and migration

1. Barkovich AJ: Abnormal vascular drainage in anomalies of neuronal migration, *AJNR* 9:939, 1988.
2. Barkovich AJ, Chuang SH, Norman D: MR of neuronal migration anomalies, *AJNR* 8:1009, 1987.
3. Barkovich AJ, Jackson DE, Boyer RS: Band heterotopias: a newly recognized neuronal migration anomaly, *Radiology* 171:455, 1989.

4. Berry M, Rogers AW: The migration of neuroblasts in the developing cerebral cortex, *J Anat* 99:691, 1965.
5. Bird CT, Gilles FH: Type I schizencephaly: CT and neuropathologic findings, *AJNR* 8:451, 1987.
6. Byrd SE, Bohan TP, Osborn RE, et al: The CT and MR evaluation of lissencephaly, *AJNR* 9:923, 1988.
7. Chi JG, Dooling EC, Gilles FH: Gyral development of the human brain, *Ann Neurol* 1:86, 1977.
8. Chuang SH, Fitz CR, Chilton SJ, et al: Schizencephaly: spectrum of CT findings in association with septooptic dysplasia. Presented at the 70th Scientific Assembly and Annual Meeting of the Radiologic Society of North America, Washington, DC, November 1984.
9. Dobyns WB, McCluggage CW: Computed tomographic appearance of lissencephaly syndromes, *AJNR* 6:545, 1985.
10. Dobyns WB, Stratton RF, Greenberg F: Syndromes with lissencephaly. 1. Miller-Dieker and Norman-Roberts syndromes and isolated lissencephaly, *Am J Med Genetics* 18:509, 1984.
11. Dobyns WB, Kirkpatrick JB, Hittner HM, et al: Syndromes with lissencephaly. II. Walker-Warburg and cerebrooculomuscular syndromes and a new syndrome with type II lissencephaly, *Am J Med Genetics* 22:157, 1985.
12. Dobyns WB, Stratton RF, Parke JT, et al: Miller-Dieker syndrome: lissencephaly and monosomy 17p, *J Pediatr* 102:552, 1983.
13. Osborn RE, Byrd SE, Naidich TP, et al: MR imaging of neuronal migrational disorders, *AJNR* 9:1101, 1988.
14. Page LK, Brown SB, Gargano FP, et al: Schizencephaly: a clinical study and review, *Child's Brain* 1:348, 1975.
15. Parrish ML, Roessmann U, Levinsohn MW: Agenesis of the corpus callosum: a study of the frequency of associated malformations, *Ann Neurol* 6:349, 1979.
16. Sidman RL, Rakic P: Neuronal migration, with special reference to developing human brain: a review, *Brain Res* 62:1, 1973.
17. Yakovlev PI, Wadsworth RC: Schizencephalies: a study of the congenital clefts in the cerebral mantle. I. Clefts with fused lips, *J Neuropathol Exp Neurol* 5:116, 1946.
18. Yakovlev PI, Wadsworth RC: Schizencephalies: a study of the congenital clefts in the cerebral mantle. II. Clefts with hydrocephalus and lips separated, *J Neuropathol Exp Neurol* 5:169, 1946.
19. Zimmerman RA, Bilaniuk LT, Grossman RI: Computed tomography in migratory disorders of human brain development, *Neuroradiology* 25:257, 1983.

Dysgenesis of the corpus callosum

The term *dysgenesis* reflects a spectrum of abnormalities of the corpus callosum varying from complete agenesis to hypogenesis or hypoplasia.[11] To understand the MRI findings and associated anomalies it is important to consider the embryology of the corpus callosum. At about the seventh to tenth week, a thickening of the lamina terminalis, called the lamina reuniens of His, occurs.[1,6] A groove (the sulcus medianus telencephali medii) develops in the superior surface of the lamina reuniens and becomes filled with cells—the commissural plate. Developing axons in both cerebral hemispheres are induced to cross from side-to-side through the commissural plate to form the corpus callosum. The interhemispheric projection of the first axons is preceded by microcystic degeneration in the plate and physiological death of astrocytes.[13]

The anterior portion of the corpus callosum forms first, followed by elongation and posterior growth to form the genu, body, splenium, and rostrum. By approximately 20 weeks this process is complete. The pathogenesis of callosal agenesis is related to two aspects of the commissural plate. If this plate is not available to guide axonal passage, the corpus callosum does not develop.[16] Also, failure of the physiological degeneration results in a glial barrier to axonal passage, and the primordial callosal fibers are then deflected posteriorly within their hemisphere of origin and either form the bundles of Probst or disappear.[19] Another theory proposes that persistence of the meninx primitiva (the precursor of the subarachnoid space) in the commissural plate both prevents development of the corpus callosum and promotes maldevelopment such as lipomas.[18]

The timing of an insult during the formation of the corpus callosum also determines the extent of the abnormality. In partial agenesis the genu may be present while the body, splenium, and rostrum are absent. If the splenium and rostrum are intact and the genu and body absent, a secondary destructive process such as anoxia or infarction may have taken place after the corpus callosum was completely developed.[2,6,11] Recent investigation suggests that in some cases atypical callosal agenesis exists when the splenium is present and the body and genu are absent. In these cases, however, the apparent splenium is actually an enlargement of the hippocampal commissure.[5] A similar pattern of callosal dysgenesis is present in the holoprosencephalies.

Callosal agenesis or dysgenesis is seen in a wide array of anomalies including Chiari II malformation, Dandy-Walker malformation, sphenoethmoidal cephaloceles, septooptic dysplasia, cleft lip and palate, acrocephalosyndactyly (Apert's syndrome), hypertelorism, ocular anomalies (coloboma of optic disc), neuronal heterotopias, dysmyelinating diseases[2,6,12,15] and anomalies of the limbic system.[4] Aicardi's syndrome, seen only in females, consists of agenesis of the corpus callosum with lacunar chorioretinopathy, mental retardation, and infantile spasms. Microphthalmia and choroidal coloboma may be present,[3,8] along with cerebellar hypoplasia, subependymal nodules, and occasional choroid plexus papillomas.[10]

MRI fully delineates the wide range of callosal anomalies (Fig. 3-34). Sagittal images demonstrate the extent of dysgenesis. As stated earlier, if an insult occurs early, there may be complete agenesis or hypogenesis with only the genu present. The medial parietal and occipital gyri and sulci radiate from the midline perpendicular to the expected course of the corpus[7] and are well seen on sagittal MR images. The lateral ventricles are parallel and widely separated as the third ventricle rises superiorly (Fig. 3-34). Colpocephaly may be seen in as many as 40% of patients.[11] The foramina of Monro are elongated. Together with the laterally placed frontal horns in the coronal plane, the anterior horns, the third ventricle, and foramen form a "trident" or "steer" appearance (Figs. 3-34 and 3-35). In the newborn infant ultrasonography may also help in the diagnosis of agenesis of the corpus callosum (Fig. 3-36). The bundles of Probst may be seen along the medial borders of the widely spaced lateral ventricles (Fig. 3-34). Azygous anterior cerebral arteries occur in many patients with callosal agenesis. Also, the internal cerebral veins are widely separated because of the high-riding third ventricle.

Two not infrequent accompaniments of callosal agenesis are interhemispheric cysts and lipomas. A paramedian interhemispheric cyst may communicate with the lateral or

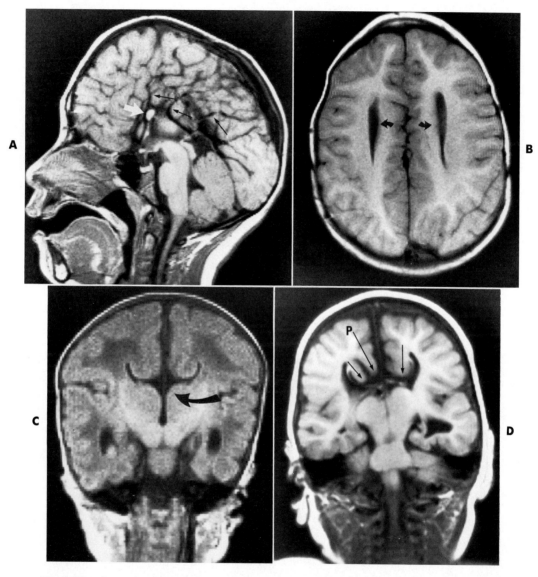

Fig. 3-34 Agenesis of the corpus callosum. All images are short TR/short TE (650/20 msec). **A,** Sagittal image shows that only the genu of the corpus callosum is present *(white arrow).* The gyri radiate toward the expected location of the corpus callosum similar to the spokes of a wheel *(black arrows).* **B,** The lateral ventricles are widely spaced *(arrows).* **C,** The appearance of the high-lying third ventricle and the lateral ventricles *(arrow)* is that of a trident or "longhorn steer." **D,** The cingulate gyri folds inward *(arrows).* Probst bundles indent the medial wall of the lateral ventricles *(P).*

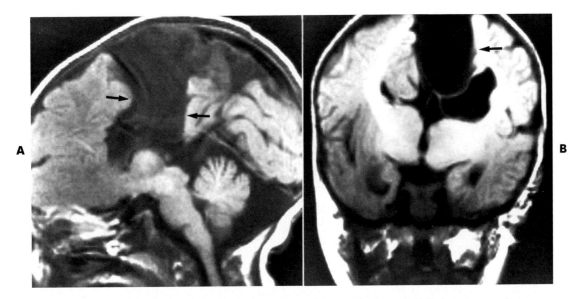

Fig. 3-35   Agenesis of the corpus callosum with interhemispheric cyst. Both images are short TR/short TE (650/20 msec.) **A** and **B,** There is complete absence of the corpus callosum. The lateral ventricles are widely separated. A large interhemispheric cyst *(arrows)* arises above the superiorly displaced third ventricle, along one side of the falx. Asymmetrical ventricular dilatation is also present.

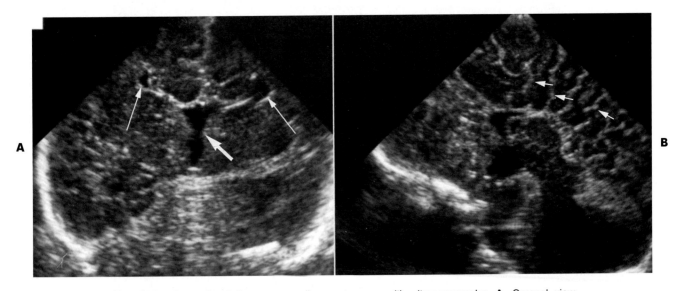

Fig. 3-36   Agenesis of the corpus callosum as seen with ultrasonography. **A,** Coronal view demonstrates separation of the lateral ventricles *(small arrows)* and a high-riding third ventricle *(large arrow).* **B,** Sagittal view demonstrates radially oriented sulci *(arrows).* (Courtesy Dr. Deborah ter Meulen, New England Medical Center Hospitals.)

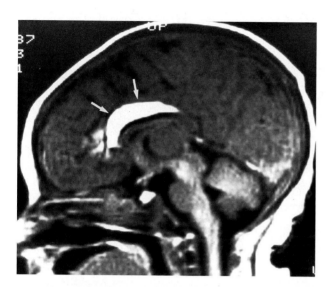

Fig. 3-37   Pericallosal lipoma. Short TR/short TE (650/20 msec) image. Pericallosal lipomas are often associated with agenesis of the corpus callosum. The lipoma is commonly in the midline and is located above the corpus callosum (or its expected location), occupying the region of the cingulate gyrus. Here the lipoma *(arrows)* curves posteriorly, following the shape of the cingulate gyrus and corpus callosum to the expected position of the splenium.

third ventricle (Fig. 3-35). It is of variable size and lies predominantly on one side of the falx.[17] When large, the cyst may displace the hemispheres. Lipomas of the interhemispheric fissure are pericallosal in location and usually do not involve the corpus callosum itself. This is one of the most common intracranial sites for lipoma. MRI demonstrates a pericallosal lesion of high signal on T1-weighted images (Fig. 3-37), with associated callosal dysgenesis in 40% of patients. These lipomas may arise from inclusion of primitive mesenchyme, may be caused by persistence of the primitive mesenchyme,[18] or may be part of a spectrum of midline craniofacial dysraphism in which encephaloceles, cutaneous lipomas and midline facial clefts are present[14] Lipomas may also occur incidentally[9] and are usually seen within or adjacent to the cisterns. Subarachnoid lipomas have been noted in the quadrigeminal, ambient, chiasmatic, interpeduncular, cerebellopontine, and sylvian cisterns. Cerebral malformations of various types are found in approximately half the patients with lipomas.[18]

REFERENCES
Dysgenesis of the corpus callosum

1. Abbie AA: The origin of the corpus callosum and the fate of the structures related to it, *J Comparative Neurol* 70:9, 1939.
2. Aicardi J, Goutieres F: The syndrome of absence of the septum pellucidum with porencephalies and other developmental defects, *Neuropediatrics* 12:319, 1981.
3. Aicardi J, Lefebevre J, Lerique A: Spasms in flexion, callosal agenesis, ocular abnormalities: a new syndrome, *Electroenceph Clin Neurophysiol* 19:609, 1965.

4. Atlas SW, Zimmerman RA, Bilaniuk LT, et al: Corpus callosum and limbic system: neuroanatomic MR evaluation of development anomalies, *Radiology* 160:355, 1986.
5. Barkovich AJ: Apparent atypical collosal dysgenesis: analysis of MR findings in six cases and their relationship to holoprosencephaly, *AJNR* 11:333, 1990.
6. Barkovich AJ, Norman D: Anomalies of the corpus callosum: correlation with further anomalies of the brain, *AJNR* 9:493, 1988.
7. Davidson HD, Abraham R, Steiner RE: Agenesis of the corpus callosum: magnetic resonance imaging, *Radiology* 155:371, 1985.
8. Denslow GT, Robb RM: Aicardi's syndrome: a report of four cases and review of the literature, *J Pediatr Ophthalmol Strabasimus* 16:10, 1979.
9. Faerber EN, Wolpert SW: The value of computed tomography in the diagnosis of intracranial lipomata, *J Comput Assist Tomogr* 2:297, 1978.
10. Hall-Craggs Harbord MG, Finn JP, et al: Aicardi syndrome: MR assessment of brain structure and myelination, *AJNR* 11:532, 1990.
11. Jinkins JR, Whittermore AR, Bradley WG: MR imaging of callosal and corticocallosal dysgenesis, *AJNR* 10:339, 1989.
12. Kendall BE: Dysgenesis of the corpus callosum, *Neuroradiology* 25:239, 1983.
13. Loeser JD, Alvord EL Jr: Agenesis of the corpus callosum, *Brain* 91:553, 1968.
14. Manz HJ, Phillips TM, Rowden G, et al: Unilateral megalencephaly, cerebral cortical dysplasia, neuronal hypertrophy, and heterotopia: cytomorphometric, fluorometric, cytochemical, and biochemical analyses, *Acta Neuropathol* 45:97, 1979.
15. Parrish ML, Roessmann U, Levinsohn MW: Agenesis of the corpus callosum: a study of the frequency of associated malformations, *Ann Neurol* 6:349, 1979.
16. Silver J, Lorenz SE, Washton D, et al: Axonal guidance during development of the great cerebral commissures: description and experimental studies in vivo on the side of preformed glial pathways, *J Comp Neurol* 210:10, 1982.
17. Swett HA, Nixon GW: Agenesis of the corpus callosum with interhemispheric cyst, *Radiology* 114:641, 1975.
18. Truwit CL, Barkovich AJ: Pathogenesis of intracranial lipoma: an MR study in 42 patients, *AJNR* 11:665, 1990.
19. Zaki W: Le processes degeneratif au cours du developement du corps calleux, *Arch Anat Micr Morphol Exp* 74:133, 1985.

ARACHNOID CYSTS

Arachnoid cysts are congenital or acquired CSF-filled collections that occur in the middle cranial fossa (50% to 66%), in the suprasellar and quadrigeminal regions (10%), or in the posterior fossa (Figs. 3-24 and 3-25) or over the frontal convexities (5%).[1] They represent 1% of all atraumatic intracranial masses. Two types have been described: (1) a dilated, circumscribed, expanded subarachnoid space that arises as an aberration in the formation of the subarachnoid space[2] and (2) an intraarachnoid cyst, formed by splitting and duplication of the arachnoid membrane.[4] Middle cranial fossa arachnoid cysts may be associated with temporal lobe agenesis[3] (Fig. 3-38). Suprasellar cysts, usually due to an optochiasmatic arachnoidits (Fig. 3-39), may cause obstructive hydrocephalus, as may retrocerebellar cysts. Quadrigeminal plate cysts (Fig. 3-40) lie between the quadrigeminal plate and the splenium of the corpus callosum.

Common clinical signs and symptoms, depending on location, include headaches, seizures, increased pressure (hydrocephalus), and, rarely, focal deficit. The most common intracranial masses of infancy are cystic (Dandy-Walker, porencephalic cyst, arachoid cyst). Although the cysts are usually detected by US or CT, MRI can better delineate those lesions that may require surgical interven-

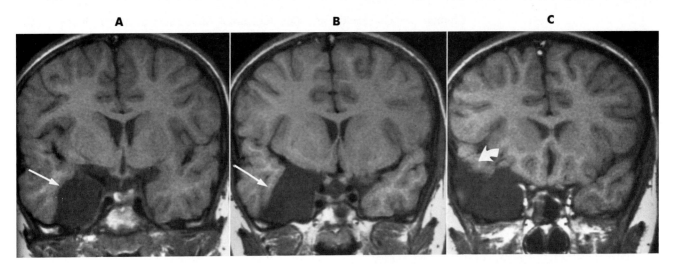

Fig. 3-38   Middle cranial fossa arachnoid cyst. **A** and **B,** Coronal images (short TR/short TE, 650/20 msec) demonstrate a CSF intensity lesion in the middle cranial fossa *(arrows)*. **C,** There is associated temporal lobe hypogenesis *(arrow)*.

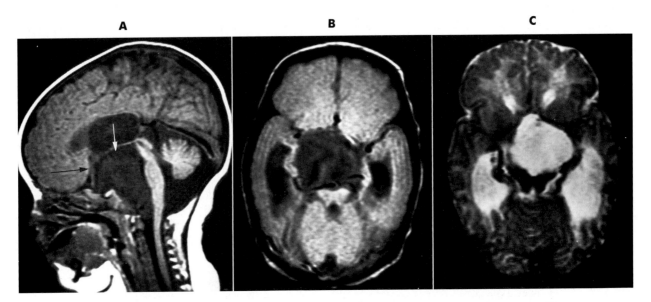

Fig. 3-39   A suprasellar cyst *(arrows)* causes mass effect on the third ventricle and brain stem with obstructive hydrocephalus. **A** and **B,** Short TR/short TE sagittal and axial images. **C,** Long TR/long TE image.

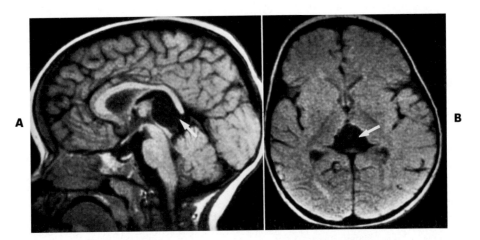

Fig. 3-40   A quadrigeminal region cyst is seen behind the third ventricle, displacing the quadrigeminal plate and splenium of the corpus callosum *(arrows)*. **A,** Sagittal short TR/short TE image. **B,** Axial short TR/short TE image.

tion. The characteristic findings of arachnoid cysts on CT and MRI are CSF-density masses that follow CSF-intensities throughout the sequences. Enhancement with iodine or gadolinium is unusual unless there is an inflammatory or reactive component. Particularly in the latter case, cystic tumor must be ruled out.

REFERENCES
Arachnoid cysts

1. Gandy SE, Heier LA: Clinical and magnetic resonance features of primary intracranial arachnoid cysts, *Ann J Neurol* 21:342, 1987.
2. Naidich TP, McClone DG, Radkowski MA: Intracranial arachnoid cysts, *Pediatr Neurosci* 12:112, 1985.
3. Robertson SJ, Wolpert SM, Runge VM: MR imaging of middle cranial fossa arachnoid cysts: temporal lobe agenesis syndrome revisited, *AJNR* 10:1007, 1989.
4. Starkman SP, Brown TC, Linnell EA: Cerebral arachnoid cysts, *Neuropathol Exp Neurol* 17:484, 1958.

Developmental disorders of the pituitary gland

Samuel M. Wolpert

With the evolution of MRI there has been a dramatic improvement in imaging of the pituitary gland, the hypothalamus, and the infundibulum, as well as the determination of their relationships to other suprasellar and parasellar structures. As a result MRI has become an important tool for investigating a number of developmental abnormalities of the pituitary gland and the hypothalamopituitary axis. In this section the development of the gland and its normal and abnormal appearances are presented.

The anterior and posterior lobes of the pituitary gland develop separately and from different origins. The anterior pituitary gland (adenohypophysis) develops from Rathke's cleft, which becomes separated from the oropharynx at 6 weeks of age. Cells of the anterior pituitary proliferate until the lobe constitutes 90% of the total gland at midgestation and 78% at term.[3] The posterior pituitary (neurohypophysis) develops as a downgrowth of the hypothalamus. The infundibulum can be identified at 6 weeks, and a rudimentary posterior lobe is seen at 34 months.[3] Fetal histochemical studies have shown considerable differentiation and activity of the pituitary cells during gestation. On T1-weighted imaging the pituitary gland at birth has a uniformly high signal involving both the anterior and posterior lobes, as compared with the adjacent brain.[14] Possibly the rapid differentiation of the gland in utero with an accompanying increase in protein synthetic activity could account for the short T1 values. With growth of the infant the high signal intensity of the anterior lobe disappears, but the posterior pituitary remains as a high intensity structure. This differential hyperintensity is quantitatively evident by 18 days[13] and is visible by the age of 6 weeks. Possibly the decrease in intensity of the anterior pituitary gland is the result of a reduction of its high synthetic protein activity to normal. The hyperintensity of the posterior pituitary is probably caused by its phospho-

lipid content,[10] although another theory attributes the high intensity to vasopressin and its neurophysin-carrier protein.[7] The bright signal of the posterior pituitary gland is seen in between 90% and 100% of healthy subjects.[5,7] Rarely, even in patients without pituitary dysfunction, is the posterior pituitary gland seen on MRI as ectopically situated in the region of the hypothalamus,[4] although this is controversial.[1]

The normal posterior pituitary hyperintensity may be absent in patients with central diabetes insipidus, pituitary dwarfism, and sella and parasellar tumors.[6,8,9] Patients with central diabetes insipidus may have an underlying abnormality such as germinoma, hypothalamic glioma, or histiocytosis. Gd-DTPA administration may be indicated in patients with unexplained diabetes insipidus to detect these processes (see Chapters 2 and 7 and Fig. 2-50), and MR imaging in such patients may show thickening of the infundibulum.[12] Absence of the normal posterior pituitary hyperintense signal with its ectopic location in the hypothalamus has been demonstrated in over 40% of patients with idiopathic growth hormone deficiency.[2] The gland is much more likely to be ectopically situated if there are multiple hormone deficiencies than if an isolated growth hormone deficiency is present. Kuroiwa et al.[11] found an association of an ectopic pituitary gland and perinatal asphyxia in patients with pituitary dwarfism.

REFERENCES
Developmental disorders of the pituitary gland

1. Abrahams JJ: Ectopia of the posterior gland or lipoma, *AJNR* 12:579, 1991 (letter to the editor).
2. Abrahams JJ, Trefelner E, Boulware S: Idiopathic growth hormone deficiency: MR findings in 35 patients, *AJNR* 12:155, 1991.
3. Asa SL, Kovacs K: Functional morphology of the human fetal pituitary. In Sommers SG, Rosen PP: *Pathology annual*, Norwalk, CT, 1984, Appleton-Century-Crofts.
4. Benshoff ER, Katz BH: Ectopia of the posterior pituitary gland as a normal variant: assessment with MR imaging, *AJNR* 11:709, 1990.
5. Columbo N, Berry I, Kucharczyk J, et al: Posterior pituitary gland: appearance on MR images in normal and pathologic states, *Radiology* 165:481, 1987.
6. El Gammal T, Brooks BS, Hoffman WH: MR imaging of the ectopic bright signal of posterior pituitary regeneration, *AJNR* 10:323, 1989.
7. Fujisawa I, Asato R, Nishimura K, et al: Anterior and posterior lobes of the pituitary gland: assessment by 1.5 T MR imaging, *J Comput Asst Tomogr* 11:214, 1987a.
8. Fujisawa I, Nishimura K, Asato R, et al: Posterior lobe of the pituitary in diabetes insipidus: MR findings, *J Comput Asst Tomogr* 11:221, 1987b.
9. Kelly WM, Kucharczyk W, Kucharczyk J, et al: Posterior pituitary ectopia: an MR feature of pituitary dwarfism, *AJNR* 9:453, 1988.
10. Kucharczyk W, Lenkinski RE, Kucharczyk J, et al: The effect of phospholipid vesicles on the NMR relaxation of water: an explanation for the MR appearance of the neurohypophysis? *AJNR* 11:693, 1990.
11. Kuroiwa T, Okabe Y, Hasuo K, et al: MR imaging of pituitary dwarfism, *AJNR* 12:161, 1991.
12. Tien RD, Newton TH, McDermott MW, et al: Thickened pituitary stalk on MR images in patient with diabetes insipidus and Langerhans' cell histiocytosis, *AJNR* 11:703, 1990.
13. Triulza F, Scotti G, Beccaria L, et al: MRI T1-weighted anterior pituitary hyperintensity in newborns, Presented at XIV Symposium Neuroradiologicum, London, 1990.
14. Wolpert SM, Osborne M, Anderson ML, et al: The bright pituitary gland: a normal MR appearance in infancy, *AJNR* 9:1, 1988.

NORMAL DEVELOPMENT OF BONE MARROW OF THE SKULL

Normally with aging there is a progressive conversion of red to yellow bone marrow (see Chapter 10). Red marrow is manifested by MRI on T1-weighted images as low signal intensity in the clivus and in the diploic space of the calvarium.[1]

The conversion from red to yellow bone marrow initially occurs in the presphenoid portion of the sphenoid bone and is first seen between the latter months of the first year of life and age 2.[1] This conversion is apparent on MRI as an increased signal intensity on T1-weighted images. At about 3 years of age high signal intensity areas are seen in the basiocciput, basisphenoid, and calvarium. These areas are patchy at first but coalesce with time. It is important to appreciate these normal appearances because they serve as visual aids in the detection of abnormal bone, for example, as found in leukemia and the chronic anemias (see Chapter 10).

NORMAL DEVELOPMENT OF BRAIN IRON

There are certain sites in the brain where nonhemic iron preferentially accumulates.[2] In decreasing order of frequency the sites are the globus pallidus, red nucleus, substantia nigra, subthalamic nucleus, dentate nucleus of cerebellum, and putamen. There is no detectable ferric iron in the brain at birth. Iron stains demonstrate iron in the globus pallidus at 6 months followed by the substantia nigra at 9 to 12 months, the red nucleus at 18 to 24 months, and the dentate nucleus at 3 to 7 years.[2,3]

By MRI the iron accumulation appears as areas of decreased intensity on T2-weighted scans (T2 shortening). The changes are better demonstrated on high-field than on low-field magnets. The changes on iron stains occur much earlier than they become evident on MRI scans. The T2 shortening is noticeable in the globus pallidus, substantia nigra, and red nucleus at 9 to 10 years of age.[1] Similar changes occur in the dentate nuclei of the cerebellum at about age 15 (see Chapters 1 and 2).

REFERENCES
Normal development of bone marrow of the skull

1. Barkovich AJ: Normal development of the neonatal and infant brain. In Barkovich AJ, editor: *Pediatric neuroimaging*, New York, 1990, Raven.

REFERENCES
Normal development of brain iron

1. Barkovich AJ: Normal development of the neonatal and infant brain. In Barkovich AJ, editor: *Pediatric neuroimaging*, New York, 1990, Raven.
2. Drayer B, Burger P, Darvin R., et al; Magnetic resonance imaging of brain iron, *AJNR*, 7:373, 1986.
3. Seitelberger F: Pigmentary disorders. In Minckler J, editor: *Pathology of the nervous system*, New York, 1972, McGraw-Hill.

4 · Metabolic and Degenerative Disorders

Samuel M. Wolpert
Mary L. Anderson
Edward M. Kaye

Metabolic disorders are conditions in which there is an abnormality in one or more metabolic pathways, producing disease or impairing function.[2] The disorders occur at the cellular or subcellular level, and structural anomalies are minimal. The great majority of the disorders are hereditary, most being autosomal recessive. Diagnosis is important because early recognition can lead to successful treatment; even those conditions that cannot be treated have genetic familial implications.

A genetic disorder has a predictable result. It may result from complete failure of synthesis of a specific enzyme, production of an abnormal enzyme, or lack of an activator or protective protein necessary for formation of an enzyme. Metabolic disorders should be suspected in the following situations: (1) unexplained abnormalities such as acidosis or hyperammonemia, (2) intolerance to certain classes of foods, (3) severe mental retardation with no other acceptable explanation, (4) familial clustering of mental retardation or a neurological disorder, and (5) clinical features characteristic of a specific metabolic disease.

The majority of these autosomal recessive disorders are present at birth, but symptoms may not occur until much later. If the only manifestation is delayed development, this will probably not be recognized until 6 to 12 months of age or later. Some disorders such as Wilson's disease do not become symptomatic until later in life.

Metabolic diseases of childhood can be classified in different ways. The ideal radiological classification would

Table 4-1 Changes in metabolic diseases

	White matter		Basal ganglia		Cerebellum		Cortex	Other
	CT	MRI	CT	MRI	CT	MRI	CT or MRI	
Phenylketonuria	LD	T2>						Microcephaly, migrational anomalies
Homocystinuria								Arterial and venous thrombosis, infarcts, atrophy, bony changes
Nonketotic hyperglycinemia	LD	T2>			Atrophy			Atrophy
Maple syrup urine disease	LD	T2>	LD	T2>	LD	T2>		
Glutaric aciduria 1	LD	T2>	LD	T2>			Frontal and temporal atrophy	
Other acidurias	LD	T2>	LD	T2>			Atrophy	Subdural collections
Urea cycle metabolism disorders	LD	T2>					Atrophy	Subdural collections
Oculocerebrorenal syndrome	LD	T2>					Atrophy	Calvarial scalloping
Galactosemia	LD	T2>						Reversible edema (?)
Mucopolysaccharidosis	LD	T2>	LD	T2>				See Table 4-2
Metachromatic leukodystrophy	LD (especially frontally)	T2>						Megalencephaly, no enhancement
Krabbe's disease	LD	T2>	HD	T2< T1>	HD	T2< T1>	Atrophy	Pontine and internal
Anderson-Fabry disease			LD	T2>				capsule involvement
GM₁ gangliosidosis	LD	T2>	LD			Atrophy	Atrophy	Megalencephaly, delayed myelination, vertebral body beaking, thickened long bones, spatulate ribs
GM₂ gangliosidosis	LD		LD					Megalencephaly, thalamic hyperdensity in Sandhoff
Leigh's disease	LD	T2>	LD	T2>			T2>	Brain stem often involved
Kearns-Sayre syndrome	LD, Calcification	T2>	LD, Calcification	T2>	LD	T2>	Atrophy	Extrapyramidal tracts T2>, Brain stem and thalamus involved
MELAS syndrome	LD	T2>	Calcification	T2>	Atrophy	T2>	LD T2>	Angiography: capillary blush, infarcts; CT: enhancement, single photon emission computed tomography changes
MERRF syndrome	LD				LD		LD	Atrophy
Menkes' syndrome	LD		Calcification		Atrophy		Atrophy	Extracerebral hematomas and effusions, tortuous arteries, bony changes

Disease	CT	MRI	Other findings	Comments
Marinesco-Sjögren syndrome			Atrophy	
Infantile bilateral striatal necrosis	LD	T1<; T2>		
Zellweger syndrome		T2>		Disorders of neuronal migration
Neonatal leukodystrophy	LD			
Adrenoleukodystrophy	LD with CE periatrial usually T2> calcifications	T2>	LD (infants)	White matter CE in pseudoneonatal variant; Gd-DTPA enhancement of zone 2, corpus callosum involvement
Adrenomyeloneuropathy		T1<; T2>	Atrophy	
Schilder's disease		LD with CE; T2>	Atrophy	Mimicks MS or tumor
Neuronal ceroid lipofuscinosis				
Alpers' syndrome				
Huntington's chorea				Caudate head atrophy
Hallervorden-Spatz disease	LD; HD	T1<; T2<	T2>	Iron, melanin
Fahr's disease	Calcification	T1<	Calcification	
Wilson's disease	LD	T2>	T2>; Atrophy	
Cockayne's syndrome	Calcification	T2>	Atrophy	Brain stem T2>; Microcephaly; Enlarged fourth ventricle, brain stem atrophy
Friedreich's ataxia			Atrophy	
Olivopontocerebellar atrophy			Atrophy	Enlarged fourth ventricle, brain stem atrophy
Ataxia-telangiectasia			Atrophy	
Pelizaeus-Merzbacher syndrome	T2>	T2<		Hypomyelination, conatal and classic types; Megalencephaly
Canavan's disease	LD	T1<; T1>; T2>; T2<		
Alexander's disease	LD (f)	T2>; LD with CE; T2> (f)		Megalencephaly; Occasional subependymal HD on CT CE (see text)

<, Hypointensity; >, hyperintensity; LD, low density; HD, high density; CE, contrast enhancement; f, frontal preponderance.

categorize the diseases by the locations in which the pathological processes occur, that is, white matter, gray matter, or basal ganglia, and then use the location of the process to indicate the correct diagnosis. Unfortunately most of the conditions are not confined to single locations in the brain, and considerable overlap occurs (Table 4-1). Megalencephaly may accompany some of the metabolic diseases and should be the first differential feature considered when attempting to attain a diagnosis in a patient in whom a metabolic disease is suspected. Diseases in which megalencephaly occurs include maple syrup urine disease, Canavan's disease, Alexander's disease, and lysosomal disorders (Tay-Sachs disease, gangliosidoses, mucopolysaccharidoses, and metachromatic leukodystrophy).[1] Furthermore, certain patterns may help in establishing a differential diagnosis. Alexander's disease is characterized by frontal white matter lesions; adrenoleukodystrophy by occipital white matter lesions. Contrast enhancement occurs in the margins of the lesions in both conditions. Most of the other metabolic conditions manifest with nonspecific white matter lesions. Basal ganglia calcification is seen in Kearns-Sayre syndrome and Cockayne's syndrome, mitochondrial cytopathies, MELAS syndrome and MERRF syndrome, Fahr's disease, and Krabbe's disease. Thus, only a few neurodegenerative disorders exhibit distinctive features, and in most cases a combined neurological, biochemical, and radiological approach is necessary to establish the correct diagnosis.

This chapter is organized according to specific enzyme deficiencies, although in a number of diseases the deficient enzyme is not as yet known. Such diseases are classified by location. Only those errors of metabolism in which radiographic, CT, or MRI abnormalities have already been described will be presented.

REFERENCES

1. DeMyer W: Megalencephaly: Types and differential diagnosis. In Swaiman KF, editor: *Pediatric neurology: principles and practice*, St Louis, 1989, Mosby–Year Book.
2. Golden GS: Metabolic disorders. In Golden GS, editor: *Textbook of pediatric neurology*, New York, 1987, Plenum.

Amino acid disorders

PHENYLKETONURIA

Phenylketonuria results from the failure of phenylalanine hydroxylase to convert phenylalanine to tyrosine. Clinically the infants are normal at birth, but during the first 2 months of life, vomiting, which at times is projectile, and irritability are frequent. Delayed intellectual development becomes apparent before 1 year of age. Seizures, taking the form of infantile spasms, may occur. Tissue damage results from the continued exposure of the brain to high phenylalanine concentration during critical periods of active organ growth. Pathologically delayed migration of neuroblasts and cortical heterotopic gray matter and defective white matter myelination in the centrum semiovale and cerebellum occur.[17] On CT scans low-density areas are seen in the white matter

bilaterally.[1] Microcephaly is often present as well. Periventricular white matter high signal intensities are seen on T2-weighted scans[3] (Fig. 4-1). The MRI abnormalities have been shown to respond to dietary therapy.[26]

HOMOCYSTINURIA

Homocystinuria is an inborn error of methionine metabolism transmitted as an autosomal recessive trait. The condition is caused by a deficiency of cystathionine β synthase and manifested by multiple thromboembolic episodes, ectopia lentis, and mental retardation. When the thromboembolic events occur in the CNS, small infarcts may result. Hemiplegia and ultimately a picture resembling pseudobulbar palsy may occur. The prevalence is approximately 1:200,000 newborns.[24]

Pathologically the disease is characterized by abnormalities in collagen and elastin formation.[19] Homocystine-induced vascular injury is characterized by patchy endothelial desquamation.[9] In addition, thickened intima, frayed media muscle fibers, and fragmented elastica have been described.[19]

Radiographs reveal biconcavity of the posterior aspects of the vertebral bodies: "codfish vertebra."[25] In addition, scoliosis and osteoporosis become apparent in late childhood. Metaphyseal spicules, enlargement of the carpal bones, and selective retardation of the development of the lunate bone also occur.[21] Vascular thromboses, both arterial and venous, occur in 26% of patients.[29] Sagittal sinus and deep cerebral vein occlusions with infarction have been shown by CT and cerebral angiography.[22] Death may occur from coronary or renal artery occlusion, cerebrovascular accidents, or pulmonary embolism.

NONKETOTIC HYPERGLYCINEMIA

Nonketotic hyperglycinemia is a heritable disorder of amino acid metabolism in which large quantities of glycine accumulate in the plasma, urine, and CSF.[10] Clinical manifestations include seizures, abnormal muscle tone, and reflexes associated with severe developmental delay.[13] At autopsy vacuolation and decreased volume of the myelinated white matter, perhaps caused by myelinolysis, are seen.[23] CT demonstrates mild cerebral and cerebellar atrophy and deep hemisphere lucencies.[28] On MRI decreased or absent myelination within the supratentorial white matter is seen, whereas the myelination of the brain stem and cerebellum progresses normally.[20] An abnormally thin corpus callosum may also be seen on the MRI scan.[4] The cerebral atrophy, spongy myelinopathy, and retarded myelination found in this disease are similar to that found in cases of methylmalonic and proprionic acidemia, maple syrup urine disease, and phenylketonuria.

MAPLE SYRUP URINE DISEASE

Maple syrup urine disease, which has a prevalence of approximately 1:200,000 newborns,[24] is caused by a defect in the ability to decarboxylate the branched-chain amino acids valine, leucine, and isoleucine. Consequently their keto-acid metabolites accumulate in the urine, serum, and

A   B   C

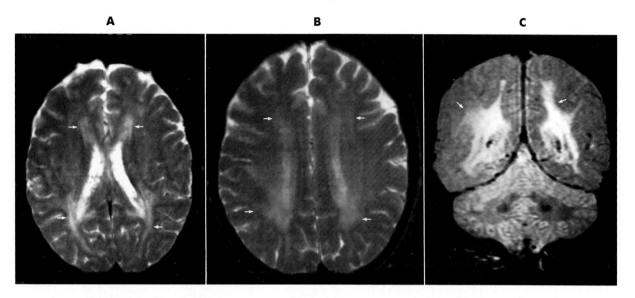

Fig. 4-1   MRI scans of phenylketonuria in a 35-year-old woman. High signal intensities are seen in the paraventricular and supraventricular areas on T2-weighted axial (spin echo, 3600/80 msec) *(arrows, **A** and **B**)* and coronal (spin echo, 3000/60 msec) *(arrow, **C**)* scans. (Courtesy G. Stimac, Seattle.)

CSF.[7] Clinically the disease is manifest by convulsions, stupor, coma, opisthotonus, and respiratory difficulties. Pathologically the cytoarchitecture of the cortex is generally immature with fewer than normal cortical layers. Also the number of oligodendrocytes and amount of myelin are less than normal.[17]

On CT symmetrical, well-defined low density areas occur in the white matter of both the cerebrum and the cerebellum.[15] Low densities may also occur in the globus pallidus and the thalami.[27] On T2 MRI high intensity changes have been described in the white matter of the cerebrum and cerebellum, and in the basal ganglia in the same areas involved on the CT scan.[27] After initiation of dietary therapy the CT abnormalities may improve, supporting the concept that early diagnosis and treatment are important for achieving maximum brain development.[15]

GLUTARIC ACIDURIA, TYPE I

In glutaric aciduria type I progressive CNS degeneration commences during the latter part of the first year of life. The disease is an autosomal recessive inborn error of lysine, hydroxylysine, and trytophan metabolism.[8] Diffuse low density changes in the white matter and frontal and temporal lobe atrophy have been observed on CT[30] and MRI scans.[2] On MRI high intensity areas are also seen in the white matter in a similar location to abnormalities found on CT (Fig. 4-2). Basal ganglia lesions may also be present.

METHYLMALONIC AND PROPIONIC ACIDURIAS

A number of disorders of intermediary metabolism, manifested by intermittent episodes of vomiting, lethargy, ketosis, and acidosis and with radiological abnormalities, have been recently described. Although the enzymatic

lesions responsible for methylmalonic and propionic acidurias are not related, the lesions are grouped together here for convenience.

Both methylmalonic and propionic aciduria are autosomal recessive disorders of aminoacid metabolism involving the conversion of propionate to succinate. The neurological abnormalities can in most patients be attributed to the attendant ketosis. The cerebral pathological abnormalities are similar to those found in phenylketonuria—retarded myelination and spongy degeneration of the white matter.[17] Leukoencephalopathy (decreased white matter density) with diffuse loss of cerebral substance and ventricular enlargement is seen on CT.[6] Basal ganglia lucencies may also be seen.[12]

DEFECTS IN THE UREA CYCLE METABOLISM

Five inborn errors of metabolism occur in the conversion of ammonia to urea. These include argininosuccinicaciduria, citrullinuria, hyperargininemia, ornithine transcarbamylase deficiency, and carbamyl phosphate synthetase deficiency. Radiographic abnormalities have been reported in cases of ornithine transcarbamylase deficiency in which CT has shown diffuse low density of the cerebral white matter with small ventricles.[5,11] With prolonged survival cerebral atrophy occurs and the ventricles increase in size. Extracerebral fluid collections may also develop.

OCULOCEREBRORENAL SYNDROME

Oculocerebrorenal syndrome (Lowe's syndrome) is characterized by severe mental retardation, myopathy, and congenital glaucoma or cataract. Biochemically the disease, which is autosomally recessive, is marked by aminoaciduria, renal tubular acidosis, and hypophosphatemic rickets.[14] Neuropathologically, parenchymal vacuolation with

A   B   C

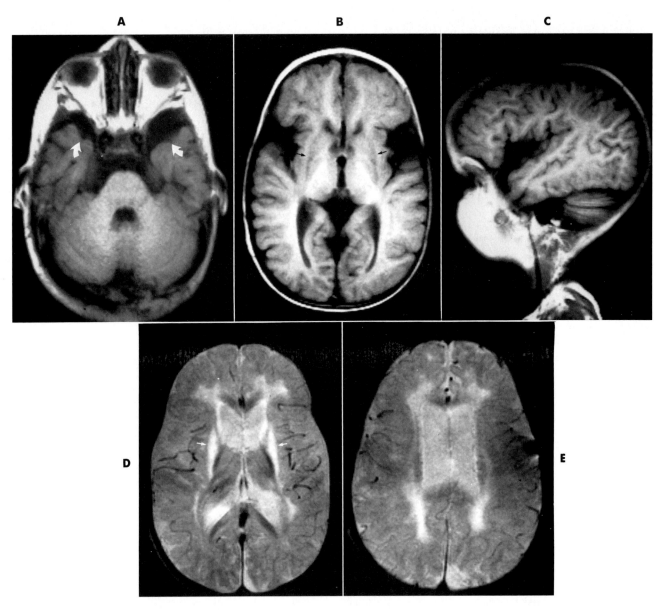

D   E

Fig. 4-2   MRI scans of glutaric aciduria type 1 in a 2-year-old girl. Temporal lobe atrophy is noted on axial and sagittal T1-weighted scans (spin echo, 600/17 msec) *(arrows,* **A** to **C***)*. Note also low signal intensities *(arrows)* on T1-weighted scan **(B)** and high intensity signal on T2-weighted (spin echo, 3000/70 msec) scan *(arrows,* **D***)* in both putamina. High intensity signals are also seen in frontal and occipital periventricular white matter **(E).**

rarefaction of the molecular layer of the cerebral cortex has been described.[16] CT scans demonstrate marked scalloping of the calvarium, especially in the occipital regions, together with mild, generalized ventricular dilatation and extensive periventricular decreased density.[18] Patchy, irregular, high intensity areas are seen on T2 MRI in the periventricular white matter.[18]

REFERENCES
Amino acid disorders

1. Behbehani AW, Krtsh H, Shulte FJ: Cranial computerized tomography in phenylketonuria, *Neuropediatrics* 12:295, 1981.
2. Bergman I, Finegold D, Gartner JC, et al: Acute profound dystonia in infants with glutaric acidemia, *Pediatrics* 83:228, 1989.
3. Brismar J, Aqeel A, Gascon G, et al: Malignant hyperphenylalaninemia: CT and MR of the brain, *AJNR* 11:135, 1990.
4. Dobyns WB: Agenesis of the corpus callosum and gyral malformations are frequent manifestations of nonketotic hyperglycinemia, *Neurology* 39:817, 1989.
5. Faerber EN: Degenerative and metabolic diseases. In Faerber EN, editor: *Cranial computed tomography in infants and children,* Philadelphia, 1986, JB Lippincott.
6. Gebarski SS, Gabrielsen TO, Knake JE, et al: Cerebral CT findings in methylmalonic and propionic acidemias, *AJNR* 4:955, 1983.
7. Golden GS: Metabolic disorders. In Golden GS, editor: *Textbook of pediatric neurology,* New York, 1987, Plenum.
8. Goodman SI, Norenberg MD, Shiles RH: Glutaric aciduria: clinical and laboratory findings in two brothers, *J Pediatr* 90:746, 1977.
9. Harker LA, Slichter SJ, Scott CR, et al: Homocystinemia: vacular injury and arterial thrombosis, *N Engl J Med* 291:537, 1974.
10. Hayasaka K, Tada K, Fueki N, et al: Nonketotic hyperglycinemia: analyses of glycine cleavage system in typical and atypical cases, *J Pediatr* 110:873, 1987.
11. Kendall B, Kingsley DPE, Leonard JV, et al: Neurological features and computed tomography of the brain in children with ornithine carbamoyl transferase deficiency, *J Neurol Neurosurg Psychiatry* 46:28, 1983.
12. Korf B, Wallman JK, Levy HL: Bilateral lucency of the globus pallidus complicating methylmalonic acidemia, *Ann Neurol* 20:364, 1986.
13. Langan TJ, Pueschel SW: Nonketotic hyperglycinemia, *Curr Prob Pediatr* 13:1, 1983.
14. Lowe CU, Terry M, MacLachlan EA: Organic-aciduria, decreased renal ammonia production, hydrophthalmos and mental retardation: a clinical entity, *Am J Dis Child* 83:164, 1952.
15. Mantovani JF, Naidich TP, Prensky AL, et al: MSUD: presentation with pseudotumor cerebri and CT abnormalities, *J Pediatr* 96:279, 1980.
16. Martin MA, Sylvester PE: Clinicopathological studies of oculocerebrorenal syndrome of Lowe, Terry and MacLachlan, *J Ment Defic Res* 24:1, 1980.
17. Menkes JH: Metabolic diseases of the nervous system. In Menkes JH, editor: *Textbook of child neurology,* ed 3, Philadelphia, 1985, Lea & Febiger.
18. O'Tuama L, Laster DW: Oculocerebrorenal syndrome: case report with CT and MR correlates, *AJNR* 8:555, 1987.
19. Perry TL: Homocystinuria: other metabolic disorders with nervous system involvement. In Vinken PJ, Bruyn GW: *Handbook of clinical neurology,* Amsterdam, 1981, North Holland.
20. Press GA, Barshop B, Haas R, et al: Abnormalities of the brain in nonketotic hyperglycinemia: MR manifestations, *AJNR* 10:315, 1989.
21. Schedewie H, Willich E, Grobe H, et al: Skeletal findings in homocystinuria: a collaborative study, *Pediatr Radiol* 1:12, 1973.
22. Schwab FJ, Peyster RG, Brill CB: CT of cerebral venous thrombosis in a child with homocystinuria, *Pediatr Radiol* 17:244, 1987.
23. Shuman RM, Leech RN, Scott CR: The neuropathology of the nonketotic and ketotic hyperglycinemias: three cases, *Neurology* 28:139, 1978.
24. Stanbury JB, Wyngaarden JB, Frederikson DS, et al: Inborn errors of metabolism in the 1980s. In Stanbury, Wyngaarden JB, Frederikson DS, et al, editors: *The metabolic basis of inherited disease,* ed 5, New York, 1983, McGraw-Hill.
25. Thomas PS, Carson NAJ: Homocystinuria: the evolution of skeletal changes in relation to treatment, *Ann Radiol* 21:95, 1978.
26. Thompson AS, Smith I, Brenton D, et al: Neurological deterioration in young adults with phenylketonuria, *Lancet* 336:602, 1990.
27. Uziel G, Savoiardo M, Nardocci N: CT and MRI in maple syrup urine disease, *Neurology* 38:486, 1988.
28. Valavanis A, Schubiger O, Hayek J: Computed tomography in nonketotic hyperglycinemia, *Comput Tomogr* 5:265, 1981.
29. Wilcken B, Turner G: Homocystinuria in New South Wales, *Arch Dis Child* 53:242, 1978.
30. Yager JY, McClarty BM, Seshia SS: CT-scan findings in an infant with glutaric aciduria type 1., *Dev Med Child Neurol* 30:808, 1988.

Carbohydrate metabolism disorders
GALACTOSEMIA

In children with galactosemia, an autosomal recessive disorder, the conversion of galactose to glucose-1-phosphate is defective.[3] The disease is manif st by the development of cataracts, failure to thrive, vomiting, diarrhea, and hepatomegaly. In one CT report decreased attenuation throughout the white matter with relative sparing of the basal ganglia was described.[2] These changes dramatically resolved after 20 months of milk restriction. The low density was thought to be probably caused by intracerebral edema.[1]

REFERENCES
Carbohydrate metabolism disorders

1. Belman AL, Moshe SL, Zimmerman RD: Computed tomographic demonstration of cerebral edema in a child with galactosemia, *Pediatrics* 78:606, 1986.
2. Marano GD, Sheils WS, Gabriele OF, et al: Cranial CT in galactosemia, *AJNR* 8:1150, 1987.
3. Menkes JH: Metabolic diseases of the nervous system. In Menkes JH, editor: *Textbook of child neurology,* ed 3, Philadelphia, 1985, Lea & Febiger.

Disorders of lysosomal enzymes
MUCOPOLYSACCHARIDOSES

Lysosomes are cytoplasmic vesicles containing enzymes that degrade the products of cellular catabolism. The number of types and variants of the mucopolysaccharidoses have expanded greatly in recent years. Several of them affect the CNS, presenting as progressive degenerative disorders with resultant mental retardation. In all these conditions degradation of the mucopolysaccharoids is defective because of the absence of lysosome hydrolyases. As a result, the mucopolysaccharides accumulate in many different organs in the body.

Table 4-2　Abnormalities of the brain in patients with mucopolysaccharidoses

	All mucopolysaccharidoses	Hurler	Hunter	Scheie	Sanfilippo	Morquio	Maroteaux-Lamy
Macrocephaly	+						
Thick cranial meninges		+		<Hurler*			
White matter low density		+	+	+	+		+
T2 high intensity		+	+	+	+		+
Communicating hydrocephalus		+	+	+			
Atrophy		+			+	+	
Suprasellar arachnoid cyst		+		+			
White matter cavities		+	+	+			+
Basal ganglia/thalamic low density		+		+			
Atlantoaxial subluxation						+	+
Thick spinal meninges		+	+		+	+	+
Gibbus/kyphus		+				+	
Kyphoscoliosis		+				+	
Platyspondyly		+				+	

*Thick cranial meninges also occur in Scheie's disease but less so than with Hurler's disease.

Hurler's disease, Hunter's disease, Hurler-Scheie disease, Sanfilippo's B syndrome, Brailsford-Morquio disease, Maroteaux-Lamy syndrome

Macrocrania is a feature of many of the mucopolysaccharidoses. This may be due to vault thickening by mucopolysaccharide deposits and be evident on skull radiography and on CT. Megalencephaly may be caused by mucopolysaccharide deposits in the brain. Thickening of the skull may also result from inner table bone deposition after shunt relief of the hydrocephalus.[28]

Imaging studies of the brain in patients with mucopolysaccharidoses usually demonstrate white matter changes and hydrocephalus (Table 4-2). In Hurler's disease, a disease with a prevalence of approximately 1:100,000 newborns,[26] there are widespread changes in the CNS.[14] The disease is transmitted through an autosomal recessive inheritance pattern. The leptomeninges are edematous and thickened. Accumulating mucopolysaccharides produce partial obstruction of the subarachnoid spaces, which, in conjunction with a narrowed foramen magnum, results in communicating hydrocephalus.[28] Arachnoid cysts may also occur. Although the neurons are swollen and vacuolated, particularly in the cerebral cortex, the density of the gray matter is normal on CT. Low density areas are seen in the white matter,[11] particularly around the dilated frontal horns but also in the parietal white matter. The latter correlates well with the pitting and cavitation around blood vessels caused by an excessive concentration of foam cells within the Virchow-Robin spaces.[29] Greatly dilated periadventitial spaces filled with viscous fluid and mesenchymal elements may also explain the low attenuation of the white

matter.[6] Increased signal in the white matter on T2-weighted MR images[10,23] correlate with the CT findings.

Hydrocephalus and white matter changes may also be present in Hunter's disease and Sanfilippo's B syndrome. The prolonged signal in the white matter on T2-weighted MRI in Hunter's disease probably represents dilated perivascular spaces.[17] Ventriculomegaly is also usually present. Hunter's disease is distinguished from the other mucopolysaccharidoses by transmission through an X-linked recessive inheritance. Hunter's disease has a prevalence of approximately 1:150,000 newborns.

The ventricular and white matter changes in Hurler-Scheie disease are similar to those in Hurler's and Hunter's diseases, although the leptomeningeal changes are usually less prominent than those in Hurler's disease.[6] Low density changes may be seen on CT in the basal ganglia and thalamus (Fig. 4-3, A) Patients with Scheie's disease may survive into the third decade. Suprasellar arachnoid cysts are seen in some patients with Scheie's disease.[20]

Large ventricles and wide sulci suggestive of cerebral atrophy may also be seen in patients with Sanfilippo's disease[17] (Fig. 4-3, B and C) and in patients with Morquio's syndrome.[19] The changes in patients with the latter disease appear to become more pronounced with increasing age. Subcortical hyperintense areas may also be noted on MRI scans in patients with Sanfilippo's disease (Fig. 4-3, C).

Spinal cord compression can occur in Morquio's disease (Fig. 4-4) and in Maroteaux-Lamy syndrome.[3,7] One of two basic mechanisms may account for this: (1) laxity of the transverse odontoid ligament may allow atlantoaxial subluxation, particularly if there is hypoplasia or aplasia of the odontoid process[3]; (2) thickening of the spinal meninges may cause spinal cord compression. The thickening is also

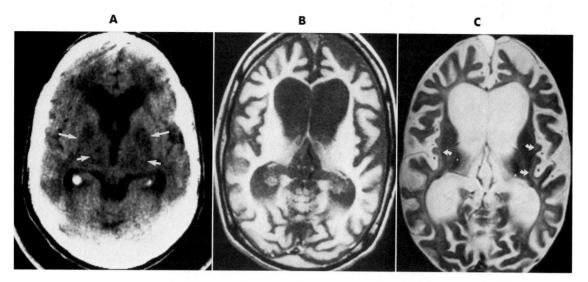

Fig. 4-3 A, Nonenhanced CT scan of a 28-year-old woman with Hurler-Scheie disease demonstrates low density changes in the basal ganglia, thalami *(arrows),* and white matter. Note also the ventriculomegaly. **B** and **C,** A 15-year-old girl with Sanfilippo disease. Note the enlarged lateral ventricles and wide sulci indicative of cerebral atrophy on both the T1-weighted (spin echo, 600/20 msec) and T2-weighted (spin echo, 2800/90 msec) images. A subcortical hyperintense stripe is also seen on the T2-weighted image *(C, arrows). (A* courtesy G. Stimac, Seattle; **B** and **C** courtesy A. Osborn, University of Utah, Salt Lake City.)

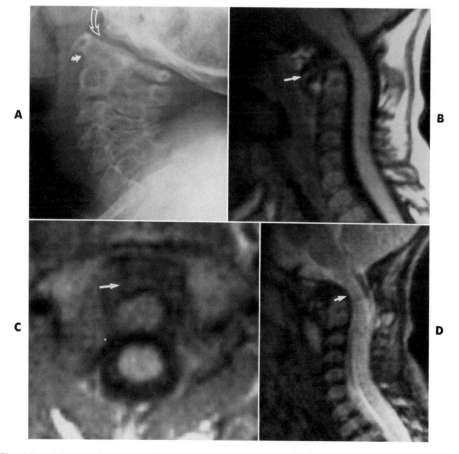

Fig. 4-4 A 6-year-old boy with hypotonia. **A,** Lateral cervical spine image demonstrates atlantoaxial *(solid arrow)* and atlantooccipital *(open arrow)* subluxation. **B** and **C,** T1-weighted MRI scans confirm the atlantoaxial subluxation *(arrows).* **D,** Angulation and minimal compression of the upper cervical cord is also seen on the T2-weighted image *(arrow).*

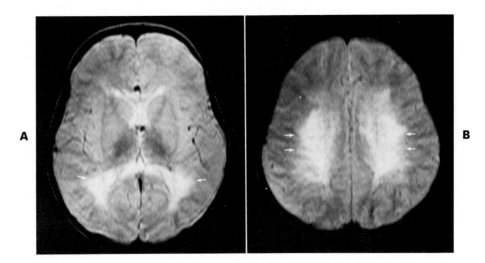

Fig. 4-5   A and **B,** A 2-year-old girl with metachromatic leukodystrophy presenting with weakness and abnormal nerve conduction studies. T2-weighted images (spin echo, 3000/70 msec) demonstrate increased signal in periatrial and supraventricular white matter *(arrows)*.

very common in Hurler's, Hunter's and Sanfilippo's B diseases. Whatever the mechanism, the clinical problem is best evaluated by MRI.

Radiographic changes in the skeleton are extensive in mucopolysaccharidoses and have been described by Caffey.[5] Among the abnormalities are swelling of the diaphysis of the humerus, shortening of the ulna and the radius, epiphyseal irregularity and thickening, and irregularity of the metacarpal bones. Changes present in the lower extremity are less marked. The anterior ends of the ribs are often splayed, and the anterior ends of the clavicles may be widened.

In Morquio's syndrome spine radiographs are distinctive and show platyspondyly and a characteristic central beak protruding from the anterior ends of the vertebral bodies. Anterior wedging may result in varying degrees of kyphosis or kyphoscoliosis, which may also produce spinal cord compression.[3] Beaking and kyphosis may also be seen in other mucopolysaccharidoses, but less so than in Morquio's disease and Hurler's disease (see Chapter 9).

SPHINGOLIPIDOSES
Metachromatic leukodystrophy

Metachromatic leukodystrophy is an autosomal recessive disorder due to deficiency of the enzyme arylsulfatase-A.[9] As a result metachromatic lipid material, galactosylceramide sulfatide, accumulates in the peripheral and central nervous system, mainly in the white matter. The number of oligodendrocytes is diminished, diffuse demyelination occurs, and the metachromatic granules accumulate either free in the tissues or within glial cells and macrophages. The prevalence of the disease is 1:100,000 newborns.[26] The disease may be classified into infantile, juvenile, and adult forms with 80% of cases occuring in childhood. The disorder is characterized by a disorder of gait, impairment

of speech, spasticity, and the gradual occurrence of intellectual deterioration. Optic atrophy occurs, and the disease is inexorable, death occurring within 6 months to 4 years after the onset of symptoms.

The CT appearances are those of moderate ventricular enlargement and low density lesions, progressing anteriorly to posteriorly within the white matter.[8,24] Contrast enhancement is not seen. There is a slight preponderance for the demyelinating process to occur in the frontal lobes.[24] Diffuse confluent high signal intensities are seen in the white matter on T2-weighted MRI[21] (Fig. 4-5).

Globoid cell dystrophy (Krabbe's disease)

There are three types of globoid cell dystrophy (Krabbe's disease): infantile, late infantile, and adult. The disease is autosomal recessive and is characterized by psychomotor deterioration, irritability, optic atrophy, and cortical blindness. Gait difficulty is seen in the older infant. Convulsions may occur later in the disease.[15] The disease is caused by a deficiency in galactosylceramide-B-galactosidase and has a prevalence of 1:50,000 births in Sweden but is much lower elsewhere.[26] Pathologically there is extensive demyelination of the white matter of the cerebrum, cerebellum, spinal cord, and their cortical projection fibers. In the areas of recent demyelination, mononuclear epitheloid cells and large multinucleated globoid cells are seen around the smaller blood vessels. It is not the mere presence of these globoid cells but their large number that is the distinguishing feature.

CT findings may be normal early in the course of the disease, but abnormal white matter low density areas subsequently appear[2] (Fig. 4-6, *A*). Later in the disease cerebral atrophy with large ventricles and wide sulci are seen. As expected, MRI demonstrates high intensity signal changes in the white matter consistent with prolonged T2

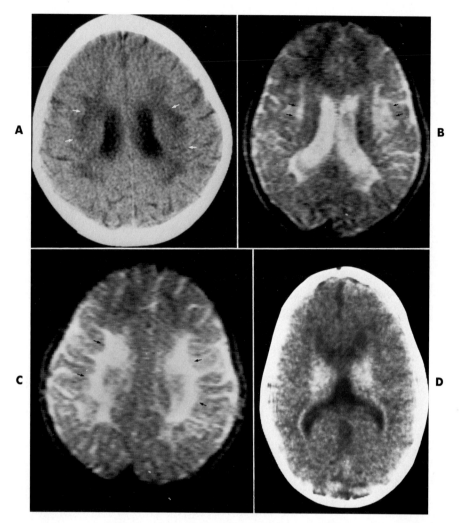

Fig. 4-6   **A,** CT scan in a boy with Krabbe's disease demonstrates low densities in the periventricular white matter *(arrows).* **B** and **C,** T2-weighted MRI scans demonstrate high intensities in the deep white matter *(arrows).* **D,** In another patient with Krabbe's disease, a 3-month-old girl, note the symmetrical high density areas in the thalami on the CT scan. (**A-C** courtesy Brownsworth R, et al: *Pediatr Neurol* 1:242, 1985; **D** courtesy E.S.K. Kwan: *AJNR* 5:453, 1984.)

values on T2-weighted scans[21] (Fig. 4-6, *B* and *C*). The white matter changes are thought to represent either edema from the abnormal accumulation of the cytotoxic substrates of galactosylceramide such as psychosine, which is highly toxic, or demyelination.[27]

High density lesions on CT have also been described in the thalami, corona radiata, and cerebellum.[12] (Fig. 4-6, *D*). These areas may also show markedly shortened T1 and T2 values, that is, slight increase in signal intensity on T1-weighted and decrease in intensity on T2-weighted scans, suggesting a paramagnetic effect.[1] These changes, although claimed to be specific for Krabbe's disease, are also seen in Hallervorden-Spatz disease (see below). Krabbe's disease is rapidly progressive and fatal.

Anderson-Fabry disease

Anderson-Fabry disease occurs in childhood and adolescence and causes lancinating pains and dysesthesias of the extremities. Later on a diffuse vascular involvement leads to hypertension, renal damage, cardiomegaly, myocardial ischemia, and thrombotic infarcts of the brain. The disease is inherited as an X-linked recessive trait with the primary deficit residing in the enzyme alpha-galactosidase. Lacunar pontine, pallidal, and internal capsule infarcts have been seen on CT and MRI scans.[16] Angiography is usually negative.

GM₁ gangliosidosis

The clinical pict/ure in GM$_1$ gangliosidosis, an autosomal recessive condition, is characterized by hypoactivity in a hypotonic infant sometimes accompanied by macrocephaly. The disease is caused by a deficiency in beta-galactosidase, which is needed to cleave the galactase moiety from the GM$_1$ molecule. As a result an abnormal accumulation of the GM$_1$ galactoside from a normal value of 20% of the brain's gangliosides to 80% to 90% may occur. Thoracolumbar kyphosis provides the basis for the characteristic radiographic changes of anterior beaking of the vertebral bodies.

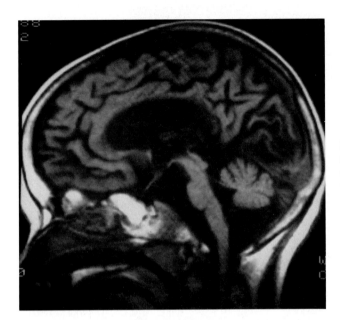

Fig. 4-7 Sagittal MRI scan (spin echo, 650/20 msec) in a 6-year-old girl with GM₁ gangliosidosis demonstrates cerebral and cerebellar atrophy as well as ventriculomegaly. Note also enlargement of interpeduncular and prepontine cisterns.

A   B   C

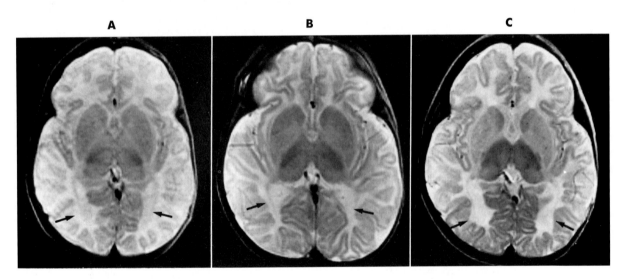

Fig. 4-8 Axial scans, all with spin echos of 3000/90 msec. Note the persistent high intensity white matter changes *(arrows)* at ages 2 months **(A)**, 5 months **(B)**, and 1 year **(C)** in a child with GM₁ gangliosidosis. Normally the white matter should not retain its hyperintensity relative to gray matter as myelination progresses and by the age of 1 year should be hypointense.

Periosteal cloaking of the long bones, spatulate ribs, and a shoe-shaped sella turcica are also seen.[22] White matter low densities have been described on CT scans in some patients[11] and cerebral atrophy in others.[13] Cerebral and cerebellar atrophy also may be seen on MRI (Fig. 4-7) along with delayed myelination (Fig. 4-8).

GM₂ gangliosidosis (Tay-Sachs and Sandhoff diseases)

Tay-Sachs disease, which is found chiefly in Jewish children of Ashkenazi descent with a prevalence of 1:3000 births,[26] is characterized by motor regression and a cherry-red spot in the retina.[14] Hexosaminidase A has been identified as the deficient enzyme. The inheritance pattern is autosomal recessive. Pathologically the brain is atrophic in the early stages, but later its weight is 20% to 50% greater than normal with broad cortical gyri and edematous, necrotic white matter.[18] CT may show moderate ventricular dilatation with symmetrical low attenuation in the cerebral white matter and basal ganglia.[11]

In Sandhoff disease both hexosaminidase A and B are deficient. The clinical syndrome is similar to that of Tay-Sachs disease. The thalamus may be hyperdense on nonenhanced CT and hypointense on T2 MRI.[4,25]

REFERENCES
Disorders of lysosomal enzymes

1. Baram TZ, Goldman AM, Percy AK: Krabbe's disease: specific MRI and CT findings, *Neurology* 36:111, 1986.
2. Barnes DM, Enzmann DR: The evolution of white matter disease as seen on computed tomography, *Radiology* 138:379, 1981.
3. Blaw ME, Langer LO: Spinal cord compression in Morquio-Brailsford disease, *J Pediatr* 74:593, 1969.
4. Brismar J, Brismar G, Coates R, et al: Increased density of the thalamus on CT scans in patients with GM_2 gangliosidoses, *AJNR* 11:125, 1990.
5. Caffey J: Gargoylism: (Hunter-Hurler disease, dysostosis multiplex, lipochondrodystrophy) prenatal and postnatal bone lesions and their early postnatal evolution, *Am J Roentgen* 67:715, 1952.
6. Dekaban AS, Constantopoulos G, Herman M, et al: Mucopolysaccharoidosis type V (Scheie's syndrome): a postmortem study by multidisciplinary technique with emphasis on the brain, *Arch Pathol Lab Med* 100:237, 1976.
7. Edwards MK, Harwood-Nash DC, Fitz CR, et al: CT metrizamide myelography of the cervical spine in Morquio's syndrome, *AJNR* 3:666, 1982.
8. Faerber EN: Degenerative and metabolic diseases. In Faerber EN, editor: *Cranial computed tomography in infants and children*, Philadelphia, 1986, JB Lippincott.
9. Golden GS: Metabolic disorders. In Golden GS, editor: *Textbook of pediatric neurology*, New York, 1987, Plenum.
10. Johnson M, Desai S, Hugh-Jones K, et al: Magnetic resonance imaging of the brain in Hurler's syndrome, *AJNR* 5:816, 1984.
11. Kingsley DPE, Kendall BE: Demyelinating and neurodegenerative diseases in childhood: CT appearances and their differential diagnosis, *J Neuroradiol* 8:243, 1981.
12. Kwan E, Drace J, Enzmann D: Specific CT findings in Krabbe's disease, *AJNR* 5:453, 1984.
13. Ludwig B, Kishikawa T, Wende S, et al: Cranial computed tomography in disorders of complex carbohydrate metabolism and related storage disorders, *AJNR* 4:431, 1983.
14. Menkes JH: Metabolic disorders of the nervous system. In Menkes JH, editor: *Textbook of child neurology*, ed 3, Philadelphia, 1985, Lea & Febiger.
15. Menkes JH: Heredodegenerative diseases. In Menkes JH, editor: *Textbook of child neurology*, ed 3, Philadelphia, 1985, Lea & Febiger.
16. Moumdjian R, Tampieri D, Melanson D, et al: Anderson-Fabry disease: A case report with MR, CT, and cerebral angiography, *AJNR* 10 supp:69, 1989.
17. Murata R, Nakajima S, Tanaka A, et al: MR imaging of the brain in patients with mucopolysaccharidosis, *AJNR* 10:1165, 1989.
18. Myrianthopoulos NC: GM_2 gangliosidosis. Type 1 (Tay-Sachs disease): lipidoses, mucolipidoses, and mucopolysaccharidoses. In Vinken PJ, Bruyn GW: *Handbook of clinical neurology*, Amsterdam, 1981, North Holland.
19. Nelson J, Grebbel FS: The value of computed tomography in patients with mucopolysaccharidosis, *Neuroradiology* 29:544, 1987.
20. Neuhauser EBD, Griscom NT, Gilles FH, et al: Arachnoid cysts in the Hurler-Hunter syndrome, *Ann Radiol* 11:434, 1967.
21. Nowell MA, Grossman RI, Hackney DB, et al: MR imaging of white matter diseases in children, *AJNR* 9:503, 1988.
22. O'Brien JS: Disorders of lysosomal enzymes: GM_1 gangliosidosis. In Stanbury JB, Wyngaarden JB, Frederikson DS, et al: *The metabolic basis of inherited disease*, ed 5, New York, 1983, McGraw-Hill.
23. Rauch RA, Friloux LA, Lott IT: MR imaging of cavitary lesions in the brain with Hurler-Scheie syndrome, *AJNR* 10:suppl1, 1989.
24. Schipper HI, Seidel D: Computed tomography in late-onset metachromatic leukodystrophy, *Neuroradiology* 26:39, 1984.
25. Stalker HP, Han BK: Thalamic hyperdensity: a previously unreported sign of Sandhoff disease, *AJNR* 10 suppl:82, 1989.
26. Stanbury JB, Wyngaarden JB, Frederikson DS, et al: Inborn errors of metabolism in the 1980s. In Stanbury JB, Wyngaarden JB, Frederikson DS, et al., editors: *The metabolic basis of inherited disease*, ed 5, New York, 1983, McGraw-Hill.
27. Swennerholm L, Vanier MT, Mansson JE: Krabbe's disease: a galactesylsphingosine (psychosine) lipidosis, *J Lipid Res* 21:53, 1980.
28. Watts RWE, Spellacy E, Kendall BE: Computed tomography studies in patients with mucopolysaccharidoses, *Neuroradiology* 21:9, 1981.
29. Winters PR, Harrad MJ, Molenich-Heetred SA, et al: a-L-iduronidase deficiency and possible Hurler-Scheie genetic compound, *Neurology* 26:1003, 1976.

Respiratory oxidative metabolic disorders (mitochondrial cytopathies)

Within the last 5 years a number of previously thought disparate and unrelated diseases have all been shown to result from defects in the major enzyme complexes of the respiratory chain. Since all the disorders are caused by abnormalities of mitochondrial function, they are considered under the heading of *mitochondrial cytopathies*. When the conditions involve, as they often do, the brain and muscles, the term *mitochondrial encephalopathy* has been coined.[32] The clinical presentation of these defects is extremely variable, with a spectrum from neonatal death to severe lactic acidosis to hypotonia in adults.[27]

Unfortunately, similar symptoms and signs may result from different biochemical defects, and conversely the same apparent biochemical lesion may induce a disparity of clinical presentations.[21] In general, the disorders manifest impairment of muscle function, congenital lactic acidosis, or progressive neurological dysfunction. Several relatively distinct clinical syndromes have been recognized.

LEIGH'S DISEASE

Otherwise known as subacute necrotizing encephalopathy, Leigh's disease is more prevalent in males. The disorder has been associated with a deficiency of cytochrome *c* oxidase,[27] defects in the pyruvate dehydrogenase complex, and defects in the electron transport chain (NADH coenzyme Q to reductase). Current opinion is that the disease results from a wide spectrum of mitochondrial disorders. The condition that manifests itself in the first 2 years of life is characterized pathologically by foci of necrosis and capillary proliferation within the basal ganglia, spinal cord, and brain stem, particularly the periaqueductal, periventricular, and tegmental gray matter.[9] The condition mimics Wernicke's encephalopathy except that the mamillary bodies are spared in Leigh's disease and the blood thiamine level is normal.

CT abnormalities include low density areas in the basal ganglia, especially in the putamen,[16] although cases of basal ganglia sparing with white matter involvement have also been described.[26] MRI offers a sensitive alternative to CT for lesion localization, and high intensity lesions in the brain stem, basal ganglia (especially putamina), cortex, and medulla have been described on T2-weighted images[8,15,19] (Figs. 4-9 and 4-10). Involvement of the white matter has also been seen on MRI scanning[8] (Fig. 4-10, *D*). The pattern of hyperintense lesions on T2-weighted images involving the basal ganglia and brain stem, with predomi-

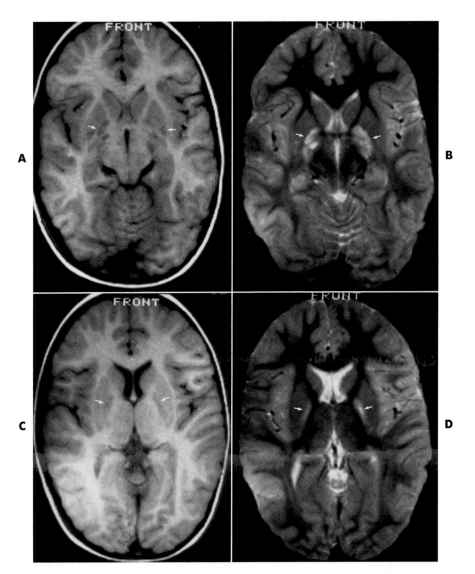

Fig. 4-9   Axial T1-weighted (spin echo, 650/20 msec) **(A** and **C)** and T2-weighted (spin echo, 3000/990 msec) **(B** and **D)** scans in a 5-year-old boy with Leigh's disease demonstrate low signal intensities **(A** and **C)** in the globus pallidi *(arrows)* that become high signal intensities **(B** and **D)** *(arrows).*

nant involvement of the putamen, is thought to be highly specific for Leigh's disease.[20] Whereas the changes involving the basal ganglia can also be seen in other conditions such as toxic encephalopathies and cerebral anoxia, the striking involvement of the brain stem nuclei is helpful in excluding these other diseases.[8] Agenesis of the corpus callosum has also been reported in patients with Leigh's disease[6] and in other metabolic diseases. The cause for the association is unknown.

KEARNS-SAYRE SYNDROME

Kearns-Sayre syndrome is a childhood disease that may be inherited as an autosomal dominant disorder, is more common in females, and is characterized by the triad of ophthalmoparesis, conduction heart block, and pigmentary degeneration of the retina. Muscular weakness with hypotonia, short stature, and mental deterioration often occur as well.[21] Biochemical abnormalities include elevated serum pyruvate, as well as deficiencies of the mitochondrial enzymes. Pathological studies have revealed spongy degeneration of the brain stem, white matter, basal ganglia, cortex, and thalamus. CT findings include symmetrical low densities in the white matter[7] and lentiform nuclei, as well as cerebral atrophy.[12] Low density areas in the midbrain and pons have also been reported and represent a particularly ominous sign.[25] Basal ganglia calcification, and occasionally white matter calcification, may accompany the low densities.[31]

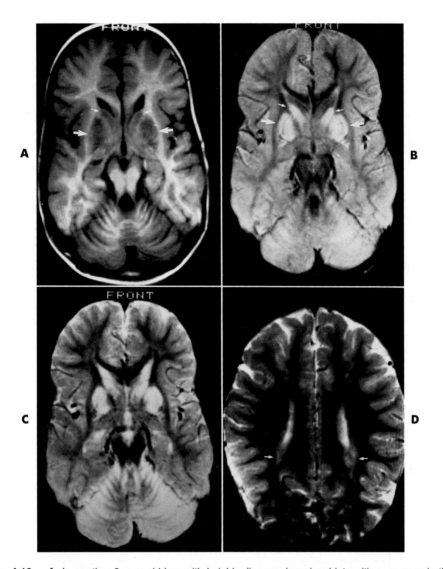

Fig. 4-10   **A,** In another 3-year-old boy with Leigh's disease, low signal intensities are seen in the heads of the caudate nuclei *(small arrows)* and putamina *(large arrows)* (spin echo, 650/20 msec). **B** and **C,** On the proton density **(B)** (spin echo, 3000/45 msec) and T2-weighted **(C)** (spin echo, 3000/90 msec) images, these areas are increased in intensity *(B, arrows).* **D,** Periventricular high intensity areas are also seen in periatrial areas bilaterally on a T2-weighted image. Cerebellar atrophy is also seen on axial T1-weighted image **(A).**

In a case report of the syndrome, high intensity lesions were seen on T2-weighted MRI scans in the dentate nuclei of the cerebellum, the superior cerebellar peduncles and substantia nigra, ventral lateral nucleus of the thalamus, medial aspect of the globus pallidus, and the white matter around the central sulcus.[10] These lesions correspond anatomically to the extrapyramidal pathways.

MELAS SYNDROME

MELAS syndrome (mitochondrial *m*yopathy, *e*ncephalopathy, *l*actic *a*cidosis, and *s*trokelike episodes), recently identified as a separate disease entity, is clinically characterized by dwarfism, vomiting, seizures, and recurrent strokes.[18] Important negative criteria, separating the condition from Kearns-Sayre syndrome, are lack of ophthalmoplegia, retinal degeneration, heart block, and myoclonus. NADH coenzyme Q reductase deficiency is possibly one cause of the syndrome.[18] The CT findings include focal low density areas, ventricular dilatation, and basal ganglia calcification. Cortical enhancement may be seen on postcontrast enhancement CT scans.[17] The low density areas, considered the result of infarction, occur predominantly in the parietal and occipital lobes.[3] On MRI high intensity lesions on T2-weighted scans have been seen in the cerebellar hemispheres and the temporal lobes, as well as in the parietal and occipital lobes[3,28] (Fig. 4-11). In a re-

A   B   C

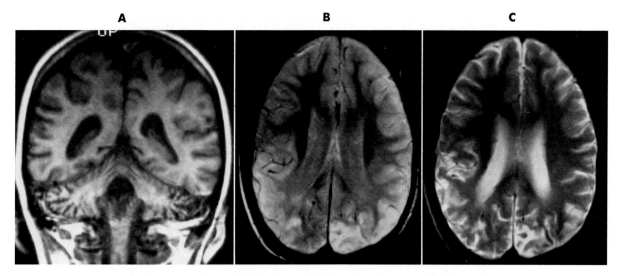

Fig. 4-11   MRI scans in a 14-year-old girl with MELAS syndrome demonstrating cerebellar atrophy on coronal T1-weighted image **(A)** (spin echo, 650/20 msec). On proton density **(B)** (spin echo, 3000/45 msec) and T2-weighted **(C)** (spin echo, 3000/90 msec) images, high intensity areas mimicking infarcts are seen in the posterior parietal cortex and subcortical areas *(arrows)*.

port on arteriography, a capillary blush and early venous filling without arterial occlusive changes were described. The blush corresponded well to the cortical enhancement seen on the CT scans.[17] Cerebellar atrophy has also been reported.[23,35] Single photon emission computed tomography of the brain utilizing I[123]-iodoamphetamine has shown both increased and decreased activity in parts of the brain which subsequently show the characteristic CT findings.[22]

MERRF SYNDROME

MERRF syndrome (*m*yoclonic *e*pilepsy with *r*agged *r*ed *f*ibers) is yet another recently identified mitochondrial disorder. The disease is characterized by myoclonic jerks and ataxia and is contrasted with the Kearns-Sayre syndrome by the absence of ophthalmoplegia and retinal degeneration.[21] The CT scan in one case report demonstrated basal ganglia calcification.[14] A positron emission tomography study carried out in an adult patient demonstrated a marked decrease in glucose utilization in all gray matter structures, with a preponderance of metabolic alterations in the posterior cortical regions and thalamus and a relative sparing of anterior cortical areas and basal nuclei.[11] Cerebral and cerebellar white matter degeneration may also occur.

MENKES' DISEASE

Menkes', or kinky-hair, disease is a lesion of the gray matter transmitted as a sex-linked disorder. Only males are affected, and the condition may be recognized at birth. Most patients die before 2 years of age.[13] The disease is characterized by a defect in the absorption of orally

administered copper. Scalp hair is sparse, coarse, stubby, and devoid of pigment. The prevalence is 1:100,000 newborns.

Because of the deficiency of copper, a variety of pathological changes are set in motion. The arteries are tortuous with irregular lumina and frayed, split intimal lining. As a result of infarction and edema, diffuse low density areas may be seen by CT.[29] Because of the brain tissue loss and accompanying severe cortical atrophy, bridging cortical veins may be torn with resulting extracerebral hematomas. Extracerebral effusions may also occur after severe brain atrophy and can be seen on CT or MRI[13,29] The tortuous intracranial arteries can also be seen on CT[13] and on MRI.[5,13] Cerebral arteriography is distinctive.[1,2] The cerebral arteries are elongated and excessively tortuous (Fig. 4-12) with considerable delayed flow. Similar changes are seen on abdominal arteriography. Radiographs of the long bones demonstrate symmetrical metaphyseal spurring and diaphyseal periosteal reactions.[34] These changes progress up to the age of 6 months and disappear at the age of 12 months. The ribs are flared, and the skull contains numerous wormian bones.

MARINESCO-SJÖGREN SYNDROME

Marinesco-Sjögren syndrome is a rare autosomal recessive condition characterized by the triad of congenital cataracts, congenital progressive ataxia, and mental retardation.[4,33] Since a myopathy is associated in the majority of the cases, the syndrome has been classified in this chapter under the mitochondrial encephalopathies, although the precise enzymatic deficiency and the microscopic confirmation that the mitochondria are at fault have not yet been

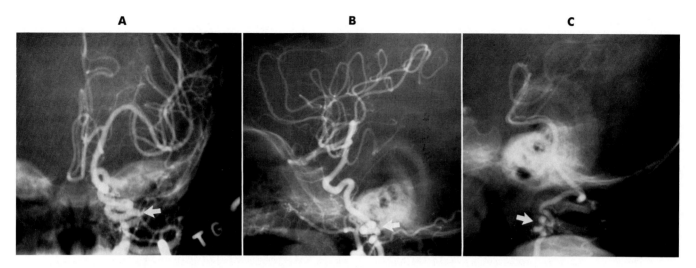

Fig. 4-12   Left carotid **(A** and **B)** and left vertebral **(C)** angiograms in a 3-month-old boy with Menkes' disease demonstrate marked tortuosity of the cervical internal carotid artery *(arrows)* as well as elongation of the internal carotid and proximal anterior and middle cerebral arteries. **C,** Vertebral angiogram shows similar elongation of the extracranial vertebral artery *(arrow)*, basilar, and posterior cerebral arteries.

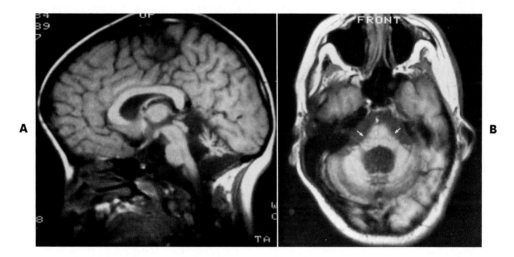

Fig. 4-13   Sagittal **(A)** and axial **(B)** T1-weighted (spin echo, 65/20 msec) MRI scans demonstrate marked cerebellar atrophy involving the hemispheres and vermis in a 11-year-old boy with Marinesco-Sjögren syndrome. Atrophy of the middle cerebellar peduncle *(arrows)* is also seen in **B.** No olivary atrophy was noted in this case. Note also the enlarged fourth ventricle caused by cerebellar atrophy.

established. Cerebellar atrophy together with olivary atrophy is seen pathologically and is evident on CT scans[36] and on T1-weighted MRI scans (Fig. 4-13). No abnormalities are seen supratentorially.

INFANTILE BILATERAL STRIATAL NECROSIS

A mitochondrially inherited progressive condition, infantile hereditary striatal necrosis is transmitted with a non-mendelian inheritance.[24] Clinically the disease is manifest by dystonia, some intellectual impairment, and muscle weakness. There is a close genetic relationship between infantile bilateral striatal necrosis and Leber's optic atrophy.

Bilateral symmetrical putaminal low densities are seen on the CT scan.[30] The caudate nuclei may be similarly involved. In one patient MRI demonstrated T1 hypointensities and T2 hyperintensities in the basal ganglia.[30]

REFERENCES
Respiratory oxidative metabolism disorders

 1. Adams PC, Strand RD, Bresnan MJ, et al: Kinky-hair syndrome: serial study of radiological findings with emphasis on the similarity to the battered child syndrome, *Radiology* 112:401, 1974.
 2. Ahlgren P, Vestemark S: Menkes' kinky-hair disease, *Neuroradiology* 13:159, 1977.
 3. Allard JC, Tilak S, Carter AP: CT and MR of MELAS syndrome, *AJNR* 9:1234, 1988.
 4. Andersen B: Marinesco-Sjögren syndrome: spinocerebellar ataxia, congenital cataract, somatic and mental retardation, *Dev Med Child Neurol* 7:249, 1965.
 5. Blaser SI, Berns UH, Ross JS, et al: Serial MR studies in Menke's disease, *J Comput Assist Tomogr* 13:113, 1989.
 6. Carleton CC, Collins CH, Schimpff RD: Subacute necrotizing encephalopathy (Leigh's disease): two unusual cases, *South Med J* 69:1301, 1976.
 7. Coulter DL, Allen RJ: Abrupt neurological deterioration in children with Kearns-Sayre syndrome, *Arch Neurol* 38:247, 1981.
 8. Davis PC, Hoffman JC, Braun IF, et al: MR of Leigh's disease (subacute necrotizing encephalomyelopathy), *AJNR* 8:71, 1987.
 9. Dayan AD, Ockenden BG, Crome L: Necrotizing encephalomyelopathy of Leigh: neuropathological findings in eight cases, *Arch Dis Child* 45:39, 1970.
10. DeMange P, Gia HP, Kalifa G, et al: MR of Kearns-Sayre syndrome, *AJNR* 10suppl:91, 1989.
11. DeVolder A, Ghilain S, deBarsy TH, et al: Brain metabolism in mitochondrial encephalomyelopathy. A PET study, *J Comput Assist Tomogr* 12:854, 1988.
12. Egger J, Kendall BE: Computed tomography in mitochondrial cytopathy, *Neuroradiology* 22:73, 1981.
13. Faerber EN, Grover WD, DeFilipp GJ, et al: Cerebral MR of Menkes' kinky-hair disease, *AJNR* 10:190, 1989.
14. Federico A, Cornelio F, Di Donato S, et al: Mitochondrial encephaloneuromyopathy with myoclonus epilepsy, basal nuclei calcification, and hyperlactacidemia, *Ital J Neurol Sci* 9:65, 1988.
15. Geyer CA, Sartor KJ, Prensky AJ, et al: Leigh disease (subacute necrotizing encephalopathy): CT and MR in five cases, *J Comput Assist Tomogr* 12:40, 1988.
16. Hall K, Gardner-Medwin D: CT scan appearances in Leigh disease (subacute necrotizing encephalomyelopathy), *Neuroradiology* 16:48, 1978.
17. Hasuo K, Taimura S, Yasumai K, et al: Computed tomography and angiography in MELAS (mitochondrial myopathy, encephalopathy, lactic acidosis and strokelike episodes): report of three cases, *Neuroradiology,* 29:393, 1987.
18. Kobayashi M, Morishita H, Sugiyama N, et al: Two cases of NADH coenzyme Q reductase deficiency: relationship to MELAS syndrome, *J Pediatr* 110:223, 1987.
19. Koch TK, Yee MH, Hutchinson HT, et al: Magnetic resonance imaging in subacute necrotizing encephalomyelopathy (Leigh disease), *Ann Neurol* 19:605, 1986.
20. Medina L, Chi TL, De Vivo DC, et al: MR findings in patients with subacute necrotizing encephalomyelopathy (Leigh syndrome): correlation with biochemical defect, *AJNR* 11:379, 1990.
21. Menkes JH: Genetic disorders of mitochondrial function, *J Pediatr* 110:255, 1987.
22. Morita K, Ono S, Fukunaga M, et al: Increased accumulation of N-isopropyl-p-(123I)-iodoamphetamine in two cases with mitochondrial encephalomyopathy with lactic acidosis and strokelike episodes (MELAS), *Neuroradiology* 31:358, 1989.
23. Nishizawa M, Tanaka K, Shinozawa K, et al: A mitochondrial encephalomyopathy with cardiomyopathy: a case revealing a defect of complex I in the respiratory chain, *J Neurol Sci* 78:189, 1987.
24. Novotny EJ, Singh G, Wallace DC: Leber's disease and dystonia, *Neurology* 36:1053, 1986.
25. Okamoto T, Mizanuk K, Iida M, et al: Ophthalmoplegia-plus: its occurrence with periventricular diffuse low density on computed tomography scan, *Arch Neurol* 38:423, 1981.
26. Paltiel HJ, O'Gorman AM, Meagher-Villemure, et al: Subacute necrotizing encephalomyelopathy (Leigh disease): CT study, *Radiology* 162:115, 1987.
27. Robinson BH, De Meirleir L, Glerum M, et al: Clinical presentation of mitochondrial respiratory chain defects in NADH coenzyme Q reductase and cytochrome oxidase: clues to pathogenesis of Leigh disease, *J Pediatr* 110:216, 1987.
28. Rosen L, Phillipo S, Enzmann DR: Magnetic resonance imaging in MELAS syndrome, *Neuroradiology* 32:168, 1990.
29. Seay AR, Bray PF, Wing SD, et al: CT scans in Menke's disease, *Neurology* 29:304, 1979.
30. Seidenwurm D, Novotny E, Marshall W: MR and CT in cytoplasmically inherited striatal degeneration, *AJNR* 7:629, 1986.
31. Seigel RS: Computed tomography in oculocraniosomatic disease (Kearns-Sayre syndrome), *Radiology* 130:159, 1979.
32. Shapira Y, Harel S, Russell A: Mitochondrial encephalomyopathies: a group of neuromuscular disorders with defects in oxidative metabolism, *Isr J Med Sci* 13:161, 1977.
33. Skre H: Spinocerebellar ataxia, oligophrenia, and congenital cataracts (Marinesco-Sjögren syndrome). In Myrianthopoulos NC: Neurologic directory. Part I. In Vinken PJ, Bruyn GW: *Handbook of clinical neurology,* Amsterdam, 1981, North Holland.
34. Wesenberg RL, Gwinn JL, Barnes GR: Radiological findings in the kinky-hair syndrome, *Radiology* 92:500, 1969.
35. Wessel K, Poremba M, Pfeiffer J, et al: Mitochondrial encephalomyopathy: clinical aspects, CT morphology, and neuropathology, *Fortschr Neurol Psychiatr* 56:154, 1988.
36. Yoshimoto Y: Neurootological findings in a case of Marinesco-Sjögren syndrome with nystagmus, *Auris Nasus Larynx* 14:171, 1987.

Disorders of peroxisomes

Peroxisomal disorders are characterized by biochemical defects in the oxidation of fatty acids in organelles called peroxisomes, which are the site for a number of different enzymes. The enzyme deficiencies lead to disorders involving multiple organ systems.

A current classification of the disorders divides them into the following three groups[7]:

Group 1—Deficiencies of multiple enzymes: Zellweger cerebrohepatorenal syndrome, neonatal leukodystrophy, hyperpipecolic acidemia, infantile Refsum's syndrome, rhizomelic chondrodysplasia punctata

Group 2— Reduction in multiple enzymes: pseudo-Zellweger syndrome

Group 3— Reduction in a single enzyme: x-linked adrenoleukodystrophy

In the following discussion only those conditions in which MRI or CT changes have been seen will be described.

ZELLWEGER SYNDROME

Patients with Zellweger syndrome have serious abnormalities in nearly every organ, characteristic dysmorphic features, and disturbance in neuronal migration.[7] Histopathologically, heterotopic gray matter, pachygyria, and polymicrogyria occur together with a general decrease in white matter volume. Dysmyelination or faulty formation of myelination also occurs. MRI reflects the histological abnormalities: pachygyria, periventricular heterotopias, and hypomyelination may be seen on T2 MRI.[13]

NEONATAL LEUKODYSTROPHY

Neonatal leukodystrophy is characterized by severe hypotonia and seizures and profound psychomotor disturbance. The infants, who ultimately become blind and deaf, have normal adrenal function but hypoplastic adrenal glands.[8] CT may show progressive, white matter hypodensities consistent with demyelination, particularly in the periventricular area, centrum semiovale, and cerebellum.[13] Pseudoneonatal leukodystrophy is a recently described variant of the disease.[9] CT may also show extensive white matter hypodensities with bilateral centrum semiovale contrast enhancement.[9] In one report MRI demonstrated posterior cerebral white matter, internal capsule, and brain stem abnormalities.[13]

RHIZOMELIC CHONDRODYSPLASIA PUNCTATA

Marked retardation of myelination, presumedly caused by lack of development, has been described on MRI in this rare condition.[13]

ADRENOLEUKODYSTROPHY COMPLEX

Adrenoleukodystrophy (ALD) complex, recently classified as among the peroxisomal disorders,[7] consists of three closely related variants: adrenoleukodystrophy, adrenomyeloneuropathy, and adrenoleukomyeloneuropathy, all characterized by X-linked recessive inheritance and all occurring in the first to fourth decades of life. A fourth type that is autosomal recessive occurs in infancy.[8] Each of these

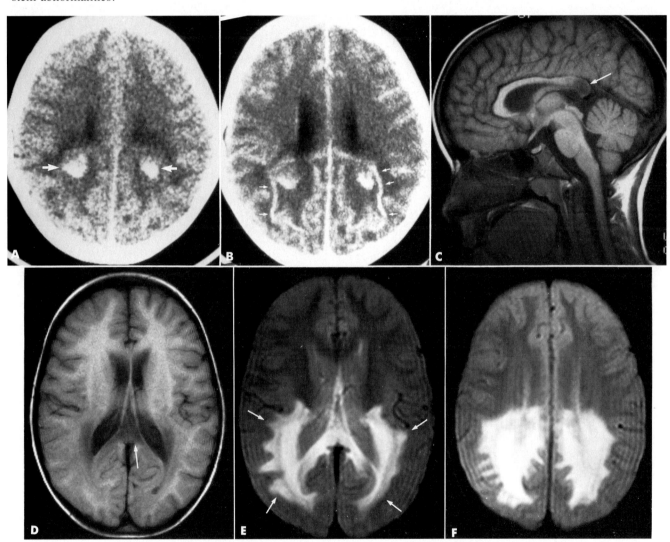

Fig. 4-14   A, Nonenhanced CT scan demonstrates low density areas bilaterally in the periatrial white matter with central high density areas *(arrows)* in a 5-year-old boy with adrenoleukodystrophy. **B,** Contrast-enhanced scan shows enhancement of margins of the low density areas *(arrows)*. **C** and **D,** T1-weighted sagittal and axial scans of a second patient, a 6-year-old boy (spin echo, 800/17 msec), demonstrate low signal areas in the splenium of the corpus callosum *(arrows)*. **E** and **F,** T2-weighted axial scans show high intensity areas in periatrial areas in the white matter bilaterally *(arrows)*. (All images with spin echoes of 3000/90 msec.)   *Continued.*

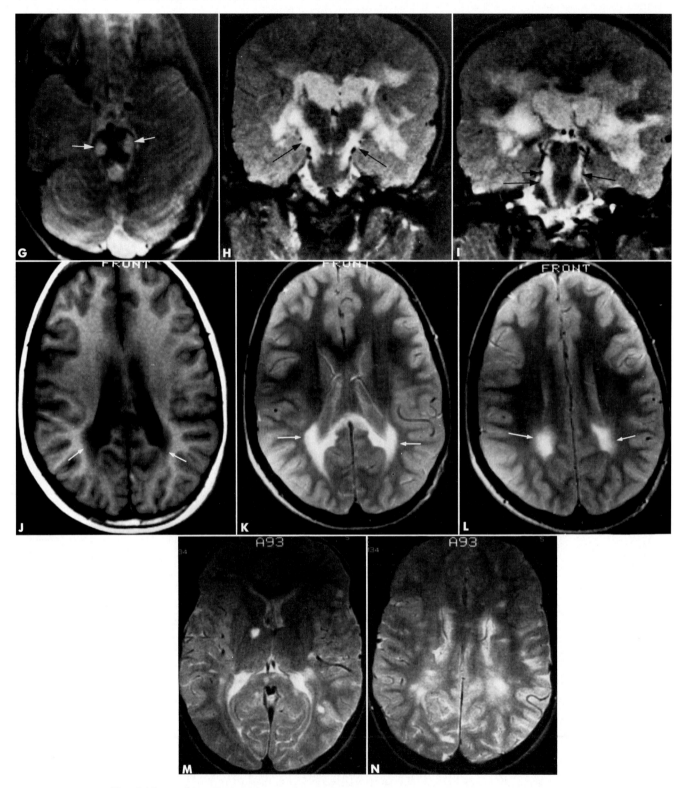

Fig. 4-14, cont'd. **G,** Axial image shows bilateral hyperintense signals in the laterally located corticospinal tracts *(arrows)*. **H,** Coronal image displays hyper intense signals in the cerebral peduncles bilaterally *(arrows.)*. Note also the involvement of the white matter as well as the internal capsules. The lateral geniculate bodies (immediately lateral to the cerebral peduncles) appear to be uninvolved. **I,** A further coronal image, 6 mm posteriorly, demonstrates the lower extent of the involved peduncles with the lesions located in the dorsolateral corticospinal tracts. The ventromedial corticospinal tracts are spared. A 12-year-old boy with adrenoleukomyeloneuropathy. **J,** T1-weighted scan (spin echo, 650/20 msec) demonstrates periatrial white matter low intensity lesions *(arrows)* that appear as high intensity lesions on proton density images **(K** and **L)** (spin echo, 3000/45 msec). **M** and **N,** A 12-year-old child with multiple sclerosis. Note the multiple periventricular high intensity lesions bilaterally in the basal ganglia periatrial area, left subcortical area, and periventricular white matter (spin echo, 2500/80 msec). **J-L** from Runge VM: Clinical magnetic resonance imaging, Philadelphia, 1990, JB Lippincott; **M** and **N** courtesy Dr. G. Stimac, Seattle.)

disorders has in common an excess of very long-chain fatty acids in the plasma and in the tissues.

The diseases are manifested by a combination of behavioral changes, impaired hearing, parietal lobe dysfunction, visual impairment, seizures, and, in approximately half of the patients, adrenal insufficiency. Males are selectively affected. Death occurs in about 3 years. Adrenoleukomyeloneuropathy (ALMN), seen in older children, young adults, and carriers, is characterized by peripheral neuropathy, impotence, and sphincter disturbance.[4]

Pathologically in ALD there is severe destruction of the myelin in the cerebral white matter accompanied by a large accumulation of lymphocytes, particularly at the margins of the lesion. In those patients with myeloneuropathy, the white matter involvement is milder and the lesions in the peripheral nerves and spinal cord are those of a distal axonopathy.

CT changes are distinctive but not pathognomonic. Typically there is a decrease in the attenuation of the periventricular, periatrial white matter. The posterior cingulum and corpus callosum are also heavily involved. Contrast enhancement may occur in the margins of the lesion (Figs. 4-14, A and B). These abnormal zones are caused by disruption of the blood-brain barrier corresponding to active demyelination and often progress posteriorly to anteriorly.[5] In atypical cases frontal lobe involvement, predominantly unilateral, and white matter calcification and mass effect occur.[5] In such cases differentiation from a neoplasm may be difficult if not impossible. Seldom are the gray matter structures such as the lentiform nuclei or the thalamus involved. Involvement of the brain stem is similarly uncommonly seen on CT but is seen on MRI. Cerebellar demyelination appears to be more pronounced in neonatal ALD than in childhood ALD.[2]

Schaumberg[11] described three distinct histopathological zones in ALD.[11] Zones 1 and 2 were at the leading frontal edge of the lesions where the myelin destruction was particularly severe (zone 1) and a vigorous perivascular response occurred (zone 2). The enhancement seen on CT appears to correspond to zone 2. In zone 3 gliosis is the main histological feature. DiChiro et al.[3] described a type of adrenoleukodystrophy in which there was marked enhancement of the white matter of the internal capsule, anterior corpus callosum, and cingulate gyrus.[3]

On MRI, as a result of white matter demyelination and concomitant edema, high intensity signal intensities are seen on the more T2-weighted images.[5,14] Involvement of the splenium of the corpus callosum, medial and lateral geniculate bodies, cerebellar white matter and brain stem corticospinal tracts can be seen on the MRI scan[12] (Fig. 4-14, C to I). Because of the clear distinction on MRI between normal and abnormal white matter, specific auditory and visual pathway structural disease may be identified and correlated with the clinical findings. Enhancement of zone 2 after gadolinium administration has also been reported.[12] Cerebral MRI in cases of ALMN can demonstrate white matter high intensity changes on T2-weighted images[9,13] (Fig. 4-14, J to L). Reversal of early MRI changes has been reported after bone marrow transplantation.[1]

Involvement of the internal capsule, cerebellar peduncles, cerebellar white matter, and brain stem tracts has also been described on MRI in patients with adrenomyeloneuropathy.[13] In contrast to x-linked adrenoleukodystrophy, not only the dorsolateral tracts but also the more ventromedial corticospinal tracts are involved.

Adrenoleukodystrophy should be distinguished from the disease originally ascribed to Schilder in 1912, inflammatory myelinoclastic diffuse sclerosis, which most likely is an acute form of multiple sclerosis. In this condition CT and MRI demonstrate extensive bihemispheric white matter lesions with mass effect, as well as fluctuating contrast enhancement[6] (Fig. 4-14, M and N). In another case report, the disease presented as a unilateral mass and mimicked a tumor on both CT and MRI scans.[10]

REFERENCES
Disorders of peroxisomes

1. Auborg P, Blanche S, Jambaque I, et al: Reversal of early neurologic and neuroradiologic manifestations of x-linked adrenoleukodystrophy by bone marrow transplantation, *N Engl J Med* 322:1860, 1990.
2. Auborg P, Scotto J, Rocchiccioli F: Neonatal adrenoleukodystrophy, *J Neurol Neurosurg Psychiatr* 49:77, 1986.
3. DiChiro G, Eiben RM, Manz HJ, et al: A new CT pattern in adrenoleukodystrophy, *Radiology* 137:687, 1980.
4. Griffin JW, Goren E, Schaumberg H, et al: Adrenomyeloneuropathy: a probable variant of adrenoleukodystrophy. 1. Clinical and endocrinologic aspects, *Neurology* 27:1107, 1977.
5. Kumar AJ, Rosenbaum AE, Naidu S, et al: Adrenoleukodystrophy: correlating MR imaging with CT, *Radiology* 165:497, 1987.
6. Mehler MF, Rabinowich L: Inflammatory myelinoclastic diffuse sclerosis (Schilder's disease), *AJNR* 10:176, 1989.
7. Moser HW: Peroxisomal disorders, *J Pediatr* 108:89, 1986.
8. Percy AK: The inherited neurodegenerative diseases of childhood: clinical assessment, *J Child Neurol* 2:82, 1987.
9. Poll-Thé B, Roels F, Ogier H: A new peroxisomal disorder with enlarged peroxisomes and a specific deficiency of acyl-Co A-oxidase (pseudoneonatal adrenoleukodystrophy), *Am J Hum Genet* 42:422, 1988.
10. Rodesch G, Avni EF, Parizel P, et al: Maladie de Schilder: considerations neuroradiologiques, *J Neuroradiol* 15:386, 1988.
11. Schaumberg HH, Powers JM, Raine CS, et al: Adrenoleukodystrophy: a clinical and pathological study of 17 cases, *Arch Neurol* 32:577, 1975.
12. van der Knapp MS, Valk J: MR of adrenoleukodystrophy: histopathologic correlations, *AJNR* Suppl10:12, 1989.
13. van der Knaap M, Valk J: The MR spectrum of peroxisomal disorders, *Neuroradiology* 33:30, 1991.
14. Young IR, Randell CP, Kaplan PW, et al: Nuclear magnetic resonance (NMR) imaging in white matter disease of the brain using spin-echo sequences, *J Comput Assist Tomogr* 7:290, 1983.

Diseases of gray matter

NEURONAL CEROID LIPOFUSCINOSIS

Neuronal lipofuscinosis is autosomal recessive in childhood but may be autosomal dominant in adulthood. The course of the disease is considerably slower in the adult form than in the infantile form.[4] Seizures, myoclonus, involuntary movements, and dementia characterize the condition. In the younger group of patients the brain shows

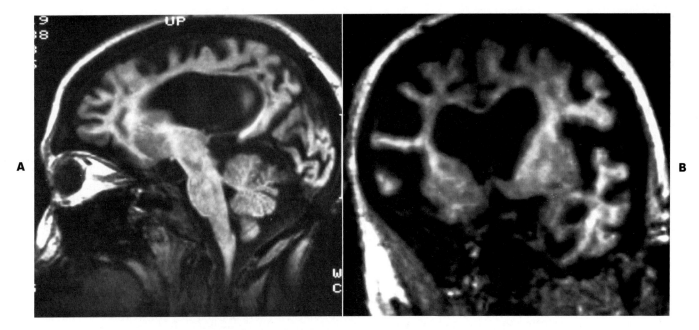

Fig. 4-15   A and B, Sagittal and coronal three-dimensional gradient echo (40/15/50°) MRI scans in a 24-year-old woman with neuronal ceroid lipofuscinosis demonstrate marked cortical atrophy with ventriculomegaly.

almost complete loss of neurons in the cerebral and cerebellar cortex.[4] Autofluorescent lipopigments accumulate within the viscera, brain, and retina. Ophthalmoscopic examination is characteristic, demonstrating macular degeneration and optic disc atrophy. The radiological changes are nonspecific. Cerebral atrophy, manifested by symmetrical enlargement of the subarachnoid spaces and the lateral and third ventricles, is seen on CT scans of children older than 14 years.[3,5] Cerebellar atrophy may also occur.[2] The scans are usually normal in the younger patients. The atrophy is also evident on MRI scans (Fig. 4-15).

ALPERS' SYNDROME

Under the eponym of Alpers' syndrome are included a group of autosomal recessive transmitted diseases affecting primarily the cerebral gray matter. Clinically the children have seizures, intellectual deterioration, and spasticity. Many of the conditions are actually cases of lactic acidosis or mitochondrial myopathy, suggesting that the diseases should be classified under the mitochondrial cytopathies. CT demonstrates diffuse cerebral atrophy.[1]

REFERENCES
Diseases of gray matter
1. Diebler C, Dulac O: Inherited metabolic diseases. In Diebler C, Dulac O, editors: *Pediatric neurology and neuroradiology,* Berlin, 1988, Springer-Verlag.
2. Dunn DW: CT in ceroid lipofuscinosis, *Neurology* 37:1025, 1989.
3. Lagenstein I, Schwendemann G, Kuhne D, et al: Neuronal ceroid lipofuscinosis: CCT findings in 14 patients, *Acta Pediatr Scand* 70:857, 1981.
4. Siakotos AN: Neuronal ceroid lipofuscinosis: lipidoses, mucolipidoses, and mucopolysaccharidoses. In Vinken PJ, Bruyn GW: *Handbook of clinical neurology,* Amsterdam, 1981, North Holland.
5. Valavanis A, Friede RL, Schubiger O, et al: Computed tomography in neuronal ceroid lipofuscinosis, *Neuroradiology* 19:35, 1980.

Diseases of the basal ganglia

HUNTINGTON'S DISEASE

Huntington's disease is usually seen in adults, but about 5% of patients are younger than 14 years of age.[5] The disease progresses rapidly in children, death usually occurring within 8 years of onset. Seizures are seen in about half the children affected. Rigidity, decreased facial expression, and reduction of voluntary movements are prominent, as in adults.

CT scans may demonstrate ventricular dilatation, particularly in the region of the head of the caudate nuclei.[13] Positron emission tomography[18] using fluorodeoxyglucose as a measure of cerebral glucose metabolism appears to be a sensitive diagnostic tool demonstrating decreased glucose utilization when the CT scan may appear normal.[7]

HALLERVORDEN-SPATZ DISEASE

Hallervorden-Spatz disease is characterized by progressive impairment of gait, slowing and diminution of voluntary movements, dysarthria, and mental deterioration. The disease is familial and usually begins before 10 years of age. Pathologically, symmetrical destruction of the globus pallidus, putamen, and part of the substantia nigra occurs and is demonstrated on CT by bilateral low densities.[3,10] Together with the destruction an abnormal pigment is deposited in the globus pallidus, reticular zone of the substantia nigra, and red nucleus. The pigment contains iron and is related to neuromelanin. In some patients the abnormal pigment is evident on CT and MRI. On CT the pigment causes high density lesions.[19] On MRI a decreased signal intensity is seen particularly on T2-weighted images.[9,12,17,18]

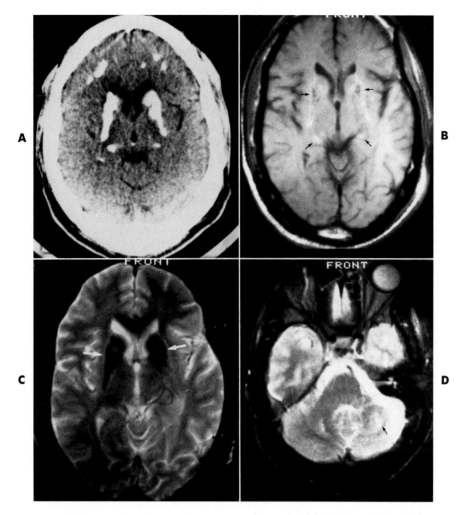

Fig. 4-16   Axial CT scans in a 48-year-old man with Fahr's disease demonstrate marked globus pallidi and subcortical calcification **(A). B,** Axial T1-weighted MRI scan (spin echo, 650/20 msec) shows low signal intensities *(anterior arrows)* in the center of high intensity areas involving the globus pallidi. Areas of calcification on the CT scans in the lateral geniculate areas also appear as high intensity areas on T1-weighted scans *(posterior arrows)*. High intensity areas in the globus pallidi on the T1-weighted scan are of a low intensity on a T2-weighted scan **(C)** (spin echo, 3000/90 msec) **D,** Increased signal intensity is also seen in the dentate nuclei of the cerebellum on a T2-weighted scan.

FAHR'S DISEASE

Fahr's disease is not a single entity but rather is a group of genetically and clinically distinct disorders that share the characteristics of calcific deposits within the basal ganglia.[10] An autosomal recessive transmission is seen in some cases; others are autosomal dominant. Mental deterioration and growth retardation occur. Pathologically the calcium is deposited within the capillaries and media of the larger blood vessels, and is also seen within the basal ganglia, cortex, and dentate nuclei.

The calcification that is readily apparent on CT is always evident in the basal ganglia and is also often seen in the subcortical white matter, as well as in the dentate nuclei in the more severe cases[8] (Fig. 4-16, *A*). Calcification of the basal ganglia may also be seen in a number of other well-delineated conditions such as in disorders of calcium metabolism including hypoparathyroidism, pseudohypoparathyroidism, and hyperparathyroidism. In addition, basal ganglia calcification can be seen in tuberous sclerosis (close to the foramen of Monro), toxoplasmosis, cytomegalic inclusion disease, HIV encephalitis, Cockayne's disease, Down's syndrome, and as a consequence of perinatal asphyxia. The differential diagnosis of basal ganglia calcification as seen on CT has been reviewed by Harrington et al.[6] and is further discussed on p. 149.

In a case report of Fahr's disease as studied by MRI, varying signal intensities were seen in different parts of the brain where the CT demonstrated the presence of calcium.[14] Absence of signal was noted on both the T1- and the T2-weighted images in the dentate nuclei and in the basal ganglia. However, high intensity signals on T1-weighted studies, thought to result from protein or mucopolysaccharides bound to calcium, were found on T1-weighted studies in calcified periventricular lesions in the white matter. Similar changes have been seen in one of our cases (Fig. 4-16, *B* to *D*).

WILSON'S DISEASE (HEPATOLENTICULAR DEGENERATION)

Wilson's disease is an inborn error of copper metabolism associated with cirrhosis of the liver and degenerative changes in the basal ganglia. The vast majority of patients show markedly diminished concentrations of ceruloplasmin, a protein that binds copper in the serum. As a result of this deficiency copper accumulates in the liver and leads to postnecrotic cirrhosis. In the brain spongy degeneration of the putamen leads to the formation of small cavities, which also occur in the frontal cortex.[10] Lesser changes are seen in the brain stem, dentate nuclei, substantia nigra, and convolutional white matter.

The disease, which has a prevalence of 1:50,000 births,[15] is transmitted as an autosomal recessive condition. The disease usually presents in the second or third decade of life with hepatic symptoms; neurological disorders appear later in the course of the disease. Dystonia, drooling, gait disturbances, impaired speech, and tremors are often severe. The diagnosis is established through the combination of family history of hepatic or neurological involvement, progressive extrapyramidal symptoms during the first or second decade of life, abnormal liver function, cupriuria, and absent or decreased serum ceruloplasmin. The presence of a Kayser-Fleischer ring in the eye is diagnostic.

Hypodense areas in the basal ganglia, atrophy, or both were seen on CT in the majority of the 60 patients studied in one series.[20] Cerebellar atrophy was also seen. In a series of 22 patients who had MRI studies the majority had high intensity lesions in the basal ganglia on T2-weighted studies.[16] The putamen and the caudate nuclei were the most commonly affected structures, followed by atrophy and subcortical white matter lesions. Whereas the caudate, putamen, and thalamus were symmetrically involved, the white matter lesions were usually asymmetrical. Lesions were also found in the tegmentum, tectum, pons, and cerebellum. Dystonia correlated with the putaminal lesions; dysarthria correlated with combined lesions of the putamina and the caudate nuclei.

COCKAYNE'S SYNDROME

Cockayne's syndrome, probably transmitted as an autosomal recessive trait, consists of microcephaly, cachexia, dwarfism, retinitis pigmentosa, deafness, premature aging, and progressive encephalopathy.[2] Neuropathological studies reveal perivascular calcifications in the basal ganglia and cerebellum together with a patchy demyelination similar to that seen with Pelizaeus-Merzbacher syndrome.[11] The CT appearances include cerebral atrophy and basal ganglia calcification.[4] White matter high intensity changes on MRI scans have also been described,[1] further suggesting that Cockayne's syndrome should be classified among the leukodystrophies.

REFERENCES
Diseases of the basal ganglia

1. Boltshauser E, Yalcinkaya C, Wichman W, et al: MRI in Cockayne's syndrome type I, *Neuroradiology* 31:276, 1989.
2. Cockayne EA: Dwarfism with retinal atrophy and deafness, *Arch Dis Child* 11:1, 1936.
3. Dooling EC, Richardson EP, Davis KR: Computed tomography in Hallervorden-Spatz disease, *Neurology* 30:1128, 1980.
4. Faerber EN: Degenerative and metabolic diseases. In Faerber EN, editor: *Cranial computed tomography in infants and children,* Philadelphia, 1986, JB Lippincott.
5. Golden GS: Metabolic disorders. In Golden GS, editor: *Textbook of pediatric neurology,* New York, 1987, Plenum.
6. Harrington MG, MacPherson P, McIntosh WB, et al: The significance of the incidental finding of basal ganglia calcification on computed tomography, *J Neurol Neurosurg Psychiatry* 44:1168, 1981.
7. Kuhl DE, Phelps ME, Markham CH, et al: Cerebral metabolism and atrophy in Huntington's disease determined by 18FDG and computed tomographic scan, *Ann Neurol* 12:425, 1982.
8. Kuroiwa Y, Mayron MS, Boller F, et al: Computed tomographic visualization of extensive calcinosis in a patient with idiopathic familial basal ganglia calcification, *Arch Neurol* 39:603, 1982.
9. Littrup PJ, Gebarski SS: MR imaging of Hallervorden-Spatz disease, *J Comput Assist Tomogr* 9:491, 1985.
10. Menkes JH: Heredodegenerative diseases. In Menkes JH, editor: *Textbook of child neurology,* ed 3, Philadelphia, 1985, Lea & Febiger.
11. Moosy J: The neuropathology of Cockayne's syndrome, *J Neuropathol Exp Neurol* 26:654, 1967.
12. Mutoh K, Okuno T, Ito M, et al: MR images of a group 1 case of Hallervorden-Spatz disease, *J Comput Assist Tomogr* 12:851, 1988.
13. Osborne JP, Munson P, Burman D, et al: Huntington's chorea: report of three cases and review of the literature, *Arch Dis Child* 57:99, 1982.
14. Scotti G, Scialfa G, Tampieri D, et al: Case report: MR imaging in Fahr's disease, *J Comput Assist Tomogr* 9:790, 1985.
15. Stanbury JB, Wyngaarden JB, Frederikson DS, et al: Inborn errors of metabolism in the 1980s. In Stanbury JB, Wyngaarden JB, Frederikson DS, et al, editors: *The metabolic basis of inherited disease,* ed 5, New York, 1983, McGraw-Hill.
16. Starosta-Rubinstein S, Young AB, Young AB, et al: Clinical assessment of 31 patients with Wilson's disease: correlation with structural changes on magnetic resonance imaging, *Arch Neurol* 44:365, 1987.
17. Swaiman KF, Smith SA, Trock GL, et al: Sea-blue histiocytes, lymphocytic cytosomes, movement disorder and 59Fe-uptake in basal ganglia: Hallervorden-Spatz disease or ceroid storage disease with abnormal isotope scan? *Neurology* 33:301, 1983.
18. Tanfani G, Mascalchi M, Dal Pozzoli GC, et al: MR imaging in a case of Hallervorden-Spatz disease, *J Comput Assist Tomogr* 11:1057, 1987.
19. Tennison MB, Bouldin TW, Whaley RA: Mineralization of the basal ganglia detected by CT in Hallervorden-Spatz syndrome, *Neurology* 38:154, 1988.
20. Williams FJB, Walshe JM: Wilson's disease: an analysis of the cranial computerized tomographic appearances found in 60 patients and the changes in response to treatment with chelating agents, *Brain* 104:735, 1981.

Diseases of the cerebellum, brain stem, and spinal cord

FRIEDREICH'S ATAXIA

Friedreich's ataxia is an abnormality, usually autosomal recessive, of unknown etiology consisting of axonal degeneration, demyelination, and gliosis of the long ascending and descending tracts in the spinal cord.[1] Less often the brain stem and cerebellum are involved. Ataxia is a prominent sign and is more marked in the legs than in the arms. In about two thirds of the patients the fourth ventricle is increased in area but not in width, possibly because of atrophy of the dentate nuclei with degeneration of the efferent fibers.[2] Atrophy of the cerebellar hemispheres and vermis also occurs.

OLIVOPONTOCEREBELLAR ATROPHIES

Olivopontocerebellar atrophies are characterized by progressive cerebellar ataxia, tremor, speech impairment, extrapyramidal signs, and cranial nerve palsies. The most commonly encountered form begins between 17 and 30 years of age.[1] There is also a type of olivopontocerebellar degeneration manifested in the first year of life. Neuronal loss occurs in the cerebellar cortex, basis pontis, inferior olivary nucleus, and cranial nerve nuclei X and XII. The spinal cord is usually normal. CT scans demonstrate

enlargement of the fourth ventricle and of the cerebellopontine angle cisterns.[2] These CT changes reflect the degeneration of the pontine nuclei and the middle cerebellar peduncles. Severe paracerebellar atrophy also occurs. The cerebellar degeneration can also easily be determined on MRI scans (Fig. 4-17).

ATAXIA-TELANGIECTASIA

Ataxia-telangiectasia is a rare disorder. However, after posterior fossa tumors it represents the most common cause of progressive ataxia in children under age 10.[1] Cerebellar cortical atrophy and demyelination of the posterior column and dorsal spinocerebellar tracts also occur and are evident on the CT scan. The diagnosis is established by the combination of cerebellar signs, conjunctival telangiectasias, an elevated alpha-fetoprotein, and reduced IgA and IgE immunoglobulins.

REFERENCES
Diseases of the cerebellum, brain stem, and spinal cord

1. Menkes JH: Heredodegenerative diseases. In Menkes JH, editor: *Textbook of child neurology*, ed 3, Philadelphia, 1985, Lea & Febiger.
2. Ramos A, Quintana F, Drez C, et al: CT findings in spinocerebellar degeneration, *AJNR* 8:635, 1987.

Diseases of the white matter

PELIZAEUS-MERZBACHER DISEASE

Pelizaeus-Merzbacher disease is a rare x-linked recessive demyelinating disorder that begins in the neonatal period and is usually fatal in 5 to 7 years. The disease most often occurs in boys and young adults and is characterized by a defect in myelin maturation due to a lack of myelin-specific proteolipid protein responsible for differentiation and survival of oligodendrocytes.[8] Since on rare occasions the disease is seen in females or is sporadic in occurrence, the mode of inheritance is not completely understood.[19] Clinically, poor head control, congenital nystagmus with head shaking, cerebellar ataxia (including intention tremor), and scanning speech occur. The disease progresses slowly.

The use of CT in the diagnosis of the disease is of limited value, although decreased density of the white matter has been described.[6] MRI is more sensitive than CT in showing high intensity signal changes in the white matter on T2-weighted images, indicative of poor myelination[6,13,16] (Fig. 4-18). The appearance on the MRI scan may help differentiate between the conatal type of the disease, in which no myelination is seen even in the brain stem and pons, and the classic type of the disease, in which the brain stem, diencephalon, cerebellum, and subcortical white matter show a good state of myelin preservation but myelination is absent elsewhere.[19] Decreased basal ganglionic and thalamic signals on T2-weighted images, possibly the result of a nonspecific increased iron deposition in these structures, have also been reported.[17]

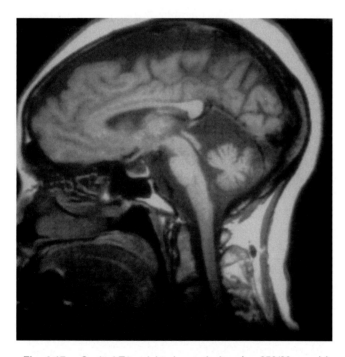

Fig. 4-17   Sagittal T1-weighted scan (spin echo, 650/20 msec) in a 20-year-old patient with olivopontocerebellar degeneration demonstrates marked cerebellar and pontine atrophy, particularly involving the superior vermis. Note also wide superior cerebellar and prepontine cisterns.

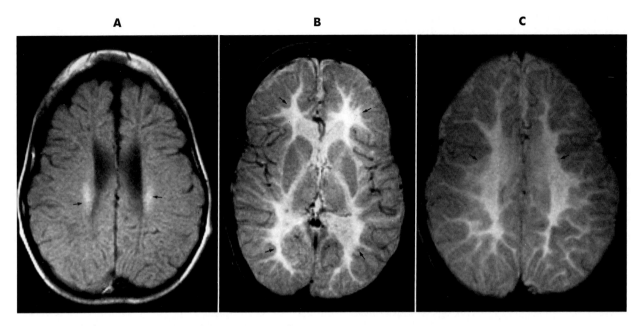

Fig. 4-18   A 10-year-old with Pelizaeus-Merzbacher disease and infantile onset of symptoms. **A,** T1-weighted scan (spin echo, 600/17 msec) shows normal myelination in the posterior coronal radiata *(arrows)* but not in the periventricular white matter elsewhere. Myelination was not present in the pons. **B** and **C,** T2-weighted scans (spin echo, 3000/70 msec) show high signal areas *(arrows)* in the white matter bilaterally.

CANAVAN'S DISEASE

Symptoms in Canavan's disease, a rare autosomal recessive disease that primarily affects Jewish children, appear between the second and fourth months of life and include failure of intellectual development, optic atrophy, and hypotonia. A significant macrocrania ensues, and death usually occurs before age 5 years.[4] The metabolic defect has been identified, and the disease is now thought to be caused by an accumulation of N-acetylaspartic acid in the urine, plasma, and human brain due to a deficiency in N-acetylaspartylase.[10]

The main pathological findings are in the white matter, which is replaced by a fine network of fluid-containing cystic spaces that give a characteristic spongy appearance (spongiform leukodystrophy). There is an increase in the brain weight because of increased water content with an absence of myelin. These changes provide the basis for the CT appearances of symmetrical low density areas within the cerebral white matter.[9,14] The U fibers are often involved. In the younger, more severe cases the basal ganglia and thalami may also be involved[7] (Fig. 4-19). Ultrasonography can demonstrate increased sonolucency and multiple anechoic lesions.[12] Diffuse white matter high intensity signals have been reported on T2-weighted studies.[2,11] In one of our patients MRI scans demonstrated high intensities in the white matter on T1-weighted images, which were of low intensity on T2-weighted images (paramagnetic effect) (Fig. 4-19, *B* to *E*). Possibly these changes represent mineralization, abnormal pigmentation, or hemorrhage.

ALEXANDER'S DISEASE

Alexander's disease usually occurs in infancy but may appear in later childhood or adult life.[15] Clinically the disease is manifested by irritability, vomiting, psychomotor retardation, spasticity, seizures, and macrocephaly. A definite pattern of inheritance has not as yet been established, and all cases develop sporadically.[3] A characteristic pathological feature is the presence of Rosenthal fibers in the frontal white matter, basal ganglia, thalamus, and hypothalamus.[3] White matter demyelination also occurs, accounting for the CT appearances of symmetrical decrease in white matter density, often most prominent in the frontal regions,[5] and also the MRI appearances of high intensity changes on T2-weighted scans in the same region[1] (Fig. 4-20, *A* and *B*). Low density areas can also be seen in the caudate and lentiform nuclei and anterior limbs of the internal capsule.[5] Well-defined stripes of high density may be present subependymally and also involve the fornices and corpus striatum.[18] Abnormal enhancement after contrast administration has been described in the basal ganglia, periventricular regions, and optic radiations[5]; in one reported case the enhancement corresponded to the location of the Rosenthal fibers.[3] Megalencephaly is seen in younger patients.

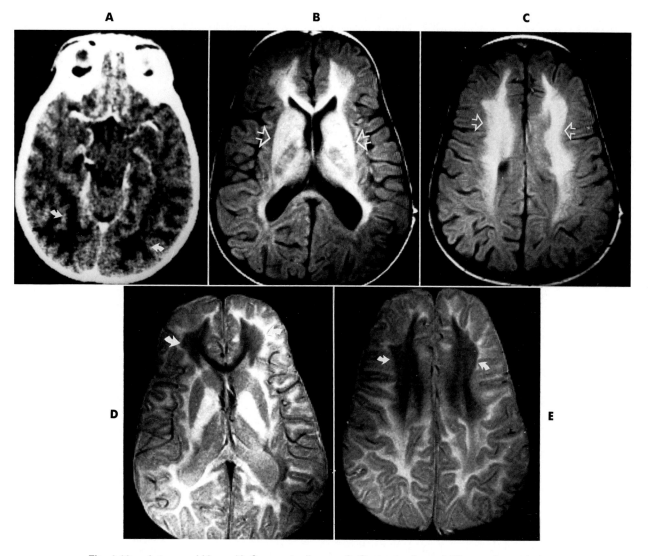

Fig. 4-19   A 4-year-old boy with Canavan's disease. **A,** Contrast-enhanced CT scan demonstrates diffuse bilateral white matter low density areas particularly in the periatrial white matter *(arrows.)* **B** and **C,** T1-weighted (spin echo, 700/19 msec) MRI scans show high intensity areas diffusely in the white matter and basal ganglia *(arrows)*. **D** and **E,** T2-weighted scans (spin echo, 3000/70 msec) show low signal intensity areas predominantly anteriorly, where T1-weighted scans demonstrate high intensities. The appearances indicate a paramagnetic effect. Elsewhere the white matter is of high intensity on the T2-weighted images, which may indicate fluid accumulation, demyelination, or both.

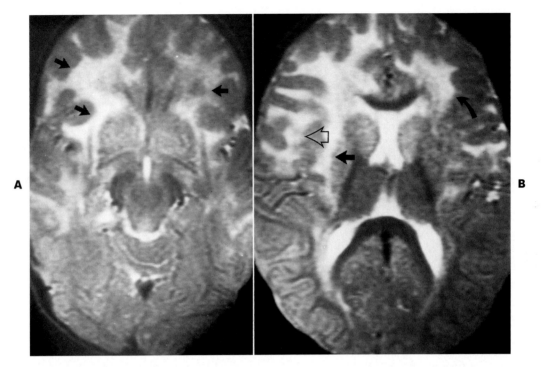

Fig. 4-20   An 18-year-old man developmentally delayed since birth with Alexander's disease (all with spin echoes of 2500/80 msec). **A,** Note the hyperintense areas in both frontal lobes, particularly on the right side where the U fibers are also involved *(arrows).* **B,** Similar changes are evident on a higher scan at the level of the lateral ventricles where involvement of the right external capsule *(straight arrow),* the U fibers *(open arrows),* and the white matter of both frontal lobes *(curved arrow)* is again seen. (Courtesy Dr. A. Osborn, Salt Lake City.)

REFERENCES
Diseases of the white matter

 1. Barkovich AJ: Metabolic and destructive brain disorders. In Barkovich AJ, editor: *Pediatric neuroimaging,* New York, 1989, Raven.
 2. Brismar J, Brismar G, Gascow G, et al: Canavan disease: CT and MR imaging of the brain, *AJNR* 11:805, 1990.
 3. Farrell H, Chuang S, Becker LE: Computed tomography in Alexander's disease, *Ann Neurol* 15:605, 1984.
 4. Golden GS: Metabolic disorders. In Golden GS: *Textbook of pediatric neurology,* New York; 1987, Plenum.
 5. Holland IM, Kendall BE: Computed tomography in Alexander's disease, *Neuroradiology* 20:103, 1980.
 6. Journel H, Roussey M, Gandon Y, et al: Magnetic resonance imaging in Pelizaeus-Merzbacher disease, *Neuroradiology* 29:403, 1987.
 7. Kingsley DPE, Kendall BE: Maladies démyélinisantes et neurodégénératives de l'enfance: Aspects tomodensitométriques et diagnostic différential, *J Neuroradiol* 8:243, 1981.
 8. Koeppen AH, Ronca NA, Greenfield EA, et al: Defective biosynthesis of proteolipid protein in Pelizaeus-Merzbacher disease, *Ann Neurol* 21:159, 1987.
 9. Lane B, Carroll BA, Pedley TA, et al: Computerized cranial tomography in cerebral diseases of white matter, *Neurology* 28:533, 1978.
10. Matalon R, Michals K, Sebesta D, et al: Aspartoacyclase deficiency and N-acetylaspartic aciduria in patients with Canavan's disease, *Am J Med Genet* 29:463, 1988.
11. McAdams HP, Geyer CA, Done SL, et al: CT and MR imaging of Canavan disease, *AJNR* 11:397, 1990.
12. Patel PJ, Kolawole TM, Mahdi AH, et al: Sonographic and computed tomographic findings in Canavan's disease, *Br J Radiol* 59:1226, 1986.
13. Penner MW, Li KC, Gebarski SS, et al: MR imaging of Pelizaeus-Merzbacher disease, *J Comput Assist Tomogr* 11:591, 1987.
14. Rushton AR, Shaywitz BA, Duncan CD, et al: CT in the diagnosis of Canavan's disease, *Ann Neurol* 10:57, 1981.
15. Russo LS, Aron A, Anderson PJ: Alexander's disease: a report and reappraisal, *Neurology* 26:607, 1976.
16. Shimomura C, Matsui A, Choh H, et al: Magnetic resonance imaging in Pelizaeus-Merzbacher disease, *Pediatr Neurology* 4:124, 1988.
17. Silverstein AM, Hirsh DK, Trobe JD, et al: MR imaging of the brain in five members of a family with Pelizaeus-Merzbacher disease, *AJNR* 11:495, 1990.
18. Trommer BL, Naidich TP, Del Cento MC, et al: Noninvasive CT diagnosis of infantile Alexander's disease: pathologic correlations, *J Comput Assist Tomogr* 7:509, 1983.
19. van der Knaap MS, Valk J: The reflection of histology in MR imaging of Pelizaeus-Merzbacher disease, *AJNR* 10:99, 1989.

Addendum: Basal ganglia calcifications and lucencies on CT as correlated with MRI

Often, patients with a suspected metabolic or neurodegenerative disorder will have a cerebral CT scan carried out early in the course of their diagnostic evaluation. In many of the metabolic disorders already discussed, as well as in a number of neurodegenerative disorders to be discussed below, calcifications or lucencies (low densities) will be seen in the basal ganglia. A discussion on the CT appearances with MRI correlations in these diseases is therefore considered necessary.

Table 4-1 shows that calcifications in the basal ganglia are seen in a number of metabolic diseases including Fahr's disease and Cockayne's disease, as well as in the mitochondrial cytopathies (Kearns-Sayre, MELAS, and MERRF syndromes). Lucencies are seen in the basal ganglia in maple syrup urine disease, methylmalonic aciduria, GM_1 and GM_2 gangliosidoses, Leigh's disease, Kearns-Sayre, MELAS, and MERRF syndromes, infantile bilateral striatal necrosis, and Hallervorden-Spatz, Wilson's, Canavan's, and Alexander's diseases. Both calcifications and lucencies are also seen in a number of nonmetabolic or degenerative conditions. Therefore the presence of calcifications or lucencies in the basal ganglia is of little differential value. However, when the neuroradiological, including both the CT and MRI appearances, and clinical presentations are considered together, the correct diagnosis may be suggested.

BASAL GANGLIA CALCIFICATIONS[6,11]

1. *Endocrine*—parathyroid disease
2. *Congenital/developmental*—tuberous sclerosis, Down's syndrome[18]
3. *Inflammatory*—cytomegalic inclusion disease, encephalitis (measles, chicken pox, and rubella) toxoplasmosis, cysticercosis, AIDS
4. *Toxic/anoxic*—Carbon monoxide intoxication, lead intoxication, birth anoxia, therapeutic radiation, methotrexate therapy
5. *Miscellaneous*—renal tubular acidosis and osteopetrosis, progressive encephalopathy with basal ganglia calcifications

Parathyroid disease

Calcification occurs in the basal ganglia in up to 50% of patients with hypoparathyroidism.[4] Idiopathic hypoparathyroidism can commence in childhood, but the diagnosis is usually not made until adulthood. Calcification of the basal ganglia and dentate nucleus can also occur in both pseudohypoparathyroidism and pseudo-pseudohypoparathyroidism. Basal ganglia calcification is more frequent in the former (44%) then in the latter disease (8%).[17] The intracranial calcification develops in late childhood or early adulthood. Rarely, basal ganglia calcification occurs in hypothyroidism.

Tuberous sclerosis

The features of tuberous sclerosis are considered in Chapter 8.

Down's syndrome

Bilateral basal ganglia calcification has been reported in up to 45% of patients with Down's syndrome and has been seen in patients as young as 8 years of age.[18] The calcification, thought to be a manifestation of the early aging that is considered to be a feature of Down's syndrome, occurs typically in the globus pallidus. Pathologically the calcification occurs in and around vessel walls and is associated with an amyloid angiopathy.

Inflammatory, toxic, and anoxic conditions

Basal ganglia calcification can occur in a number of inflammatory, toxic, and anoxic conditions. The inflammatory causes are considered in Chapter 5 and the toxic and anoxic conditions in Chapter 6.

Radiation therapy

Radiation therapy has a number of effects on the pediatric brain.[7] Generalized volume loss or atrophy is the most frequently reported abnormality, although in many patients chemotherapy or other drug administration may be contributory. Calcification is not seen as frequently as atrophy and occurs usually at the subcortical gray-white junction as well as in the basal ganglia. The calcification is a result of a radiation-induced vasculopathy with perivascular calcification (mineralizing angiopathy). The MRI appearance of radiation-induced leukoencephalopathy is discussed in Chapters 6 and 7.

Renal tubular acidosis and osteopetrosis

Basal ganglia calcification has been seen in patients with renal tubular acidosis and osteopetrosis.[16] The disease is thought to be caused by a deficiency in carbonic anhydrase II, a zinc metalloenzyme that catalyzes the reversible hydration of carbon dioxide. The disease appears to be transmitted as an autosomal recessive condition and probably should be classified as a metabolic disease. It is characterized clinically by developmental delay.

Progressive encephalopathy with basal ganglia calcifications and CSF lymphocytosis

In 1984 Aicardi and Goutiéres described eight infants belonging to five families with a syndrome characterized by a progressive encephalopathy beginning in the first year of life and leading rapidly to death or to a behavioral vegetative state.[1] In every case CT demonstrated bilateral, symmetrical, nonenhancing lenticular nuclei calcific densities, areas of decreased density in the white matter, and progressive central and cortical atrophy. Possibly the condition is transmitted as a mendelian autosomal recessive condition, but this has not been confirmed.

Correlation with MRI

It is well known that calcifications appear as high density lesions on CT scans. It is less well known that, although calcifications on MRI are either not detected or appear as low intensity areas, on occasion an appearance of hyperintensity may be revealed on T1-weighted images.[8] The explanation for this effect is not yet well established but may be because of the presence of paramagnetic substances such as manganese in the calcium salt or to hydration and paramagnetic effects of the calcium salts.[12]

In cases where calcification is not detected on spin-echo MRI, gradient-echo acquisition scans may detect the lesions as areas of signal loss.[3] The loss can be attributed to variations in static local magnetic susceptibilities created by the presence of diamagnetic calcium crystal deposits causing rapid dephasing of protons due to $T2^*$ decay (see Chapter 1). This effect is eliminated or markedly decreases in standard spin-echo sequences where the effect of the local gradient variations are intentionally rephased by the 180° pulse.

BASAL GANGLIA LUCENCIES

1. Toxic
2. Anoxic
3. Infections

Intoxications

Basal ganglia lucencies are seen on the CT scan after exposure to carbon monoxide gas, massive hydrogen sulfide inhalation, methanol poisoning, and cyanide poisoning.[2,9,14,15] In all these conditions the changes are thought to be caused by the relatively large metabolic demand of the basal ganglia for oxygen, associated with their vulnerability that is attributed to their border-zone location between the major cerebral artery distributions.[5] White matter hypodensity may also occur.[14] The basal ganglia lesions may enhance after contrast administration. When the lesions are present in patients with carbon monoxide inhalation, the prognosis is poor. Areas of mild hypointensity on T1-weighted images and of high intensity on T2-weighted images may also be seen on MRI scans (see Chapter 6).

Patients with central pontine myelinolysis due to rapidly treated hyponatremia may also have basal ganglia lesions, particularly involving the putamina, that are hypointense or isointense on T1-weighted images and hyperintense on T2-weighted images. Central pontine myelinolysis is further discussed in Chapters 5 and 7.

Anoxic brain damage

In cases of severe cerebral hypoxia as occurs with perinatal hypoxia and near drowning, similar low density basal ganglia lesions are seen on CT scans as those seen in patients after toxin ingestion. Identical changes can occur in children with severe hypoglycemia (see Chapter 6).[13]

Infections

Basal ganglia hypodensities on CT have been described in children after encephalitis associated with a lymphocytic meningitis.[10] The associated infectious agent is unknown (see Chapter 5).

Correlation with MRI

The basal ganglia lucencies seen on CT scans are generally caused by edema or gliosis. On MRI these conditions appear as low intensity areas on T1-weighted scans and high intensity areas on T2-weighted scans. Often the high intensity is isointense with CSF on T2-weighted images. Distinction from a CSF-containing cavity is generally possible on the proton-density image where areas of edema or gliosis are brighter than CSF (see Chapter 1).

REFERENCES
Basal ganglia calcifications and lucencies on CT as correlated with MRI

1. Aicardi J, Goutiéres F: A progressive familial encephalopathy in infancy with calcifications of the basal ganglia and chronic cerebrospinal fluid lymphocytosis, *Ann Neurology* 15:49, 1984.
2. Aquilonious SM, Bergstrom K, Enoksson P, et al: Cerebral computer tomography in methanol intoxication, *J Comput Assist Tomogr* 4:425, 1980.
3. Atlas SW, Grossman RI, Hackney DB, et al: Calcified intracranial lesions: detection with gradient-echo acquisition rapid MR imaging, *AJNR* 9:253, 1988.
4. Bennett JC, Maffly RH, Steinbach HL: The significance of bilateral basal ganglia calcification, *Radiology* 72:1954.
5. Bianco F, Floris R: Transient disappearance of bilateral low-density lesions of the globi pallidi in carbon monoxide intoxications and MRI, *J Neuroradiol* 15:381, 1988.
6. Cohen CR, Duchesnau PM, Weinstein MA: Calcification of the basal ganglia as visualised by computed tomography, *Radiology* 134:97, 1980.
7. Davis PC, Hoffman JCJ, Pearl GS, et al: CT evaluation of effects of cranial radiation therapy in children, *AJR* 147:587, 1986.
8. Dell LA, Brown MS, Orrison WW, et al: Physiologic intracranial calcification with hyperintensity on MR imaging: case report and experimental model, *AJNR* 9:1145, 1988.
9. Finelli PF: Case report: changes in the basal ganglia following cyanide poisoning, *J Comput Assist Tomogr* 5:755, 1981.
10. Goutières F, Aicardi J: Acute neurological dysfunction associated with destructive lesions of the basal ganglia in children, *Ann Neurol* 12:328, 1982.
11. Harrington MG, Macpherson P, McIntosh WB, et al: The significance of the incidental finding of basal ganglia calcification on computed tomography, *J Neurol Neurosurg Psychiatry* 44:1168, 1981.
12. Henkelman R, Watts J, Kucharezyk W: High signal intensity on MR images of calcified brain tissue, *Radiology* 179:199, 1991.
13. Kaiser MC, Pettersson H, Harwood-Nash DC, et al: Case report: computed tomography of the brain in severe hypoglycaemia, *J Comput Assist Tomogr* 5:757, 1981.
14. Kim KS, Weinberg PE, Suh IH, et al: Acute carbon monoxide poisoning: computerized tomography of the brain, *AJNR* 1:399, 1982.
15. Matsuo F, Cummins JW, Anderson RE: Neurological sequelae of massive hydrogen sulfide inhalation, *Arch Neurol* 36:451, 1979.
16. Ohlsson A, Cumming WA, Paul A, et al: Carbonic anhydrase II deficiency syndrome: recessive osteopetrosis with renal tubular acidosis and cerebral calcification, *Pediatrics* 77:371, 1986.
17. Steinbach HL, Young OA: The roentgen appearance of pseudohypoparathyroidism (PH) and pseudo-pseudohypoparathyroidism (PPH): differentiation from the syndromes associated with short metacarpals, metatarsals, and phalanges, *Radiology* 97:49, 1966.
18. Takashima S, Becker LE: Basal ganglia calcification in Down's syndrome, *J Neurol Neurosurg Psychiatry* 48:61, 1985.

5 · Intracranial Inflammatory Processes

Samuel M. Wolpert
Edward M. Kaye

Infections of the fetal nervous system differ in their manifestations from those in the adult nervous system in two aspects[1]: (1) infections occurring in the first two trimesters of fetal life may cause congenital malformations, and (2) biologically the fetal nervous system has the capacity to repair damaged brain and compensate for missing tissue, unlike the developed nervous system, which responds to infections by gliosis. Congenital malformations are discussed in Chapter 3. This chapter is concerned with infections acquired in late pregnancy, during birth, in the neonatal period, and during childhood.

Bacterial, viral, and opportunistic infections of the pediatric central nervous system are the most important causes of intracranial infections in childhood. Of these, bacterial meningitis is probably the most common and often the most serious. Other bacterial processes such as epidural and subdural empyema, brain abscess, infections of the central nervous system secondary to extraneural infections (for example, mycotic aneurysms from bacterial endocarditis), and recurrent infections from an otherwise occult cranial or spinal osteomyelitis, sinusitis, or mastoid infection are considerably less frequent. Viral infections such as cytomegalic virus disease, congenital varicella, and herpes encephalitis are also less common than bacterial meningitides. The AIDS epidemic is changing the pattern of intracranial infection, and opportunistic agents involving the central nervous system are becoming more prevalent.

Neuroradiology plays a major role in the identification and assessment of intracranial infections in the pediatric age group. Computed tomography (CT) remains an excellent initial test, identifying as it does so effectively the periventricular calcification, which is a feature of the TORCH group of infections. Ultrasonography (US) or CT can easily identify hydrocephalus caused by either an abscess blocking CSF outflow or meningitis causing an adhesive arachnoiditis. Cerebritis, abscess, or both can be easily detected by CT. The excellent soft tissue contrast obtained with magnetic resonance imaging (MRI) may detect subtle intracranial inflammatory changes not seen on US or CT, including small leptomeningeal collections (obscured by bone on CT) and infections of brain substance (for example, encephalitis).[13] Cerebral angiography is necessary to diagnose intracerebral mycotic aneurysms.

Bacterial infections

MENINGITIS

Meningitis may produce headache, backache, fever, irritability, lethargy, occasional febrile seizures, stiff neck, stiff back, or signs of elevated intracranial pressure. In the neonatal period (first month of life) enterobacteria, listeria monocytogenes, and beta-streptococci are the most frequent cause of meningitis; in infancy and childhood meningococci, *Hemophilus influenzae, Neisseria meningitidis,* and pneumococcus are the primary organisms causing meningitis. The organisms may reach the meninges by one of a number of different routes: (1) direct hematogenous spread, (2) passage through the choroid plexus, (3) rupture of superficial cortical abscesses, or (4) contiguous spread from adjacent structures such as the ear or sinuses.[1] Neuropathologically the meninges are lined by a purulent exudate that involves the base of the brain and may extend over the convexity of the brain. In the neonatal period choroid plexitis with ventriculitis may also occur.

Often at the early stage of the disease symptoms are nonspecific and diagnosis is delayed until neurological complications such as convulsions, coma, bulging of the fontanelle, and macrocephaly occur. The perivascular, or Virchow-Robin, spaces provide access for organisms into the brain.[15] Cerebral edema is a characteristic feature of the acute stage of neonatal bacterial meningitis, and the ventricles may be slitlike. Initially in the neonatal period the CT scan may show areas of extensive hypodensity that may be difficult to distinguish from the normal hypodensity of the developing brain. As the meningitis evolves, enlargement and occasional enhancement of the subarachnoid spaces may occur[3] (Fig. 5-1). According to Bilaniuk and colleagues, the enhancement is caused by vascular enlargement and extravasation of the contrast into the subarachnoid space from newly formed capillaries.[3] Also, a mild hydrocephalus, usually transient, may occur. Similarly, if an MRI scan is carried out in a patient with meningitis, enhancement of the meninges often occurs after Gd-DTPA administration.[6] (Fig. 5-2). On occasion, however, the enhancement may be difficult to distinguish from that occuring after any neurosurgical procedure, such as a shunt placement for hydrocephalus.

Neuroimaging (US or CT) need not be obtained in all patients with meningitis but should be obtained in those with an unfavorable clinical course including depressed consciousness, persistent full fontanelle, prolonged fever, focal neurological deficits, and seizures.[15]

COMPLICATIONS

Complications of meningitis may include seizures, focal deficits, increased intracranial pressure, or recurring fever. US or CT is sufficient for diagnosis and management in most cases and is also used to rule out mass effect before lumbar puncture for CSF analysis and culture.

Hydrocephalus

One of the more frequent complications of leptomeningitis is the development of a communicating hydrocephalus due to blockage of the basal cisterns or other CSF pathways by the purulent exudate. On CT or US the hydrocephalus becomes apparent through ventricular enlargement (Fig. 5-1), sometimes accompanied by enlargement of the basal cisterns.[4,7] Secondary hydrocephalus is relatively frequent in pneumococcal, streptococcal, and *Escherichia coli* meningitis, but infrequent in meningococcal and *Hemophilas*

influenzae meningitis. Ventricular dilatation secondary to obstruction of CSF flow should be distinguished from that due to loss of brain substance. Since both hydrocephalus and atrophy are usually present concurrently, this distinction may be difficult.[16]

Infarction

Cerebral infarcts have been described in 30% of neonatal patients with bacterial meningitis[9] and can rapidly evolve into porencephalic cysts.[8] The infarcts are related to an associated vasculitis, which is an almost invariable accompaniment of neonatal meningitis.[2] Involvement of the veins is severe, and, despite arterial involvement, arterial occlusions are infrequent, although segmental narrowing of major intracranial arteries has been demonstrated angiographically[10] and infarcts have been seen on MRI scans.[14] The infarcts are usually caused by cortical and subependymal venous thrombosis and may be large and multiple. They may also occur in older children.[9]

Abscess

Intracerebral abscesses are usually of hematogenous origin[9] and rarely follow meningitis except in the premature infant, in which case the offending organism is usually *Citrobacter* (see Brain Abscess, p. 165). The abscesses often develop in a region of infarction and may rupture into the ventricles. On CT the abscesses appear as low density mass lesions with margin enhancement after the administration of intravenous contrast material.

Ventriculitis

Ventriculitis, that is, inflammatory exudate and bacteria in the ventricular fluid and ependymal lining, is a particularly common feature of neonatal meningitis.[16] The critical events are bacteremia and infection of the choroid plexus and lateral ventricles. On CT there is focal contrast enhancement of the ventricular walls.[5] US shows intraventricular echogenicity. The intact ventricular walls appear to be a barrier against penetrating infection of the adjacent white matter. However, in the hydrocephalic infant it is postulated that the enlarged extracellular spaces adjacent to the ventricle promote the spread of infection to the adjacent white matter.[12] The process leads to edematous periventricular cavities that may coalesce, enlarge, and compress the ventricles. On US or CT pseudoloculation of the ventricles is seen. Ependymal scarring with ventricular loculation may result. MRI scans after Gd-DTPA administration may show enhancement of the ventricular walls.[14]

Subdural effusion

Seldom seen in the newborn period, subdural effusions are more frequently seen at the age of 2 to 3 months or later. Usually they do not require surgical management except when they are large or purulent. CT is more reliable than US in the diagnosis of subdural effusions. The effusions, which are usually bilateral, are evident as low density extraaxial fluid collections in the frontal or parietal regions

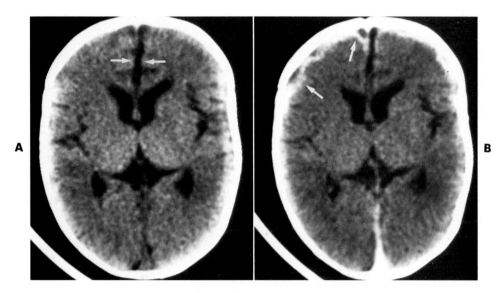

Fig. 5-1   CT scans in a 2-month-old girl. **A,** There is moderate enlargement of the lateral ventricles and some widening of the interhemispheric fissure *(arrows).* **B,** Note the prominence of the sylvian fissures and the surface contrast enhancement over the frontal lobes *(arrows).*
Diagnosis: Hemophilus influenzae meningitis and communicating hydrocephalus.

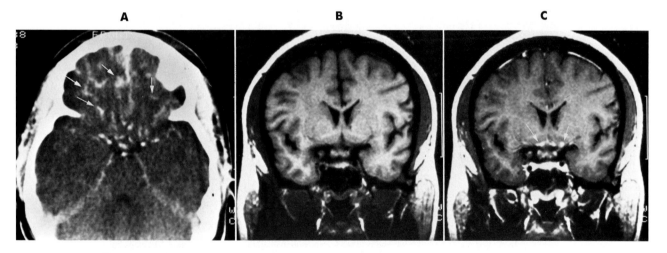

Fig. 5-2   CT and MRI scans in an adult with meningitis following sarcoid infection. **A,** CT scan after contrast administration demonstrates irregular enhancement in the basal meninges *(arrows).* Coronal T1 MRI before gadolinium administration **(B)** and after gadolinium enhancement **(C)** demonstrate enhancement of the basal meninges *(arrows).* (Same case as illustrated in Fig. 5-21.)

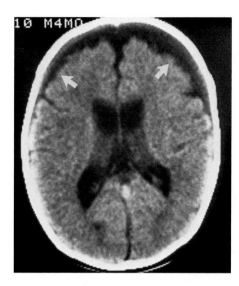

Fig. 5-3   Nonenhanced CT scan in a 4-month-old infant demonstrates enlargement of both lateral ventricles, as well as widening of the extracerebral spaces anteriorly extending into the hemispheric fissure *(arrows)*.
Diagnosis: Bilateral subdural effusions (postmeningitis).

(Figs. 5-3 and 5-4). Contrast enhancement is common but does not distinguish effusion from empyema and is therefore not usually indicated. The collections may be indistinguishable from a wide subarachnoid space after loss of brain parenchyma. Increase in head size confirms the diagnosis.

Subdural and epidural empyema

Infected subdural effusions rarely lead to the development of subdural empyemas as a complication of meningitis. More commonly, subdural and epidural empyemas arise denovo from sinus or otomastoid infection. They are considered later in this chapter (see Intracranial Suppuration, p. 165). By CT the lesions are usually unilateral and evident as crescent-shaped hypodense or isodense areas adjacent to the cortex with a peripheral rimlike enhancement after intravenous contrast administration with underlying cerebral edema.[11] In this context the lesions are usually neurosurgical emergencies because of the tendency for rapid subpial extension and brain involvement with subsequent edema, infarction, and potential herniation. Although not recommended for routine evaluation, MRI studies following gadolinium-DTPA administration may

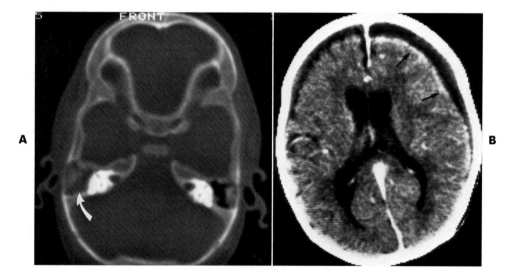

Fig. 5-4   CT scans in a 9-month-old child. **A,** Axial scan through the skull base demonstrates erosion and opacification of the right mastoid air cells *(arrow).* **B,** Contrast-enhanced scan at the level of the lateral ventricles demonstrates bilateral subdural effusions with enhancement of the cortical surface particularly on the left side *(arrows).* Note also the slight ventricular enlargement.
Diagnosis: Pneumococcal meningitis with erosive mastoiditis, bilateral subdural effusions, and communicating hydrocephalus.

demonstrate inflammatory exudates otherwise not seen following contrast-enhanced CT scans.

Cerebral atrophy and encephalomalacia

Cerebral atrophy constitutes one of the more prevalent complications of meningitis. It is manifested by loss of both gray and white matter. Radiologically, enlargement of the ventricles and widening of the sulci are seen. Occasionally, widespread necrosis with or without cystic change (that is, encephalomalacia) may occur.

Venous thrombosis

Cortical, deep vein, and dural sinus thrombosis may follow meningitis (see p. 168).

Recurrent meningitis

In patients in whom infectious meningitis is a recurrent problem, a parameningeal focus needs to be suspected and diagnosed if possible. Possible sites include the mastoid air cells, nasal sinuses, occult cranial and spinal infections, or dysraphism with dermal sinuses. A CSF leak, through either the nose or ear, may also be a source for recurrent infections. The leak is evaluated by CT cisternography using a water-soluble contrast agent or by radionuclide cisternography (RC). CT provides better special resolution and specificity, although RC may be more sensitive. Recurrent noninfectious or chemical meningitis may be related to intracranial or intraspinal epidermoid or dermoid cysts.

REFERENCES
Bacterial infections
1. Barkovich A: Infections of the nervous system. In Barkovich A: *Pediatric neuroimaging,* New York, 1990, Raven.
2. Berman PH, Banker BQ: Neonatal meningitis: a clinical and pathological study of 29 cases, *Pediatrics* 38:6, 1966.
3. Bilaniuk LT, Zimmerman RA, Brown L, et al: Computed tomography in meningitis, *Neuroradiology* 16:13, 1978.
4. Bodino J, Lylyc P, Del Valle M, et al: Computed tomography in purulent meningitis, *Am J Dis Child* 136:495, 1982.
5. Brown LW, Zimmerman RA, Bilaniuk LT: Polycystic brain disease complicating neonatal meningitis: documentation of evolution by computed tomography, *J Pediatr* 94:757, 1979.
6. Chang KH, Han MH, Roh JK, et al: Gd-DTPA–enhanced MR imaging of the brain in patients with meningitis: comparison with CT, *AJNR* 11:69, 1990.
7. Cockrill HH, Dreisbach J, Lowe B, et al: Computed tomography in leptomeningeal infections, *AJR* 130:511, 1978.
8. Diebler C, Dulac O: Infectious diseases of the central nervous system. In Diebler C, Dulac O, editors: *Pediatric neurology and neuroradiology,* Berlin, 1987, Springer-Verlag.
9. Friede RL: Cerebral infarcts complicating neonatal meningitis: acute and residual lesions, *Acta Neuropathol* 23:245, 1973.
10. Gado M, Axley J, Appleton DB, et al: Angiography in the acute and post-treatment phases of *Hemophilus influenzae* meningitis, *Radiology* 110:439, 1974.
11. Jacobson PL, Farmer TW: Subdural empyema complicating meningitis in infants: improved prognosis, *Neurology* 31:190, 1981.
12. Naidich TP, McLone DG, Yamanouchi Y: Periventricular white matter cysts in a murine model of gram-negative ventriculitis, *AJNR* 4:461, 1983.
13. Schroth G, Kretzschmar K, Gawehn J, et al: Advances of magnetic resonance imaging in the diagnosis of cerebral infections, *Neuroradiology* 29:120, 1987.
14. Smith RR, Kuharik MA: Inflammation and infection of the brain. In Cohen MD, Edwards MK: *Magnetic resonance imaging of children,* Philadelphia, 1990, BC Decker.
15. Snyder RD: Bacterial infection of the nervous system. In Swaiman KF: *Pediatric neurology: principles and practice,* St Louis, 1989, Mosby–Year Book.
16. Volpe JJ: Bacterial and fungal intracranial infections. In Volpe JJ: *Neurology of the newborn,* ed 2, Philadelphia, 1987, WB Saunders.

Viral and parasitic infections

Viral infections of the CNS may affect the embryo, occur during delivery, or be acquired in infancy or childhood. The viruses may attack specific CNS cells or affect entire regions of the brain.[9] For instance, rabies tends to involve the hypothalamus, brain stem, and limbic system; herpes simplex virus type 1 involves the basal frontal and temporal lobes; herpes simplex type 2 produces a generalized encephalitis; varicella attacks the cerebellum; mumps affects the brain stem; and poliomyelitis involves the anterior horn cells of the spinal cord. The clinical and imaging (when present) characteristics of these diseases are then appropriate to the areas involved. Almost all virus infections of the CNS are associated with an immune host response, and the neurological disorders are a result of both the direct viral effect and the host reaction.

The clinical expression of the neurological disease can be acute, subacute, or chronic. Herpes encephalitis is an example of an acute viral neurological disease, and subacute sclerosing encephalitis an example of a subacute disease. Both diseases have implications in neuroimaging. Both hemorrhagic leukoencephalitis and disseminated encephalomyelitis have been called *acute,* not because of the acuity of clinical presentation but because of the rapid course of the disease. Characteristic imaging changes are seen in both. Acquired rubella manifests as a chronic infection. Chronic neuroviral disorders appear years after the contraction of congenitally acquired infections such as rubella and cytomegalic disease. On occasions an encephalitis may occur as a sequel to a prophylactic vaccination, known as *postvaccinal encephalomyelitis.* This disorder may be caused by both a viral invasion of the nervous system and an antigen-antibody reaction.[4]

Most viral infections in infancy result from the transplacental passage of microorganisms, usually consequent to infection within the maternal blood stream. Infections due to herpes simplex is an exception to this rule, because most such cases are contracted around the time of birth, as either an ascending infection just before birth or during passage through an infected birth canal.[27]

In addition to the perinatal-acquired viral infections a host of viruses and nonviruses are known to attack the embryo and cause an embryogenic encephalopathy. The TORCH group of microbes (*t*oxoplasmosis, *o*ther enteroviruses, varicella, mumps, measles, *r*ubella, *c*ytomegalic inclusion disease and *h*erpes simplex) have a special virulence in the developing nervous system. HIV needs to be added to the TORCH acronym. For most of these diseases CT with or without contrast enhancement (or US in the neonate) is usually adequate for diagnosis, and MRI is usually not necessary.

MUMPS

CNS involvement has been observed in up to 6.5% of patients with mumps, usually as an aseptic meningitis.[18] Hydrocephalus may occur after a variable latent period of between months and years.[22] The use and advantages of MRI over CT in demonstrating mumps encephalitis have been described by Tarr et al.,[24] who found MRI to be more sensitive than CT in the detection of an associated encephalitis.

RUBELLA

Both rubella and measles may cause leukoencephalitis. In those few children in whom a progressive downhill course occurs, diffuse edematous low density of the white matter associated with progressive cerebral atrophy is seen on the CT scan.[5] In cases of congenital rubella, microcephaly may result. Although rare, intracranial calcifications may occur.

CYTOMEGALIC VIRUS DISEASE

Cytomegalic virus infection is the most common and serious of the congenital infections. Maternal infection is very common, occurring in 3% to 6% of unselected pregnant women.[23] Nearly 50% of infants whose mothers are infected during pregnancy develop the infection, usually transplacentally.

In patients with cytomegalic virus infections, pathologically a number of different processes occur together or in varying degrees. Meningoencephalitis characterized by parenchymal brain necrosis has a predilection for the periventricular region of the lateral ventricles and accounts for periventricular calcification (mineralizing microangiopathy). The appearances are similar to those of toxoplasmosis. Calcification and the resulting atrophy, multicystic encephalomalacia, or hydranencephaly are readily seen on CT[2] (Fig. 5-5) and often with US. Microcephaly, which is related to the encephaloclastic effects of the virus, may cause a disturbance of germinal matrix proliferation in the developing brain and may account for the decrease in cellular count found in the disease.[15] This teratogenic effect may also explain the polymicrogyria seen in many infants with the infection. On MRI paraventricular cystic structures, usually bilateral and adjacent to the occipital horns, are noted[3] (Fig. 5-6). The calcification may be bright on T1-weighted images (Figs. 5-5, C and D). Pachygyria and neuronal heterotopia have also been seen in patients with cytomegalic virus disease as a result of intrauterine infection.[25]

HERPES SIMPLEX ENCEPHALITIS

Herpes simplex virus is responsible for one of the most frequent forms of perinatal and childhood encephalitis.

Although less common than cytomegalic encephalitis, essentially all cases of neonatal herpes simplex infections are symptomatic, which is often not the case with cytomegalic disease. The increased incidence of neonatal herpes simplex infection appears to be linked to the increase in the incidence of genital herpes simplex infection in adults.

The disease is acquired at the time of birth through direct contact with the infant's skin, eye, or oral cavity.[27] Since herpes simplex virus type 2 usually infects the maternal genital tract, the majority of infections in infants and young children are of this type. Herpes simplex virus type I usually occurs in older children and adults. Pathologically a diffuse meningoencephalitis occurs with multifocal necrosis accompanied by a considerable degree of brain swelling. In contradistinction to the more regional adult form of the disease, the frontal and temporal lobes are not usually primarily involved in infantile herpes, although exceptions occur (Fig. 5-7). Multicystic encephalomalacia and microcephaly may result.[6]

Herpes simplex encephalitis may be present before abnormalities can be seen on CT or US, and therapy should not depend on an abnormal study. A normal CT scan has no prognostic value.[1] As the disease evolves, the scan demonstrates patchy areas of low density in the cerebral parenchyma (Fig. 5-8), often commencing in the parietal lobes and subsequently affecting the temporal and occipital lobes. The gyri may be hyperintense on an nonenhaced scan, possibly because of an intrinsic hypervascularity, the previous administration of contrast material with prolonged contrast retention, or calcification.[17] The contrast enhancement, which is usually asymmetrical (Figs. 5-7 and 5-8), may be intense and prolonged.[11] Ventricular compression due to cerebral edema may be initially observed with subsequent rapid evolution of areas of encephalomalacia (Fig. 5-9). Because of the increased sensitivity of MRI to early cerebral edema as compared to CT, MRI may be the preferred test[16,20] (Fig. 5-10). MRI demonstrates abnormal decreased signal on T1-weighted scans and increased signal on T2-weighted scans. Both the white and gray matter may be involved. Hemorrhagic changes may also be detected in the margin of the lesion.[21] Gd-DTPA enhancement is patchy and irregular.[21] MRI may not be as helpful in the young infant as in the older child because the high intensity changes on T2-weighted scans may not be easily separated from the normal "watery" immature white matter.

ACUTE LEUKOENCEPHALITIS

Acute disseminated encephalomyelitis (ADEM) is one of the commonest forms of infectious or postinfectious encephalopathy in childhood. It is characterized by nonspecific symptoms and signs such as drowsiness, fever, seizures, pyramidal and extrapyramidal signs, nystagmus, cranial nerve abnormalities, and akinetic mutism. The disease is often associated with a viral prodrome or is postviral or postvaccinal. It is usually self-limiting, running a 2- to 3-week course.[5]

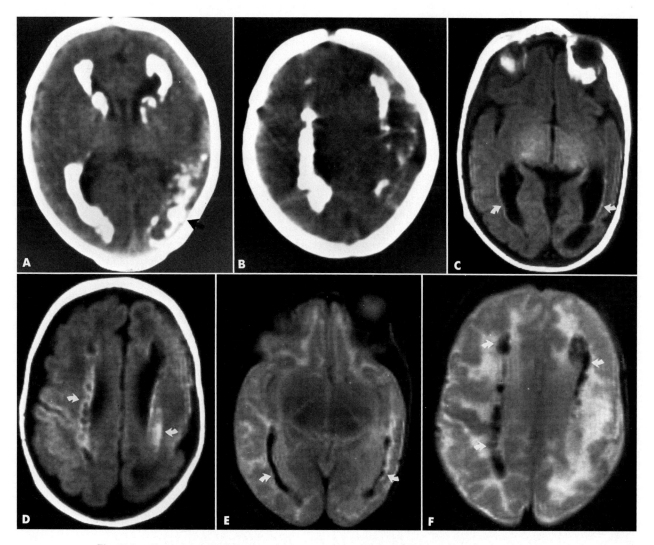

Fig. 5-5 Nonenhanced CT scans in a 15-day-old infant. **A,** Note the marked subependymal calcification surrounding both anterior horns and both occipital horns. Calcification also exists in the left parietal cortex *(arrow).* **B,** Supraventricular calcification is present at a higher level. **C,** Short TR/short TE MRI scan demonstrates slight enlargement of the occipital horns together with thin high intensity subependymal lesions bilaterally *(arrows).* **D,** At a higher level high intensity areas are apparent bilaterally in the subependymal regions (compare with **B**). **E,** Long TR/long TE MRI scan in same level as shown in **C.** Note the bilateral low intensity lesions surrounding both occipital horns *(arrows).* **F,** Scan at same level as that in **D.** Note the bilateral low intensity lesions particularly on the right side *(arrows).*

Diagnosis: Cytomegalic virus infection. The high intensity areas seen on the short TR/short TE scans may be caused by a proteinaceous matrix within the calcification that causes T1 shortening. The low intensity areas seen on the long TR/long TE scans are probably caused by the lack of mobile protons within the calcium. See p. 149.

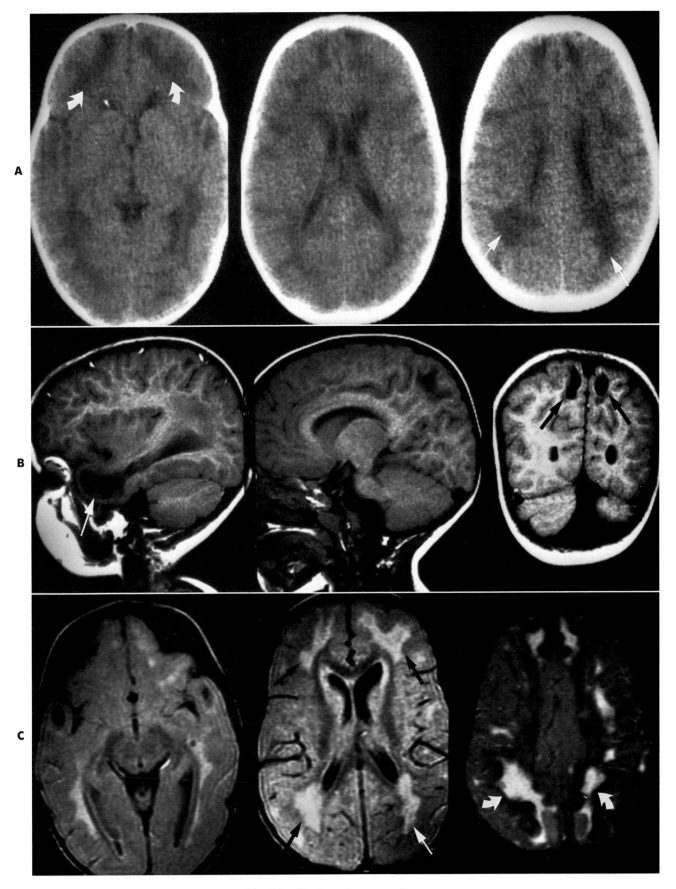

Fig. 5-6   For legend see opposite page.

Fig. 5-6   CT and MRI scans in a 4-year-old girl. **A,** Nonenhanced CT scans. Low density areas are present in both frontal lobes and in the centrum semiovale and periatrial regions bilaterally *(arrows).* **B,** MRI scans. Short TR/short TE images, sagittal *(left* and *center)* and coronal *(right),* demonstrate low intensity areas in the right temporal lobe, as well as in the parietal lobes bilaterally *(arrows).* **C,** Long TR/short TE images demonstrate increased signal in the periatrial regions bilaterally and in the supraventricular areas frontally and bilaterally *(arrows).* The child demonstrated gross motor and language delay together with hepatosplenomegaly and cytomegalic inclusion virus infection. The levels of the three CT scans in **A** approximately match those of the three MRI scans in **C.**
Diagnosis: Cytomegalic virus disease (presumptive).

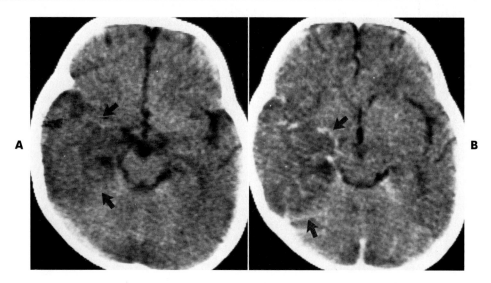

Fig. 5-7   CT scans in a 6-month-old infant. **A,** Nonenhanced CT image demonstrates a low density area in the right temporal lobe *(arrows).* **B,** Following contrast administration marginal enhancement surrounds the low density area *(arrows).*
Diagnosis: Herpes encephalitis type 2.

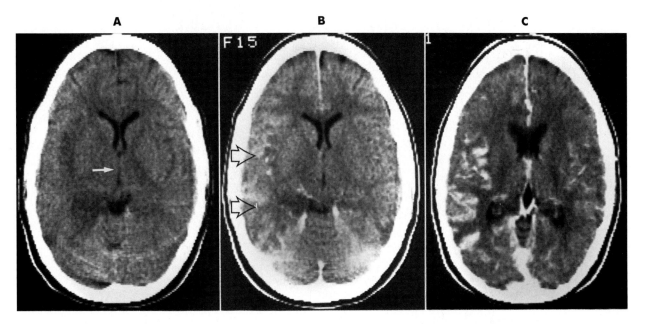

Fig. 5-8   CT scans in a 16-year-old. **A,** Note the slight compression of the third ventricle *(arrow)* and minimal compression of the anterior horn. The sylvian fissure is effaced on the right side. **B,** Following contrast administration there is subtle enhancement of the right temporal lobe *(arrows).* **C,** Scan obtained after contrast enhancement 2 weeks later demonstrates marked enhancement of the right temporal and parietal lobes.
Diagnosis: Herpes encephalitis.

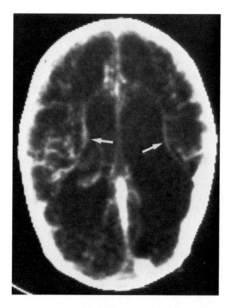

Fig. 5-9   Contrast-enhanced CT scan. Note the massive enlargement of the lateral ventricles *(arrows)* with marked destruction of the surrounding brain in a 7-week-old child.
Diagnosis: Herpes encephalitis.

Usually the CT scan is normal, but on occasion low density areas attributed to edema may be seen in the white matter. In children with a favorable outcome the low density areas disappear, but in children with an unfavorable outcome progressive cerebral atrophy may result.[5] Rarely the aqueduct may be occluded when the disease follows congenital rubella infection.[19] MRI is the imaging method of choice, often showing poorly marginated, multifocal white matter lesions mimicking multiple sclerosis.[8] (Fig. 5-11). When the lesions are symmetrical they additionally involve the basal ganglia, thalami, and cerebellum. If no new lesions appear on follow-up examination, the diagnosis of acute disseminated encephalomyelitis rather than multiple sclerosis can be made.[12] Acute hemorrhagic encephalomyelitis occurs less frequently than ADEM and generally runs a more fulminating course, although recovery has been observed (Fig. 5-12).

SUBACUTE SCLEROSING PANENCEPHALITIS

Subacute sclerosing panencephalitis (SSPE) is a slowly progressive and usually fatal encephalitis probably caused by the measles virus. It typically starts with mental or behavioral abnormalities, progressing to myoclonic jerks, convulsions, tremors, coma, and death. The disease usually

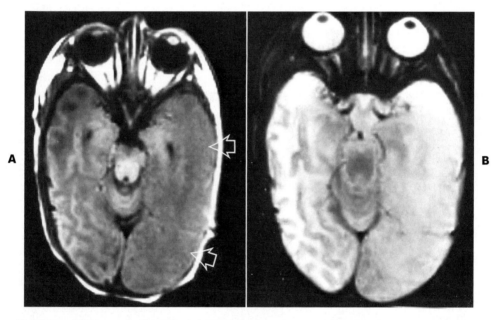

Fig. 5-10   MRI scans. **A,** Short TR/short TE image demonstrates a diffuse low intensity area involving the left temporal and occipital lobes *(arrows)*. **B,** Long TR/long TE image at same level as that shown in **A**. There is an ill-defined high intensity area involving the left temporal and occipital lobes. Note the effacement of the sulci and lack of white-gray matter differentiation on both **A** and **B**.
Diagnosis: Herpes encephalitis in a 3-week-old infant.

lasts from 1 to 3 years. Neuropathological studies demonstrate gray matter gliosis and perivascular lymphocytic infiltration. Demyelination of variable degrees is seen in the white matter. Pathological changes are also found in the basal ganglia, pons, and thalamus.

CT findings are usually normal in the first weeks after onset, and then low density lesions may appear in the white matter and basal ganglia.[7] These features may be seen only after 1 month into the course of the disease.[5] Lateral ventricular dilatation, cortical atrophy, as well as brain stem and cerebellar atrophy are seen late in the disease.[13] Areas of increased intensity on T2-weighted images have been reported in the cerebellum, anterior pons, and in the white matter of the temporal, occipital, and parietal lobes bilaterally.[26]

PROGRESSIVE MULTIFOCAL LEUKOENCEPHALOPATHY

Progressive multifocal leukoencephalopathy (PML), caused by papovavirus, has become one of the most common viral demyelinating disorders.[10] The disease affects immunocompromised patients or those infected with the AIDS virus. The lesions are hypodense on CT and hyperintense on T2 MRI and occur in the subcortical white

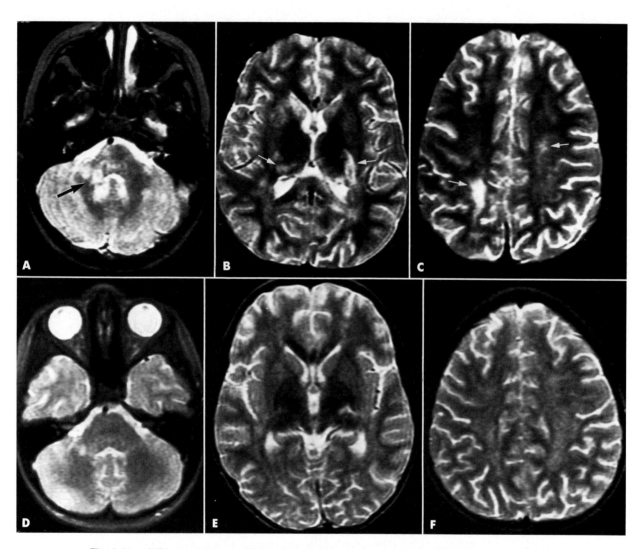

Fig. 5-11   MRI scans (all long TR/long TE studies) of a 7-year-old with headaches, neck stiffness, and seizure after vaccination. Note the high intensity lesions in the middle cerebellar peduncles (**A,** *arrows*), both posterolateral thalami (**B,** *arrows*), and both centra semiovale (**C,** *arrows*). **D-F,** 1 week later after steroid therapy all the lesions have almost completely resolved, indicating a favorable prognosis.
Diagnosis: Acute disseminated encephalomyelitis.

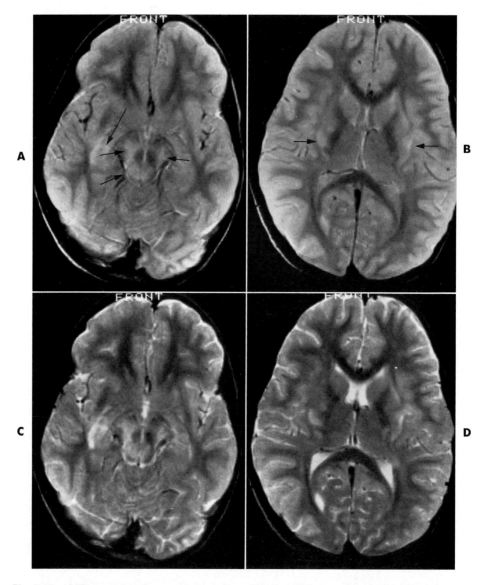

Fig. 5-12   MRI scans in a 6-year-old girl. **A,** Long TR/short TE image. Note the high intensity areas in the tegmentum and tectum of the midbrain *(arrows),* as well as in the hippocampal region on the right side *(long-tailed arrow).* **B,** Long TR/short TE image. Note the high intensity areas in the putamina bilaterally *(arrows).* **C,** Long TR/long TE scans at same level as that shown in **A.** Again note the high intensity areas in the tectum and tegmentum of the midbrain, as well as in the hippocampus on the right side. **D,** Scan at same level as that shown in **B.** Note the high intensity lesions in the putamina bilaterally with extension into the external capsule on the left.
Diagnosis: Acute hemorrhagic leukoencephalitis in a 6-year-old girl.

matter.[14] Enhancement of the margins of the lesions may occur after Gd-DTPA administration.[10]

TOXOPLASMOSIS

Infection with *Toxoplasma gondii* has become particularly prevalent with the AIDS epidemic and is a relatively frequent finding in the adult patient. Toxoplasmosis represents one of the significant infections occurring during intrauterine life and results from the transplacental passage of the parasite, usually in the third trimester. The neuroimaging appearances grossly correlate with the time of fetal infection. If the infection occurs in the first half of pregnancy, enlargement of the third and lateral ventricles is constant[5] and may be marked. Multiple periventricular calcifications symmetrically line the ventricles and may also occupy the basal ganglia (Fig. 5-13). Microophthalmia and ocular calcifications (chorioretinitis) may also be evident. Multiple porencephalic cysts may appear. With infection in the last trimester, ventricular dilatation and intracerebral calcification are unusual. The pathological basis for the imaging findings include multifocal, necrotizing, granulomatous meningoencephalitis with perivascular and parenchymal necroses. Since the toxoplasmosis inflammation has a predilection for the periventricular region and since the *Toxoplasma* organisms enter the ventricular system to cause periventricular arteritis or thrombophlebitis and necrosis, an aqueductal block can occur, resulting in hydrocephalus. If the multifocal necrotizing encephalitis is overwhelming, microcephaly may result. When toxoplasmosis affects the fully developed brain, the lesions are seen as cystic or solid

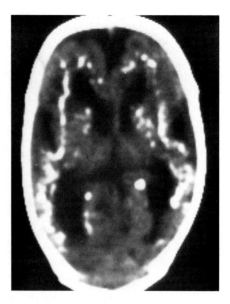

Fig. 5-13   CT scan in a 2-month-old infant. Diffuse bifocal periventricular and basal ganglia calcification is seen. Note also the dilated ventricles.
Diagnosis: Congenital toxoplasmosis

intracerebral masses (Figs. 5-14 and 5-15) and are of low intensity on T1-weighted and high intensity on T2-weighted scans. Toxoplasmosis lesions may also be seen as hyperechoic areas on US, which may be valuable as a screening test (Fig. 5-16).

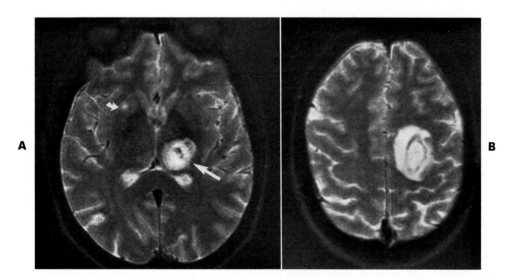

Fig. 5-14   MRI scans. **A,** Axial long TR/long TE images demonstrate high intensity lesion with central low intensity in the basal ganglia on the left side *(straight arrow).* A second high intensity lesion is seen in the anterior putamen on the right side *(curved arrow).* **B,** A third lesion with a central high intensity, surrounding low intensity, and outer high intensity representing edema is noted in the left centrum semiovale.
Diagnosis: Toxoplasmosis.

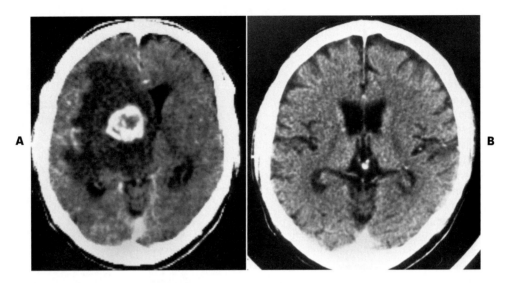

Fig. 5-15   CT scans. **A,** Note the contrast-enhancing lesion with a central lucency and marked surrounding edema in the right cerebral hemisphere. There is obliteration of the right anterior horn with marked displacement of the ventricular system to the left side. **B,** Following treatment there is complete resolution of the lesion. The patient was treated with sulfadiazine and pyrimethamine with dramatic response.
Diagnosis: Toxoplasmosis.

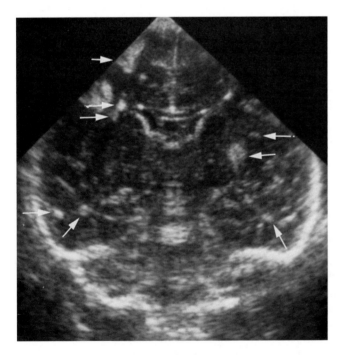

Fig. 5-16   Coronal ultrasound study in a 7-day-old infant who has positive blood titres for toxoplasmosis, demonstrating multiple hyperechoic areas bilaterally *(arrows).*

REFERENCES
Viral and parasitic infections

1. Arvin AM, Yeager AS, Brahn FW, et al: Neonatal herpes simplex infection in the absence of mucocutaneous lesions, *J Pediatr* 100:715, 1982.
2. Bale JF, Bray PF, Bell WE: Neuroradiologic abnormalities in congenital cytomegalovirus infection, *Pediatr Neurol* 1:42, 1985.
3. Boesch CL, Issakainen J, Kewitz G, et al: Magnetic resonance imaging of the brain in congenital cystomegalovirus infection, *Pediatr Radiol* 19:19, 1989.
4. Croft P: Parainfectious and postvaccinal encephalomyelitis, *Postgrad Med J* 45:392, 1969.
5. Diebler C, Dulac O: Infectious diseases of the central nervous system. In Diebler C, Dulac O, editors: *Pediatric neurology and neuroradiology,* Berlin, 1987, Springer-Verlag.
6. Dublin AB, Merten DF: Computed tomography in the evaluation of herpes simplex encephalitis, *Radiology* 125:133, 1977.
7. Duda EE, Huttenlocker PR, Patronas NJ: CT of subacute sclerosing panencephalitis, *AJNR* 1:35, 1980.
8. Dunn V, Bale JF, Zimmerman RA, et al: MRI in children with postinfectious disseminated encephalomyelitis, *Magn Reson Imag* 4:25, 1986.
9. Dyken P: Viral diseases of the nervous system. In Swaiman K: *Pediatric neurology: principles and practice,* St Louis, 1989, Mosby–Year Book.
10. Edwards MK: Metabolic, endocrine, and iatrogenic lesions of the brain. In Cohen MD, Edwards MK: *Magnetic resonance imaging of children,* Philadelphia, 1990, BC Decker.
11. Junck L, Enzmann DR, DeArmond SJ, et al: Prolonged brain retention of contrast agent in neonatal herpes simplex encephalitis, *Radiology* 140:123, 1981.

12. Kesselring J, Miller DH, Robb SA, et al: Acute disseminated encephalomyelitis. MRI findings and the distinction from multiple sclerosis, *Brain* 113:291, 1990.

13. Krawiecki NS, Dyken PR, El Gammal T, et al: Computed tomography of the brain in subacute sclerosing panencephalitis, *Ann Neurol* 15:489, 1984.

14. Levy JD, Cottingham KL, Campbell RJ, et al: Progressive multifocal leukomalacia and magnetic resonance imaging, *Ann Neurol* 19:399, 1986.

15. Naeye RL: Cytomegalic inclusion disease: the fetal disorder, *Am J Clin Pathol* 47:738, 1967.

16. Neils EW, Lukin R, Tomsick TA, et al: Magnetic resonance imaging and computerized scanning of herpes simplex encephalitis, *J Neurosurg* 67:592, 1987.

17. Noorbehesht B, Enzmann DR, Sullender W, et al: Neonatal herpes simplex encephalitis: correlation of clinical and CT findings, *Radiology* 162:813, 1987.

18. Russell RR, Donald JC: The neurological complications of mumps, *Br Med J* II:27, 1958.

19. Sarwar M, Azar-Kia B, Schechter MM, et al: Aqueductal occlusion in the congenital rubella syndrome, *Neurology* 24:198, 1974.

20. Schroth G, Kretzschmar K, Gawehn J, et al: Advances of magnetic resonance imaging in the diagnosis of cerebral infections, *Neuroradiology* 29:120, 1987.

21. Smith RR, Kuharik MA: Inflammation and infection of the brain. In Cohen MD, Edwards MK: *Magnetic resonance imaging of children*, Philadelphia, 1990, BC Decker.

22. Spataro RF, Lin SR, Horner FA, et al: Aqueductal stenosis and hydrocephalus: rare sequelae of mumps virus infection, *Neuroradiology* 12:11, 1976.

23. Stagno S, Pass RF, Britt WJ, et al: Consequences of primary maternal CMV infection (P-CMV), *Pediatr Res* 19:305, 1985.

24. Tarr RW, Edwards KM, et al: MRI of mumps encephalitis: comparison with CT evaluation, *Pediatr Radiol* 17:59, 1987.

25. Titelbaum DS, Hayward JC, Zimmerman RA: Pachygyric-like changes: topographic appearance at MR imaging and CT and correlation with neurologic status, *Radiology* 173:663, 1989.

26. Tsuchiya K, Yamauchi T, Furui S, et al: MR imaging vs. CT in subacute sclerosing panencephalitis, *AJNR* 9:943, 1988.

27. Volpe JJ: Viral, protozoan, and related intracranial infections. In Volpe JJ: *Neurology of the newborn*, ed 2, Philadelphia, 1987, WB Saunders.

Intracranial suppuration

BRAIN ABSCESS

In the premature infant brain abscesses usually occur in the deep white matter. The infectious agent is most often *Citrobacter,* an endotoxic bacterium that causes cerebral necrosis in the setting of hypoperfusion of the white matter.[8] The mass effect of the abscess is generally less marked than its volume would indicate, suggesting that the abscess results from the superinfection of an infarct.[2] Cranial US may be as useful as CT in the early diagnosis and will show a hypoechoic center.[4] Occasionally, listeria monocytogenes is the offending agent, producing granulomatous involvement of the meninges, choroid plexus, and subependymal regions; abscesses may result.

In childhood abscesses are usually hematogenous or result from thrombophlebitis associated with infection in adjacent structures. The abscesses most often arise at the junction of the white and gray matter, usually in the cerebral hemispheres and rarely in the cerebellum.[6] Commonly associated conditions include the following:

1. Uncorrected or palliated congenital cyanotic heart disease
2. Suppurative pulmonary infection (for example, cystic fibrosis, now relatively uncommon)
3. Sinus or otomastoid infection
4. Trauma to the sinus or otomastoid region
5. Surgery
6. Sepsis
7. Endocarditis
8. Immunodeficiency (for example, agammaglobulinemia, HIV) or immunosuppression (transplant and the like)

Because of incomplete development, the mastoids and sinuses are rare sources for brain abscess in the first year of life.

In infants older than 2 years of age, cyanotic heart disease (CHD) had been a leading cause of brain abscesses, particularly "uncorrected" or palliated CHD. Early definitive surgical correction of the heart defect and antibiotic prophylaxis have greatly reduced the incidence. Infections of the middle ear and mastoid may cause cerebellar or temporal lobe abscesses or empyema, and infections of the frontal sinuses may cause frontal lobe abscesses or empyema (Fig. 5-17). The brain stem is rarely involved. Abscesses commonly involve or extend into the white matter because of its poorer vascularization relative to gray matter. This often results in delayed and incomplete formation of a capsule on the white matter side with a predilection for microabscess formation or rupture into the ventricular system. The pathological basis for the CT appearance of cerebritis and abscess has been described.[5] Cerebritis represents the earliest stage of abscess formation. In the initial stage of cerebritis CT demonstrates a low density area with ill-defined margins as a result of both the lesion and associated edema.[17] After injection of contrast material irregular dense zones may appear. At a later stage an enhancing ring appears that may not necessarily indicate encapsulation[1] (Figs. 5-17 and 5-18). Within 4 to 6 weeks encapsulation occurs and is evident on the CT scan as a heterogenous area of low density with ill-defined margins and a clear mass effect.[2] Edema and mass effect may be less pronounced in patients whose immune responses are compromised or suppressed (for example, steroids). Ring enhancement is present (Figs. 5-17 and 5-18); the ring is thicker on the cortical side than on the ventricular side because of the higher vascularity of the cortex as compared with the white matter. Because a ring may be present in both cerebritis and in the abscess stage, it may not always be easy to determine when surgical intervention is necessary. The abscesses may be multiple or multiloculated. With cerebellar abscesses there may be marked obstructive hydrocephalus. With cerebellar and temporal lobe abscesses the middle ear and mastoid may be opaque on CT.[2] If medical therapy is chosen, the lesion should progressively become smaller but the ring enhancement may persist for 2 to 3 months.

Features corresponding to those seen on the CT scan are also seen on the MRI scan. On T1-weighted images the ring

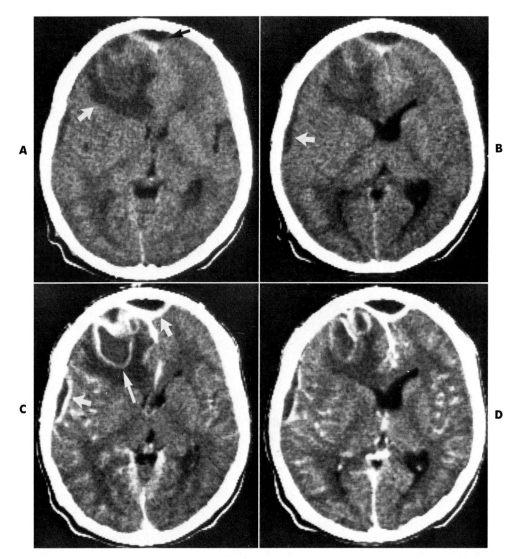

Fig. 5-17   CT scans in a 13-year-old. **A,** Nonenhanced scan. Note the large area of low density in the right frontal lobe *(white arrow)* and a central area of slightly higher density. The ventricular system is displaced to the left. An extraaxial fluid collection is present anteriorly *(black arrow)*. **B,** Scan 1 cm higher than scan in **A.** Again, the low density area is seen in the right frontal lobe with a central area of relatively higher density. Note the low density area extraaxially in the midline in the frontal region and a second extraaxial low density in the right parietal area *(arrow)*. **C,** Contrast-enhanced scan at same level as that in **A** demonstrates marked ring enhancement in the right frontal region *(short arrows)* together with enhancement of the margins of the extraaxial fluid collections anteriorly and over the right parietal cortex *(arrow)*. **D,** Note the posterior displacement of the falx indicating the epidural location of the fluid collection. Contrast-enhanced scan at same level as that in **B** demonstrates similar appearances to those shown in **C.**
Diagnosis: Right frontal lobe abscess, right parietal subdural empyema, and right frontal epidural empyema. (Note: the extraaxial parietal lesion could be in either the subdural or epidural space.)

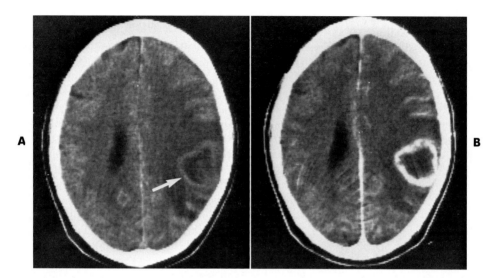

Fig. 5-18   CT scans. **A,** Nonenhanced scan. There is a left parietal low density lesion with a surrounding higher density ring *(arrow).* Surrounding the ring white matter low density indicative of edema is evident. **B,** Following contrast administration the ring lesion is markedly enhanced.
Diagnosis: Cerebral abscess together with marked surrounding edema and ventricular compression.

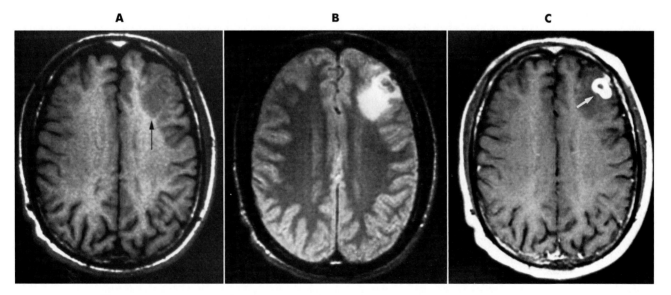

Fig. 5-19   MRI scans. **A,** Short TR/short TE image. Note the low intensity lesion at the gray-white matter interface in the left frontal lobe *(arrow).* **B,** Long TR/short TE image. The lesion is of a high intensity because of surrounding edema. The abscess itself is seen as a low intensity area within the high intensity region. **C,** Study after Gd-DTPA administration using short TR/short TE image. Note the ring-enhancing lesion *(arrow)* with surrounding low intensity indicating edema.
Diagnosis: Cerebral abscess.

is mildly hyperintense, and on T2-weighted images the ring is hypointense relative to white matter (Fig. 5-19). There may be a progressive decrease in the signal on later echoes, possibly because of a paramagnetic effect. The ring is present in all mature and chronic abscesses but absent in cases of acute cerebritis.[9] In addition, vasogenic edema surrounds the abscess cavity and is evident as a hypointense halo on T1-weighted images and a hyperintense area on T2-weighted images. The abscess center demonstrates T1 lengthening relative to brain (hypointensity) and T2 prolongation relative to brain (hyperintensity). Identical features also occur in cystic or necrotic neoplasms.

Neuroimaging also plays a significant role in the treatment of children with brain abscesses. Stereotactic devices are now available using either CT- or MRI-compatible frames for the development of coordinates for the draining of abscesses under local anesthesia. If a craniotomy is necessary for the drainage of an abscess, US guidance can help detect the abscess in the operating room.

SUBDURAL EMPYEMA

Incompletely treated sinusitis or otitis in the young child may lead to subdural empyemas, usually secondary to a phlebitis (see Fig. 5-17). Other causes of subdural empyemas are postoperative infection of a craniotomy cavity, posttraumatic infection of an extraaxial hematoma, or any other cause of intracranial infection. In the infant the empyema may rarely follow meningitis. Pus may collect along the tentorium and falx. The lesions are evident on CT as low density or isodense areas with margin enhancement over the convexity of the brain or parasagittally alongside the falx.[15] The medial border (toward brain) is concave, which is a distinguishing feature from the rare epidural abscess, which usually has a convex border medially.[14] A subdural empyema may have an accompanying epidural abscess or be associated with a brain abscess. Mass effect due to cerebral edema and associated cerebritis is frequent and may be progressive. Therefore subdural empyema is usually considered a neurosurgical emergency. In the case of combined brain abscess and extracerebral suppuration, antibiotics may reach the subdural/epidural pus but not the brain abscess if the blood-brain barrier is not broken. Follow-up imaging therefore may show more rapid resolution of the extracerebral process but persistence or slower evolution of the intracerebral process.

MRI plays a significant role in the determination of loculations of pus, and frequently such pockets may be evident on MRI scans but not on CT scans.[16] The lesions are mildly hyperintense relative to CSF and hypointense relative to white matter on T1-weighted images and hyperintense relative to both CSF and white matter on T2-weighted scans. Edema, mass effect, and reversible cortical hyperintensity on T2-weighted images also are seen on the MRI scan.

On occasion CT or MRI may not adequately differentiate a subdural empyema from an effusion that develops after

Hemophilus influenzae infection. The bilaterality of subdural effusions may be a helpful hint, since subdural empyemas are almost always unilateral and associated with a neighboring source of infection.[11]

VENOUS THROMBOSIS

Thrombosis of the dural venous sinuses or cortical veins may follow sepsis, meningitis, or infections of contiguous sites, particularly if the patient is dehydrated. We have also encountered full-term neonates with venous sinus thrombosis and no identifiable cause. The CT diagnosis of sagittal sinus thrombosis can be difficult to make because of the potential for the overdiagnosis of the "empty delta" as representative of thrombus within the sinus. The empty delta sign refers to a filling defect within the sinus as demonstrated by CT scans of the sagittal sinus on axial views following contrast administration[18] (Fig. 5-20). This appearance is not always pathological; a high splitting sinus or adjacent epidural lesions may mimic a sinus thrombosis.[13] Other diagnostic difficulties include compartmentalization of the sinus and also subarachnoid blood, which may simulate a delta sign with high attenuation blood along the dural leaves. On occasion a sinus thrombosis can appear on CT as a high density linear structure with subsequent enhancement on a postcontrast scan.[3,7] Sinus thrombosis may also be suspected if parasagittal infarcts and hemorrhages and enlarged medullary veins appear after contrast administration.[13]

MRI can also detect intravascular thrombosis. The appearances parallel those of intracranial hematomas except for absence of the hemosiderin peripheral rim of hypointensity on long TR/long TE images.[10] Infarcts, either bland or hemorrhagic, in the high convexity of the brain are often associated with superior sagittal sinus thrombosis and are easily detected by MRI scans (Fig. 5-20). Edema or infarction of deeper structures (brain stem, basal ganglia, thalamus) may occur after thrombosis of the internal cerebral vein or straight sinus. After gadolinium-DTPA administation, enhancement of the falx adjacent to the thrombosed sinus can occur as a result of an associated thrombophlebitis.

On occasion it may be difficult to use MRI to separate the low intravascular signal of normal flowing blood from that of acute thrombus, or to distinguish the high intravascular signal of slowly flowing blood from subacute thrombus. A number of methods are available for making the distinction; for example, if a high intensity signal is present in the sinus in two planes at right angles to each other (for example, sagittal and coronal, or axial and coronal) and the signals are of equal intensity, an intravascular thrombus is almost certainly present. Phase-contrast MRI angiography using flow-sensitive gradient echo imaging can also suggest a diagnosis of intravascular thrombus and distinguish it from flowing blood.[12] Gradient echo imaging also is particularly sensitive to flowing blood that is of a high intensity, whereas thrombus has moderate or low signal intensity.

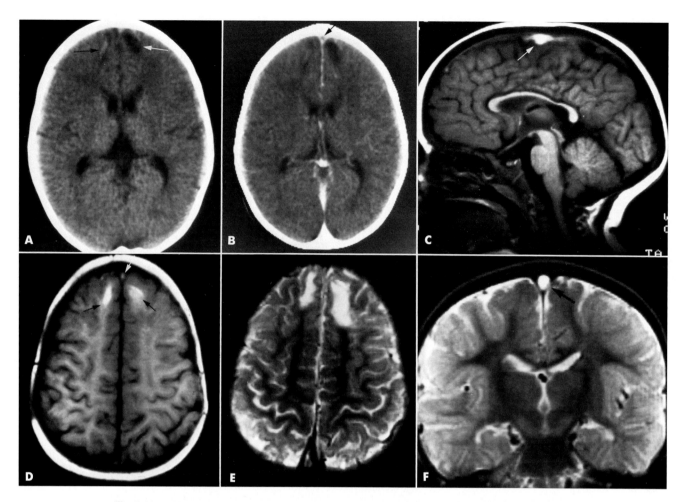

Fig. 5-20   CT scans. **A,** Note the left frontal low density area *(white arrow)* and the high density area indicative of hemorrhage in the right frontal lobe *(black arrow).* **B,** Scan at same level as that in **A.** Following contrast administration a lucency is apparent anteriorly within the sagittal sinus *(arrow).* MRI scans. **C,** Short TR/short TE sagittal scan demonstrates a high intensity signal area in the superior sagittal sinus *(arrow).* **D,** The high intensity signal is also seen on the axial scan anteriorly *(white arrow).* Note also the bilateral high intensity areas indicative of hemorrhages (black arrows), probably within infarcts (hemorrhagic infarcts). **E,** Long TR/long TE image demonstrates high signal intensity areas due to the hemorrhages. **F,** Coronal long TR/long TE image demonstrates a high signal within the superior sagittal sinus caused by thrombosis *(arrow).*
Diagnosis: Superior sagittal sinus thrombosis with hemorrhagic venous infarcts.

REFERENCES
Intracranial suppuration

1. Britt RH, Enzmann DR, Yeager AJ: Neuropathological and CT findings in experimental brain abscess, *J Neurosurg* 55:580, 1981.
2. Diebler C, Dulac O: Infectious diseases of the central nervous system. In Diebler C, Dulac O, editors: *Pediatric neurology and neuroradiology,* Berlin, 1987, Springer-Verlag.
3. Eick JJ, Miller KD, Bell KA, et al: Computed tomography of deep cerebral venous thrombosis in children, *Radiology* 140:399, 1981.
4. Enzmann DR, Britt RH, Lyons B, et al: High resolution ultrasound evaluation of experimental brain abscess evolution: comparison with computed tomography and neuropathology, *Radiology* 142:95, 1982.
5. Enzmann DR, Britt RH, Yeager AS: Experimental brain abscess evolution: computed tomographic and neuropathologic correlation, *Radiology* 130:113, 1979.
6. Fischer EG, McLennon JE, Suzuki Y: Cerebral abscess in children, *Am J Dis Child* 135:746, 1981.

7. Ford K, Sarwar M: Computed tomography of dural sinus thrombosis, *AJNR* 2:539, 1981.
8. Foreman SD, Smith EE, Ryan NJ, et al: Neonatal *Citrobacter* meningitis: pathogenesis of cerebral abscess formation, *Ann Neurol* 16:655, 1984.
9. Haimes AB, Zimmerman RD, Morgello S, et al: MR imaging of brain abscesses, *AJNR* 10:279, 1989.
10. Kwan ESK, Wolpert SM, Scott RM, et al: MR evaluation of neurovascular lesions after endovascular occlusion with detachable balloons, *AJNR* 9:523, 1988.
11. Moseley IF, Kendall BE: Radiology of intracranial empyemas, with special reference to computed tomography, *Neuroradiology* 26:333, 1984.
12. Pernicone JR, Siebert JE, Potchen EJ, et al: Three-dimensional phase-contrast MR angiography in the head and neck: preliminary report, *AJNR* 11:457, 1990.

13. Rao KVG, Knipp HC, Wagner EJ: Computed tomographic finding in cerebral sinus and venous thrombosis, *Radiology* 140:391, 1981.
14. Sarwar M: Current status of neuroradiologic interpretation of CNS inflammatory disease, *Curr Prob Diag Radiol* 9:1, 1980.
15. Smith HP, Hendrick EB: Subdural empyema and epidural abscess in children, *J Neurosurg* 58:392, 1983.
16. Weingarten K, Zimmerman RD, Becker RD, et al: Subdural and epidural empyemas: MR imaging, *AJNR* 10:81, 1989.
17. Weisberg LA: Cerebral computerized tomography in intracranial inflammatory disorders, *Arch Neurol* 37:137, 1980.
18. Zilkha A, Diaz AS: Computed tomography in the diagnosis of superior sagittal sinus thrombosis, *J Comput Assist Tomogr* 4:124, 1980.

Subacute and chronic infections

TUBERCULOSIS

Although the overall incidence of tuberculosis has declined, it remains a common disease in many parts of the world. The disease may become manifest as a meningitis or as a discrete tuberculoma. Tuberculous meningitis is rare before 3 months of age, but the incidence is high in the first 5 years of life.[23] Cranial nerve deficits, particularly those involving the sixth cranial nerve, result from basilar meningitis.

On CT tuberculous meningitis demonstrates cisternal, sulcal, and meningeal enhancement often with obstructive hydrocephalus.[18] The legacy of a basal tuberculous meningitis may be calcification.[6] Infarcts due to basal arteritis can also occur.[6] The arteritis can be demonstrated by arteriography and may represent an unusual cause of moyamoya syndrome.[13] Two distinct CT appearances of tuberculoma have been described by Whelan and Stern.[27] The lesions may appear as enhancing nodular areas or as contrast-enhancing rings with central lucent areas. This latter lesion represents caseating granuloma. When tuberculomata enlarge, they may adhere to the dura and simulate a meningioma.[27] Calcification is rare in intracranial tuberculomata. MRI, although rarely indicated, is an excellent tool for detecting meningitis, with the inflamed and thickened meninges enhancing remarkably after the administration of gadolinium.[1,4]

Infarctions caused by occlusion of the central perforating arteries from the basal meningitis are particularly well defined by MRI.[22] Tuberculomas may have a specific appearance on MRI scans.[9,26] The central core of caseation is slightly decreased in infants on the T1-weighted image but markedly increased on T2-weighted images. Surrounding this area is a dense capsule isointense on T1-weighted images and markedly hypointense on T2-weighted images. Surrounding the lesions is the typical hyperintensity on T2-weighted scans, indicative of edema.

SARCOIDOSIS

In 5% of patients with sarcoidosis, the central nervous system, particularly the cranial nerves, meninges, and hypothalamus, is involved. Both the meninges and the brain parenchyma are infiltrated. The granulomas appear on CT to be of a high density, which may enhance on postcontrast

scans.[11,17] Typically the lesions are well circumscribed with minimal surrounding edema. Basal cisternal enhancement also occurs. Communicating hydrocephalus is a common finding, although aqueduct or fourth ventricular outlet obstruction may also appear.[12] In infants, obstructive hydrocephalus and noncaseating granulomas throughout the central nervous system are rare manifestations of sarcoidosis. Hyperintense lesions on long TR/long TE images is the usual pattern, although the appearances can be greatly variable.[11] Hypothalamic involvement is easily seen on the sagittal plane MRI scan. Enhancement may also occur after gadolinium-DTPA administration (Fig. 5-21).

FUNGAL INFECTIONS

Fungal involvement of the brain may be of two types[1]: that produced by pathogens and that produced by saprophytes in patients with reduced resistance to infection (for example, patients with AIDS, diabetes, leukemia, and lymphoma and those receiving long-term antibiotic treatment, steroids, cytotoxic drugs, or immunosuppressive agents). The latter group of infections are known as opportunistic.

Cryptococcosis (torulosis), candidiasis, and aspergillosis

Cryptococcosis, candidiasis, and aspergillosis are the most frequently encountered mycoses.[28] Cryptococcosis is global in distribution and is the most prevalent fungal infection of the CNS.[14] Cryptococcosis neoformans, an encapsulated yeast fungus, may cause meningitis, granulomas, or abscesses. Granulomas may cause mass lesions with consequent papilledema, cranial nerve palsies, and hemiparesis. Hydrocephalus, necessitating shunting, occurs in a high percentage of patients.[21] The mass lesions may be seen by CT or MRI scans.

Meningitis, abscesses, and miliary granulomas occur independently or together in patients with candidiasis. *Candida* can invade the walls of the blood vessels and produce vasculitis with thrombus formation with resultant infarction and hemorrhage. *Candida* meningitis enhances remarkably after the infusion of intravenous contrast. *Candida* abscesses have thicker walls than pyogenic abscesses.[1]

The intracerebral vessels are usually thrombosed in cases of aspergillosis. Infarction or a mycotic aneurysm with hemorrhage from erosion of the fungus through the vessel wall into surrounding brain parenchyma may occur.

Coccidiomycosis, histoplasmosis, and blastomycosis

Coccidiomycosis is endemic in the southwestern United States. As with the other meniningitides, the basal cisterns enhance remarkably after contrast administration. Hydrocephalus is almost always present. Granulomas and leptomeningitis are seen after infection with histoplasma and *Blastomyces*. Prominent enhancement of the basal subarachnoid cisterns has been demonstrated.[7] Early encephalitic changes can be seen on MRI scans when the CT scan is normal.[15]

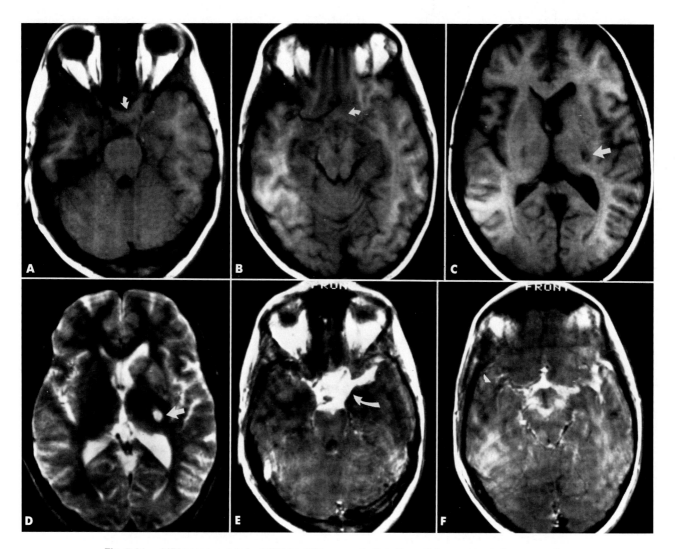

Fig. 5-21   MRI scans: axial short TR/short TE scans. **A,** Note the soft tissue mass in the suprasellar cistern obliterating the optic chiasm *(arrow).* **B,** The mass is also in the suprasellar cistern *(arrow).* **C,** A low intensity area is apparent in the left globus pallidus posteriorly *(arrows),* presumedly resulting from an infarct following occlusion of some of the lenticulostriate arteries. **D,** Long TR/long TE image demonstrates a high intensity lesion in the posterior left globus pallidus *(arrow)* corresponding to the low intensity lesion in **C. E,** Short TR/short TE scans. Following Gd-DTPA administration marked enhancement of the basal cisterns occurs with extension into the left sylvian fissure. **F,** Scan at the same level as that in **B.** Note the extensive enhancement of the basal cisterns with extension into the left sylvian fissure.
Diagnosis: Sarcoidosis with infarct in left globus pallidus. (From Carollo BR, Runge VM: Brain: vascular disease. In Runge VM: *Clinical magnetic resonance imaging,* Philadelphia, 1990, JB Lippincott.)

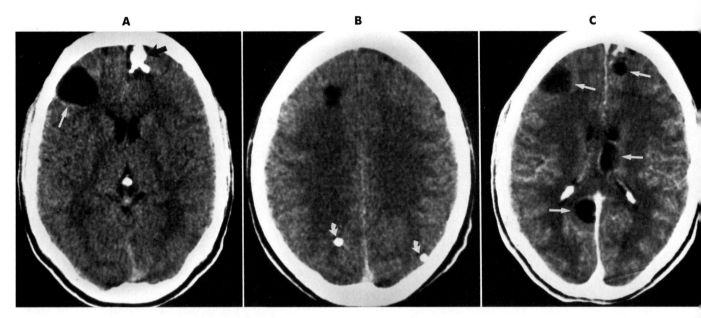

A   **B**   **C**

Fig. 5-22   CT scans. **A,** Nonenhanced scan. Note the well-defined low density lesion with discrete margins in the right frontal lobe *(white arrow).* There is no evidence of ventricular displacement. Note also the calcified lesion in the left frontal lobe *(black arrow).* **B,** At a higher level two calcified lesions are evident: one in the posterior centrum semiovale on the right side and the other in the left occipital cortex *(arrows).* **C,** Contrast-enhanced scan at the level of the lateral ventricle demonstrates four cystic lesions *(arrows):* one in the left frontal lobe (adjacent to the calcified lesion), the second in the right frontal lobe, the third in the right occipital lobe, and the fourth in the body of the left lateral ventricle. None of the lesions enhanced.
Presumed diagnosis: Cerebral cysticercosis.

PARASITIC INFECTIONS
Hydatid disease

Hydatid disease of the brain is rare but is seven times more frequent in children than in adults.[3] In most cases of brain infection an associated cyst can be demonstrated elsewhere in the body, most often in the liver.

Hydatid cysts in the brain grow slowly, which probably explains the usual mild associated neurological deficits.[25] The CT scan is essential to demonstrate single or multiple lesions. The lesions appear as well defined round or oval masses with a density close to that of CSF. There may be slight enhancement of the walls of the lesions.[16] The cyst may destroy the squama of the skull.[6]

Cysticercosis

Cysticercosis is a parasitic disease presenting with either seizures or an encephalitic picture in which humans serve as the intermediate host of *Taenia solium.* The larvae have a predilection for the central nervous system, with the brain being involved in the majority of patients. The lesions may be meningobasal, parenchymal, intraventricular, spinal, or multifocal.[6] The parenchymal lesions usually are cystic or solitary with a density on CT close to that of CSF and may be as large as 6 cm in diameter[2] (Fig. 5-22). Other lesions may appear solid and may enhance slightly.[6] Calcifications

appear after a number of years. There may be only one or two areas of calcification, which are scattered, small, and located at the junction of gray and white matter. Intraventricular lesions may cause obstructive hydrocephalus due to blockage at the foramen of Monro or aqueduct of Sylvius. The meningobasal lesions may enhance.[29] MRI may demonstrate a low signal focus with signal properties paralleling ventricular CSF, and a high intensity mural nodule on both T1- and T2-weighted sequences contouring the scolex,[20,24] although low intensity lesions may also be seen on T2-weighted scans (Fig. 5-23). The calcified lesions generally are not visible on MRI. In cysticercotic encephalitis, as the parasites begin to degenerate, proteins from the scolex combine with the vesicle's fluid within the lesion to produce a cyst discernible only on T2-weighted images.[5] Severe brain edema may accompany the encephalitis and be seen on the MRI scan.

LYME DISEASE

Lyme disease is a multisystem inflammatory disease caused by the spirochete *Borrelia burgdorferi.* It is transmitted to the ixodid tick, using the whitetail deer and the white-footed mouse as the reservoir.[8] Neurological manifestations include encephalopathy, neuropathy, meningitis, and cranial neuropathies.[10] The disease has been reported in children as young as 7 years of age.[10]

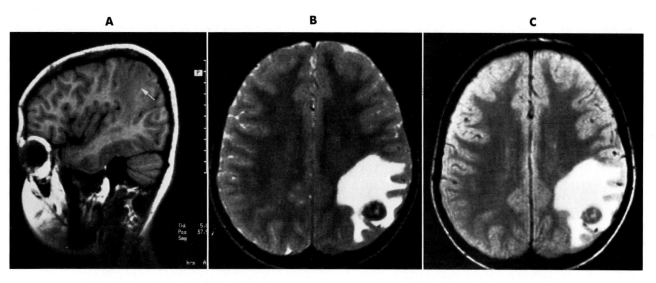

Fig. 5-23 A 10-year-old from South America with a seizure disorder. **A,** Sagittal short TR/short TE image demonstrates a low intensity lesion in the left parietal lobe *(arrow)*. Long TR/short TE **(B)** and long TR/long TE **(C)** images demonstrate a central lesion with a lower intensity than gray matter and marked surrounding edema.
Diagnosis: Cysticercosis.

Radiologically, lesions have been identified by CT and MRI in the frontal, temporal, parietal and occipital lobes and in the thalamus, corpus callosum, and pons. On CT scans low density focal lesions that may enhance have been reported.[8] On MRI the lesions are seen as multifocal isointensity or low intensity areas on T1-weighted scans and as high intensity areas on T2-weighted scans.[8,10] Gadolinium enhancement may occur.[19] The lesions simulate multiple sclerosis, acute disseminated encephalomyelitis, as well as inflammatory or infectious processes including vasculitis.

REFERENCES
Subacute and chronic infections

1. Barkovich A: Infections of the nervous system. In Barkovich A: *Pediatric neuroimaging,* New York, 1990, Raven.
2. Byrd SE, Locke GE, Bigger S, et al: The computed tomographic appearance of cerebral cysticercosis in adults and children, *Radiology* 144:819, 1982.
3. Carcassonne M, Aubrespy P, Dor V, et al: Hydatid cysts in childhood, *Prog Pediatr Surg* 5:1, 1973.
4. Chang KH, Han MH, Roh JK, et al: Gd-DTPA–enhanced MR imaging of the brain in patients with meningitis: comparison with CT, *AJNR* 11:69, 1990.
5. Del Brulto OH, Zenbeno MA, Salgado P, et al: MR imaging of cysticercotic encephalitis, *AJNR* 10:518, 1989.
6. Diebler C, Dulac O: Infectious diseases of the central nervous system. In Diebler C, Dulac O, editors: *Pediatric neurology and neuroradiology,* Berlin, 1987, Springer-Verlag.
7. Enzmann DR, Britt RH, Yeager AS: Experimental brain abscess evolution: computed tomographic and neuropathologic correlation, *Radiology* 130:113, 1979.
8. Fernandez RE, Rothberg M, Ferencz G, et al: Lyme disease of the CNS: MR imaging findings in 14 cases, *AJNR* 11:479, 1990.
9. Gupta RK, Jena A, Sharma A, et al: MR imaging of intracranial tuberculomas, *J Comput Assist Tomogr* 12:280, 1988.
10. Halperin JB, Luft BJ, Anand AK, et al: Lyme neuroborreliosis: central nervous system manifestations, *Neurology* 39:753, 1989.
11. Hayes WS, Sherman JH, Stern BJ, et al: MR and CT evaluation of intracranial sarcoidosis, *AJNR* 8:841, 1987.
12. Lukin RR, Chambers AA, Soleimanpour M: Outlet obstruction of the fourth ventricle in sarcoidosis, *Neuroradiology* 10:65, 1975.
13. Mathew NT, Abraham S, Crowdy S: Cerebral angiographic features in tuberculous meningitis, *Neurology* 20:1015, 1970.
14. Meloff KL: Fungal, rickettsial, and parasitic diseases of the nervous system. In Swaiman KF: *Pediatric neurology: principles and practice,* St Louis, 1989, Mosby–Year Book.
15. Mikhael MA, Rushovich AM, Ciric I: Magnetic resonance imaging of cerebral aspergillosis, *Comput Radiol* 9:85, 1985.
16. Ozgen T, Erbengi A, Burton V, et al: The use of CT in the diagnosis of cerebral hydatid cysts, *J Neurosurg* 50:339, 1979.
17. Powers WJ, Miller EM: Sarcoidosis mimicking glioma: case report and review of intracranial sarcoid mass lesions, *Neurology* 31:907, 1981.
18. Price HI, Danziger A: Computed tomography in cranial tuberculosis, *AJR* 130:769, 1978.
19. Rafto SE, Milton WJ, Galetta SL, et al: Biopsy-confirmed CNS Lyme disease: MR appearance at 1.5 T, *AJNR* 11:482, 1990.
20. Rhee RS, Kumasaki DY, Sarwar M, et al: MR imaging of intraventricular cysticercosis, *J Comput Assist Tomogr* 11:598, 1987.
21. Richardson PM, Mohandas A, Arumugasamy N: Cerebral cryptococcosis in Malaysia, *J Neurol Neurosurg Psychiatry* 39:330, 1976.

22. Schoeman J, Hewlett R, Donald P: MR of childhood tuberculous meningitis, *Neuroradiology* 30:473, 1988.
23. Snyder RD: Bacterial infection of the nervous system. In Swaiman KF: *Pediatric neurology: principles and practice,* St Louis, 1989, Mosby–Year Book.
24. Suss RA, Maravilla KR, Thompson J: MR imaging of intracranial cysticercosis: comparison with CT and anatomopathologic features, *AJNR* 7:235, 1986.
25. Vaquero J, Jiminez C, Martinez R: Growth of hydatid cysts evaluated by CT scanning after presumed cerebral hydatid embolism, *J Neurosurg* 57:837, 1982.
26. Venger BH, Dion FM, Rouah E, et al: MR imaging of pontine tuberculoma, *AJNR* 8:1149, 1987.
27. Whelan MA, Stern J: Intracranial tuberculoma, *Radiology* 138:75, 1981.
28. Whelan MA, Stern J, and de Napoli RA: The computed tomographic spectrum of intracranial mycosis: correlation with histopathology, *Radiology* 141:703, 1981.
29. Zee CS, Segall HD, Miller C, et al: Unusual neuroradiological features of intracranial cysticercosis, *Radiology* 137:397, 1980.

Mycotic aneurysms

Compared with congenital saccular aneurysms, intracranial mycotic aneurysms occur more frequently in children than in adults. The aneurysms follow bacterial and fungal infections. Approximately 3% to 15% of patients with bacterial endocarditis develop mycotic aneurysms, and rupture with hemorrhage is often the primary event. Children with a right-to-left intracardiac shunt or an artificial cardiac valve and those with rheumatic heart disease are at particular risk, along with intravenous drug users and patients with an immune deficiency.

The pathogenesis of aneurysmal formation is direct spread of the infection through the arterial wall due to involvement of the vasa vasorum. The aneurysms are most often located on the peripheral cerebral vasculature, most often in the distribution of the middle cerebral artery.[9] Angiographically, they often are fusiform rather than saccular in appearance (Fig. 5-24). Mycotic aneurysms are multiple in approximately 20% of cases[4,9] (see Chapter 6).

Acquired immunodeficiency syndrome

Between 30% to 50% of children with human immunodeficiency virus (HIV) infection also have a progressive encephalopathy characterized by an inability to achieve developmental milestones.[12] The incubation period from infection to clinical manifestation of the disease is relatively short, with the majority of children contracting the disease by the age of 2 years,[10] although a case with an incubation period of 5½ years has been reported.[6] Neuropathological studies of the brain have shown inflammatory cell infiltration and calcification of small- and medium-sized vessels, particularly in the basal ganglia.[11] Demyelination may also occur. Unlike in adults with AIDS, opportunistic infection and neoplasia in children are rare.

In patients with HIV encephalitis CT scans characteristically demonstrate diffuse cerebral atrophy with secondary ventriculomegaly and symmetrical bilateral calcification of the basal ganglia and the white matter adjacent to the frontal horns.[1] Contrast enhancement of the basal ganglia also can occur.[1] The basal ganglia calcification and enhancement may be unilateral early on in the disease, becoming bilateral later.[3] Whereas the calcifications can be seen in children with HIV infection but without TORCH infection, Post et al. have described patients with both cytomegalovirus (CMV) infection and AIDS[7] who had periventricular calcifications, presumedly caused by CMV infection. The central and cortical parenchymal loss may also be seen on MRI scans.

CNS infections are another common complication of AIDS. In one report[2] the infectious organisms found included *Hemophilus influenzae, Escherichia coli, Streptococcus pneumoniae, Pseudomonas,* and *Salmonella.* Mass lesions due to other opportunistic infections (for example, toxoplasmosis) or neoplasia are much rarer in children than in adults, although a case report of a primary lymphoma in a 9-month-old child has been reported.[8] Cerebral mass lesions in children with AIDS are usually caused by primary lymphoma.[5] CT shows multicentric hyperdense lesions that enhance after contrast administration. MRI is probably more sensitive than CT for demonstrating intracranial lesions such as lymphomas in patients with AIDS (see Chaper 7). Toxoplasma encephalitis has also been described in children with AIDS.[5] Progressive multifocal leukoencephalopathy is another disease that may affect children with AIDS (see p. 161).

REFERENCES
Mycotic aneurysms and acquired immunodeficiency syndrome

1. Belman AL, Lantos G, Horoupian D, et al: AIDS: Calcification of the basal ganglia in infants and children, *Neurology* 36:1192, 1986.
2. Bradford BF, Abdenour GE, Frank JL, et al: Usual and unusual radiologic manifestation of acquired immunodeficiency syndrome (AIDS) and human immunodeficiency virus (HIV) infection in children, *Radiol Clin North Am* 26:341, 1988.
3. Epstein LG, Berman CZ, Sharer LR, et al: Unilateral calcification and contrast enhancement of the basal ganglia in a child with AIDS encephalopathy, *AJNR* 8:163, 1987.
4. Frazee JA, Cahan LD, Winter J: Bacterial intracranial aneurysms, *J Neurosurg* 56:443, 1982.
5. Haney PJ, Yale-Loehr AJ, Nussbaum AR, et al: Imaging of infants and children with AIDS, *AJR* 152:1033, 1989.
6. Maloney MJ, Cox F, Wray BB, et al: AIDS in a child 5½ years after transfusion, *N Engl J Med* 312:1256, 1985.
7. Post MJD, Curless RG, Gregorios JB, et al: Reactivation of congenital cytomegalic inclusion disease in an infant with HTLV III associated immunodeficiency: a CT pathologic correlation, *J Comput Assist Tomogr* 10:533, 1986.
8. Price DB, Inglese CM, Jacobs J, et al: Pediatric AIDS: neurologic and neurodevelopmental findings, *Pediatr Radiol* 18:445, 1988.
9. Roach MR, Drake CA: Ruptured cerebral aneurysms caused by microorganisms, *N Engl J Med* 273:240, 1965.
10. Scott GB, Hutto C, Makuch RW, et al: Survival in children with perinatally acquired immunodeficiency virus type 1 infection, *N Engl J Med* 321:1791, 1989.
11. Sharer LR, Epstein LA, Cho ES, et al: Pathologic features of AIDS encephalopathy in children: evidence for LAV/HTLV III infection of brain, *Human Pathol* 17:271, 1986.
12. Ultmann MH, Belman AL, Ruff HA, et al: Developmental abnormalities in infants and children with acquired immune deficiency syndrome (AIDS) and AIDS-related complex, *Dev Med Child Neurol* 27:563, 1985.

A   B   C

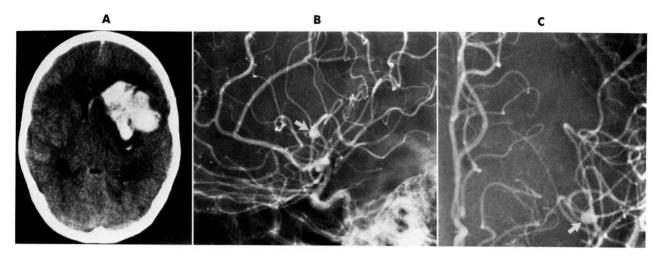

Fig. 5-24   A 14-year-old with aortic valvular disease and seizure disorder. **A,** CT scan demonstrates a hemorrhage in the left parietal lobe. **B** and **C,** Left carotid angiography demonstrates an aneurysm *(arrows)* originating from a sylvian branch of the left middle cerebral artery.
Diagnosis: Mycotic aneurysm with hemorrhage.

Other intracranial inflammations

REYE'S SYNDROME

Reye's syndrome (encephalopathy and fatty degeneration of the liver) is characterized by a prodromal viral illness followed by protracted vomiting, stupor, coma, and signs of elevated intracranial pressure. The syndrome is much more common in children than in adults and is fairly evenly distributed throughout infancy and childhood until about 15 years, after which the incidence decreases rapidly.[5] The blood lactate and ammonia levels parallel the severity of the encephalopathy. Acetylsalicylate ingestion is a possible causative factor.

Cerebral edema is a prominent factor associated with the coma and provides the basis for the CT observation of a diffuse white matter low density with ventricular compression.[8] If the child survives, the scan may demonstrate an atrophic picture with ventricular dilatation and prominent cisterns and fissures.

MULTIPLE SCLEROSIS

Multiple sclerosis may occur in children, although not nearly with the same incidence as in adults.[1,4] MRI is an excellent way to depict the lesions, which in children have the same periventricular, multifocal appearance with sharply angled lateral margins as seen in adults. Cerebellar and brain stem lesions are much more common in adolescents than in adults.[6]

The lesions, which on CT scanning are of low density, have a low signal intensity on T1-weighted scans and a high signal intensity on T2-weighted scans (see Fig. 4-14, *M* and *N*). Some of the lesions enhance after Gd-DTPA administration, particularly during the acute phase of the disease. Characteristically, older lesions may resolve and new lesions appear during the course of the disease. As in the adults there is no correlation between the severity of the symptoms and the extent of the disease as seen on the MRI scan.[6,7] This demyelinating disease may appear clinically and by neuroimaging as a single mass lesion that is difficult to distinguish from a neoplasm because of mass effect and enhancement.

CENTRAL PONTINE MYELINOLYSIS

Central pontine myelinolysis (CPM) is a demyelinating disorder of uncertain origin that primarily affects the pons. The disorder primarily affects adults, but it has been reported in children as young as 3 years of age.[10] It usually occurs in the setting of hyponatremia, particularly if corrected too rapidly.

CT scanning demonstrates low density areas in the pons. These areas are also seen on MRI scans as high signal areas on T2-weighted images.[9] The pontine lesion is centrally located, with sparing of a rim of tissue peripherally. Extrapontine areas of myelinolysis may also occur in the putamina[2] and would then need to be distinguished from other lesions due to ischemia and the effects of radiation therapy[3] (see Chapter 7).

REFERENCES
Other intracranial infections

1. Bye AME, Kendall B, Wilson J: Multiple sclerosis in children: a new look, *Dev Med Child Neurol* 27:215, 1985.
2. Dickoff DJ, Raps M, Yahr MD: Striatal syndrome following hyponatremia and its rapid correction: a manifestation of extrapontine myelinolysis confirmed by magnetic resonance imaging, *Arch Neurol* 45:112, 1988.
3. Edwards MK: Metabolic, endocrine, and iatrogenic lesions of the brain. In Cohen MD, Edwards MK: *Magnetic resonance imaging of children,* Philadelphia, 1990, BC Decker.
4. Haas G, Schroth G, Krageloh-Mann I, et al: Magnetic resonance imaging of the brain of children with multiple sclerosis, *Dev Med Child Neurol* 29:586, 1985.
5. Huttenlocher PR: Reye's syndrome. In Swaiman KF: *Pediatric neurology: principles and practice,* St Louis, 1989, Mosby–Year Book.
6. Osborn AG, Harnsberger HR, Smoker WRK, et al: Multiple sclerosis in adolescents: CT and MR findings, *AJNR* 11:489, 1990.
7. Paty DW, Oger JJF, Kastrukoff LF, et al: MRI in the diagnosis of multiple sclerosis: a prospective study with comparison of clinical evaluation, evoked potentials, oligoclonal banding, and CT, *Neurology* 38:180, 1988.
8. Russell EJ, Zimmerman RD, Leeds NE, et al: Reye's syndrome: computed tomographic documentation of disordered intracerebral structure, *J Comput Assist Tomogr* 3:217, 1979.
9. Takeda K, Sakuta M, Saeki F: Central pontine myelinolysis diagnosed by magnetic resonance imaging, *Ann Neurol* 17:310, 1985.
10. Valsamis MP, Peress NS, Wright LD: Central pontine myelinolysis in childhood, *Arch Neurol* 25:307, 1971.

6 · Vascular Diseases and Trauma

Mary L. Anderson
Samuel M. Wolpert
Edward M. Kaye

Vascular diseases in infants and children differ in pathogenesis, clinical presentation, and outcome depending on the age of the patient at the onset of the disease. The differences depend on the developing vascular system, which continues to change even into adulthood. In this chapter lesions occurring before or at term are initially considered, and vascular lesions occurring in older children are subsequently discussed.

Vascular diseases in infants

HYPOXIC-ISCHEMIC ENCEPHALOPATHY

Hypoxic-ischemic brain injury is an important cause of morbidity and mortality in the perinatal period. Neurological sequelae of this injury include cerebral palsy, developmental retardation, and seizures.[19] Hypoxemia refers to diminished oxygen content in the blood, and ischemia refers to a decrease in cerebral blood flow. Perinatal asphyxia, along with its sequelae, is a major cause of hypoxic-ischemic injury. The asphyxia may be caused by intrauterine factors, meconium aspiration, hyaline membrane disease, recurrent apneic episodes, or cyanotic heart disease.

A variety of cerebral lesions are caused by ischemia and differ according to both the gestational age at the time of asphyxia and the duration of the insult. These lesions include periventricular leukomalacia (usually occurring before term), parasagittal injury, diffuse cerebral injury with neuronal necrosis, and multifocal cerebral injury (usually occurring at full term). The predominant lesions found in the different age groups are as follows:

Preterm	Term
Periventricular leukomalacia	Parasagittal or watershed cerebral injury
Selective neuronal necrosis	Selective neuronal necrosis
Focal and mutifocal ischemic cerebral necrosis	Focal and multifocal ischemic cerebral necrosis
Periventricular hemorrhagic lesions	Status marmoratus of basal ganglia and thalamus

An important factor in the cause of cerebral ischemia is the alteration of cerebral blood flow (CBF). Initially after an asphyxic episode, CBF is increased and cerebral vascular autoregulation is lost. Normally, autoregulation allows constant CBF independent of variations in systemic blood pressure (SBP)[38] The loss of autoregulation in the newborn allows the development of a pressure-passive circulation in which CBF varies directly with changes in SBP. A later effect of asphyxia is a drop in SBP caused by a decrease in the cardiac output with subsequent diminution of CBF. The resulting cerebral insult then depends on the duration of the insult and on the gestational age at the time of the insult. Fetuses or infants between 24 and 26 weeks' gestational age develop enlarged ventricles because of incorporation of

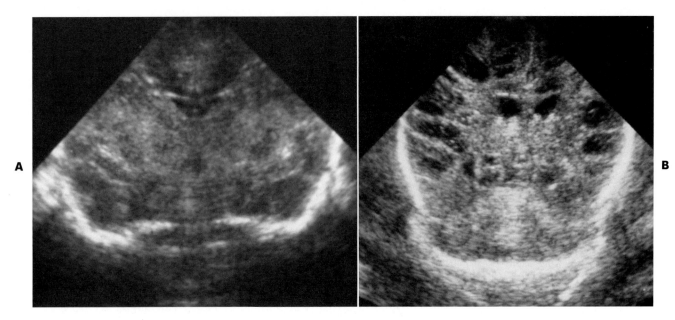

Fig. 6-1   A, A 7-day-old infant who had suffered birth asphyxia with persistently low Apgar scores. Coronal sections at level of anterior body of lateral ventricles. Diffusely echogenic brain is evident with loss of definition of gray and white matter planes. Initially this appearance may be caused by cerebral edema (bright brain appearance) but later may represent diffuse infarct. **B,** Scan taken 14 days after the anoxic insult shows multiple cystic spaces within the white matter consistent with cystic encephalomalacia. (Courtesy Dr. Roy McCauley, New England Medical Center Hospitals, Boston.)

periventricular cavities into the ventricles.[7] As the gestational age at the time of asphyxia increases, periventricular gliosis (periventricular leukomalacia) becomes more prevalent. In infants born around term the cortex and subcortical white matter are most severely involved with areas of ischemic necrosis and gliosis.

Periventricular leukomalacia

Periventricular leukomalacia (PVL) is an ischemic lesion of periventricular white matter occurring principally in preterm fetuses and in premature infants who survive more than a few days and in whom there is evidence of cardiorespiratory disturbance. The lesion results from diminished cerebral perfusion, generally as a result of systemic hypotension. Before the seventh month of gestation the periventricular white matter is thought to be a border zone of arterial perfusion between the ventriculopedal penetrating branches of the middle cerebral artery and the ventriculofugal posterior choroidal branches of the posterior cerebral artery. A recent histopathological study, however, has refuted the existence of ventriculofugal arteries and a deep white matter arterial border zone.[30] In the premature infant this periventricular border zone is susceptible to decreased cerebral blood flow. Because of a lack of autoregulation in the immature brain, compensatory mechanisms are not present to improve the flow. Furthermore the white matter just before and at term is a site for intense metabolic activity

with considerable oxygen demand and vulnerability to hypoxia.[15] Therefore infarction occurs in the deep cerebral white matter adjacent to the lateral ventricles.[34] The cerebral cortex is spared because of its collateral blood supply by meningeal intraarterial anastamoses, which are present in the preterm brain and do not regress until approximately term. Pathological findings can vary from small areas of necrosis at the angles of the ventricles to an extensive cystic lesion extending from the ventricles to the cortex. The most common sites for PVL are at the level of the occipital radiations at the trigones of the lateral ventricles and at the level of the cerebral white matter around the foramen of Monro.

Both US (Fig. 6-1) and CT can assist in the diagnosis of PVL by demonstrating hyperechoic areas and low density lesions, respectively.[13] However, the sonographic sensitivity for moderate or mild disease is low, with many false-negative studies resulting.[12] CT is of less value during the neonatal period than in later infancy and childhood[10] because of the difficulties of distinguishing pathological low densities from the natural low density of the neonate's developing brain. In older infants and young children the CT findings may show lateral ventriculomegaly (often similar in appearance to colpocephaly) with poor gray-white matter differentiation. The outlines of the bodies and trigones of the lateral ventricles are irregular, and often prominent deep sulci and subcortical gray matter directly abutting the ventricles are also evident on the CT scan.[13]

MRI of the brain demonstrates areas of decreased signal on T1-weighted images and increased signal on proton density and T2-weighted images indicative of the white matter involvement[11] (Figs. 6-2, 6-3, and 6-4). Areas of gliosis not appreciated by the CT scan may also be seen on MRI studies. However, in the young infant (less than 6 months) the high water content of preterm and term brain makes the detection of cerebral edema caused by infarct or PVL difficult or impossible to detect. Due to normally delayed myelination, high signal areas adjacent to the atria of the lateral ventricles are apparent on T2-weighted MRI scans of infants. Distinguishing normal from PVL may be difficult except that in the normal patient a band of white matter is usually seen between the bright signal areas and the ventricles. This normal band is often absent in PVL.[4]

On occasion PVL becomes hemorrhagic, which then may be confused with periventricular hemorrhagic infarction following germinal matrix and intraventricular hemorrhage. (see pp. 184 and 185).

Parasagittal or watershed injury

Injury of the cortex and subcortical white matter in specific areas is a characteristic lesion in the asphyxiated term fetus and term newborn. The systemic hypotension coupled with the loss of autoregulation accompanying perinatal asphyxia affects the vascular border zones between the terminal branches of the anterior cerebral, middle cerebral, and posterior cerebral arteries resulting in parasagittal parietooccipital and frontotemporal cortical and subcortical injury. The vascular development that occurs during the deepening of cerebral sulci causes the penetrating medullary arteries to bend acutely in the depths of the sulci, creating a triangular relatively avascular zone at the depth of the sulcus and affecting the basal aspects of the gyri.[36] This triangular zone becomes an end arterial zone that is most susceptible to hypoxic-ischemic injury. Bilateral, often symmetrical, wedge-shaped hemorrhagic infarcts occurring between the distributions of the anterior, middle, and posterior cerebral arteries are seen on CT.[32] The lesions have also been documented by technetium-enhanced brain scans,[41] and we have also seen them on MRI. Ulegyria, mushroom-shaped gyri, result and may be identified on MRI. The gyri appear narrow near the bases (atrophy) and wide at the apices.[5] Lesions have also been noted on positron-emission tomography scans.[42]

Diffuse injury with selective neuronal necrosis

Primarily as a result of inadequate cerebral perfusion, diffuse cerebral injury involving the cerebral cortex, cerebellar cortex, thalamus, and brain stem may occur in both term and preterm infants.[17,18] The reason that these groups of neurons are selectively vulnerable is not well understood; presumedly neurons in vascular border zones are susceptible to injury as are those with higher metabolic requirements. Also, mature neurons in structures such as the basal ganglia, cranial nerve nuclei, and thalami are more vulner-

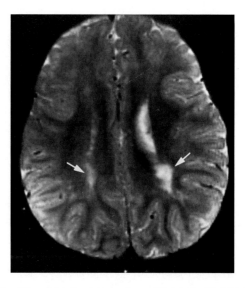

Fig. 6-2 T2-weighted axial scan in an 18-month-old child demonstrates high intensity lesions bilaterally *(arrows)* lateral to the occipital horns.
Diagnosis: Periventricular leukomalacia.

able to injury than more primitive neural elements. Pathologically, selective neuronal necrosis and gliosis result, and the CT demonstrates diffuse or patchy low density areas in the white and gray matter.[1,24] MRI demonstrates hypointense areas on T1-weighted scans and hyperintense areas on T2 images that may be difficult to distinguish from the normal developing brain. Ultrasonography demonstrates hyperechoic areas in the brain.[26] This distribution of necrosis and gliosis has also been reported following severe hypotension and hypoglycemia in infants.[14] When the ischemia is less severe and is caused by partial asphyxia, the basal ganglia appear to bear the brunt of the cerebral insult. If the ischemia occurs at the stage of basal ganglia myelination, status marmoratus results[35] (see following discussion). If the insult occurs later in the infant's life, bilateral symmetrical necrosis of the globi pallidi or putamina results (Fig. 6-5).

Status marmoratus

One of the least common types of hypoxic-ischemic encephalopathy, seen more often in term infants than in preterm infants and involving the basal ganglia and thalamus, is known as status marmoratus. The lesion is characterized by neuronal loss, gliosis, and hypermyelination; the hypermyelination produces the marbled appearance of the disease. The hypermyelination may result from the hypervascularity of the basal ganglia and thalamus that occurs in some infants after anoxic episodes.[39] The hypermyelination has been noted to occur as early as 8 months of life and is usually not fully developed until after the first year of life. The hypervascularity appears on CT as high density or abnormal enhancement in an anoxic infant within weeks of delivery.[35] Whether or not the hypervas-

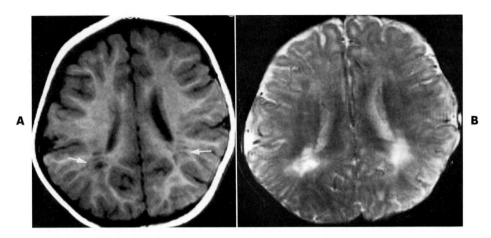

Fig. 6-3   T1-weighted **(A)** and T2-weighted **(B)** scans in a 1-year-old child demonstrate low intensity lesions *(arrows)* in the T1-weighted image **(A)** and high intensity lesions on the T2-weighted image **(B)**. *Diagnosis:* Periventricular leukomalacia.

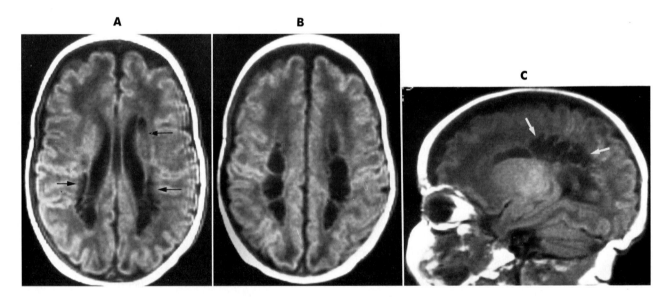

Fig. 6-4   **A,** T1-weighted scan at the level of the ventricles show low intensity lesions adjacent to the frontal and occipital horns *(arrows)*. **B,** Scan at a higher level shows the lesions are separate from the lateral ventricles. **C,** Sagittal scan above the left lateral ventricle demonstrates low intensity lesions *(arrows)* on the T1-weighted image. This 2-month-old infant suffered asphyxia at birth. *Diagnosis:* Periventricular leukomalacia.

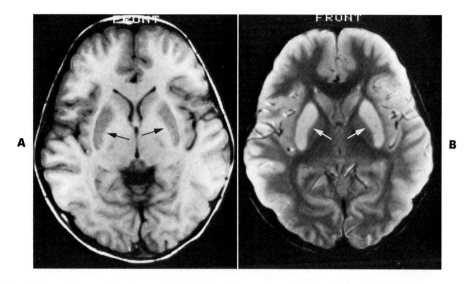

Fig. 6-5 MRI scans in a 6-year-old child who became hypointensive during abdominal surgery. The axial T1-weighted scan **(A)** demonstrates low intensity lesions in both putamina, which are of a high intensity on the T2-weighted scan **(B)**. Appearances are caused by hypoxic-ischemic changes.

cularity represents a stage in the development of status marmoratus is unknown. The high density may also be caused by hemorrhage or calcification, which occurs in the necrotic basal ganglia neurons and in the vessel walls. MRI may show hypointensity on T1-weighted images and hyperintensity on T2-weighted images. T1 hyperintensity with or without T2 hypointensity may indicate hemorrhage, mineralization, or hypermyelination.

Cerebral calcification due to hypoxic-ischemic insult is well known, occurs most often in premature infants, and is caused by a break in the cell membrane allowing extracellular calcium to move into the intracellular compartment.[3] The calcification occurs in the periventricular white matter or in the basal ganglia (Figs. 6-6 and 6-7). In severe cases the dentate nuclei may also be involved. MRI may detect the calcification as a low or absent signal. On occasion high intensity signals may be present on T1-weighted images (Fig. 6-7). Iron deposited in the basal ganglia following severe ischemic-anoxic episodes causes a low signal on T2-weighted images.[9]

Focal or multifocal ischemic cerebral injury

Focal or multifocal cerebral necrosis may result from either venous or arterial occlusions. Usually the middle cerebral artery (MCA) is involved, particularly in term infants, whereas multiple small infarcts are seen in premature infants.[20] Large lesions tend to become cystic (Fig. 6-8) and can on occasion communicate with the lateral ventricles (Fig. 6-9). The tendency toward tissue dissolution is probably because of the high water content and relative paucity of myelinated fibers and the lack of glial response in the immature brain.

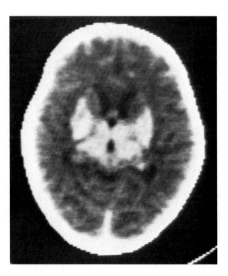

Fig. 6-6 CT scan in a newborn full-term infant, who was flaccid at birth without spontaneous movements, demonstrates bilateral hyperdensities in both thalami, globi pallidi, and putamina. The hyperdensities were also present in the brain stem and in the cortex. At autopsy, astrocytic gliosis involved the brain stem, basal ganglia, and cerebral hemispheres. Sparse calcifications appeared in the basal ganglia; the CT appearances are therefore probably the result of a combination of the excessive glial reaction together with the calcification.

Diagnosis: Anoxic encephalopathy with status marmoratus.

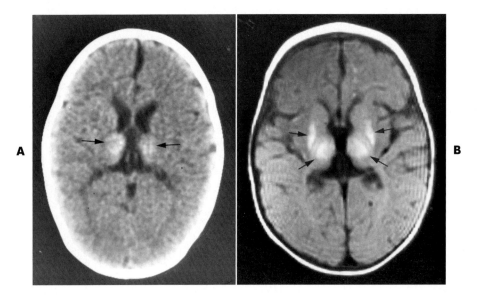

Fig. 6-7   A, CT scan in a full-term infant, born after fetal distress, obtained at the age of 3 months demonstrates high density lesions bilaterally, presumed due to calcification in the thalami. **B,** T1-weighted MRI scan demonstrates high intensity lesions involving the thalami and the putamina *(arrows)*. These areas were of a lower intensity than gray matter on a T2-weighted image (not shown). Calcification can paradoxically be of high signal intensity on T1-weighted scans.

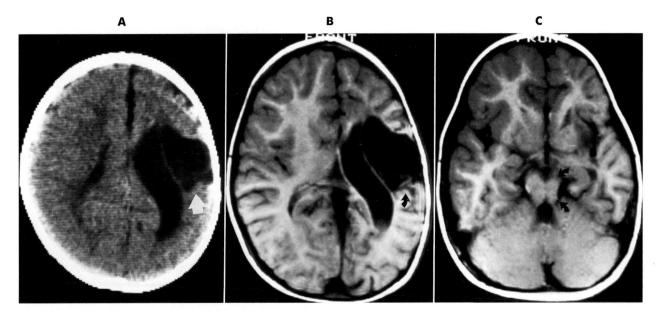

Fig. 6-8   A, CT scan in a 2-year-old child with a right hemiparesis demonstrates a well-defined low density lesion in the distribution of branches of the left middle cerebral artery. Note also the enlarged left lateral ventricle and generalized hemiatrophy of the left cerebral hemisphere. **B** and **C,** T1-weighted MRI scans show the infarct as a well-defined left parietal lobe lesion *(arrows)* associated with ipsilateral ventricular dilatation and cerebral hemiatrophy. **C,** Scan at the level of the ponto-mesencephalic junction demonstrates atrophy of the left cerebral peduncle *(arrows)* due to Wallerian degeneration.

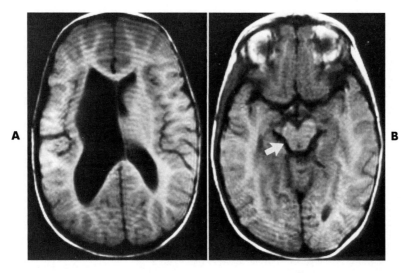

Fig. 6-9   T1-weighted scan in a 1-year-old demonstrates marked unilateral enlargement of the right lateral ventricle **(A)** with Wallerian degeneration of the ipsilateral mesencephalon **(B,** *arrow*).

The most common cause of focal or multifocal injury is thromboembolism of placental origin or consequent to disseminated intravascular coagulation, neonatal polycythemia, or involuting fetal vessels.[2,7,14] Also, focal ischemic injury, again in the territory of the MCA, may surprisingly follow a diffuse hypoxic-ischemic insult. The CT and MRI findings are distinctive (Fig. 6-8). A porencephalic cyst may occur as a single unilateral cavity that may or may not communicate with the lateral ventricle (Fig. 6-9), or there may be massive bilateral loss of tissue[29,33] (Fig. 6-10). Hydranencephaly or multicystic encephalomalacia may also result. Focal cystic lesions have been demonstrated on CT in approximately 50% of infants with congenital hemiparesis.[8] In many of these cases Wallerian degeneration is a result of axonal and myelin sheath dissolution due to axonal death along the pathways of nerve conduction from the cell body. MRI is an excellent technique for imaging this type of degeneration particularly when it involves the corticospinal tract.[22]

INTRACRANIAL HEMORRHAGE

Several types of intracranial hemorrhage are found in preterm and term infants. The major types are periventricular (germinal matrix), intraventricular, subdural, subarachnoid, and intracerebellar hemorrhage.[20] Each type has different clinical and prognostic features.

Germinal matrix hemorrhage

Germinal matrix (GM) hemorrhage resulting in intraventricular hemorrhage is the most common type of hemorrhage in the preterm infant and carries the most serious prognosis. It usually is found in infants with gestational

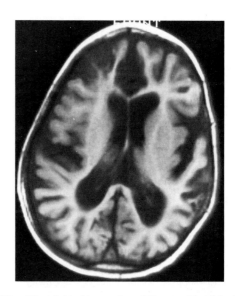

Fig. 6-10   T1-weighted image in a 3½-year-old child with microcephaly demonstrates marked bilateral cortical atrophic changes with dilatation of the lateral ventricles and the interhemispheric fissure.

ages less than 32 weeks (< 1500 g), although it may also occur in term infants. The germinal matrix is present in the subependymal region of the fetal brain and is the origin of neuronal and glial development. It is richly vascularized with arterial supply from the deep perforating branches of the anterior, middle, and posterior cerebral arteries. The rich capillary network drains into the deep venous system.

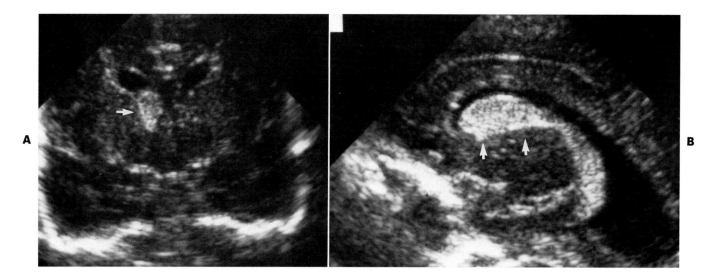

Fig. 6-11   Premature, 18-day-old infant with grade I subependymal hemorrhage. **A,** Coronal section at level of thalamocaudate groove showing a hyperechoic area of hemorrhage *(arrow)* beneath the mildly dilated right lateral ventricle. **B,** Parasagittal section through right lateral ventricle. An ovoid hyperechogenic area of hemorrhage *(arrows)* is seen in the subependymal area over the head of the caudate nucleus and thalamus. (Courtesy Dr. Roy McCauley, New England Medical Center Hospitals, Boston.)

With posterior to anterior regression of the germinal matrix occurring between the twenty-fourth and twenty-eighth weeks of gestation, the blood supply to the germinal matrix gradually diminishes. Residual germinal matrix located over the head of the caudate nucleus at 28 weeks is the most common location for GM hemorrhage.[19,23]

The hemorrhage may be associated with respiratory distress (hyaline membrane disease); fluctuations in cerebral blood flow in a pressure-passive circulation; increased blood pressure from asphyxia, hypercarbia, blood transfusions, volume expansion; and systemic complications such as surgery, seizures, and pneumothoraces.[39]

The hemorrhage destroys the germinal matrix and neuronal precursor cells (neuroblasts). Rupture into the ventricular system is common and has been reported in up to 80% of autopsied infants.[24,40] The intraventricular hemorrhage may cause ventricular dilatation and disruption of the ependymal lining. The hemorrhage mixes with cerebrospinal fluid, spreads throughout the ventricular system, and enters the subarachnoid space. Blockage of the arachnoid villi or an obliterative arachnoiditis may lead to a communicating hydrocephalus. Less frequently, a noncommunicating hydrocephalus may occur if blood clots or ependymal debris block a portion of the ventricular system such as the foramen of Monro, the cerebral aqueduct, or the outlet foramina of the fourth ventricle.

Volpe[39] has devised the following grading system to characterize the extent of GM hemorrhage:

1. *Grade I hemorrhages* are limited to the germinal matrix (little or no intraventricular involvement).

2. *Grade II hemorrhages* extend into the ventricles but are not associated with ventricular dilatation.
3. *Grade III hemorrhages* rupture into the ventricles and are associated with hydrocephalus.
4. *Grade IV hemorrhages* are associated with hemorrhagic parenchymal involvement.

Grade IV hemorrhages were thought to represent direct extension of the GM/intraventricular hemorrhage into the parenchyma. However, it is currently believed that periventricular parenchymal hemorrhages occur as the result of hemorrhagic venous infarctions or hemorrhagic periventricular leukomalacia. The hemorrhages usually occur on the side of the largest ventricle that is dilated with hemorrhage.[28,40] Venous obstruction occurs as a result of compression of the deep venous system by both the dilated, blood-filled ventricle and the subependymal hemorrhage, resulting in hemorrhagic venous infarction. The long-term sequela of the hemorrhages is the formation of parenchymal cysts.

The clinical syndromes associated with periventricular and intraventricular hemorrhages are varied. The hemorrhage may be clinically silent, may be manifested in a saltatory stepwise fashion with diminished level of consciousness, hypotonia, and subtle abnormal eye movements, or may appear abruptly with coma, seizures, apnea, and decerebrate posturing.

Preterm infants have a high incidence of germinal matrix hemorrhages and are now routinely screened for intracranial abnormalities so that treatment, if necessary, can be initiated quickly. Since many infants are systemically

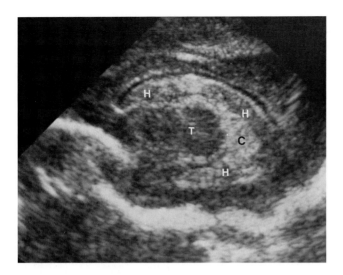

Fig. 6-12   Grade III intracranial hemorrhage. Parasagittal image of right lateral ventricle showing a thin rim of CSF outlining a thick clot that fills the moderately dilated ventricles. *T,* Thalamus; *C,* choroid plexus; *H,* intraventricular hemorrhagic clot. A subependymal hemorrhage was present on the opposite site. (Courtesy Dr. Roy McCauley, New England Medical Center Hospitals, Boston.)

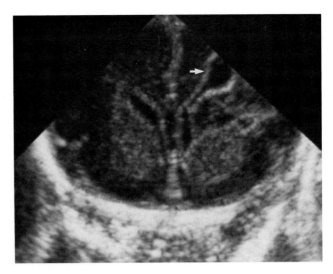

Fig. 6-13   A 26-day-old infant who had a grade IV hemorrhage into the left frontal white matter shortly after birth. Coronal image is at level of frontal horns. A porencephalic cyst *(arrows)* communicates with the upper lateral corner of the left frontal horn. (Courtesy Dr. Roy McCauley, New England Medical Center Hospitals, Boston.)

unstable, portable cranial ultrasonography (US) is the ideal method for the evaluation of these patients. The sagittal and coronal images demonstrate GM hemorrhage as a focal region of increased echogenicity in the subependymal region of the inferior frontal horn of the lateral ventricle at the caudothalamic groove (Fig. 6-11). Intraventricular hemorrhage is also readily apparent as echogenic material filling the ventricular system (Fig. 6-12). Serial US is important in the evaluation of the progressive development of hydrocephalus, since the usual signs of splitting of the sutures, bulging fontanelle, and increasing head circumference may be delayed. US also easily demonstrates porencephalic cysts (Fig. 6-13). Parenchymal hemorrhages are apparent on US as areas of increased echogenicity that may have mass effect. These are usually located dorsal and lateral to the external angles of the lateral ventricles.

CT also depicts the hemorrhages (Fig. 6-14). After the first 3 days following a neonatal hemorrhage, MRI may be better than either CT or US at identifying hemorrhage.[27] Hemorrhages may become imperceptible on CT scans, whereas the high signal of hemorrhage on MRI scans can persist for many weeks. Intracranial abnormalities including hemorrhagic and nonhemorrhagic complications have also been described in the newborn infant with severe respiratory insufficiency following extracorporeal membrane oxygenation (ECMO).[37] Hemorrhages are usually located in the cerebral parenchyma and are not necessarily related to the side of the bypass procedure. This type of hemorrhage is probably related to either the underlying asphyxia, which alone is associated with intracranial hemorrhage, or to

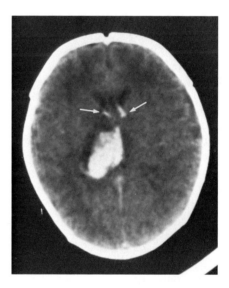

Fig. 6-14   Nonenhanced CT scan demonstrates germinal matrix and thalamic hemorrhages that ruptured into both lateral ventricles *(arrows).*

ECMO-related factors, including systemic heparin administration, thrombocytopenia, and the increased venous pressure following ligation of the internal jugular vein.

Epidural hemorrhage

Epidural hemorrhages during the neonatal period in infancy are uncommon but may occur in the infratentorial or supratentorial compartments. These hemorrhages are not usually associated with skull fractures and may be venous rather than arterial in origin.[21]

Subdural hemorrhage

Subdural hemorrhages in infancy are usually caused by tearing of the falx or tentorial veins and the dural venous sinuses as a result of severe head molding during delivery[20] or obstetrical trauma. The hemorrhage may occur in the posterior fossa and produce brain stem or cerebellar compression, or may be supratentorial and cause hemispheric displacement. Intratentorial hemorrhages may also occur. CT or MRI are excellent tests for demonstrating the site of the hemorrhage and the extent of the injury (see Figs. 6-22, 6-23, and 6-24).

Subarachnoid hemorrhage

Subarachnoid hemorrhage (SAH) in the infant is usually of venous origin and results from the rupture of small vessels in the leptomeningeal plexus or rupture of bridging veins within the subarachnoid space.[31] The hemorrhages are caused by trauma or hypoxia, and the diagnosis is made by either CT or lumbar puncture. Characteristically the hemorrhage lies posteriorly in the interhemispheric fissure[16] and is diagnosed by CT as a hyperdense area that may require differentiation from straight or superior sagittal sinus thrombosis, slow venous circulation, or neonatal polycythemia. Interhemispheric SAH tends to be evident on contiguous scans, whereas sinus thrombosis may appear on only one scan. MRI is not as sensitive as CT for diagnosing subarachnoid hemorrhage.

Intracerebellar hemorrhage

Cerebellar hemorrhages in infancy generally have a poor prognosis. The hemorrhages arise from traumatic laceration of the cerebellum, disruption of major posterior fossa veins, extension from an initial intraventricular hemorrhage, or, less frequently, massive subarachnoid hemorrhage into the cerebellum.[20] Although US is portable and more readily available for the critically ill infant, CT is often more reliable for diagnosing a posterior fossa hemorrhage. Seriously ill infants are often not candidates for MRI, although MRI is more sensitive to and more specific for subacute hemorrhage than either US or CT. MRI more precisely dates the hemorrhage because of its sensitivity to the breakdown products of hemoglobin. The multiplanar capability of MRI also demonstrates and characterizes extraaxial collections better than does CT or US.

REFERENCES
Vascular diseases in infants

1. Adsett DB, Fitz CR, Hill A: Hypoxic-ischemic cerebral injury in the term newborn: correlation of CT findings with neurological outcome, *Dev Med Child Neurol* 27:155, 1985.
2. Amit M, Camfield PR: Neonatal polycythemia causing multiple cerebral infarcts, *Arch Neurol* 37:109, 1980.
3. Ansari MO, Chincanchan CA, Armstrong DL: Brain calcification in hypoxic-ischemic lesions: an autopsy review, *Pediatr Neurol* 6:94, 1990.
4. Baker L, Stevenson D, Enzmann D: End-stage periventricular leukomalacia, *Radiology* 168:809, 1988.
5. Barkovich AJ: Metabolic and destructive brain disorders. In Barkovich AJ: *Pediatric neuroimaging*, ed 1, New York, 1989, Raven.
6. Barkovich AJ, Truwitt CL: Brain damage from perinatal asphyxia: correlation of MR findings with gestational age, *AJNR* 11:1087, 1990.
7. Barmada MA, Moosey J, Sherman RM: Cerebral infarct with arterial occlusion in neonates, *Ann Neurol* 6:495, 1979.
8. Cohen ME, Duffner PK: Prognostic indicators in hemiparetic cerebral palsy, *Ann Neurol* 9:353, 1981.
9. Dietrich RB, Bradley WG: Iron accumulation in the basal ganglia following severe ischemic-anoxic insults in children, *Radiology* 168:203, 1988.
10. Flodmark O, Fitz CR, Harwood-Nash DC: CT diagnosis and short-term prognosis of intracranial hemorrhage and hypoxic ischemic brain damage in neonates, *J Comput Assist Tomogr* 4:775, 1980.
11. Flodmark O, Lupton B, Li D, et al: MR imaging of periventricular leukomalacia in childhood, *AJNR* 10:111, 1989.
12. Flodmark O, Poskitt KJ, Whitfield MF, et al: Inability of neurosonography to diagnose periventricular leukomalacia (PVL), Twenty-seventh Meeting of the American Society of Neuroradiology, Orlando, Fla, 1989.
13. Flodmark O, Roland EH, Hall A, et al: Periventricular leukomalacia, *Radiology* 162:119, 1987.
14. Friede RL: *Developmental neuropathology*, New York, 1975, Springer-Verlag.
15. Gilles FH: The developing human brain: growth and epidemiologic neuropathology. In Gilles FH, Leviton A, Dooling EC: *The developing human brain: growth and epidemiologic neuropathology*, Boston, 1983, John Wright.
16. Govaert P, Van de Velde E, Vanhaesebrouck P, et al: CT diagnosis of neonatal subarachnoid hemorrhage, *Pediatr Radiol* 20:139, 1990.
17. Griffith AD, Lawrance KM: The effect of hypoxia and hypoglycemia on the brain of the newborn human infant, *Dev Med Child Neurol* 16:308, 1974.
18. Grunnet ML, Curtess RG, Bray PF, et al: Brain changes in newborn infants from an intensive care unit, *Dev Med Child Neurol* 16:320, 1974.
19. Hambleton G, Wigglesworth JS: Origin of intraventricular hemorrhage in the preterm infant, *Arch Dis Child* 51:651, 1976.
20. Hill A, Volpe JJ: Stroke and hemorrhage in the premature and term neonate. In Edwards MSD, Hoffman HJ: *Cerebral vascular disease in children and adolescents*, Baltimore, 1989, Williams & Wilkins.
21. Kaye EM, Cass PR, Dooling E, et al: Chronic epidural hematomas in childhood: increased recognition and nonsurgical management, *Pediatr Neurol* 1:255, 1985.
22. Kuhn MJ, Johnson KA, Davis KR: Wallerian degeneration: evaluation with MR imaging, *Radiology* 168:199, 1988.
23. Larroche JC: Intraventricular hemorrhage in the premature infant, *Adv Perinat Neurol* 1:115, 1979.
24. Leech RW, Kohnen P: Subependymal and intraventricular hemorrhages in the newborn, *Am J Pathol* 77:1974.
25. Lipp-Zwahlen AE, Deonna T, Chrzanowski R, et al: Temporal evolution of hypoxic-ischemic brain lesions in asphyxiated full-term newborns as assessed by computerized tomography, *Neuroradiology* 27:138, 1985.
26. Martin DJ, Hill A, Fitz CK, et al: Hypoxic-ischemic cerebral injury in the neonatal brain: a report of sonographic features with computed tomography correlation, *Pediatr Radiol* 13:307, 1983.
27. McArdle CB, Richardson CJ, Hayden CK, et al: Abnormalities of the neonatal brain: MR imaging. Part I. Intracranial hemorrhage, *Radiology* 163:387, 1987.
28. McMenamin JB, Shackelford GD, Volpe JJ: Outcome of neonatal intraventricular hemorrhage with periventricular echodense lesions, *Ann Neurol* 15:1984.
29. Naidich TP, Chakera TMH: Multicystic encephalomalacia: CT appearance and pathological correlation, *J Comput Assist Tomogr* 8:63, 1984.
30. Nelson MD, Gonzalez-Gomez I, Gilles FH: The search for human telencephalic ventriculofugal arteries, *AJNR* 12:215, 1991.
31. Pape KE, Wigglesworth JS: Specific hemorrhagic lesions of the newborn brain. In Pape KE, Wigglesworth JS: *Hemorrhage, ischemia, and the perinatal brain*, Lavenham, Suffolk, 1979, Lavenham Press.

32. Pasternak JF: Parasagittal infarction in neonatal asphyxia, *Ann Neurol* 21:202, 1987.
33. Raybaud C: Destructive lesions of the brain, *Neuroradiology* 25:265, 1983.
34. Sherman RM, Seledrik LJ: Periventricular leukomalacia: A 1-year autopsy study, *Arch Neurol* 37:231, 1980.
35. Shewmon DA, Fine M, Masdeau JC, et al: Postischemic hypervascularity of infancy: a stage in the evolution of ischemic brain damage with characteristic CT scan, *Ann Neurol* 9:358, 1981.
36. Takashima S, Armstrong DL, Becker LE: Subcortical leukomalacia, relationship to development of the cerebral sulcus and its vascular supply, *Arch Neurol* 35:470, 1978.
37. Taylor GA, Fitz CR, Miller MK, et al: Intracranial abnormalities in infants treated with extracorporeal membrane oxygenation: imaging with US and CT, *Radiology* 165:675, 1987.
38. Volpe JJ: Hypoxic-ischemic encephalopathy: biochemical and physiological aspects. In Volpe JJ: *Neurology of the newborn*, Philadelphia, 1987, WB Saunders.
39. Volpe JJ: Hypoxic-ischemic encephalopathy: neuropathology and pathogenesis. In Volpe JJ: *Neurology of the newborn*, Philadelphia, 1987, WB Saunders.
40. Volpe JJ: Intraventricular hemorrhage in the premature infant—current concepts. Part 1. *Ann Neurol* 25:3, 1989.
41. Volpe JJ, Pasternak JF: Parasagittal cerebral injury in neonatal hypoxic-ischemic encephalopathy, *J Pediatr* 91:472, 1977.
42. Volpe JJ, Herscovitch P, Perlman JM, et al: Positron emission tomography in the newborn: extensive impairment of regional cerebral blood flow with intraventricular hemorrhage and hemorrhagic intracerebral involvement, *Pediatrics* 72:589, 1983.

Vascular diseases in children

Four types of vascular diseases affect children: (1) arteritis and arteriopathy presenting as acute hemiplegia, (2) arterial and venous infarction excluding arteriopathy, (3) vascular lesions such as malformations, aneurysms, vein of Galen malformations, and (4) angiodysplasias.[7] Whereas CT or MRI is valuable in the initial work-up of the patient, angiography often remains the examination of choice to define subtle detail such as altered vascular morphology.

ARTERITIS AND ARTERIOPATHY

In almost all cases of arteritis and arteriopathy the cause is not known with certainty.[7,21,49] At one time it was speculated that inflammatory vascular involvement at the skull base after nasopharyngeal infection was the origin of most cases of internal carotid artery occlusion in children. In many cases when the cause is not apparent, an arteritis is suggested as a probable cause. Internal carotid arterial occlusion also occurs in patients with Down's syndrome, neurofibromatosis, after radiation therapy and chemotherapy for intracranial tumor, autoimmune disorders, and migraine.

Moyamoya disease

A specific type of arteritis known as moyamoya disease is seen in some children and is characterized by progressive occlusion of the supraclinoid internal carotid artery and proximal anterior and middle cerebral arteries. The disease was first described by the Japanese[29] and further elucidated by Suzuki,[54] who noted the characteristic appearance of the fine collateral arterial network (basilar telangiectatic collat-

erals) that develops at the base of the brain in response to progressive arterial stenoses. Suzuki used the term *moyamoya* (Japanese for "puff of smoke" or "hazy") to describe the condition. There is a familial incidence, which in the Japanese population accounts for 7% of the patients affected. The disease may be immunologically mediated as autoantibodies have been found in some patients,[28] and the disease has been reported in children with immunodeficiency syndromes.[23] Histologically, all three layers of the arterial wall are abnormal with intimal thickening, buckling and splitting of the internal elastic lamina, as well as medial atrophy.

Moyamoya is usually limited to the arteries at the base of the brain, that is, the supraclinoid internal carotid and proximal anterior and middle cerebral arteries. Involvement is frequently bilateral. The posterior cerebral arteries are less frequently involved, and vertebrobasilar involvement is rare. The progressive occlusions result in the development of abundant collateral arteries composed of fine hypertrophied thalamoperforate and lenticulostriate arteries. Leptomeningeal and external-to-internal carotid collateralization develops, as does transdural collateralization. As the stenoses progress to complete occlusion, the leptomeningeal collateral arteries no longer fill and the penetrating basal ganglia collateral arteries further dilate to take over the blood supply to the brain.

The clinical presentation of moyamoya is often that of recurrent transient ischemic attacks, usually in a motor distribution, that eventually progresses to hemiparesis or hemiplegia. Seizures may occur, and older children may complain of headache. Some older children, adolescents, and adults may have parenchymal or subarachnoid hemorrhage due to rupture of the aneurysmally dilated basal collateral arteries.

CT findings may be normal in the early stages of moyamoya but eventually show multiple low attenuation zones compatible with infarcts. After intravenous contrast administration the moyamoya collateral arteries may appear as intense enhancement within the basal ganglia. Prominent leptomeningeal collateral arteries may also be evident. MRI may be used in place of CT to demonstrate the infarcts and atrophy. The extensive collateral network near the base of the brain may also be visualized as pinpoint and curvilinear flow voids[15] (Fig. 6-15). Angiography demonstrates the extent of the internal carotid and cerebral arterial stenoses. The entire collateral network is best visualized with bilateral angiography (Fig. 6-15), including external carotid injections.

Serial angiography can follow the progression of the stenoses and the results of surgical treatment. Treatment of moyamoya is surgically oriented and is based on improving collateral flow. An anastomotic connection of the superficial temporal artery to a distal branch of the middle cerebral artery bypasses the stenoses and provides an immediate improvement in flow to the distal middle cerebral artery branches. This procedure, however, is difficult to perform in children because of their small vessels. Some neurosur-

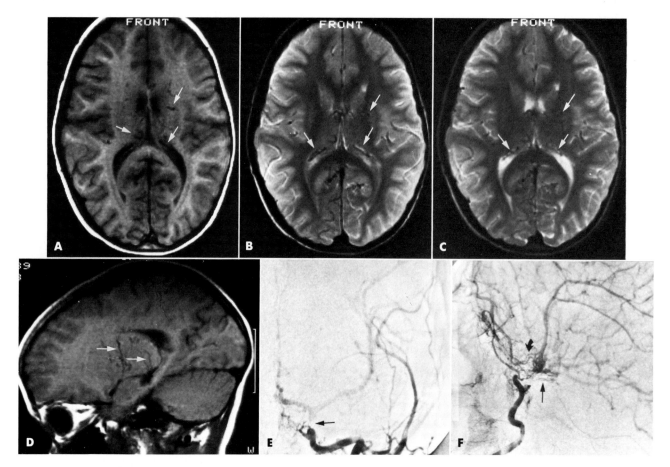

Fig. 6-15   T1-weighted **(A)**, proton density **(B)**, T2-weighted **(C)**, and sagittal T1-weighted **(D)** scans demonstrate flow voids in the basal ganglia and thalami representing collateral arteries in a 9-year-old boy with moyamoya disease. **E,** Left carotid angiography, frontal view, demonstrates marked narrowing of the terminal internal carotid artery *(arrow)*. **F,** Lateral view shows collateral basal ganglia arteries with a moyamoya pattern *(straight arrow)*. Collaterals *(curved arrow)* also arise from the ophthalmic artery.

geons advocate placing either the temporalis muscle (encephalomyosynangiosis) or the superficial temporal artery (encephaloduroarteriosynangiosis)[34] directly on the cortical surface of the brain to improve perfusion through collateral cortical revascularization. Improvement of flow has been documented with angiography and correlates with improving intelligence quotients, previously diminished from progressive ischemia. Also, the demonstrated reduction or lack of progressive increase in the size of the moyamoya collateral arteries correlates with a reduced chance of hemorrhage. Some patients may not show an improvement in radiographic flow but have shown clinical improvement.[43]

ARTERIAL AND VENOUS INFARCTION

There are many causes of arterial and venous occlusions.[43] Cerebral infarction in children may be caused by anoxia (including metabolic anoxia), emboli from congenital heart disease, and cortical venous infarction from infection or dehydration.[7] Other causes include trauma, blood dyscrasias, collagen-vascular diseases, meningitis, sickle cell

disease, and metabolic diseases such as homocystinuria or mitochondrial cytopathies[17] (see Chapter 4). A CT scan may be normal or demonstrate a low density that eventually evolves to atrophy. Occasionally the infarction is hemorrhagic. A specific cause may be found in only 60% of patients. Arteriography may demonstrate a nonspecific acute arterial occlusion (Fig. 6-16), but more often the study is normal. The MRI scan demonstrates low or isointense signal intensity on T1-weighted images and high signal intensity on T2-weighted images as a result of increased water content. MRI may also demonstrate hemiatrophy or hemihypoplasia and gliosis from presumed in utero or perinatal arterial occlusion (see Chapter 3). MRI is often more sensitive and specific than CT for hemorrhagic and multiple infarctions. The risk of arteriography is high in patients with sickle cell disease but can be decreased by maintaining good hydration and by preceding angiography with a blood transfusion to reduce the level of hemoglobin S below 20%.[47] Angiographically, many patients with sickle cell disease demonstrate arterial occlusions or irregularities, as well as segmental ectasias or aneurysms that

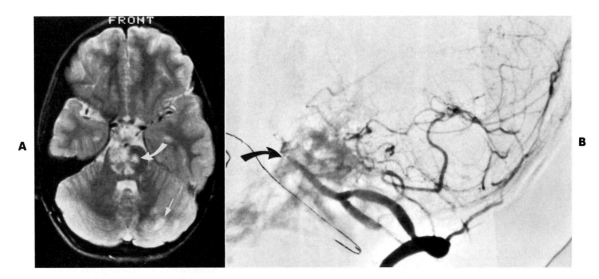

Fig. 6-16   A, T2-weighted scan demonstrates high intensity lesions in the pons *(curved arrow)* and left cerebellar hemisphere *(straight arrow)* of a 6-year-old boy with basilar artery occlusion. **B,** Lateral view of the vertebral angiogram shows an occlusion of the basilar artery at the junction of the middle and upper thirds *(arrow)* beyond the anterior inferior cerebellar arteries. The posterior cerebral arteries were filled from the internal carotid arteries. Occlusion of penetrating arteries arising from the basilar artery caused the pontine infarct. The cerebellar infarct is at the border zone between the posterior inferior and anterior inferior cerebellar arteries. (From Carollo BR, Runge VM: Brain: vascular diseases. In Runge VM: *Clinical magnetic resonance imaging,* Philadelphia, 1990, JB Lippincott.)

may produce subarachnoid hemorrhage. Occasionally, venous occlusion from sickling or stasis results in edema or infarction.

Arteritis and secondary ischemic lesions of the brain may result from radiation therapy and chemotherapy. The white matter lesions that occur may be transient or permanent, the latter including leukomalacia, mineralizing angiopathy, and atrophy.[22] Focal atrophy of the pituitary gland has also been described.[9] Radiation effects may appear as diffuse hyperintensity in the white matter without mass effect on T2-weighted images.[9] The corpus callosum is usually spared (see Chapter 7). L-Asparaginase, an enzyme used in treating acute leukemia, has been associated with intracranial sinus thrombosis in 1% to 2% of children.[42] (Cortical vein and dural sinus occlusions are considered in Chapter 5.)

VASCULAR LESIONS

Intracranial vascular lesions (angiomas) result from congenital maldevelopment of blood vessels during an early embryonic stage.[27] These lesions are subclassified into four groups: arteriovenous malformations, venous angiomas, telangiectasias (capillary angiomas), and cavernous angiomas. Categorization is based on the nature of the blood vessels and on the intervening tissue between the blood vessels. The different types may coexist in the same lesion.[10]

The main presenting symptoms of vascular lesions of the brain are bleeding, seizures, progressive neurological def-

icit, and headaches. The majority of lesions become apparent during the second or third decade of life. Primary intracranial hemorrhage after rupture of an intracerebral vascular malformation is relatively rare; most infant and childhood cerebral hemorrhages are related to trauma.

The neuroradiological investigation of a suspected intracranial vascular lesion commences with CT or MRI scans and is often followed by angiography. Often, the initial studies demonstrate an intracranial hemorrhage and the angiogram confirms the cause. Increasingly, however, because of the widespread use of CT and MRI, vascular lesions causing minor neurological deficits are discovered that are often negative by angiography.[10] These so-called "occult" vascular lesions, which occur more commonly in adults than in children, are becoming increasingly diagnosed in children through the use of MRI. They may present clinically and have imaging appearances similar to those of childhood neoplasms, and therefore deserve special attention in the differential diagnosis and management of pediatric intracranial tumors (see Chapter 7).

Arteriovenous malformations

Arteriovenous malformations (AVM) constitute the largest group of congenital vascular malformations. They are composed of a compact nidus, or tangle, of thin-walled vessels that replace the capillary bed. The nidus connects abnormally enlarged arteries to dilated thin-walled veins. Because of the lack of intervening capillaries, a direct arteriovenous shunt is created. Often the malformations are

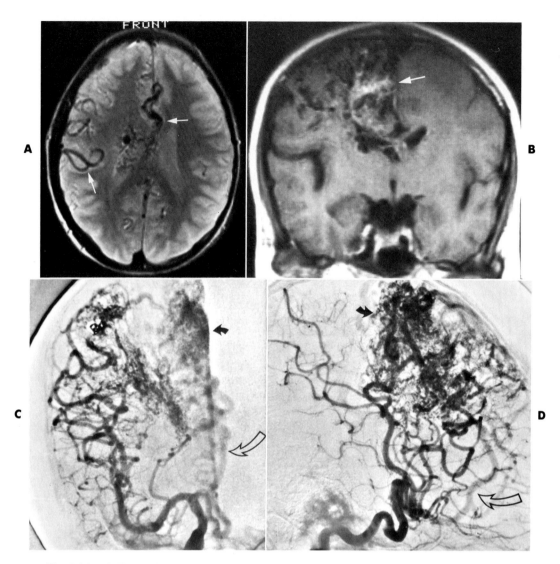

Fig. 6-17   A, Proton density scan demonstrates serpiginous vessels seen as flow defects involving the midline anterior cerebral artery and middle cerebral artery *(arrows).* **B,** Coronal T1-weighted scan demonstrates high signal intensity in the frontal lobe caused by hemorrhage from an arteriovenous malformation in this 13-year-old girl. **C** and **D,** The right carotid arteriogram demonstrates an enlarged anterior cerebral artery *(curved open arrow)* supplying an arteriovenous malformation in the parafalcine frontal lobe *(curved black arrow).*

surrounded by gliotic neural parenchyma, which is thought to result from chronic ischemia. Approximately 90% of pial AVMs are located above the tentorium and involve the cerebral hemispheres, whereas 10% are situated in the cerebellum or brain stem.[33] Approximately 20% of AVMs become symptomatic before the patient is 20 years old.[41]

When an AVM is large, either CT or MRI may demonstrate serpiginous vascular channels (arteries and veins) (Fig. 6-17) and the hemorrhage, if present. With CT intravenous contrast material is required to adequately document the serpiginous nature of the enlarged vascular

channels. MRI demonstrates these lesions without contrast enhancement as serpiginous flow voids representing the nidus and the vascular channels entering and exiting the lesions. Some motion-compensating spin echo techniques may potentially mask the detection of an AVM by eliminating or reducing the flow voids created by the moving blood, and therefore these techniques should not be used to evaluate an AVM. Advances in MRI with three-dimensional angiography and selective presaturation of feeding arteries can clearly define the vascular supply of AVMs.[8] The combination of MR angiographic and spin echo methods also provides information useful for therapeutic planning not provided by either technique alone. Arteriovenous malformations occasionally contain calcific deposits that are well seen by CT but not often by MRI. On the other hand, subtle hemosiderin deposits from an old hemorrhage may be unapparent on CT scans but generally are detected by MRI, particularly with gradient echo sequences[4,30] (see Chapter 1 and 2).

Ischemic changes from an intracerebral steal associated with arteriovenous shunting may produce gliosis and atrophy. The gliosis often appears as a high signal intensity on T2-weighted images. Angiography remains the definitive procedure to confirm, define, and characterize the arteriovenous malformation (Fig. 6-17), particularly the three features critical to treatment planning: enlarged feeding arteries, nidus, and enlarged draining veins. Serial angiography in children has demonstrated that AVMs may grow with time.

The malformations may be exclusively supplied by the dural arteries, the pial arteries, or a combination of both. Dural malformations are most commonly located in the posterior fossa and are rare in infants and children.[38,44] Children with dural-based AVMs may show signs of hydrocephalus and developmental delay; infants may have a heart murmur, macrocephaly, distended scalp veins, and cardiac failure. A thorough knowledge of the vascular anatomy of the dura mater is essential to understand the arterial supply of dural AVMs.[38]

On occasion, a significant problem during resection of an intracerebral AVM is the surgeon's inability to see the lesion adequately during surgery. Color Doppler flow ultrasound generates a two-dimensional image in which Doppler shifts can be encoded for blood flow in different directions.[46] This technique has been successful in the resection of AVMs, in differentiating hematomas from AVMs, for locating deep vascular supplies to the lesions, and for confirming resection of the lesions after surgery.

Heavy charged–particle radiosurgery and stereotactic small field megavoltage therapy have been extensively used in the treatment of cerebral AVMs, particularly for deep-seated lesions.[53] CT and MRI are necessary for obtaining contour information of the AVMs and for transferring the vascular data into a three-dimensional format for treatment planning.[11] Furthermore MRI and MR angiography are excellent modalities for assessing the response of AVMs to radiosurgery.[32]

Cavernous angiomas

Evidence from published MRI reports suggests that cavernous angiomas may be the most common type of vascular malformation of the brain, especially in the pediatric and adolescent populations. Patients may be asymptomatic or may have seizures or hemorrhage. The angiomas are composed of clusters of endothelial-lined spaces that lack large arterial feeding vessels.[35,37] Although cavernous angiomas may occur anywhere in the central nervous system, the supratentorial location is the most

common site. They occur less commonly in children than in adults but, because of MRI, are increasingly being diagnosed in children. Up to 33% of angiomas are multiple and often familial.[10]

Pathologically, small hemorrhages within and around the lesions, as well as fibrosis and calcification within the lesion, are commonly found.[35,51] Histologically, "pure" cavernous angiomas are less frequent than lesions in which a mixture of all types of angiomas are present. On CT the lesions appear as well-defined, slightly hyperdense, nodular, mottled, or ring-like masses (Fig. 6-18) and may enhance slightly after contrast administration. Calcification may occur within larger lesions.[18,35,57] These lesions may be single or multiple.

The MRI appearance is due to the visualization of hemorrhage in various stages of evolution. Often there is evidence of multiple recurrent hemorrhages. The lesions are surrounded by a ring of hypointensity, most noticeable on T2-weighted images, which represents hemosiderin within the surrounding macrophages (Fig. 6-18). Increased signal intensity is present centrally and consistent with extracellular methemoglobin. A central core of isointensity may be apparent on T1 images and could represent the stasis of blood within the vessels of the malformation or perhaps a recent hemorrhage with intracellular deoxyhemoglobin.[18,55] Intratumoral hemorrhage may display a similar appearance in the adult population.[55] A hemorrhagic tumor, however, usually is surrounded by a collar of edema, absent from most cavernous angiomas. This differentiation is more of a problem when the angioma is complicated by acute or subacute hemorrhage with surrounding edema, since most hemorrhagic neoplasms are accompanied by significant edema. The clinical history and symptoms may aid in differentiating cavernous angiomas from hemorrhagic neoplasm in this situation. Iodine enhancement with CT and gadolinium-DTPA enhancement with MRI in these lesions probably correlate with a combination of blood-brain barrier breakdown and the slow-flow blood pool effect. The slow arterial flow within these lesions accounts for the lack of visualization on angiography. Because of this, these lesions are often referred to as occult (by angiography) vascular malformations.

Venous angiomas

Venous angiomas represent a group of vascular malformations characterized by an abnormality of venous drainage of the normal brain. No abnormal arterial component is present, and there is no nidus. These malformations may occur as the result of fetal venous occlusions or perhaps because of underdevelopment of medullary venous structures, and represent pathways of collateral or alternate venous drainage. It is hypothesized that the insult causing this abnormal pattern must occur during Padget's fourth to seventh stage of development at the sixth to ninth week of fetal life.[25,48] Pathologically a cluster of radially oriented, dilated periventricular medullary veins drain into a single dilated draining vein. The draining vein is enlarged, takes a

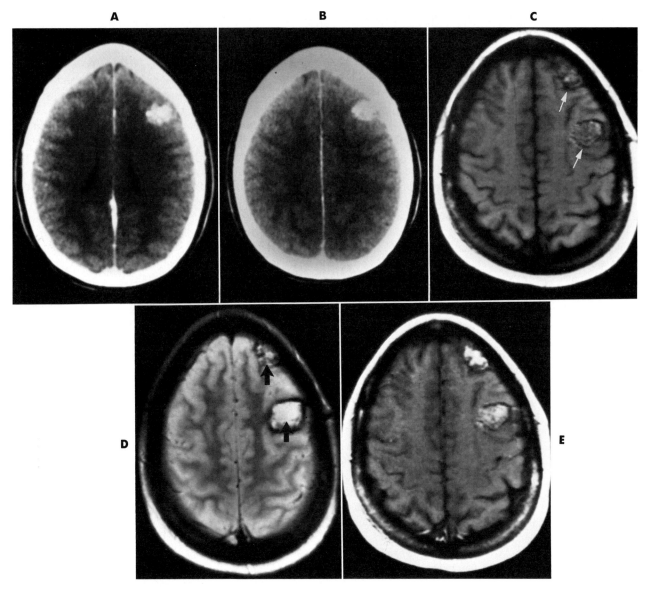

Fig. 6-18 **A,** Axial contrast-enhanced CT scan demonstrates a high density lesion in the left frontal lobe that was equally dense on the nonenhanced scan (not shown). **B,** A scan obtained 1 cm more cephalad shows a second lesion anterior to the first lesion. **C,** An axial T1-weighted scan demonstrates the two lesions on the same image (which was obtained more horizontally than the CT scans). Hemorrhage is evident on both the T1-weighted **(C)** and proton density **(D)** scans as evidenced by the high intensity material **(D,** *arrows)* within the lesions (due to extracellular methemoglobin) with surrounding low intensity rims due to hemosiderin **(C,** *arrows).* The hemosiderin rim is also seen. After Gd-DTPA administration the center of both lesions enhance because of the slow vascular flow through the lesions.
Diagnosis: Multiple cavernous angiomas (proven at surgery).

transcerebral or transcerebellar course and empties into a cortical vein, venous sinus, or into the deep venous system.[13,48] The brain surrounding these malformations is usually normal, although similar anomalous venous drainage may occur with migrational aberrations. These lesions may be found incidentally or may cause seizures or hemorrhage. Symptomatic presentation in children is rare when compared with AVMs and cavernous angiomas.

Venous angiomas with hemorrhage most commonly occur in the cerebellum or brain stem.[35,45] The transcerebral or cerebellar course that the draining vein takes is apparent on CT as an enhancing linear or serpiginous structure coursing from the ventricle to the cortex. Because of its flow characteristics, the vessel is evident on MRI as a flow void (Fig. 6-19) on spin echo sequences (especially without flow compensation techniques) or as high intensity on flow-

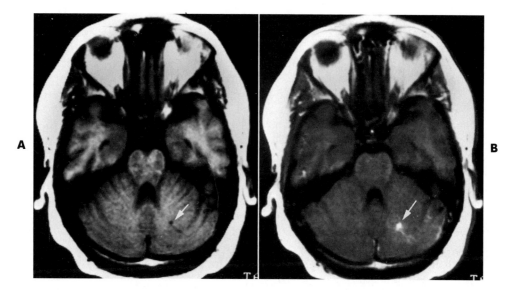

Fig. 6-19 T1-weighted scans before (**A**) and after (**B**) Gd-DTPA enhancement demonstrate a flow void on the nonenhanced scan (**A**, *arrow*), which enhances following Gd-DTPA administration (**B**, *arrow*). The appearances are caused by a venous angioma in the cerebellum of a 14-year-old girl.

sensitive gradient echo sequences. The dilated medullary veins are not always demonstrated on CT or MRI. Because of very slow flow or no flow, the veins may appear as regions of decreased signal on T1-weighted images and increased signal on T2-weighted images because of imaging of the blood pool.[5] Angiography demonstrates the nidus of the venous malformation as a radial pattern of deep white matter (medullary) veins draining into a single vein, which in turn may enter the deep or superficial venous system.

Capillary telangiectasias

Capillary telangiectasias are a group of malformations and are composed of small vessels similar to capillaries. Usually the vessels are less than 1 cm in diameter and most commonly occur in the pons. Most of these are incidental findings and rarely present with hemorrhage or other symptoms. Pathologically, hemorrhage is not found within these lesions. Telangiectasias are angiographically occult, primarily because of their small size.[35]

Aneurysms

CONGENITAL. Aneurysms rarely occur in infants or children. Between 0.5% to 4.6% of all aneurysms occur in this age group.[19,31,40] Several unique features of these aneurysms distinguish them from those occurring in adults. In contrast with the female predominance reported in adults, the pediatric male to female ratio is 2:1 to 3:1.[2,31,36] Approximately 30% to 45% are giant aneurysms,[2,19,26] which are infrequent in adults. Furthermore the distribution of aneurysms in the circle of Willis is unique, a large percentage occurring in the posterior circulation and at the internal carotid bifurcation. Also many of the aneurysms are

peripherally located along branches of the middle and posterior cerebral arteries,[2] especially those resulting from trauma or infection. Patients with certain conditions such as coarctation of the aorta, polycystic renal disease, and fibromuscular dysplasia of the renal arteries are predisposed to congenital aneurysms.[1]

The cause of pediatric intracerebral aneurysms is controversial, and discussion often centers on the question of congenital versus degenerative causes. Congenital defects in the media have been demonstrated in up to 80% of patients in autopsy studies,[16] and a congenital basis for aneurysms has been promoted by some authors who have cited the existence, although rare, of saccular aneurysms in children as an argument against a degenerative process.[36] However, Stehbens[51] has concluded that most histological reports of pediatric aneurysms contain insufficient evidence to support a congenital mechanism. Furthermore degeneration of the internal elastic lamina by hemodynamic forces is the initial pathophysiological alteration.[12]

Symptoms from rupture of aneurysms include severe headache with meningeal signs. Focal neurological symptoms such as cranial nerve palsies may herald the presentation of a giant aneurysm.[19,40] Radiologic evaluation includes nonenhanced CT, which demonstrates high density subarachnoid hemorrhage (SAH), the distribution of which may predict the location of the aneurysm. Enhanced CT may demonstrate the aneurysm itself. MRI demonstration of subarachnoid blood is unreliable because of CSF flow dynamics, as well as the higher oxygen tension of SAH in the subarachnoid space, which maintains the oxyhemoglobin state. Clotted subarachnoid hemorrhage may be detected through the identification of the degradation products

products of hemoglobin. Both CT and MRI can detect acute parenchymal hemorrhage, whereas MRI more specifically approximates the age of the hematoma through demonstration of the degradation products of hemoglobin. Giant aneurysms and thrombus within the aneurysm are well seen with MRI.[3,39,56]

Arteriography is necessary to define the aneurysm, particularly the neck and adjacent vessels, the remaining cerebral arteries to exclude additional aneurysms, and the circle of Willis and its capacity to provide collateral circulation to the hemispheres. Magnetic resonance angiography may soon play a major role in the detection and evaluation of cerebral aneurysms.

The treatment of aneurysms is generally surgical with clipping of the neck of the aneurysm and preservation of the parent vessels. Giant aneurysms that are not surgically accessible can be treated through either isolation of the aneurysm from the circulation with arterial balloon occlusion, or placement of balloons or other embolic material within the aneurysm to obliterate the lumen.

MYCOTIC. Mycotic aneurysms constitute 2% to 5% of all intracranial aneurysms. They are commonly associated with bacterial endocarditis, less commonly with distant infection with bacteremia or septicemia, mastoiditis, cavernous sinus thrombosis, sinusitis, or basilar meningitis. Mycotic aneurysms occur in 4% to 10% of patients with bacterial endocarditis, and patients with this disease may initially present with a mycotic aneurysm.[6,14] The most common clinical presentations of mycotic aneurysm are hemorrhage (either subarachnoid or parenchymal), transient ischemic attacks, or infarction.

Vessel wall infection is caused either by infected emboli, which lodge within the arteries proximal to bifurcations, or hematogenous infected emboli, which lodge within the vaso-vasorum. Subsequent degeneration of the internal elastic lamina and media allows focal expansion of the arterial wall and formation of a fusiform aneurysm. Radiologic evaluation of the patient with neurological symptoms and the clinical setting to suggest mycotic aneurysm should initially include CT (see Chapter 5) or MRI. CT is optimal for detecting subarachnoid hemorrhage.

Cerebral angiography is essential for the evaluation of mycotic aneurysms. Mycotic aneurysms tend to be fusiform and occur more peripherally than do congenital aneurysms, which are usually saccular and occur about the circle of Willis. Mycotic aneurysms are usually located within the middle cerebral arterial distribution, although they have also been found in other or multiple sites throughout the cerebral circulation. Mycotic aneurysms may be multiple in up to 20% of patients,[6] and therefore complete angiography should be performed. Intravenous antibiotic therapy for 4 to 6 weeks is the cornerstone treatment of mycotic aneurysms. Serial angiography during this period may be necessary to evaluate interval change within the aneurysm. Surgical excision is advocated for aneurysms that have enlarged despite antibiotic therapy and for those that are peripherally located.

VEIN OF GALEN MALFORMATIONS. The vein of Galen malformation is defined as an arteriovenous malformation with arterial input from intracranial branches of the carotid or basilar arteries and venous drainage via an aneurysmally dilated vein of Galen. The pathogenesis in many cases may be attributed to dural venous sinus aplasia, hypoplasia, stenosis, or atresia. The malformations may be one of two types: a true aneurysm of the vein of Galen, which is usually diagnosed at birth and in which there is a direct arteriovenous fistula, and a second type, which is diagnosed at a slightly later age and is a true arteriovenous malformation with secondary enlargement of the vein of Galen. The arterial supply may arise from the posterior cerebral, superior cerebellar, anterior cerebral, middle cerebral, lenticulostriate, thalamostriate, or anterior and posterior choroidal arteries.[7]

The clinical presentation depends on the age of the patient: neonates, infants, or older children and adults. Most malformations occur in the neonatal period with high output cardiac failure secondary to a large arteriovenous fistula[50] and hydrocephalus. The arteriovenous shunt is often diminished in children and young adults because of the angiomatous network within the malformation or partial thrombosis or stenosis of the vein of Galen or other venous drainage. Infants usually show progressive hydrocephalus, which is probably caused by compression of the posterior third ventricle and cerebral aqueduct by the enlarged vein of Galen. Seizures may also occur in this group. Older children and adults often complain of headaches and may have a subarachnoid hemorrhage as a result of aneurysm rupture.

On imaging studies the aneurysmal vein of Galen appears as a spherical mass that impinges on the posterior third ventricle (Fig. 6-20). The enlarged vein appears as a hypoechoic mass on ultrasound, and the communication with the straight sinus or midline anomalous sinus suggests the diagnosis. CT demonstrates a homogeneous high density mass that enhances intensely after contrast administration. The dilated midline sinus and the arterial supply may also be apparent. The malformation appears as a hypointense region or signal void on MRI because of the flow turbulence created by the arteriovenous shunt (Fig. 6-20). Thrombus is frequently evident within the malformation, and its appearance is related to its age. Angiography remains the primary modality to define the malformation and is necessary to plan treatment. Branches of the posterior cerebral artery (choroidal arteries) and of the superior cerebellar artery usually supply the lesion (Fig. 6-20).

Therapy depends on the age of the patient and the symptoms. The neonate is the most difficult to treat because of the delicate fluid balance, the high output cardiac failure, and the risk of myocardial ischemia. Medical therapy is usually not successful in controlling heart failure, and approximately 50% of patients treated by surgery alone are impaired or die.[23] Embolotherapy directed at the arteriovenous fistula has proven successful in same cases. Both superselective arterial and transtorcular techniques have been used. Early alleviation of cardiac failure allows the

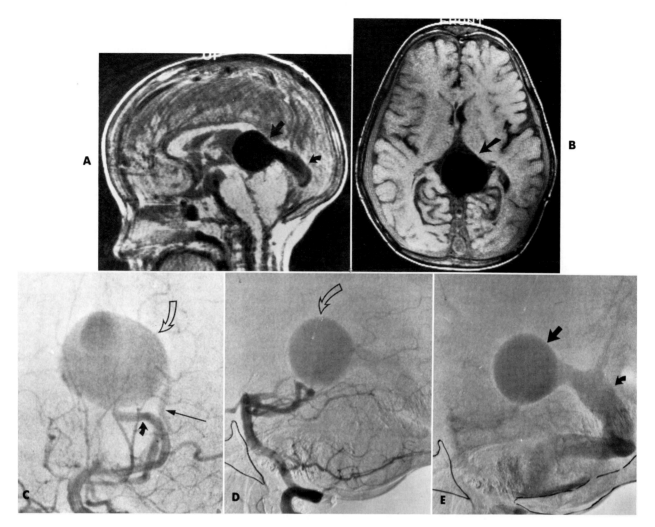

Fig. 6-20   Sagittal **(A)** and axial **(B)** T1-weighted scans demonstrate a large aneurysm of the great vein of Galen (**A**, *straight arrow*) draining into an enlarged straight sinus (**B**, *curved arrow*). **C,** The left vertebral angiogram (frontal view) demonstrates enlarged posterior cerebral *(black curved arrow)* and superior cerebellar arteries *(straight arrow)* supplying the large aneurysm *(curved arrow)*. In the lateral arterial **(D)** and venous phases **(E)** the aneurysm is again documented (**D**, *curved arrow;* **E**, *straight arrow*) draining into the enlarged straight sinus (**E**, *curved arrow*). The transverse sinus is also enlarged.

child to grow and develop for more definitive treatment later. The use of embolotherapy with isobutylcyanoacrylate or coils has reduced the morbidity and mortality in this group.[20,37]

Treatment in infants, older children, and adults is often successful with a combination of surgical and interventional techniques, achieving complete or nearly complete thrombosis of the malformations.

ANGIODYSPLASIA. See Chapters 8 and 9.

REFERENCES
Vascular diseases in children

1. Allcock JM: Aneurysms. In Newton TH, Potts DG: *Radiology of the skull and brain,* St Louis, 1974, Mosby–Year Book.
2. Amacher AL, Drake CG: The results of operating on cerebral aneurysms and angiomas in children and adolescents. I. Cerebral aneurysms, *Childs Brain* 5:151, 1979.
3. Atlas SW, Grossman RI, Goldberg HI, et al: Partially thrombosed giant intracerebral aneurysms: correlation of MR and pathological findings, *Radiology* 162:111, 1987.
4. Atlas SW, Mark AJ, Fram EK, et al: Vascular intracranial lesions: applications of gradient echo MR imaging, *Radiology* 169:455, 1988.
5. Augustyn GT, Scott JA, Olson E, et al: Cerebral venous angiomas: MR imaging, *Radiology* 156:391, 1985.
6. Bohmfalk GL, Story JL, Wissinger JP, et al: Bacterial intracranial aneurysms, *J Neurosurg* 48:369, 1978.
7. Chuang S: Vascular diseases of the brain in children. In Edwards MSD, Hoffman HJ: *Cerebral vascular disease in children and adolescents,* Baltimore, 1989, Williams & Wilkins.
8. Edelman RR, Wentz KU, Mattle HP, et al: Intracerebral arteriovenous malformations: evaluation with selective MR angiography and venography, *Radiology* 173:831, 1989.
9. Edwards MK: Metabolic, endocrine, and iatrogenic lesions of the brain. In Cohen MD, Edwards MK: *Magnetic resonance imaging of children,* Philadelphia, 1990, BC Decker.
10. El-Gohary M, El-Gohary MD, et al: Angiographically occult vascular malformations in childhood, *Neurosurgery* 20:750, 1987.

11. Fabrikant JI, Frankel KA, Phillips MH, et al: Stereotactic heavy-charged particle Bragg peak radiosurgery for intracranial arteriovenous malformations. In Edwards MSB, Hoffman HJ: *Cerebral vascular diseases in children and adolescents*, Baltimore, 1989, Williams & Wilkins.

12. Ferguson CG: Physical factors in the initiation, growth and rupture of human intracranial, saccular aneurysms, *J Neurosurg* 37:666, 1972.

13. Fierstein SB, Pribram HW, Hieshima G: Angiography and computed tomography in the evaluation of cerebral venous malformations, *Neuroradiology* 17:137, 1979.

14. Frazee JG, Story JL, Wissinger JP, et al: Bacterial intracranial aneurysms, *J Neurosurg* 53:633, 1980.

15. Fujisawa I, Asato R, Nishimura K, et al: Moyamoya disease: MR imaging, *Radiology* 164:103, 1987.

16. Glynn LE: Medical defects in the circle of Willis and their relationship to aneurysm formation, *J Pathol Bacteriol* 51:213, 1940.

17. Golden GS: Cerebrovascular disease. In Swaiman KF: *Pediatric neurology: principles and practice*, St Louis, 1989, Mosby–Year Book.

18. Gomori JM, Grossman RI, Goldberg HI, et al: Occult cerebral vascular malformations: high-field MR imaging, *Radiology* 158:707, 1986.

19. Hacker RJ: Intracranial aneurysms of childhood: a statistical analysis of 500 cases from the world literature (abstract), *Neurosurg* 10:775, 1982.

20. Halbach VV, Barkovich AJ: Anomalies of cerebral vasculature. In Barkovich JJ: *Pediatric neuroimaging*, New York, 1990, Raven.

21. Harwood-Nash DC, Fitz CR: Abnormalities of the cerebral arteries. In Harwood-Nash DC, Fitz CR: *Neuroradiology in infants and children*, St Louis, 1976, Mosby–Year Book.

22. Hecht-Leavitt C, Grossman RI, Curran SJ, et al: MR of brain radiation injury: experimental study in cats, *AJNR* 8:427, 1987.

23. Hoffman HJ, Chuang S, Hendrick B, et al: Aneurysm of the vein of Galen, *J Neurosurg* 57:316, 1982.

24. Hoffman HJ and Griebel RW: Moyamoya syndrome in children. In Edwards MSB, Hoffman HJ: *Cerebral vascular disease in children and adolescents*, Baltimore, 1989, Williams & Wilkins.

25. Huang YP, Wolf BS: Veins of the white matter of the cerebral hemispheres (the medullary veins), *AJR* 92:739, 1964.

26. Humphreys RP, Hendrick EB, Hoffman HJ: Childhood aneurysms, atypical features, atypical management, *Neurosurg* 6:213, 1985.

27. Kaplan HA, Aronson SM, Browder EJ: Vascular malformations of the brain: an anatomical study, *J Neurosurg* 18:630, 1961.

28. Kitahara T, Okamura K, Semba A, et al: Genetic and immunologic analysis on moya-moya, *J Neurol Neurosurg Psychiatry* 45:1048, 1982.

29. Kudo T: Juvenile occlusion at the circle of Willis, *Clin Neurol* 5:607, 1965.

30. Lee BC, Harzberg L, Zimmerman RD, et al: MR imaging of cerebral vascular malformations, *AJNR* 6:863, 1985.

31. Locksley HB: Report on the Cooperative Study of Intracranial Aneurysms and Subarachnoid Hemorrhage. Section V Part 1. Natural history of subarachnoid hemorrhage, intracranial aneurysms and arteriovenous malformations, *J Neurosurg* 25:219, 1966.

32. Marks MP, Delapaz RL, Fabrikant JI, et al: Intracranial vascular malformations: imaging of charged-particle radiosurgery, *Radiology* 168:447, 1988.

33. Martin NA, Edwards MSB: Supratentorial arteriovenous malformations. In Edwards MSB, Hoffman HJ: *Cerebral vascular disease in children and adolescents*, Baltimore, 1989, Williams & Wilkins.

34. Matsushima Y, Inaba Y: Moyamoya disease in children and its surgical treatment: introduction of a new surgical procedure and its follow-up angiograms, *Childs Brain* 11:155, 1984.

35. McCormack WF, Hardman JF, Boutler TR: Vascular malformations "angiomas" of the brain, with special reference to those occurring in the posterior fossa, *J Neurosurg* 28:241, 1968.

36. Meyer FB, Sundt TM, Fode NC, et al: Cerebral aneurysms in childhood and adolescence, *J Neurosurg* 70:420, 1989.

37. Mickle JP, Quisling RG: The transtorcular embolization of vein of Galen aneurysms, *J Neurosurg* 64:731, 1986.

38. Newton TH, Cronquist S: Involvement of dural arteries in intracranial arteriovenous malformations, *Radiology* 93:1071, 1969.

39. Olsen WL, Brant-Zawadzki M, Hodes, et al: Giant intracranial aneurysms: MR imaging, *Radiology* 163:431, 1987.

40. Patel AN, Richardson AE: Ruptured intracranial aneurysms in the first two decades of life: a study of 58 patients, *J Neurosurg* 35:571, 1971.

41. Perret G, Nishioka H: Report on The Cooperative Study of Intracranial Aneurysms and Subarachnoid Hemorrhage: arteriovenous malformations—an analysis of 545 cases of craniocerebral arteriovenous malformations and fistulae reported to the cooperative study, *J Neurosurg* 25:467, 1989.

42. Priest JR, Ramsay NKC, Steinherz PG, et al: A syndrome of thrombosis and hemorrhage complicating L-asparaginase therapy for childhood acute lymphotoxic leukemia, *J Pediatr* 100:984, 1982.

43. Rooney CM, Kaye EM, Scott RM, et al: Modified encephaloduroarteriosynangiosis as a surgical treatment of childhood Moyamoya disease: report of five cases, *J Child Neurol* 1990 (in press).

44. Rosenbloom S, Edwards MSB: Dural arteriovenous malformations. In Edwards MSB, Hoffman HJ: *Cerebral vascular disease in children and adolescents*, Baltimore, 1989, Williams & Wilkins.

45. Rothfus WE, Albright AL, Casey KF, et al: Cerebellar venous angioma "benign" entity? *AJNR* 5:61, 1984.

46. Rubin JM, Hatfield MK, Chandler WF, et al: Intracerebral arteriovenous malformations: intraoperative color Doppler flow imaging, *Radiology* 170:219, 1989.

47. Russell MO, Goldberg HI, Hodson A, et al: Effect of transfusion therapy on arteriographic abnormalities and on recurrence of stroke in sickle cell disease, *Blood* 63:162, 1984.

48. Saito Y, Kobayashi N: Cerebral venous angiomas: clinical evaluation and possible etiology, *Radiology* 139:87, 1981.

49. Shillito JJ: Carotid arteritis: a cause of hemiplegia in childhood, *J Neurosurg* 21:540, 1964.

50. Silverman BK, Brekz T, Craig J, et al: Congestive failure in the newborn caused by cerebral AV fistula, *Am J Dis Child* 89:539, 1959.

51. Stehbens WE: Telangiectasias, hemangiomas, arteriovenous aneurysms and allied disorders. In Stehbens WE: *Pathology of the cerebral blood vessels*, St Louis, 1972, Mosby–Year Book.

52. Stehbens WE: Intracranial berry aneurysms in childhood, *Surg Neurol* 18:58, 1982.

53. Steiner L, Lindquist C, Steiner M: Radiosurgery with focused gamma-beam irradiation in children. In Edwards MSB, Hoffman HJ: *Cerebral vascular diseases in children and adolescents*, Baltimore, 1989, Williams & Wilkins.

54. Suzuki J, Takaku A: Cerebrovascular "moyamoya" disease: disease showing abnormal netlike vessels in the base of the brain, *Arch Neurol* 20:288, 1969.

55. Sze G, Krol A, Olsen WL, et al: Hemorrhagic neoplasms: MR mimics of occult vascular malformations, *AJNR* 8:795, 1987.

56. Tsuruda JS, Halbach VV, Higashida T, et al: MR evaluation of large intracranial aneurysms using cine low flip angle gradient focused imaging, *AJNR* 9:415, 1988.

57. Vaquero J, Leunda G, Martinez R, et al: Cavernomas of the brain, *Neurosurg* 12:208, 1983.

Trauma in infants and children

Traumatic unconsciousness is uncommon in children younger than 1 year of age, particularly if the head injury is the result of a short fall (that is, from the bed or changing table).[8] Skull fractures are fairly frequent, but immediate loss of consciousness is rare. The fractures are linear and are often combined with suture diastasis. CT findings are often otherwise normal, although subarachnoid hemorrhage may be apparent. The value of CT in this setting is often limited but necessary, especially if split sutures or a full fontanelle is present, indicating elevated intracranial pressure.

Traumatic unconsciousness is more frequent in the shaken child in whom diffuse white matter injury, acute subarachnoid hemorrhage, subdural bleeding, or acute brain swelling occurs. In such cases CT is mandatory to identify the cause of the loss of consciousness and to identify brain

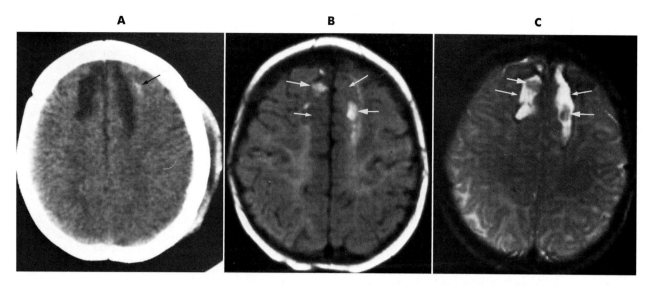

Fig. 6-21   Scans of a 6-month-old girl who fell off a changing table 3 months previously striking her head, and then had another head injury 2 weeks before these scans were obtained. **A,** Axial nonenhanced CT scan demonstrates bifrontal low density areas presumed due to encephalomalacia with a small area of high density adjacent to the left frontal low density *(arrow)*. **B,** On the T1-weighted MRI scan high intensity lesions are seen bifrontally *(large arrows)*, which are low intensity *(large arrows)* on the T2-weighted scan **(C)**. These changes probably are the result of intracellular methemoglobin. The surrounding isointense area on the T1-weighted scan **(B,** *small arrows)* is hyperintense on the T2-weighted scan **(C,** *small arrows)* and corresponds to the low density lesions seen on the CT scan. These areas probably result from the proteinaceous fluid-filled encephalomalacic cavities from old resolved hemorrhage from the first head injury. The high density area on the CT scan **(A,** *arrow)* due to recent hemorrhage is of high intensity on the T1-weighted scan **(B)** because of intracellular methemoglobin.

injury, which may require surgical management.

In the older child or teenager, traumatic unconsciousness is often caused by an acceleration/deceleration injury. CT is indicated to exclude an extracerebral hematoma. If concussion is followed by a lucid period with subsequent deterioration of consciousness, pallor, bradycardia, decerebrate posturing, or episodes of apnea, the CT scan usually shows diffuse brain swelling due to increased blood volume (hyperemic swelling), not due to edema.[35]

CONTUSION

Contusion implies bruising with microscopic hemorrhage within the brain. Two mechanisms are involved. Local trauma to the static head produces inbending with a depressed skull fracture and underlying bruising. An acceleration/deceleration force causes a to-and-fro movement of the brain across the orbital roof and sphenoid wing producing laceration and contusion of the inferior frontal lobes and anterior temporal lobes.[8] CT demonstrates an ill-defined area of increased density with surrounding low density edema and possibly mass effect. On follow-up scans areas of local encephalomalacia may ensue. In more subtle cases MRI has shown superior sensitivity for defining areas of cortical contusion and gliosis. In the subacute or chronic phase the T2-weighted spin echo scans are especially sensitive to gliosis and hemorrhage, even when the CT scan is normal.[5] The gliotic areas may follow nonhemorrhagic shear injury, also known as diffuse axonal injury, and

appear as high signal foci on T2-weighted images[13,18] (Fig. 6-21). Subacute hemorrhages are of a high intensity on both T1-weighted or T2-weighted images because of the presence of methemoglobin. On T2-weighted scans chronic injuries appear either as areas of high signal intensity (gliosis) or low signal intensity (residual hemosiderin from previous hemorrhage). Gradient echo images are particularly sensitive to chronic hemorrhage. These are displayed as areas of very low signal intensity due to the presence of hemosiderin.[28] In the chronic phase areas of macroscopic encephalomalacia are easily detected on either CT or MRI scans as CSF-filled defects.

HEMATOMA

Failure to recognize an intracranial hematoma may transform an otherwise mild injury into a fatal or permanent disabling entity.[25] Both CT and MRI are excellent tests for the diagnosis of intracranial hematomas, but CT remains the procedure of choice in the evaluation of head injury during the first 72 hours.

Epidural hematoma

Epidural hematoma is less common in children than in adults and is even rarer in infants. It has been postulated that adherence of the dura to the suture provides some fixation of the dura to the calvarium and diminishes the likelihood of separation from the inner skull surface. This theory is disputed by Choux et al.,[11] who found no attachment of the dura to the suture lines with the exception of the coronal sutures. Whereas the hematoma is often caused by an arterial tear, especially fractures across the anterior or posterior branches of the middle meningeal artery, the incidence of venous bleeding as a cause of hematoma is higher than in adults and is related to fractures across the dural venous sinuses, as is seen with posterior fossa epidural hematomas. Characteristically the CT scan demonstrates a biconvex high density lesion between the brain and the skull, sometimes limited by the attachment of the dura to the sutures. Occasionally an epidural hematoma in infants and young children may have an atypical appearance of a mixed high and low density—the high density representing clotted blood and the low density representing more fresh or hyperacute nonclotted hemorrhage. With time the contents of the hematoma appear as low density areas, and the dura displaced away from the skull may be evident after contrast administration. MRI may infrequently play a role in the diagnosis of epidural hematomas, particularly in the subacute and chronic phases and particularly those within the posterior fossa.[31] As with intracerebral hematomas, the content of subacute/chronic epidural hematomas is of high intensity on T1-weighted scans because of methemoglobin. The dural membrane may be defined as a low intensity line between the brain and the hematoma.

Subdural hematoma

As with epidural hematomas, subdural hematomas may be arterial or venous in origin; either the cortical arteries or the bridging veins from the cortex to the dural sinuses may be torn. When a subdural hemorrhage occurs in a newborn infant, as occurs with parituritional or obstetrical trauma, it probably is caused by arterial bleeding. The other clinical setting, especially in older infants and children, is usually that of a severe head injury. The CT appearance of an acute lesion is that of an extracerebral high density lesion, usually crescentic, sometimes extending into the interhemispheric fissure.[34] Newborn infants are also susceptible to subdural hematomas in the posterior fossa from tears of the tentorial arteries or veins or the great vein of Galen.[25] The rapidly expanding subdural collection can cause brain stem compression and death.[17] Immediate surgery therefore is often indicated.

If a subdural hemorrhage is of arterial origin, the presence of the hematoma is manifested early in the course of the disease. If the hemorrhage is venous, the accumulation may be slow and go undetected for weeks or months. Often such a hemorrhage occurs in the context of the battered child syndrome. With time the contents of the subdural hematoma may either spontaneously resolve or organize with the formation of neomembranes lining and encapsulating the subdural accumulation. The outer layers of these accumulations are in contact with the dura and often are richly vascularized. CT scans demonstrate a low density crescentic collection that is often bilateral in location. The vascular membranes may enhance after contrast administration.

On occasion it may be difficult to differentiate by CT an interhemispheric subdural collection from the normal falx cerebri. Usually the subdural collection is thicker than the normal falx, is asymmetrical (often extending over the tentorium), and has flat medial and convex lateral borders. Acute posterior fossa subdural hematomas are usually indicative of a severe head injury and, in contrast to convexity subdural hematomas, are usually associated with massive fractures of the occipital bone.[20]

MRI is a sensitive and often more specific test than CT for the diagnosis of subdural hematomas. The contents of subacute to chronic subdural hematomas are often hyperintense on both T1- and T2-weighted scans because of the high protein content of the fluid, although they are less hyperintense than methemoglobin on T1-weighted scans. The vascular membrane is apparent on gadolinium-enhanced MRI.[10] Small subdural hematomas (Fig. 6-22) poorly seen by CT because of bone artifact may be readily detected by MRI.

The intensity of the subdural hematoma on T1-weighted images decreases as the hematoma ages (Figs. 6-23 and 6-24). The subdural hematomas evolve in a pattern similar to intracerebral hemorrhages with the exception that hemosiderin is rarely seen in chronic hematomas, probably because of the absence of a blood-brain barrier and, as a consequence, rapid clearance or dilution of the blood products.[12] Long-standing chronic subdural hematomas are of CSF-intensity throughout the sequences and may not be distinguished from chronic hygromas (see Chapter 1). On occasion it may be difficult to differentiate bilateral chronic subdural hematomas from benign infantile subdural hygromas and external hydrocephalus, a self-limiting condition characterized by rapidly increasing head size that usually stabilizes by the age of 2 years. In the latter condition CT often demonstrates mild ventriculomegaly and enlarged low density, extracerebral spaces over the surface of the brain.[27] The wide extracerebral spaces are usually situated in the interhemispheric fissure and in the frontotemporal or frontoparietal areas and represent dilated subarachnoid spaces.[23] The dilated subarachnoid spaces and ventriculomegaly result from transient impairment of CSF absorption possibly caused by immaturity of the arachnoid villi. Occasionally, similar findings are seen after intracranial hemorrhage or infection.

MRI may assist in differentiating chronic subdural hematomas from external hydrocephalus by demonstrating cortical vein displacement toward the brain surface with subdural collections, and displacement away from the brain surface with external hydrocephalus. The subdural collections may also contain the hemoglobin breakdown products of hemorrhage, which are readily recognized by MRI (see Chapter 1). However, if the extracerebral fluid is isointense with CSF, as occurs with subdural hygromas, differentiation may be impossible. Acute subdural hygromas resulting from traumatic tearing of the arachnoid and escape of cerebrospinal fluid into the subdural space may occur in isolation or in conjunction with acute subdural hemorrhage.

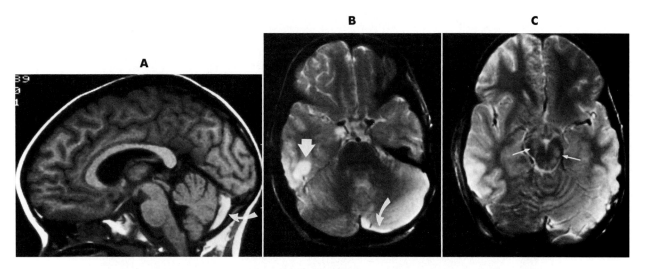

Fig. 6-22   A, Sagittal T1-weighted scan in a 5-year-old child who suffered a severe head injury with loss of consciousness demonstrates a posterior fossa subacute subdural hematoma (arrow). **B,** The hematoma is seen on the left side in the axial proton density scan *(curved arrow)* . In addition, a high intensity area is apparent in the right temporal lobe as a result of cerebral contusion *(straight arrow)*. **C,** Scan obtained through the midbrain shows high intensity lesions *(arrows)* due to contusions.

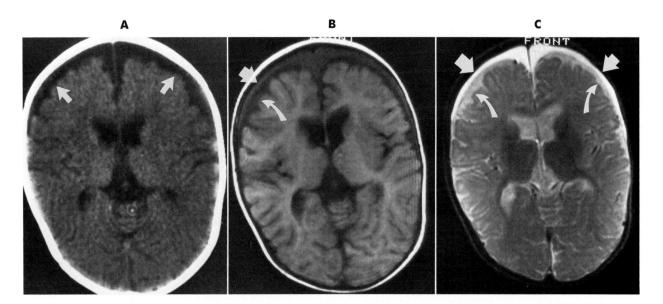

Fig. 6-23   A, Axial CT scan in a 9-month-old child who suffered head trauma a few months previously demonstrates bilateral frontal extraaxial low densities *(arrows)* extending into the interhemispheric fissure. The distinction between subdural and subarachnoid fluid collections cannot be made on the CT scan. **B,** T1-weighted MRI scan reveals two separate extraaxial compartments. The inner compartment *(curved arrow)* follows the signal intensities of CSF, and the outer compartment *(straight arrow)* is of a higher signal intensity than CSF. **C,** Similarly, T2-weighted scan shows the inner compartment *(curved arrow)* following CSF and the outer compartment *(straight arrow)* as an area of higher signal intensity. The outer fluid compartment is the result of chronic subdural hematomas, and the inner compartment is the subarachnoid space.

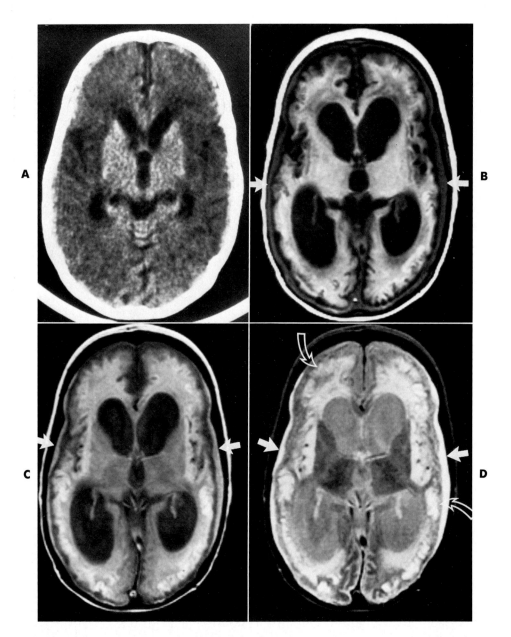

Fig. 6-24   A, CT scan in a 2-year-old infant after an episode of anoxic encephalopathy during a liver transplant. There is diffuse low density changes in the white matter bilaterally with sparing of the basal ganglia. During recovery the patient suffered unexpected head trauma, and an MRI scan was obtained. **B,** The axial T1-weighted scan demonstrates an extraaxial fluid collection of a higher intensity than brain *(arrows)* together with hydrocephalus ex vacuo. The extraaxial fluid is of a higher intensity than the ventricles on a T1-weighted image **(B),** a proton density image **(C),** and on a T2-weighted image **(D,** *arrows).* In addition, note the high intensity changes in the white matter indicative of leukomalacia, gliosis, or both **(D,** *curved arrows).* At surgery bilateral chronic subdural hematomas were evacuated from both sides.

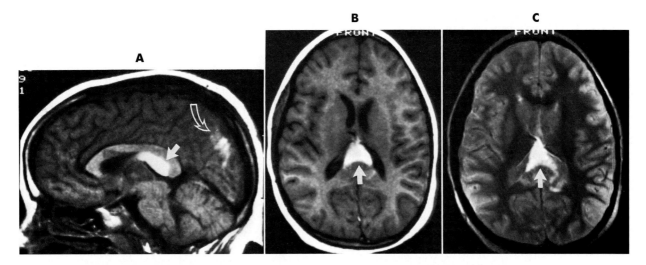

Fig. 6-25   A, Sagittal T1-weighted MRI scan in a 10-year-old child 9 days after a head injury demonstrates high intensity signals in the fornix *(straight arrow)* and in the parietooccipital cortex *(curved arrow).* **B,** Axial T1-weighted scan reveals the high intensity changes that are also of high intensity on the proton density scan (**C,** *arrow).* The appearances are those of subacute hemorrhages involving the fornix and the cerebral hemispheres.

The subdural hygroma or diluted acute subdural hematoma may appear as isodense or of low density on CT scans and mimic chronic subdural hematomas. Again, if MRI demonstrates signal abnormalities related to protein content or blood products, then more acute trauma may be suggested. Cerebral atrophy may often be distinguished from all these conditions when the atrophy is characterized by a diffuse prominence of the sulci throughout the cerebrum and the ventricles and the basal cisterns are dilated proportionately to the subarachnoid dilatation.[23]

Intracerebral hematoma

Intracerebral hematomas are an infrequent complication of trauma in infancy and childhood; in the neonatal period they appear in the subcortical areas of the brain. Such hemorrhages are distinctly less common than surface contusions.[25] The immature, incompletely myelinated brain of infants often responds to blunt head trauma with a contusional cleft of the white matter.[22] In the older child intracerebral hemorrhage may immediately follow trauma or may be delayed several days.[4] The hemorrhage may be isolated or occur in conjunction with cerebral contusion or concomitant surface hemorrhage. On a CT scan the hematoma is frequently ovoid, with the axis oriented toward the brain surface (see Fig. 6-21). Again the sensitivity of MRI in demonstrating hemorrhagic shear injuries is superior to that of CT. The signal characteristics on MRI scanning in these injuries[18] are similar to those previously described for extracerebral hematomas: areas of short T1 and prolonged T2 signals due to blood degradation products in characteristic locations such as at the corticomedullary junctions (see Fig. 6-21), in the centrum semiovale, the fornix (Fig. 6-25), and in the corpus callosum.[5]

Subarachnoid hemorrhage

CT is more sensitive than MRI in detecting acute subarachnoid hemorrhage.[7] However, on follow-up MRI scans pial or subpial hemosiderosis appearing as areas of low signal intensity may be identified at the site of a previous subarachnoid hemorrhage.[14]

INTRACEREBRAL SWELLING AND EDEMA

Blunt trauma and rapid acceleration and deceleration are responsible for the vast majority of brain injuries in infants and children.[20] Violent shaking alone, as occurs in child abuse, may also cause severe head injury. As the brain shifts within the calvarium, certain areas are relatively restricted because of fixation by the falx or tentorium, as well as by bony regions such as the sphenoid wings. The differential tissue densities of white and gray matter may also lead to abnormal strains at their interfaces.[36] As a result of these forces diffuse or focal edema, contusional hemorrhage and tear, or laceration with associated intracranial hemorrhage can occur.[20] Cerebral edema, which reflects one of the major secondary effects of CNS trauma, is often associated with coma.[9]

The cerebral swelling is caused by vasodilation with increased vascular permeability and by increased cerebral blood volume. Microscopically, if there are no other changes of cerebral injury, differentiation from hypoxic changes may be impossible to demonstrate. CT and MRI in hyperemic swelling demonstrate decreased distinction between white and gray matter, effacement of the cortical sulci, and compression of the cisterns and ventricles.[5] Obliteration of the perimesencephalic cisterns also occurs. Occasionally there is a striking but transient early phase of "enhanced" gray-white differentiation on CT. More extensive low densities may indicate edema or necrosis related to complicating hypoxic-ischemic injury (for example, from aspiration, cardiopulmonary arrest, or strangulation or suffocation in child abuse).

SKULL FRACTURE

Skull fractures occur in over one quarter of all children admitted to hospitals for treatment of head injuries.[16] The finding of a fracture has little prognostic significance[32]; its presence does not augur ill for the patient nor does its absence indicate lack of brain injury. A skull fracture, however, may confirm child abuse.

Plain films surpass CT scans in documentating the number, extent, and nature of the fractures. The fractures may be simple, consisting of a single fracture line with closely opposed margins, or complex, with a branching or stellate pattern. If the fracture results in isolation of one or more separate fragments it is considered comminuted. Comminuted fractures, which may be depressed, are best visualized by CT scans, in which the degree of underlying brain damage, if any, can be assessed. CT is more effective than MRI for the detection and characterization of skull fractures and can also alert the physician to the associated presence of an extracerebral hematoma.

Basal skull fractures can on occasion lead to cerebrospinal fluid rhinorrhea or otorrhea. The more specific methods for diagnosing such leaks are by high resolution, thin section axial or coronal CT of the paranasal sinuses or temporal bones, respectively, and CT cisternography, in which appropriate axial and coronal views of the suspected areas are obtained after the lumbar instillation of a water-soluble contrast agent.[3] Isotope cisternography may also be a sensitive method for detecting leakage. Pneumocephalus is an important finding indicating an open skull fracture, fracture into an air-containing sinus or otomastoid, or a persistent CSF leak.

An infrequent complication of head injury is the formation of a skull defect at the site of the fracture. The basic substrate is a fracture with diastasis and a dural tear. The condition is called *leptomeningeal cyst* when there is an arachnoid protrusion that increases in size because of transmitted vascular and CSF pulsations and entrapment of CSF. The increasing size of the cyst erodes the margins of the bone leading to a "growing skull fracture", a condition seen only in infants and children. Subgaleal hygroma, subdural hygroma, and cortical brain injury with atrophy are often associated findings.

BATTERED CHILD SYNDROME

In the neuroradiologic evaluation of pediatric trauma, the range of CNS injury in child abuse may be similar to that in accidental trauma. This includes skull fractures, subarachnoid hemorrhage, subdural hematomas, contusions, and shearing injuries. Certain factors, however, warrant further consideration that abuse is the underlying mechanism in pediatric injury including (1) clinical or imaging findings of injury more extensive or more severe than the history of trauma, (for example, SDHs with a history of a fall from a

chair) and (2) multiple injuries of varying age implying repeated trauma (for example old and new bone fractures).[20,21,26,30]

In this context, other findings become even more suggestive of abuse such as (1) retinal hemorrhages, (2) bilateral, multiple, or diastatic skull fractures in infancy, (3) intracranial hemorrhages of varying age, (4) an interhemispheric subdural hematoma (shaking mechanism), and (5) subdural hematoma associated with hypoxic-ischemic cerebral injury, that is, edema or infarction (shaking plus strangulation or suffocation mechanism).

CT often suffices in evaluating CNS injury in these situations. MRI, however, may further assist in the evaluation by delineating the full extent of the acute injury, by providing more accurate age assessment of the hemorrhages, in confirming nonhemorrhagic injury not shown by CT (for example, shear injury), confirming hemorrhage when the CT reveals collections of a nonspecific character (for example, subacute or chronic SDH that are low density or isodense by CT), and in evaluating the long-term sequelae of injury (for example, gliosis, encephalomalacia).

TRAUMATIC LESIONS OF THE MAJOR HEAD AND NECK VESSELS

Traumatic injuries of the major head and neck arteries and veins often occur in the young adult male population.[29] All patients who have sustained penetrating wounds or serious blunt trauma to the soft tissues of the neck should receive emergency angiography in cases of suspected carotid or vertebral arterial injury. There is little purpose in obtaining MRI scans of the neck in this group, although CT scans may be helpful if bony injury to the cervical spine is suspected. If the spinal canal is injured, information as to the condition of the contents of the canal can be obtained by MRI or myelography (assisted by CT) (see Chapter 10).

Occasionally, patients with blunt injury to the neck can sustain a stroke due to cerebral embolism. Such strokes are usually caused by cervical arterial dissections, which may be suspected on MRI scans but are best diagnosed by cerebral angiography. Cranial CT or MRI in these patients can document the extent of the cerebral damage.

Traumatic aneurysms, due to either blunt or penetrating trauma, can develop on the branches of the external carotid artery or at the base of the brain.[1] Again angiography is critical for assessment of the size and configuration of these lesions, which generally have a very poor prognosis if not treated early and effectively. Injuries of the venous sinuses can also occur in children, but because of the lower pressure in the venous system, this type of injury does not have the same ominous prognostic implications as damage of the arteries.[24]

Caroticocavernous fistulas may develop either spontaneously or as a consequence of trauma. In children these lesions are almost always traumatic in origin.[19] Whereas CT MRI, or both can demonstrate these lesions, cerebral angiography is ultimately necessary to document the lesion, establish the venous drainage patterns, assess the cerebral arterial vasculature, and plan interventional treatment.[33]

LONG-TERM EFFECTS OF TRAUMA

After severe head trauma generalized cerebral atrophic changes occur in approximately one third of survivors. The changes are manifested by generalized sulcal enlargement and ventriculomegaly,[6] occur 2 or more months after the trauma or surgery, and are caused by diffuse axonal injury.[2] The atrophy should be distinguished from posttraumatic communicating hydrocephalus, which usually develops by the end of the second posttraumatic week.[15] Focal or multifocal atrophic changes may also occur after trauma. All the above morphological changes can be well seen by MRI. In addition, the presence of hemosiderin, signifying an old posttraumatic hemorrhage, may be evident on the MRI scan years after the traumatic event.

REFERENCES
Trauma in infants and children

1. Acosta C, Williams PEJ, Clark K: Traumatic aneurysms of the cerebral vessels, *J Neurosurg* 36:531, 1972.
2. Adams JH, Graham DI, Murray LS, et al: Diffuse axonal injury due to non-missile head injury in humans: an analysis of 45 cases, *Ann Neurol* 12:557, 1982.
3. Admadi J, Weiss MH, Segall HD, et al: Evaluation of cerebrospinal fluid rhinorrhea by metrizamide computed tomographic cisternography, *Neurosurgery* 16:54, 1985.
4. Atluru V, Epstein LG, Zilker A: Delayed traumatic intracerebral hemorrhage in children, *Pediatr Neurol* 2:297, 1986.
5. Barkovich AJ: Metabolic and destructive brain disorders. In Barkovich AJ: *Pediatric neuroimaging*, ed 1, New York, 1989, Raven.
6. Bognanno JR: Trauma and mechanical disorders of the brain. In Cohen MD, Edwards MK: *Magnetic resonance imaging of children*, Philadelphia, 1990, BC Decker.
7. Bradley WG, Schmidt PG: Effect of methemoglobin formation on the MR appearance of subarachnoid hemorrhage, *Radiology* 156:99, 1985.
8. Bruce DA, Schut L: Concussion and contusion following pediatric head trauma. In McLaurin RL, Venes JL, Schut L, et al: *Pediatric neurosurgery*, Philadelphia, 1989, WB Saunders.
9. Bruce DS, Alavi A, Bilaniuk LT, et al: Diffuse cerebral swelling following head injuries in children: the syndrome of ''malignant brain edema,'' *J Neurosurg* 54:170, 1981.
10. Bydder GM: Clinical applications of gadolinium-DTPA. In Stark DD, Bradley WG: *Magnetic resonance imaging*, ed 1, St Louis, 1988, Mosby–Year Book.
11. Choux M, Grisoli F, Peragut J: Extradural hematomas in children: 104 cases, *Childs Brain* 1:337, 1975.
12. Fobben ES, Grossman RJ, Atlas SW, et al: MR characteristics of subdural hematomas and hygromas at 1.5 T, *AJNR* 10:687, 1989.
13. Gentry LR, Godersky JC, Thompson B, et al: Prospective comparative study of intermediate-field MR and CT in the evaluation of closed head trauma, *AJNR* 9:91, 1988.
14. Gomori JM, Grossman RI, Bilaniuk LT, et al: High-field MR imaging of superficial siderosis of the central nervous system, *J Comput Assist Tomogr* 9:972, 1985.
15. Gudeman SK, Kishore RRS, Becker DP, et al: Computerized tomography in the evaluation of incidence and significance of posttraumatic hydrocephalus, *Radiology* 141:597, 1981.
16. Harwood-Nash DC, Hendrick EB, Hudson AR: The significance of skull fractures in children: a study of 1187 patients, *Radiology* 101:151, 1971.
17. Hernansanz J, Munoz F, Rodriquez M, et al: Subdural hematomas of the posterior fossa in normal-weight newborns, *J Neurosurg* 61:972, 1984.
18. Hesselink JR, David CF, Gealy ME, et al: MR imaging of brain contusions: a comparative study with CT, *AJR* 150:133, 1988.
19. Hosobuchi Y: Carotid-cavernous fistulas. In Edwards MSB, Hoffman HJ: *Cerebral vascular disease in children and adolescents*, Baltimore, 1989, Williams & Wilkins.
20. Kleinman PK: Head trauma. In Kleinman PK: *Diagnostic imaging of child abuse*, Baltimore, 1987, Williams & Wilkins.
21. Kravitz H, Driessen G, Gomberg R, et al: Accidental falls from elevated surfaces in infants from birth to 1 year of age, *Pediatrics* (suppl) 44:869, 1969.
22. Lindenberg R, Freytag E: Morphology of brain lesions from blunt trauma in early infancy, *Arch Pathol* 87:298, 1969.
23. Maytal J, Alvarez LA, Elkin CM, et al: External hydrocephalus: radiologic spectrum and differentiation from cerebral atrophy, *AJNR* 8:271, 1987.
24. McLauren RL, McLennan JE: Diagnosis and treatment of head injury in children. In Youmans JR: *Neurological surgery*, Philadelphia, 1982, WB Saunders.
25. McLauren RL, Towbin R: Posttraumatic hematomas. In McLauren RL, Venes JL, Schut L, et al: *Pediatric neurosurgery*, ed 2, Philadelphia, 1989, WB Saunders.
26. Merten DF, Osborne DRS: Craniocerebral trauma in the child abuse syndrome: radiological observations, *Pediatr Radiol* 14:272, 1984.
27. Nickel RE, Gallenstein JS: Developmental prognosis for infants with benign enlargement of the subarachnoid spaces, *Dev Med Child Neurol* 29:181, 1987.
28. Norfray JF, Taveras JM: Gradient echoes: simplified, *AJNR* 10:209, 1989.
29. Samson D: Traumatic lesions of the cerebral vasculature. In Edwards MSB, Hoffman HJ: *Cerebral vascular disease in children and adolescents*, Baltimore, 1989, Williams & Wilkins.
30. Sato Y, Yuh WTC, Smith WL, et al: Head injury in child abuse: evaluation with MR imaging, *Radiology* 173:653, 1989.
31. Stark DD, Bradley WG: MRI of hemorrhage and iron in the brain. In Stark DD, Bradley WG: *Magnetic resonance imaging*, ed 1, St Louis, 1988, Mosby–Year Book.
32. Thornbury JR, Campbell JA, Masters SJ, et al: Skull fracture and the low risk of intracranial sequelae in minor head trauma, *AJR* 143:661, 1984.
33. Vinuela F, Dion J, Lylyk P, et al: Update on interventional neuroradiology, *AJR* 153:23, 1989.
34. Zimmerman RA, Bilaniuk LT: Computer tomography in pediatric head trauma, *J Neuroradiol* 8:257, 1981.
35. Zimmerman RA, Bilaniuk LT, Bruce DA, et al: Computed tomography of pediatric head trauma: acute generalized cerebral swelling, *Radiology* 126:403, 1978.
36. Zimmerman RA, Bilaniuk LT, Genneralli T: Computed tomography of cerebral injuries of the cerebral white matter, *Radiology* 127:393, 1978.

7 · Cranial and Intracranial Tumors

Patrick D. Barnes
William J. Kupsky
Roy D. Strand

NOSOLOGY

Tumors of the central nervous system (CNS) and the peripheral nervous system (PNS), or related embryonic neural crest derivatives, constitute the largest group of solid neoplasms in childhood. The World Health Organization (WHO) has classified nonneoplastic and neoplastic tumors of the nervous system into two categories: primary neuroepithelial tumors and tumors of nonneuroepithelial tissues.[4,36-38] Neuroepithelial tumors contain cell types derived from the embryonic neuroepithelial tube (for example, gliomas), whereas tumors of nonneuroepithelial tissues include those of presumed neural crest or PNS origin (for example, meningioma, nerve sheath tumors, neuroblas-

toma), as well as those of other cell types (for example, germinoma, pituitary adenoma, craniopharyngioma).

Nervous system tumors, as well as tumors of other tissues, are usually classified by *cell type* and *degree of malignancy*.[4,21,36-38,47] Determination of cell type and differentiation are based on the morphologic and functional similarity of the tumor cell to a normal adult or embryonic cell type as assessed by standard light microscopy (for example, astrocytoma, resembling the normal or reactive astrocytes of the CNS). Further clues to cell type are gathered through supplementary morphologic techniques such as electron microscopy and immunohistochemistry. Electron microscopy may be useful in recognizing cell specializations too small to be seen by light microscopy (for example, cilia and intercellular junctions in ependymoma cells). Immunohistochemical analysis may reveal proteins or other markers characteristic of the cell type (for example, glial fibrillary acidic protein [GFAP] in many glial cells, particularly astrocytes). Neoplasms, however, may be heterogeneous, may express markers not normally characteristic of the cell type, may lose differentiating characteristics with increasing malignancy, or may lack currently identifiable cell-specific markers, so some tumors cannot be definitively classified.[4,36-38] Furthermore, neoplasms may evolve with time or in response to therapeutic interventions, and sampling errors at the time of biopsy may be problematic (for example, as with stereotactic biopsy).

For tumors outside of the CNS, malignancy usually implies rapid and invasive local growth patterns and the potential for distant metastasis. The degree of malignancy, or the grade, of the tumor generally correlates with the loss of histological differentiation, that is, anaplasia.[4,5,36-38] For a variety of reasons it is often difficult to assess the prognosis for CNS tumors by histological grading. Grading systems based on degree of anaplasia to determine histological malignancy have been proposed for most CNS tumors (for example, the Kernohan system for glial tumors, which distinguishes four increasing levels of malignancy). Such systems, however, are unreliable for assessing most neuroepithelial tumors other than some astrocytomas. The WHO has attempted to simplify such systems to a twofold scheme, recognizing only differentiated and anaplastic forms of many primary CNS tumors for a rough correlation with prognosis.[37]

Using invasiveness as a criterion for establishing malignancy of tumors in the CNS has limited value because many histologically "benign" CNS tumors such as astrocytomas are usually invasive. Furthermore, neuroanatomical and surgical considerations rarely permit complete excision of tumors with normal tissue margins. Neuroanatomical location and resectability, in fact, are frequently more important prognostic factors than is histological malignancy. Lastly, although some primary CNS tumors spread within the subarachnoid space, metastatic potential beyond the CNS is generally low even when related to previous surgical intervention.[6,21,28]

Despite nosological limitations, we present a modified classification of pediatric nervous system tumors in the box on the right; the classification is based on the "Revision of the WHO Classification of Brain Tumors for Childhood Brain Tumors" proposed at the American Cancer Society Workshop Conference on Pediatric Brain Tumors in 1984.[37] Although some disagree with the revision, we have used the general outline of the revision in the neuropathological and neuroradiological discussions that follow. In addition, each tumor type is presented anatomically and clinically in the text and in the illustrations according to the major region or compartment involved (for example, cerebral hemispheric tumors, tumors about the third ventricle, posterior fossa tumors, and parameningeal tumors).

CLASSIFICATION OF BRAIN TUMORS IN CHILDREN

I. TUMORS OF NEUROEPITHELIAL TISSUE
  A. Glial tumors
    1. Astrocytic tumors
    2. Oligodendroglial tumors
    3. Ependymal tumors
    4. Choroid plexus tumors
    5. Mixed gliomas
    6. Glioblastomatous tumors
    7. Gliomatosis cerebri
  B. Neuronal tumors
    1. Gangliocytoma
    2. Anaplastic gangliocytoma
    3. Ganglioglioma
    4. Anaplastic ganglioglioma
  C. "Primitive" neuroepithelial (neuroectodermal) tumors
  D. Pineal cell tumors
    1. "Primitive" neuroectodermal tumor (pineoblastoma)
    2. Pineocytoma

II. TUMORS OF MENINGEAL AND RELATED TISSUES
  A. Meningiomas
  B. Meningeal sarcomatous tumors
  C. Primary melanocytic tumors

III. TUMORS OF NERVE SHEATH CELLS
  A. Neurilemmoma (schwannoma, neurinoma)
  B. Anaplastic neurilemmoma
  C. Neurofibroma
  D. Anaplastic neurofibroma (neurofibrosarcoma, neurogenic sarcoma)

IV. PRIMARY MALIGNANT LYMPHOMAS

V. TUMORS OF BLOOD VESSEL ORIGIN
  A. Hemangioblastoma

VI. GERM CELL TUMORS
  A. Germinoma
  B. Embryonal carcinoma
  C. Choriocarcinoma
  D. Endodermal sinus tumor
  E. Teratomatous tumors
  F. Mixed

VII. MALFORMATIVE TUMORS
  A. Craniopharyngioma
  B. Rathke's cleft cyst
  C. Epidermal cyst
  D. Dermoid cyst
  E. Colloid cyst of the third ventricle
  F. Enterogenous or bronchial cyst
  G. Cyst, NOS (not otherwise specified)
  H. Lipoma
  I. Granular cell tumor (choristoma)
  J. Hamartoma

VIII. TUMORS OF NEUROENDOCRINE ORIGIN
  A. Tumors of the anterior pituitary
  B. Paraganglioma

IX. LOCAL EXTENSIONS FROM REGIONAL TUMORS ("PARAMENINGEAL")

X. METASTATIC TUMORS

XI. UNCLASSIFIED TUMORS

Modified from Rork L, Gilles F, Davis R, et al: *Cancer* 56:1869, 1985.

CLINICAL PRESENTATIONS

The clinical presentation of an intracranial neoplasm depends, of course, on location, on whether the process is either infiltrative or acts as a mass displacing normal structures, and on whether there is vascular invasion or obstruction of the CSF pathways.[6,21,28] Consequently, common signs and symptoms include increased intracranial pressure, motor or sensory deficit, seizures, neuroendocrine disorder, headache, and, rarely, developmental delay or mental status impairment. The course is often insidious. Occasionally the symptoms or signs may be acute as a result of vascular invasion, meningeal involvement, or intratumoral hemorrhage. Episodic manifestations may include seizures or headaches.

The manifestation of intracranial neoplasms depends on the age of the patient at onset. In early infancy the symptoms may be quite nonspecific: irritability, lethargy, or failure with feeding. More compelling symptoms are vomiting, weight loss, eye deviation, focal weakness, and focal seizures. There may be developmental delay or failure to thrive. Neurological signs may include an abnormal increase in head circumference, unilateral weakness, or eye deviation. Papilledema is usually absent, even with large tumors.

In childhood and adolescence the symptoms of intracranial neoplasm often are more specific. Headache becomes a more important sign, especially when associated with other complaints or findings, such as declining school performance. Focal weakness with or without new seizure is also an important finding. In this age group epilepsy without explanation, and particularly those with focality as the hallmark, requires definitive neuroimaging. A subacute to chronic increase in intracranial pressure may be manifested by morning vomiting, gait unsteadiness, discoordination, weight loss, and subtle weakness.

More specific symptoms or signs that may direct attention to a certain region or compartment are presented within each of the following sections. Intracranial neoplasia may also be associated with neurocutaneous or other syndromes in childhood including neurofibromatosis, tuberous sclerosis, von Hippel–Lindau syndrome, Turcot syndrome, and the family cancer syndrome.[6,21,28]

NEUROIMAGING APPROACHES

Ultrasonography (US) or computed tomography (CT) detects the vast majority of intracranial masses in childhood, particularly in infancy, often because of their large size at presentation.[2,3] In the pediatric age group MRI is recommended, however, for definitive evaluation, especially for treatment planning.[1,2,10] Furthermore, MRI is the procedure of choice after infancy for evaluating clinical presentations such as increased intracranial pressure, unexplained focal seizures, neuroendocrine disorder, and posterior fossa signs when neoplasm becomes the leading consideration.[2] The multiplanar and multiparametric (T1, p, T2) capabilities of MRI along with its superior contrast resolution and lack of bony artifact make it the preferred modality for surgical, radiotherapy, and chemotherapy planning, as well as for follow-up of tumor response and treatment effects. This is particularly important for malignant and invasive tumors, tumors that tend to seed, and benign tumors in critical areas (for example, suprasellar, brain stem, and so forth).

The superior contrast sensitivity of MRI also makes it the definitive procedure for the detection of tumors often occult to CT or US (see Fig. 7-27). These include mesial or basal temporal neoplasms in unexplained partial complex seizure disorders (such as astrocytoma or ganglioglioma), periaqueductal tumors in unexplained hydrocephalus or hydrocephalus from apparent aqueductal stenosis (for example, tectal glioma), cervicomedullary junction tumors (for example, astrocytoma), and leptomeningeal neoplastic dissemination (demonstrated by gadolinium enhancement).[2] The superior anatomical delineation provided by multiplanar MRI is important for treatment planning of posterior fossa lesions regarding brain stem, cranial nerve, aqueductal, fourth ventricular, and vascular landmarks. It is also critical for evaluating perisellar tumors for optic pathway, other cranial nerve, third ventricular, carotid-cavernous, and pituitary-hypothalamic involvement. In deep or cortical cerebral masses anatomical characterization is important for delineating basal ganglia, capsular, and motor strip landmarks, language and memory areas, visual radiations, and so forth. MRI's superior tissue characterization allows improved delineation of cystic, proteinaceous, fatty, hemorrhagic, and vascular components, as well as subtle mass effect, intrinsic versus extrinsic origin, and invasion versus displacement. However, CT remains more reliable for demonstrating calcification and cortical bony involvement, especially for orbit, sinus, otomastoid, petrous temporal, skull base, and cranial calvarial lesions.[2]

Other important pretreatment imaging procedures for precise tumor localization and guidance[27,30,42] include stereotactic CT or MRI for biopsy, resection, or radiotherapy (Fig. 7-1) and intraoperative sonography (Fig. 7-2). Although gadolinium or iodine enhancement never ensures separation of tumor and edema, the enhancement may provide the high-yield biopsy target (that is, tumor core) for more reliable histopathological studies* (see Fig. 7-11).

Follow-up evaluation of tumor response and treatment effects may require a combination of CT and MRI. In the immediate postoperative period precontrast- and postcontrast-enhanced CT may be routinely preferred as a baseline study for distinguishing surgical effects from residual tumor. CT may be used primarily in follow-up for displaying resolution or stabilization of surgical effects (operative site hemorrhage, edema, and the like) or for demonstrating hydrocephalus and subsequently the need for shunting or shunt follow-up (catheter placement, subdural collections, and so forth). CT may occasionally be the procedure of choice for follow-up of completely resected neoplasms that were well delineated by CT before treatment. This is particularly appropriate for benign neoplasms, which are enhanced with iodine, and cerebral or cerebellar

---

*References 12, 16, 17, 24, 33, 45.

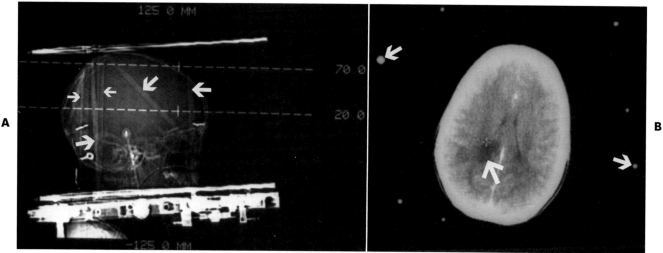

Fig. 7-1   Cerebral oligodendroglioma stereotactically localized for surgical excision with lateral scout projection image **(A)** and axial CT scan **(B)** showing coordinate bars of the stereotactic head frame *(small white arrows)* relative to the low density tumor *(large white arrow)*. The x,y coordinates of the head frame and tumor within the slice range from 20 to 70 mm are analyzed for precise computer guidance of the surgical procedure. A similar technique is employed whether for biopsy, excision, or small field radiotherapy.

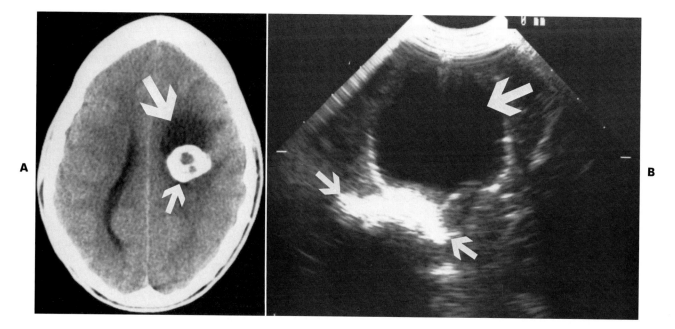

Fig. 7-2   Calcified, cystic cerebral astrocytoma demonstrated by CT **(A)** and intraoperative US **(B)**. The cystic component *(large white arrows)* is demonstrated as low density by CT **(A)** and sonolucent by US **(B)**. The calcified component *(small white arrows)* is shown as high density on CT **(A)** and echogenic with shadowing on US **(B)**.

hemispheric in location (for example, choroid plexus papilloma or cystic cerebellar astrocytoma) (see Fig. 7-12). Such lesions may be routinely followed only with contrast-enhanced CT[45] unless there are changing neurological symptoms or signs that warrant precontrast- and postcontrast-enhanced CT to rule out hemorrhage. Otherwise, MRI is recommended for follow-up of tumor response and treatment effects, especially for malignant neoplasms of any intracranial location or more benign processes in more critical locations (for example, brain stem, perisellar). Although enhancement by CT (iodine) or MRI (gadolinium) may not be a feature of some neoplasms initially, contrast administration may be needed for follow-up particularly for gliomas of mixed grading or histology and for tumors suspected of changing biological behavior after initial treatment.[17,33]

Craniospinal MRI with gadolinium enhancement is important for the evaluation of tumor seeding[17,33] (see Figs. 7-18 and 7-23). This is especially important in medulloblastoma, other primitive neuroectodermal tumors, germ cell tumors (for example, germinoma, choriocarcinoma), and undifferentiated or high grade gliomas (for example, glioblastoma). A baseline craniospinal MRI is usually done after the initial surgery and before chemotherapy and radiotherapy. After the baseline examination additional spinal imaging is not routinely done unless seeding was present initially or is suspected on follow-up. Although gadolinium enhancement is an important component of MRI for following intracranial neoplasm, a more complete MRI examination is necessary, since many tumors may demonstrate partial or no enhancement (for example, ependymoma). The following is one imaging approach suggested, for example, in a child with a medulloblastoma when time limitations are often imposed by sedation factors and when examination with gadolinium enhancement is the priority: preenhancement sagittal T1 brain sections followed by postgadolinium sagittal T1 sections, and then axial proton density and T2 sections. The preenhancement T1 images are important because a hemorrhage at the operative site may be indistinguishable from residual enhancing tumor. The high intensity enhancement of tumor on T1 images almost always carries over to the proton density and T2 images (p/T2), as discussed in Chapter 1. Moreover, at currently used gadolinium-DTPA dosages and resultant tissue concentrations, a significant T2 shortening effect has not been consistently observed.[17,33] If confusing intensity patterns appear on the postenhanced axial p/T2 images, then additional axial T1 sections may be obtained.

A preferred approach may be that which employs sagittal T1 and axial p/T2 sections preinjection followed by postinjection sagittal or axial T1 images. The proton density and T2-weighted images are of further importance to demonstrate nonenhancing tumor and edema as well as to show treatment effects, such as after radiation. Furthermore, the radiologist must be constantly aware that it may not be possible by CT or MRI (including enhancement) to distinguish tumor radionecrosis or chemonecrosis from tumor progression without serial studies (Fig. 7-18).

Metabolic, perfusion, and blood-brain barrier radionuclide imaging (SPECT or PET) may assist in this differentiation.[19,21] The inclusion of all major parameters (T1, proton density, and T2) is important because tumor-brain interfaces are usually best demonstrated with proton density and T2 images, whereas tumor-CSF interfaces are often better delineated with proton density and T1 images.

THERAPEUTIC ASPECTS OF NEUROIMAGING

As a result of improvements and advances in therapeutic approaches, greater demand is placed on neuroimaging to assess and provide more precise and reliable information regarding tumor response and treatment effects.[1-3,10,13,32,44] The major objectives of surgery are to establish the diagnosis and achieve complete or maximum excision (debulking) of the tumor without compromising vital neurological function.[42] This approach is always preferable to biopsy except in relatively inaccessible locations, such as the brain stem, since response to other treatment modalities and, ultimately, prognosis are often directly and most definitively linked to residual tumor volume.[19,21] Advancing technologies and techniques in neurosurgery include the operating microscope, laser and ultrasonic resection systems, dedicated neuroanesthesia, and sophisticated neurophysiologic monitoring. Image-based advances include computer-assisted CT and MRI stereotactic systems for biopsy, excision, and radiosurgery, as well as intraoperative ultrasonography.* Reoperation with further resection or debulking of residual or recurrent tumor is often preferred before or in place of radiotherapy.[19,21] This is especially important in younger patients (under 2 years of age) to prevent or lessen the known age-related sequelae of radiotherapy including cognitive and neuroendocrine deficits.[15,19,31] Furthermore, reoperation for resection or debulking of gross necrotic tumor is often employed after external beam radiotherapy and chemotherapy in anticipation of intracavitary implant radiotherapy (brachytherapy) to control or palliate higher grade tumors such as glioblastoma.[19]

Advances in external beam radiotherapy include computerized treatment planning using CT and MRI for whole-brain and involved-field applications, as well as computer-assisted CT or MRI stereotaxis for small-field radiosurgery and brachytherapy.[19,27,40] Radiosurgical and brachytherapy techniques are designed to deliver a higher focal dose to the tumor site while sparing normal tissue. Although chemotherapy has traditionally served as an adjunct to surgery and radiation, preradiation chemotherapy (for example, for medulloblastoma) is becoming more popular because of real and potential advantages.[19,21,23] These include better hematogenous drug penetration of tumor before radiation-induced microvascular changes take place, the potential use of these agents as radiosensitizers, and better patient tolerance to chemotherapy myelosuppression, that is, without the additive myelosuppressive effect of previous radiation. Other potential advantages are decreased morbidity

*References 9, 25, 30, 41, 42, 46.

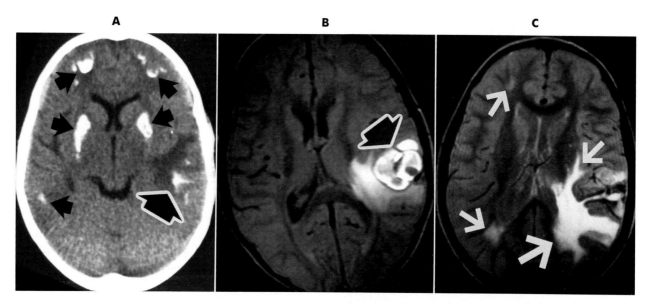

Fig. 7-3   Treatment effects after radiotherapy and chemotherapy for leukemia demonstrated by CT **(A)** as multiple calcifications *(small black arrows)* and white matter low densities. **B** and **C,** Axial p/T2 MRI fails to show the calcifications but reveals white matter high intensity abnormalities *(white arrows).* CT and MRI show temporal lobe density and intensity abnormalities *(large black arrow)* consistent with angioma and repeated hemorrhage.

from agents whose toxicity is potentiated by prior radiation, the possibility of delaying radiation until later childhood, and the reduction of radiation dosage to decrease the long-term effects.

Treatment effects revealed by neuroimaging are often those primarily related to radiotherapy.* The clinical and imaging findings are variably progressive and generally correlate with a higher radiation dosage, larger treatment volumes, and younger age.[7] The immature brain (less than 2 years of age) is especially sensitive to radiation. The effects may be manifested early or many months to years after treatment.[7,15,19,31] Clinical manifestations include the temporary "somnolence syndrome," which occurs 6 to 8 weeks after radiation. More permanent effects include cognitive deficits (learning disability, mental retardation), neuroendocrine deficiency (hypopituitarism, growth hormone deficiency), and occasionally hearing loss or visual loss, and seizure disorder or motor deficits. Moyamoya syndrome may be seen especially after radiotherapy for optic glioma in neurofibromatosis (Chapter 8). Other serious late effects are oncogenesis or radiation-induced second tumors (see Figs. 7-18 and 7-31) including meningioma, sarcomas (osteosarcoma, fibrosarcoma, and the like), gliomas, glioblastoma, thyroid carcinoma, and osteochondroma.[15,19,29,35] More recently, angiomatous-like lesions have been encountered (Fig. 7-3). All of these effects have been reported in children receiving CNS radiotherapy for leukemia (generally less than 2500 cGy) as well as in children treated for primary CNS neoplasia (usually greater

than 2500 cGy).[7,15,26] The higher dose group has manifested more profound clinical sequelae and imaging findings, although correlation between severity of clinical impairment and imaging findings has often been inconsistent from patient to patient.

The neuropathology of therapeutic irradiation includes those effects on irradiated tumor and those on the surrounding brain.* In radiation-sensitive tumors often there is extensive necrosis of the tumor center that may evolve into a fluid-filled cyst. In malignant tumors regrowth may occur about the periphery despite massive central necrosis. Irradiation may also lead to alteration of tumor cytology with the development of large, bizarre, often multinucleated cells in and around the tumor. This reactive change may be difficult to distinguish from anaplastic tumor progression. CT often shows central hypodensity with peripheral ringlike iodine enhancement and surrounding low density edema.[27] MRI often shows a T1 isointense to hypointense center that is hypointense, isointense, or hyperintense on p images, and hyperintense on T2 images. Peripheral gadolinium enhancement also occurs along with surrounding edema, which is T1 hypointense and p/T2 hyperintense. Radiation tumor necrosis may not be readily distinguished from tumor progression, as mentioned previously.

The sequelae of irradiation to the surrounding brain are divided into early delayed and late delayed effects.[7,15] Characteristically the injury is borne more by the white matter. Early delayed effects (within 3 months) may include focal demyelination, presumedly due to direct or autoim-

*References 7, 8, 11, 14, 20, 43.

*References 8, 11, 13, 14, 18, 20, 43.

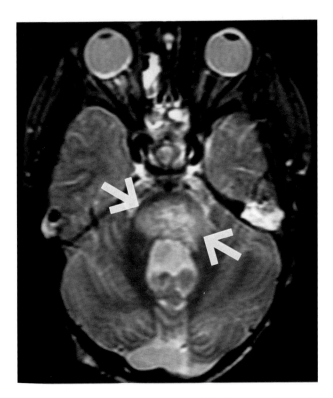

Fig. 7-4   Pontine myelinolysis after combined treatment for medulloblastoma complicated by fluid-electrolyte imbalance and shown by axial T2 MRI as a high intensity expansion of the pons (white arrows) that evolved to atrophy on follow-up MRI.

mune injury of the oligodendrocytes, and accumulations of perivascular mononuclear inflammatory cells. Late delayed effects (months to years) include coagulative necrosis of brain parenchyma (radionecrosis) with or without inflammatory cellular reaction, demyelination accompanied by loss of nerve fibers, and reactive astrocytosis occasionally with the formation of dysplastic cells. There is dystrophic mineralization of nerve cells and fibers, especially in the basal ganglia, gross atrophy related to nerve cell loss, and prominent vasculopathy. Radiation-induced vasculopathy may take the form of fibrinoid necrosis of vessel walls with fibrinous thrombi, endothelial proliferation with microvascular occlusion, perivascular fibrosis, telangiectasias, and dystrophic calcification of large and small vessels (mineralizing microangiopathy). Vasogenic edema (radiation edema) may result from blood-brain barrier disruption and produce mass effect. Injury to arachnoid granulations may result in impairment of CSF dynamics. Radiation injury to the spinal cord may produce similar changes, including coagulative necrosis, leading to the clinical picture of radiation myelopathy.

The neuroimaging findings parallel the neuropathological evolution of radiation edema or necrosis and include white matter edema, loss of differentiation between gray and white matter, hemorrhages, cystic degeneration or cavita-

tion, mass effect, and abnormal contrast enhancement* (Fig. 7-3). Ventricular and subarachnoid space dilatation are seen with impaired CSF dynamics or atrophy. White matter changes are of low density on CT and of high intensity on p/T2 MRI. In contrast to interstitial edema associated with obstructive hydrocephalus, the white matter abnormalities associated with radiation injury are often more peripheral, with scalloping along the gray matter–white matter junctions. Occasionally the appearance and distribution of radiation edema are indistinguishable from interstitial edema, tumor edema, or seeding. Neuroimaging findings of white matter involvement without iodine or gadolinium enhancement often correlate with edema or demyelination, whereas associated enhancement correlates with additional necrosis and an inflammatory response (Fig. 7-3). Pontine myelinolysis may also be a complication of radiation therapy in childhood, although it is often a complication of fluid-electrolyte imbalance or other metabolic derangement (Fig. 7-4). Calcifications are more readily demonstrated by CT than by MRI and often involve the basal ganglia, cerebral and cerebellar white matter, and brain stem[11] (Fig. 7-3). It is often difficult to separately evaluate treatment effects due to chemotherapy from those of radiotherapy in cases requiring combined treatment. Although chemotherapy toxicity may produce a variety of encephalopathies, neuroimaging is primarily used to exclude other possibilities including tumor progression and complications of myelosuppression such as hemorrhage, opportunistic infection, or the rare progressive multifocal leukoencephalopathy.[21]

---

*References 8, 11, 14, 18, 20, 43.

REFERENCES

1. Barkovich A: *Pediatric neuroimaging,* New York, 1990, Raven.
2. Barnes P: Magnetic resonance in pediatric and adolescent neuroimaging, *Neurol Clin North Am* 8:741, 1990.
3. Barnes P, Lester P, Yamanashi W: MR imaging in childhood intracranial masses, *Magn Res Imaging* 4:41, 1986.
4. Becker L: An appraisal of the WHO classification of tumors of the CNS, *Cancer* 56:1858, 1985.
5. Burger P: Malignant astrocytic neoplasm: classification, pathology, anatomy, and response to therapy, *Semin Oncol* 13:16, 1986.
6. Cohen M, Duffner P: Tumors of the brain and spinal cord. In Swaiman K: *Pediatric neurology,* St Louis, 1989, Mosby–Year Book.
7. Constine L, Konski A, Ekholm S, et al: Adverse effects of brain irradiation correlated with MR and CT, *J Radiat Oncol Biol Phys* 13:88, 1987.
8. Curnes J, Laster D, Ball M, et al: MR imaging of radiation injury to the brain, *AJNR* 7:389, 1986.
9. Davis D, Kelly P, Marsh W, et al: Computer-assisted stereotactic biopsy of intracranial lesions in pediatric patients, *Pediatr Neurosci* 14:31, 1988.
10. Davis P: Tumors of the brain. In Cohen M, Edwards M, editors: *MR imaging of children,* Philadelphia, 1990, BC Decker.
11. Davis P, Hoffman J, Pearl G, et al: CT of effects of cranial radiation therapy in children, *AJNR* 7:639, 1986.
12. Dean B, Drayer B, Bird C, et al: Gliomas: classification with MRI, *Radiology* 174:411, 1990.

13. DiChiro G, Oldfield E, Wright D, et al: Cerebral necrosis after radiotherapy and intraarterial chemotherapy of brain tumors: PET and neuropathology, *AJNR* 8:1083, 1987.
14. Dooms G, Hecht S, Brant-Zawadski M, et al: Brain radiation lesions: MR imaging, *Radiology* 158:149, 1986.
15. Duffner P, Cohen M, Thomas P, et al: Long-term effects of cranial irradiation on the CNS, *Cancer* 56:1841, 1985.
16. Earnest F, Kelly P, Scheithauer B, et al: Cerebral astrocytomas, histopathologic correlation of MR and CT contrast enhancement with stereotactic biopsy, *Radiology* 166:823, 1988.
17. Elster A, Rieser G: Gd-DTPA–enhanced cranial MR imaging in children, *AJNR* 10:1027, 1989.
18. Grossman R, Hecht-Leavitt C, Evans S, et al: Experimental radiation injury: MR imaging and spectroscopy, *Radiology* 169:305, 1988.
19. Halperin E, Kun L, Constine L, et al: *Pediatric radiation oncology,* New York, 1989, Raven.
20. Hecht-Leavitt C, Grossman R, Curran W, et al: MR of brain radiation injury, *AJNR* 8:427, 1987.
21. Heideman R, Packer R, Albright L, et al: Tumors of the CNS. In Pizzo P, Poplock D, editors: *Pediatric oncology,* Philadelphia, 1989, JB Lippincott.
22. Heinz E, Heinz T, Radtke R, et al: Efficacy of MR vs. CT in epilepsy, *AJNR* 9:1123, 1988.
23. Horowitz M, Kun L, Mulhern R, et al: Feasibility and efficacy of preirradiation chemotherapy for pediatric brain tumors, *Neurosurgery* 22:687, 1988.
24. Johnson P, Hunt S, Drayer B: Human cerebral gliomas: correlation of postmortem MR imaging and neuropathologic findings, *Radiology* 170:211, 1989.
25. Kelly P, Daumas-Duport C, Kispent D, et al: Imaging-based stereotactic serial biopsies in untreated intracranial glial neoplasms, *J Neurosurg* 66:865, 1987.
26. Kramer J, Norman D, Brant-Zawadski M, et al: Absence of white matter changes on MR imaging in children treated with CNS prophylaxis therapy for leukemia, *Cancer* 61:928, 1988.
27. Loeffler J, Rossitch E, Siddon R, et al: Stereotactic radiosurgery in treatment of intracranial malformations and tumors in children, *Pediatrics* 85:774, 1990.
28. Menkes J: *Textbook of child neurology,* ed 3, Philadelphia, 1985, Lea & Febiger.
29. Moss S, Roskwald G, Chen S, et al: Radiation-induced meningiomas in pediatric patients, *Neurosurgery* 22:758, 1988.
30. Naidich T, Quencer R, editors: *Clinical neurosonography,* New York, 1987, Springer-Verlag.
31. Packer R, Sutton L, Atkins T, et al: Cognitive function in children receiving whole-brain radiotherapy and chemotherapy, *J Neurosurg* 70:707, 1989.
32. Pierce S, Barnes P, Loeffler J, et al: Definitive radiotherapy in symptomatic optic glioma: survival and long-term effects, *Cancer* 69:45, 1990.
33. Powers T, Partain C, Kessler R, et al: CNS lesions in pediatric patients: Gd-DTPA–enhanced MR imaging, *Radiology* 169:723, 1988.
34. Radkowski M, Naidich T, Tomita T, et al: Neonatal brain tumors: CT and MR, *J Comput Assist Tomogr* 12:10, 1988.
35. Ron E, Modan B, Boice J, et al: Tumors of the brain and nervous system after radiotherapy in childhood, *N Engl J Med* 319:1033, 1988.
36. Rorke L: Classification and grading of childhood brain tumors: overview and statement of the problem, *Cancer* 56:1849, 1985.
37. Rorke L, Gilles F, Davis R, et al: Revision of the WHO classification of brain tumors for childhood, *Cancer* 56:1869, 1985.
38. Russell D, Rubinstein L: *Pathology of tumors of the nervous system,* ed 4, Baltimore, 1977, Williams & Wilkins.
39. Sage M: Blood-brain barrier: phenomenon of increasing importance to the imaging clinician, *AJR* 138:887, 1982.
40. Schad L, Boesecke R, Schlegel W, et al: Three-dimensional image correlation of CT, MR, and PET in radiotherapy treatment planning of brain tumors, *J Comput Assist Tomogr* 11:948, 1987.
41. Schmitt H, Wowra B, Sturm V: The stereotactic approach to focal lesions in the deep brain of children and adolescents, *Brain Dev* 10:305, 1988.
42. Storrs B: Stereotactic procedures in children, In McLaurin R, Schut L, Venes J, Epstein F, editors: *Pediatric neurosurgery,* ed 2, Philadelphia, 1987, WB Saunders.
43. Tsuruda J, Kortman K, Bradley W, et al: Radiation effects on cerebral white matter: MR evaluation, *AJR* 149:165, 1987.
44. Wechsler-Jentzsch K, Witt J, Fitz C, et al: Unresectable gliomas in children: tumor volume response to radiation therapy, *Radiology* 169:237, 1988.
45. Zagzag D, Goldenberg M, Brem S: Angiogenesis and blood-brain barrier breakdown modulate CT scan contrast enhancement, *AJNR* 10:529, 1989.
46. Zhang J, Levesque M, Wilson C, et al: Multimodality imaging of brain structures for stereotactic surgery, *Radiology* 175:435, 1990.
47. Zulch K: *Brain tumors: biology and pathology,* ed 3, New York, 1986, Springer-Verlag.

Cerebral hemispheric tumors

Cerebral hemispheric tumors may be manifested by focal seizures, hemiparesis, central facial palsy, rare sensory phenomena, and movement disorder or hemiplegia-hemisensory syndrome with deeper involvement.[16,38,54] The vast majority are of neuroepithelial origin (see box below) including gliomas, neuronal tumors, and primitive neuroectodermal tumors (PNET).[16,67,68] Meningeal, lymphoreticular, vascular-origin, and metastatic neoplasms are less common. Of the gliomas, astrocytomas are by far the most common, whereas choroid plexus tumors occur frequently in infancy. Nonneoplastic masses to be differentiated from neoplastic tumors include arachnoid cysts, vascular malformations, hemorrhages or infarctions, abscesses or other inflammatory masses, hamartomas, and so forth. As mentioned in previous sections, in infancy most

---

CEREBRAL HEMISPHERE TUMORS

1. **Glial tumors (IA)***
   a. Astrocytic
   b. Oligodendroglial
   c. Ependymal
   d. Choroid plexus
   e. Mixed
   f. Glioblastomatous
   g. Gliomatosis

2. **Neuronal tumors (IB)**
   a. Ganglioglioma

3. **Primitive neuroectodermal tumors (IC)**

4. **Meningeal tumors (II)**
   a. Meningioma

5. **Lymphoma (IV)**

6. **Blood-vessel origin tumors (V)**

7. **Parameningeal tumors (IX)**

8. **Metastatic tumors (X)**

---

*Parenthetical data following each tumor type are designations referring to the outline of the revision of the WHO classification, as presented in the box on p. 205.

intracranial masses or tumors are nonneoplastic and cystic (for example, arachnoid cyst, Dandy-Walker cyst). Rare neoplasia of infancy include astrocytoma, PNET, germ cell tumors (for example, teratoma), and choroid plexus tumors (papilloma, carcinoma).[3,63] Parameningeal neoplasia or other extradural processes of cranial or scalp origin may invade or extend to involve the cerebrum (for example, neuroblastoma or histiocytosis).

NEUROEPITHELIAL NEOPLASMS

Neuroepithelial neoplasms (see box on p. 205) constitute the largest group of CNS tumors occurring at all ages, as well as in childhood and adolescence.[16,38] Cells in this group of neoplasms resemble to a varying degree cells normally derived from the embryonic neural tube that give rise to the principal neuronal and glial cells composing the parenchyma of the CNS. The group includes glial cell tumors (gliomas), neuronal (ganglion cell) or mixed neuronal-glial tumors, primitive neuroectodermal tumors (PNET), and pineal cell tumors. Glial tumors make up the largest group and include astrocytomas, oligodendrogliomas, ependymomas, choroid plexus tumors, mixed gliomas, glioblastomatous tumors, and gliomatosis.

Astrocytic tumors

Astrocytic tumors account for the majority of gliomas and CNS neoplasia of childhood (40% to 50%).[16,38,67] As the name implies, astrocytomas are composed of cells resembling astrocytes, which normally serve as supporting cells in the CNS, react to injury as glial scars (gliosis), and characteristically contain glial fibrillary acidic protein (GFAP). Astrocytomas are a heterogeneous group of neoplasms and may occur anywhere within the CNS. Cerebral hemispheric astrocytomas, particularly higher-grade forms, more commonly occur in adulthood than in childhood. In contrast, astrocytomas arising in the optic system (optic gliomas), diencephalon (hypothalamus and thalamus), brain stem (brain stem glioma), and cerebellum are more prominent in children. Astrocytomas show considerable histological diversity. Subtypes of astrocytoma based on cytological appearance include fibrillary, protoplasmic, gemistocytic, pilocytic, and xanthomatous types, although many astrocytomas show mixed patterns. Except for some of the pilocytic and xanthomatous types, the patterns have little prognostic significance.[11,25,50] Most astrocytomas are infiltrative or contain areas of infiltration of CNS parenchyma and thus have indistinct boundaries, although the pilocytic and xanthomatous types more frequently grow as solid circumscribed masses.

The modified WHO classification and various authors recognize three grades of increasing malignancy: astrocytoma, anaplastic astrocytoma, and glioblastoma, which imply correspondingly worse prognoses.* Anaplastic astrocytoma is distinguished histologically from astrocytoma by greater cell density, increasing cellular and nuclear pleomorphism, mitotic activity, and hyperplasia of blood vessels. The same features are present in a greater degree in glioblastoma, along with tumor necrosis, generally considered to be the histological hallmark of high-grade astrocytic neoplasms. The heterogeneous gross appearance of most glioblastomas, which is caused by intermixed areas of solid or cystic tumor, damaged or invaded brain, tumor necrosis, and hemorrhage, inspired the term *glioblastoma multiforme*.[7,67,68] Both low- and high-grade tumors may have solid or cystic components, although cysts and calcification are more common in lower-grade tumors. High-grade, and, rarely, low-grade tumors may invade and disseminate in the subarachnoid spaces.

Grading of astrocytic neoplasms, although useful, has several important limitations. Anaplastic change in a tumor represents a spectrum rather than discrete steps, so many of the histological differences between grades are differences of degree rather than kind and are essentially matters of opinion. Astrocytic tumors are notoriously heterogeneous; anaplastic foci may be widely scattered through a tumor of otherwise low-grade appearance. Tumors may progress to higher-grade lesions, so a recurrent astrocytoma may evolve into an anaplastic astrocytoma or glioblastoma.

Among the clinicopathological variants of astrocytoma most in the cerebral hemispheres and brain stem, particularly those arising in the pons, are infiltrative astrocytomas, anaplastic astrocytomas, or glioblastomas. In contrast, astrocytomas arising in the cerebellum of children are more frequently cystic pilocytic astrocytomas (cerebellar cystic or microcystic astrocytomas), which are frequently circumscribed, grow slowly, and rarely progress to higher-grade neoplasms. Optic system gliomas and thalamic or diencephalic gliomas are also commonly pilocytic astrocytomas.

Some histological variants of astrocytoma occur almost exclusively in children or young adults.[7,67,68] The pleomorphic xanthoastrocytoma and the gigantocellular glioma usually occur as large, circumscribed or infiltrative, and often cystic, cerebral hemispheric tumors in later childhood or adolescence. These often are associated with a favorable prognosis despite the presence of considerable cytological pleomorphism. The subependymal giant cell tumor, often but not invariably encountered in the setting of tuberous sclerosis, arises in the walls of the lateral or rostral third ventricle, is usually calcified, and is composed of cells with mixed glial and neuronal characteristics.

The neuroimaging findings are often nonspecific regarding the differentiation of astrocytic tumors from other glial neoplasms or distinguishing higher-grade (malignant) from lower-grade (benign) forms.* The tumors may be cystic, solid, or a combination thereof and may or may not contain calcification (Figs. 7-5 to 7-7). The tumors are often isodense or of low density by CT with variable iodine enhancement. By MRI the astrocytic tumors are often

---

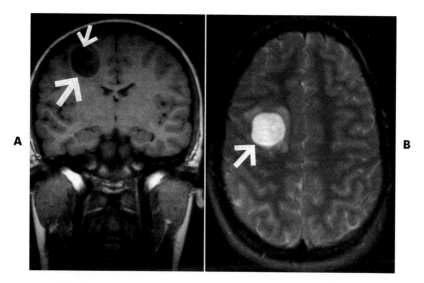

Fig. 7-5 Circumscribed frontal cerebral anaplastic astrocytoma shown by coronal T1 MRI **(A)** with isointense solid component *(large white arrow)* and low intensity cystic component *(small white arrow)*.**B,** Axial T2 MRI shows a circumscribed high intensity mass *(white arrow)* with surrounding high intensity rim (?edema).

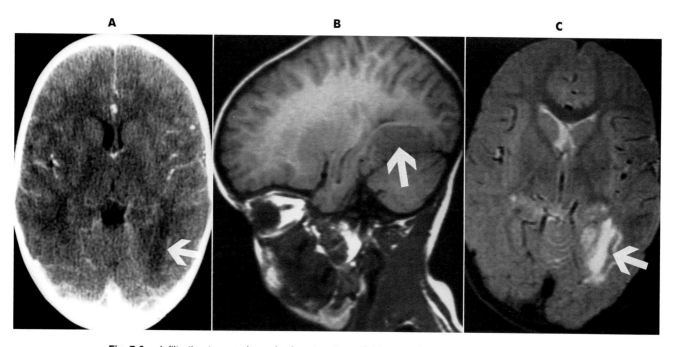

Fig. 7-6 Infiltrating temporal anaplastic astrocytoma *(white arrow)* poorly delineated by CT **(A)** as a low density, nonenhancing lesion. The tumor is isointense to hypointense on sagittal **(B)** T1-MRI but hyperintense on axial T2 MRI **(C)**

isointense or low intensity on T1 images and isointense to high intensity on proton density and T2 images[5,19] (Figs. 7-5 to 7-7). Occasionally the tumor may be of relative low intensity on p/T2 images depending on the intracellular or extracellular free water content. Gadolinium-DTPA enhancement is variable. Occasionally, imaging findings may

indicate the tendency for higher grades of malignancy (see Figs. 7-17 to 7-19) including off-midline or cerebral hemispheric location, intratumoral signal heterogeneity, irregular shape and poor margination, mass effect, edema, hemorrhage, and irregularly thick and nodular ringlike enhancement about a watery density or intensity cen-

A   B   C

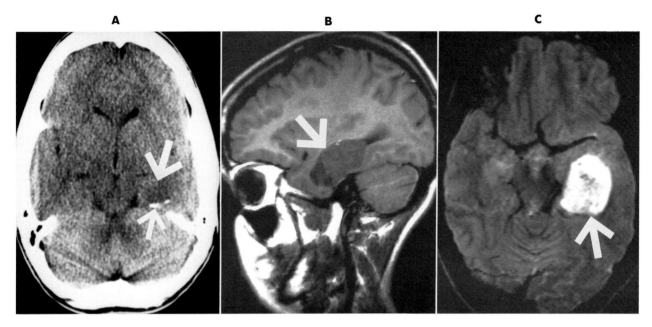

Fig. 7-7   A, Temporal calcified astrocytoma poorly shown by CT with high density calcification *(small white arrow)* near the petrous ridge and subtle low density *(large white arrow)*. **B,** Sagittal T1 MRI shows the isointense to hypointense tumor *(large white arrow)* involving the dilated temporal horn. **C,** Axial p/T2 MRI shows the tumor as isointense to hyperintense.

ter.[5,19,21,59] In general, however, enhancement has never consistently correlated with grade of malignancy nor has it served as an accurate indicator of tumor margins (tumor versus edema). It does correlate with tumor neovascularity and endothelial proliferation and often serves as a histologically high-yield guide for biopsy (that is, tumor core) in de novo cases.[18,25,82] In treated cases, however, the enhancement is often nonspecific for differentiating recurrent tumor from tumor radionecrosis or chemonecrosis (see Fig. 7-18).

Imaging difficulties with tumor diagnosis, delineation of extent, and adequacy of treatment are further dramatized by three-dimensional tumor configurations for gliomas as divided into three categories.[21,25,43,45] The first type of configuration (tumor core only) corresponds to circumscribed tissue without peripheral isolated tumor cells as may be seen with pilocytic astrocytomas (see Posterior Fossa section). The second type of configuration (tumor core plus corona) represents tumor tissue core with peripheral isolated tumor cells. Glioblastomas commonly fall into this category (Figs. 7-17 to 7-19). In the third type (tumor corona only) only isolated tumor cells are present. Many of the low-grade astrocytomas are in this latter category, and anaplastic tumors may overlap all three divisions (Figs. 7-5 and 7-6).

MRI is clearly superior to CT for demonstrating neoplastic processes that produce minor alterations in the blood-brain (tumor) barrier, allowing only slight increases in water content but not the passage of protein-bound contrast agents.[5,6,19,69,81] However, neuroimaging in general remains limited in its ability to estimate the extent of tumor cell infiltration accurately for white matter, gray matter, leptomeninges, and subarachnoid spaces, particularly when unaccompanied by edema or abnormal enhancement. Furthermore, neuroimaging is limited in its ability to differentiate edematous tumor corona from nontumor vasogenic edema or cytotoxic edema, which may be reactive and related to tumor response or treatment effects (for example, necrosis, gliosis, demyelination, edema, and so forth.) Therefore neuroimaging and especially MRI may tend to underestimate tumor extent de novo, as well as overestimate extent in treated cases.

For astrocytic tumors, as well as most other CNS neoplasia, maximum safe surgical excision or debulking is preferred to biopsy. Radiotherapy is always important in the treatment of higher-grade tumors (anaplastic, glioblastoma), as well as recurrent or symptomatic lower-grade tumors. Chemotherapy may be adjunctive or palliative. A transient slight increase in tumor volume may occur after radiotherapy. Higher-grade tumors often show faster response rates but recur earlier than lower-grade tumors, which often demonstrate slower response and later recurrence. The overall treatment results, however, are often disappointing for both higher-grade and lower-grade tumors other than the pilocytic astrocytoma.[11,36,38,61,80]

Oligodendrogliomas

Oligodendrogliomas are composed of cells resembling oligodendrocytes, the myelin-forming cells of the central nervous system, and are an uncommon finding in chil-

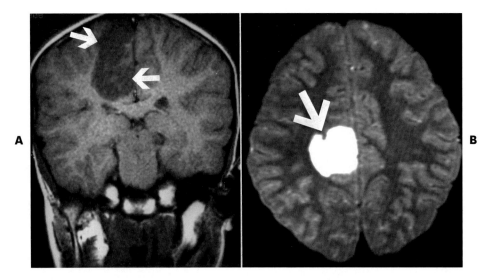

Fig. 7-8   A, Parietal cerebral oligodendroglioma *(white arrows)* shown by coronal T1 MRI as a circumscribed, noncalcified, and nonenhancing low intensity mass. **B,** On axial T2 MRI the tumor is high intensity (same as Fig. 7-1).

dren.[67,68] The majority of these tumors occur in the cerebral hemispheres, usually in a cortical or subcortical location. The well-differentiated oligodendroglioma is slow growing, may be circumscribed or infiltrative, shows proliferation of the microvasculature, and is frequently calcified. Variant forms may be seen with abundant extracellular mucoid material, gross cysts or hemorrhages, but edema is unusual. Cortical tumors may produce erosion of the cranial inner table. A tendency for invasion and spread in the leptomeninges has also been reported. Dense cellularity, prominent mitotic activity, vascular proliferation, and necrosis characterize anaplastic oligodendrogliomas, which may have similar appearances to glioblastomas.

Oligodendrogliomas may contain other glial components, most often astrocytic. The neuroimaging appearance is often that of a circumscribed uniform density or intensity mass that is more often solid than cystic[5,19,49] (Figs. 7-8 and 7-9). Calcification is common and often the dominating feature. Edema is often lacking. The tumor itself is often isodense or low density by CT. By MRI the tumor is often isointense or low intensity on T1 images, and isointense to hyperintense on proton density and T2 images (Fig. 7-8). Iodine or gadolinium enhancement produces variable results. Occasionally the tumor may be poorly marginated and have more heterogeneous density or intensity characteristics including irregular enhancement, edema, and dissemination (oligodendrogliomatosis). This may be particularly evident with mixed or anaplastic oligodendrogliomas (Fig. 7-10).

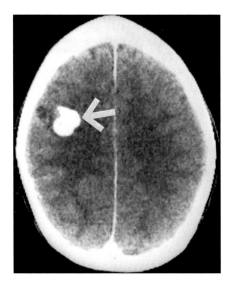

Fig. 7-9   Frontal calcified oligodendroglioma shown by CT as a predominantly high density mass *(arrow).*

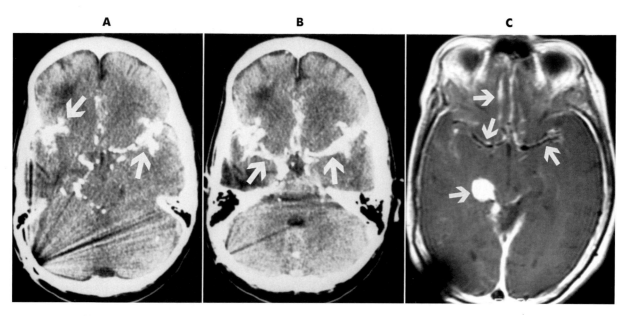

Fig. 7-10   Oligodendrogliomatosis shown by precontrast **(A)** and postcontrast **(B)** CT as calcified, enhancing high densities *(arrows)* within the basal cisterns. **C,** Axial gadolinium-enhanced MRI shows extensive high intensity enhancement *(arrows)* along the cisterns and within the right temporal lobe.

Ependymal tumors

Ependymal tumors of childhood are more common within the posterior fossa. (These are more fully discussed and illustrated in the Posterior Fossa section.) These occur infrequently in the cerebral hemispheres but typically project extraventricularly from the ependymal surface of the lateral ventricle or arise from ependymal cell rests.[67,68] Neuroimaging may demonstrate heterogeneous or occasionally homogeneous density or intensity characteristics often with calcification and cyst formation plus irregular enhancement with iodine or gadolinium[5,19,74] (Fig. 7-11). Anaplastic forms occur more commonly above the tentorium than below, although the posterior fossa anaplastic tumors tend to seed more often. Formerly referred to as ependymoma variants, subependymoma (mixed glioma) and ependymoblastoma (PNET with an ependymal cell component) are presented in their appropriate sections.

Choroid plexus tumors

Choroid plexus tumors are encountered primarily in childhood, usually in the first decade of life, and are classically tumors of infancy.[3,16,63,67,68] The choroid plexus is a focal specialization of the ventricular lining cells in the walls of the lateral and roofs of the third and fourth ventricles and in the cerebellopontine angles. It is a papillary secretory epithelium folded over a vascular and leptomeningeal core. The choroid plexus is responsible for the production of cerebrospinal fluid (CSF). The rare nonneoplastic proliferations (villous hypertrophy), as well as choroid plexus neoplasms, may result in overproduction of CSF and hydrocephalus. Developmentally, choroid plexus is formed as an infolding of vascular pia arachnoid

and ependyma. It consists of an ependymal layer and a mesenchymal stromal layer containing fibroblasts, vascular elements, and arachnoidal cell rests. Choroid plexus tumors, therefore, may originate from the ependymal layer and may be manifested as a papilloma, carcinoma, astrocytoma, ependymoma, or neuroepithelial cyst.[67,68] Tumors of mesenchymal or stromal origin include meningioma, vascular malformation, hemangioma, lipoma, and teratoma.

This discussion is directed to the two common choroid plexus neoplasms of childhood: choroid plexus papilloma and choroid plexus carcinoma (anaplastic papilloma). These are soft papillary tumors arising from the epithelial cells of the choroid plexus and often occur in the lateral ventricles, less often in the third or fourth ventricle, or the cerebellopontine angle.[67,68] Papillomas are the most common of the choroid plexus tumors, are histologically mature, resembling normal choroid plexus, and are generally circumscribed intraventricular tumors. Anaplastic papillomas (carcinomas) are malignant and invasive and arise from the choroid plexus by either anaplasia within a papilloma or de novo.[26] These resemble higher-grade adenocarcinomas and characteristically invade rather than compress the brain substance. Seeding occasionally occurs with choroid plexus tumors, particularly the carcinomas. Hydrocephalus is almost always associated with these tumors, whether as a result of CSF overproduction, tumor obstruction of CSF pathways, or impaired CSF absorption from hemorrhage. Choroid plexus tumors are hypercellular and highly vascularized neoplasms often with calcification or hemorrhage. These tumors are rarely bilateral (that is, benign, villous hypertrophy) or multiple (see Fig. 7-13).

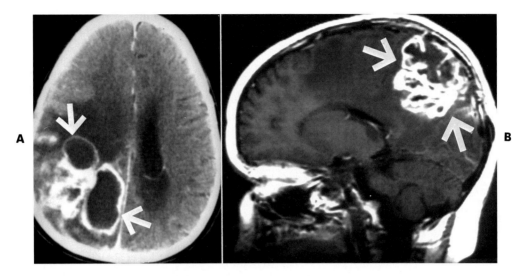

Fig. 7-11   Cerebral anaplastic ependymoma *(arrows)* shown by CT **(A)** and MRI **(B)** as a large, irregular cystic and calcified mass with marked iodine and gadolinium enhancement, plus extensive low density and low intensity edema.

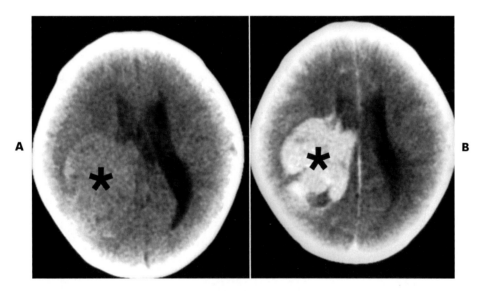

Fig. 7-12   Choroid plexus papilloma of the lateral ventricle *(asterisk)* shown by precontrast **(A)** and postcontrast **(B)** CT as an isodense to hyperdense circumscribed mass with marked iodine enhancement.

In the case of papillomas neuroimaging usually demonstrates a lateral intraventricular mass of homogeneous density or intensity with calcification, enhancement, and ventricular dilatation[5,15,19,26,42] (Figs. 7-12 and 7-13). The mass is often isodense to hyperdense by CT, isointense to hypointense on T1 MRI and isointense to hyperintense on p/T2 MRI (Fig. 7-14). Occasionally the tumor itself is of relative low intensity on p/T2 MRI. The homogeneous or occasional heterogeneous CT hyperdensity or MR hypoin-tensity may correlate with hypercellularity, hypervascularity, mineralization, or hemorrhage. Invasive papillomas or carcinomas are more often heterogeneous in CT density and MR intensity with irregular enhancement, hemorrhage, or cyst formation. The tumor often extends beyond the ventricular margin with invasion of brain and extensive edema (Figs. 7-15 and 7-16).

There is excellent survival with surgical excision of papillomas. Since the tumors are often large and produce

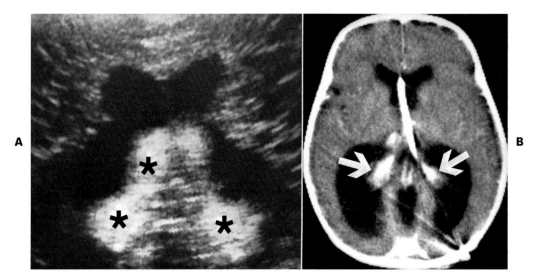

Fig. 7-13 An unusual case of choroid plexus villous hypertrophy with hydrocephalus due to CSF overproduction shown by US **(A)** as markedly echogenic intraventricular masses *(asterisks)* within the dilated sonolucent lateral ventricles, and by CT **(B)** as markedly enhancing nodules *(arrows)*.

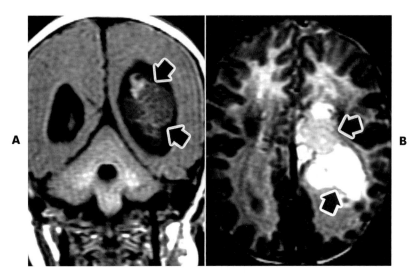

Fig. 7-14 Cystic choroid plexus papilloma *(black arrows)* and callosal agenesis in Aicardi's syndrome. Coronal **(A)** T1 MRI shows lateral intraventricular isointense to hypointense lobular and cystic mass that is of irregular isointensity to hyperintensity on axial T2 MRI **(B)**.

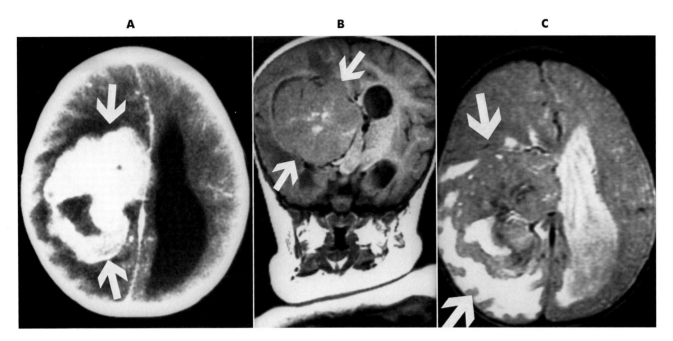

Fig. 7-15   Lateral ventricular choroid plexus carcinoma *(arrows)* shown by CT **(A)** as a large hyperdense calcified and enhancing mass that extends beyond the lateral ventricle and is associated with surrounding low density edema. Coronal **(B)** T1 MRI plus axial T2 **(C)** MRI show the tumor proper as isointense to hypointense. The internal high and low intensities probably represent a combination of abnormal vascularity, hemorrhage, and mineralization. The surrounding T1 hypointensity and T2 hyperintensity represent additional edema.

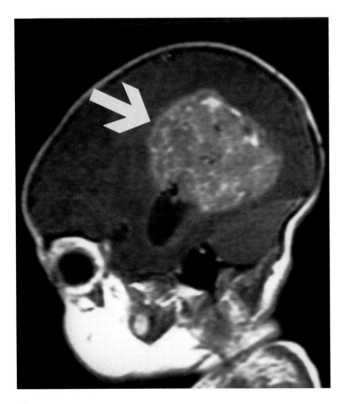

Fig. 7-16   Lateral ventricular choroid plexus carcinoma *(arrow)* demonstrated by sagittal T1 MRI as an irregularly gadolinium-enhancing tumor.

severe hydrocephalus, postresection subdural collections are a management problem especially after ventricular shunting. Total or en bloc excision is preferred, although excessive blood loss is a potential problem with these highly vascular tumors. Prolonged survival after aggressive initial and follow-up excision has been reported for patients with carcinomas.[26] This approach along with added chemotherapy may allow postponement of radiotherapy until the child is older and can better tolerate treatment. Supratentorial papilloma may be evaluated on follow-up with contrast-enhanced CT, whereas carcinoma, especially of the posterior fossa, is probably better evaluated with MRI, including gadolinium enhancement.

Mixed gliomas

Many gliomas contain roughly equal portions of different glioma types, either as segregated areas or intermixed, and the designation of *mixed glioma* has been proposed.[67,68] The specific nomenclature is derived from the recognized components in descending order of prominence. Some of the mixed gliomas encountered in childhood include oligoastrocytoma, ependymoastrocytoma, oligoastroependymoma, oligoependymoma, subependymoma, and gliofibroma. Although prognosis probably depends on the more aggressive element, grading is difficult, and the revised WHO classification restricts grading to distinguishing merely nonanaplastic and anaplastic forms of each subtype.[67]

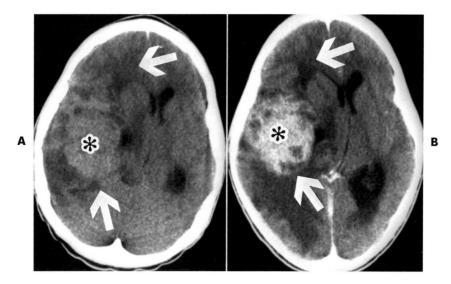

Fig. 7-17   Cerebral glioblastoma *(arrows)* shown by precontrast **(A)** and postcontrast **(B)** CT as a large, heterogeneous mass with central isodensity to hyperdensity and enhancement *(asterisk)* with more peripheral low density.

The *subependymoma* is a special type of mixed glioma composed of astrocytes and ependymal cells arising beneath the ventricular ependyma. Although commonly asymptomatic and incidental at autopsy in adults, large nonanaplastic tumors have been reported in children and have a relatively poor prognosis. *Gliofibroma* is another rare but special type of nonanaplastic mixed glioma that is composed of intermingled astrocytes and fibroblasts. Neuroimaging (MRI or CT) is usually nonspecific regarding the possible differentiation of these tumors from one another or from other CNS tumors.[5,19]

Glioblastomatous tumors

Glioblastomatous tumors are generally considered anaplastic forms of astrocytic tumors by some authorities.[67] Recognizing that many glioblastomas do not appear to arise from preexisting astrocytomas or anaplastic astrocytomas, but rather occur de novo or develop in gliomas of other types, the revised WHO classification maintains a separate category of glioblastomatous tumors.[67] These include glioblastoma multiforme, giant cell glioblastoma, and glioblastoma with a sarcomatous component (gliosarcoma).

Glioblastoma multiforme is a pleomorphic, highly cellular anaplastic tumor with endothelial proliferation and necrosis, often with mitoses and classically prominent perinecrotic pseudopalisades.[61,67,68] Recognizable glial cell types (for example, astrocytes) are often absent. These occur primarily in the cerebral hemispheres and are the most malignant of neuroepithelial tumors, including seeding potential and poor survival.

Glioblastoma may occur as part of the cancer family syndrome or may be induced by radiation. The giant cell variant (monstrocellular or giant cell glioblastoma) is the anaplastic version of the gigantocellular glioma and combines excessive cell size, pleomorphism, and a variably prominent connective tissue component with the other typical features of glioblastoma. Gliosarcoma is the malignant form of a mixed glial and mesenchymal neoplasm.

Again, the neuroimaging findings are diverse and range from a circumscribed mass to a diffuse process. Often these are large, heterogeneous, solid or cystic, and usually enhancing tumors with mass effect, edema, or hemorrhage[5,19,21,59] (Figs. 7-17 to 7-19). Calcification is occasionally present. Irregular nodular ring enhancement with a necrotic center and surrounding vasogenic edema is often characteristic. Occasionally the giant cell glioblastoma may appear innocent as a cyst and mural nodule (Fig. 7-20).

Gliomatosis cerebri

The term *gliomatosis cerebri* refers to the rare entity of diffuse infiltrative glioma that involves either multiple sites or large areas of the CNS, usually the cerebral hemispheres.[67,68] Grossly and microscopically, gliomatosis cerebri resembles diffuse astrocytoma, although foci of frank glioblastoma may occur. Although postmortem examination has traditionally been required to confirm this rare diagnosis, the increasing availability of high-quality neuroimaging has facilitated the diagnosis during life. Gliomatosis cerebri occurs, and may even predominate, in children or young adults. The term should not be used as a synonym for diffuse leptomeningeal or intraventricular spread of malignant glioma, which has sometimes been referred to as secondary meningeal and ventricular gliomatosis. Neuroimaging often underestimates the extent of tumor involvement even after contrast enhancement[5,19] (Figs. 7-21 to 7-23).

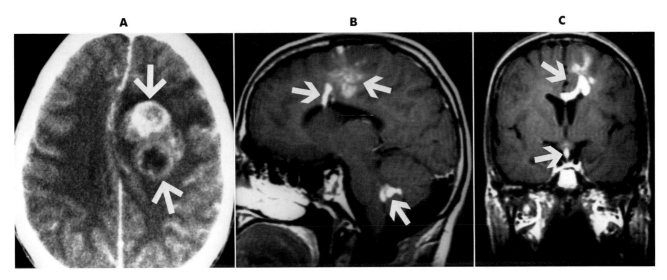

Fig. 7-18   Cerebral glioblastoma years after cranial irradiation for leukemia. **A,** contrast CT shows irregular nodular and ring enhancement with surrounding low density and mass effect *(arrows)* extending across the midline. Sagittal **(B)** and coronal **(C)** T1 MRI after gadolinium administration shows irregular enhancement in the primary tumor site *(upper white arrows)* after small field radiotherapy. Abnormal enhancement is also present in the suprasellar region (**(C)** *(lower white arrow)* and posterior fossa (**B,** *lower white arrow*) consistent with tumor dissemination.

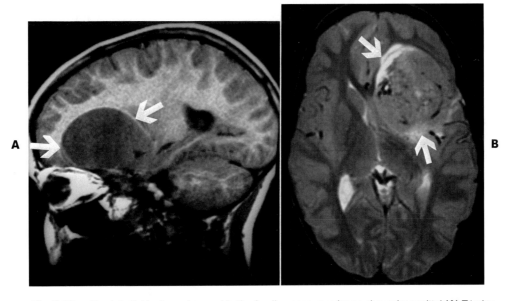

Fig. 7-19   Frontal glioblastoma *(arrows)* in the family cancer syndrome shown by sagittal **(A)** T1 plus axial T2 MRI **(B)** as a heterogeneous, isointense to hypointense tumor. Internal high and low intensities probably represent a combination of abnormal vascularity, hemorrhage, and necrosis. Additional peritumoral edema is best shown as a high intensity rim on the axial T2 image **(B).**

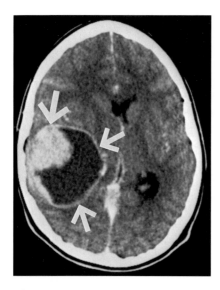

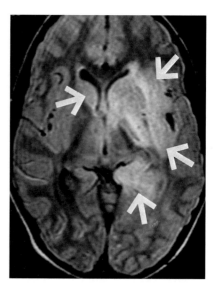

Fig. 7-20   Circumscribed cerebral gigantocellular glioblastoma shown by contrast CT as a rim-enhancing cyst *(small arrows)* with enhancing mural nodule *(large arrow)*.

Fig. 7-21   Gliomatosis cerebri *(arrows)* shown by axial proton density MRI as bilateral high intensity temporal and basal ganglia abnormalities.

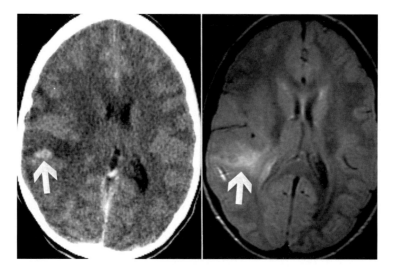

Fig. 7-22   Gliomatosis cerebri-anaplastic astrocytoma *(arrows)* underestimated by contrast CT **(A)** and p/T2 MRI **(B).** Diffuse and extensive cerebral and meningeal infiltration was present at postmortem examination.

Neuronal tumors

Neuronal tumors contain neoplastic neurons and represent an important group of neoplasms in children and adolescents, particularly in the setting of epilepsy from temporal lobe tumors.[16,67,78] Because many neoplasms with demonstrable neuronal elements also contain glial components, classification may be difficult. The category of *tumors of neurons or bipotential precursors* has been suggested to indicate the common origin of neuronal and glial cells from the embryonic neuroepithelium and to imply

that the cell of origin of neuron-containing tumors retains the capability of neuronal or glial differentiation. The WHO similarly includes neuronal tumors as a subcategory of tumors of neuroepithelial tissue and distinguishes five categories based on the presence or absence of a prominent glial component (ganglioglioma and gangliocytoma, respectively), the presence of anaplasia (anaplastic ganglioglioma or gangliocytoma), and the presence of primitive neurons or neuronal precursors (ganglioneuroblastoma and neuroblastoma).[7] The proposed revision of the WHO

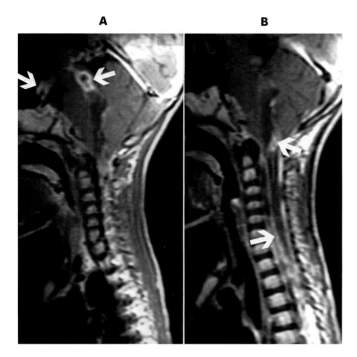

A   **B**

Fig. 7-23   Diffuse leptomeningeal nonanaplastic astrocytoma presenting as communicating obstructive hydrocephalus. **A** and **B**, Sagittal T1 images after gadolinium administration show multifocal intracranial and intraspinal enhancement including optic-hypothalamic **(A)**, tectal **(A)**, cisterna magna **(B)**, and cervico-thoracic perimedullary **(B)**.

classification groups the neuroblast-containing tumors with other primitive neuroectodermal tumors and thus recognizes only four types of neuronal tumors: gangliocytoma, ganglioglioma, and anaplastic forms of each.[67]

Neuron-containing tumors, typically arising in the cerebral hemispheres, are often circumscribed but may be infiltrative. Many also contain a prominent reactive connective tissue component, areas of calcification, or cysts.[67,68] By definition, *gangliocytoma* consists largely or exclusively of neoplastic differentiated neurons and lacks a significant glial component. *Ganglioglioma* implies the presence of a glial component, whether astroglial or oligodendroglial, which may be segregated from or intermixed with the neuronal component or even predominate. Both gangliocytoma and ganglioglioma are typically slowly growing tumors. In small biopsy specimens and in the absence of evidence of a growing mass, the distinction between neoplasm and hamartoma or other neuroglial malformation may be difficult or impossible to make. An unusual form of malformative lesion of the cerebellar cortex, the dysplastic gangliocytoma of Lhermitte and Duclos, and rare similar lesions of cerebral cortex are probably not true neoplasms, although the former may present as a mass lesion.[67,68] In neuron-containing tumors the presence of cellular anaplasia or other features associated with rapid growth (dense cellularity, mitoses, necrosis, vascular hyperplasia) defines the anaplastic gangliocytoma and anaplastic ganglioglioma and implies a worse prognosis. Such tumors may overlap

with glioblastoma multiforme or forms of PNET such as the rare ganglioneuroblastoma (see subsequent discussion).

Neuroimaging of gangliocytoma often reveals a relatively uniform density or intensity abnormality with little or no mass effect and no abnormal enhancement[1,5,19] (Fig. 7-24). The tumor is often isodense or high density by CT with T1 isointensity to hypointensity, proton density isointensity to hyperintensity, and T2 isointensity to hypointensity by MRI. Gangliogliomas are more commonly cystic and calcified and usually demonstrate iodine or gadolinium enhancement[5,14,19,24] (Figs. 7-25 to 7-27). Precontrast CT often shows isodense or hyperdense tumor matrix, whereas MRI shows T1 isointensity to hypointensity with p/T2 isointensity to hyperintensity. The density or intensity character of the cyst component varies with the fluid content and may have a CSF appearance, proteinaceous fluid appearance, or hemorrhagic features. Surgical resection is the primary mode of therapy for neuronal tumors. Radiotherapy is reserved for incompletely resected tumors that are symptomatic, for demonstrated regrowth or recurrence, especially for the ganglioglioma with a prominent glial component, and for anaplastic tumors.[36,38]

Primitive neuroectodermal tumors

The generic term *primitive neuroectodermal tumor* (PNET) was proposed by Hart and Earle to encompass the rare undifferentiated or poorly differentiated tumor arising in the cerebral hemispheres of children or young adults that resembled the cerebellar medulloblastoma but could not be classified into other recognized diagnostic entities.[7,16,67,78] Since then the term has been expanded to encompass not only histologically similar CNS tumors arising in other locations (for example, the pineoblastoma) but also tumors outside the CNS of uncertain histogenetic relationship to CNS tumors or to any tumor showing an undifferentiated or embryonal component. The term *PNET* thus has at least three different meanings: (1) as Hart and Earle's supratentorial undifferentiated tumor; (2) as a generic term for largely undifferentiated CNS tumors with neuroectodermal features in any location, encompassing the entities previously known as medulloblastoma, cerebral neuroblastoma, ependymoblastoma, and pineoblastoma; and (3) as a term for non-CNS "small, round, blue cell tumors" not classifiable into one of the other major diagnostic categories.[7,16,67,68]

The original WHO classification proposed a category of *poorly differentiated and embryonal tumors* encompassing the five subcategories of glioblastoma, medulloblastoma, medulloepithelioma, primitive polar spongioblastoma, and gliomatosis cerebri.[7] The proposed revision assigned glioblastoma and gliomatosis cerebri to the category of glial tumors and proposed a separate category of primitive neuroectodermal tumors (PNET), uniting the medulloblastoma, the PNET of Hart and Earle, the neuroblastoma, and similar tumors from locations other than the pineal region.[67] In view of its characteristic resemblance to embryonic neural tube, the rare medulloepithelioma was assigned to a

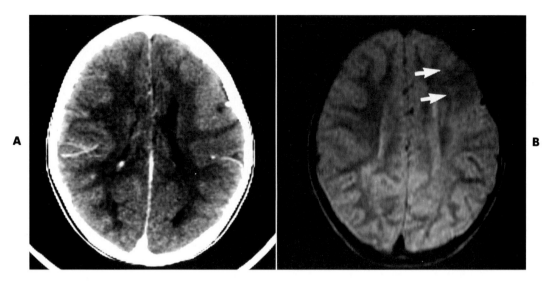

Fig. 7-24   Cerebral gangliocytoma *(arrows)* shown by CT **(A)** and MRI **(B)** as an isodense to hyperdense and isointense to hypointense abnormality. (From Altman N: *AJNR* 9:917, 1988.)

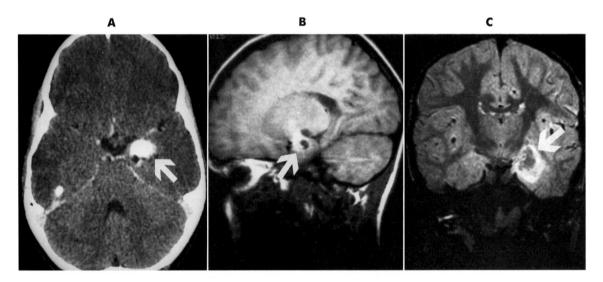

Fig. 7-25   Temporal calcified ganglioglioma producing focal seizures *(arrows)* shown by CT **(A)** as a high density mass. **B,** Sagittal T1 MRI shows abnormal high and low intensities. **C,** Coronal p/T2 MRI demonstrates central hypointensity with surrounding hyperintensity.

separate subcategory, whereas the other non-pineal PNETs were classified as *PNET NOS* (''not otherwise specified'') or *PNET with specified differentiation,* depending on the absence or presence of evidence of differentiation along any neuroepithelial line.

At The Children's Hospital of Boston the term *PNET* has been used for consistency of definition as a generic name for otherwise unclassifiable neoplasms resembling primitive neuroectodermal tissue. In view of the disproportionately high frequency of PNET in the cerebellum, the designation *medulloblastoma* has been retained for the usual cerebellar tumor. In the case of the rare CNS tumor showing widespread evidence of differentiation along a particular line or with a characteristic histological appearance, a specific name has been applied when possible; for example, neuroblastic differentiation (central neuroblastoma or ganglioneuroblastoma), ependymal differentiation (ependymoblastoma), glial differentiation (embryonic glioma), or primitive neuroepithelium (medulloepithelioma). PNETs in other locations, except for the pineal gland and retina, are

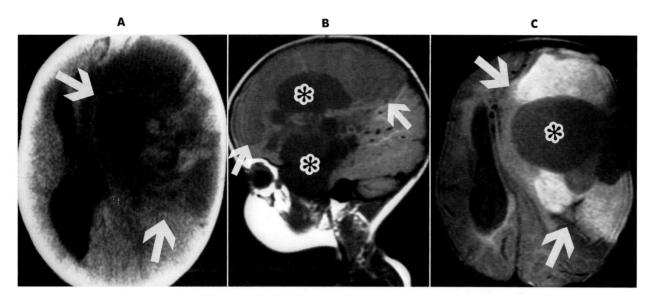

Fig. 7-26   Desmoplastic ganglioglioma *(arrows)* of infancy shown by CT **(A)** as a huge, mixed isodense to hypodense left hemispheric mass with marked rightward shift and contralateral ventricular dilatation. Sagittal T1 **(B)** and axial proton density **(C)** MRI shows areas correlating with solid *(arrows)* and cystic *(asterisks)* tumor components.

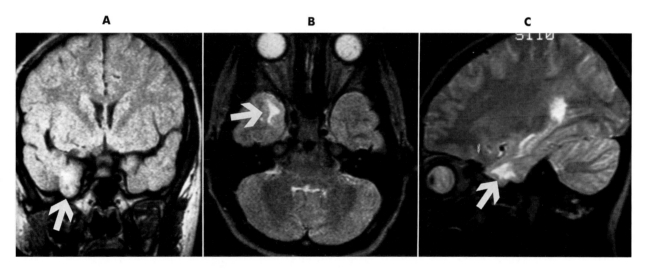

Fig. 7-27   Temporal ganglioglioma with seizures and negative CT. The tumor is shown by coronal proton density MRI **(A)**, and axial **(B)** and sagittal **(C)** T2 MRI as a basal temporal high intensity lesion *(arrows)*.

denominated PNET NOS if no definite evidence of differentiation is noted by routine light microscopic, immunohistochemical, or electron microscopic techniques, or as PNET with specified differentiation, as suggested in the proposed revision of the WHO classification.[67]

Neuroimaging of cerebral PNET often reveals a large hemispheric mass with calcification or cyst, occasional hemorrhage, but with variable edema[2,5,19,33] (Figs. 7-28 and 7-29). CT may demonstrate a homogeneous isodense to hyperdense tumor or a heterogeneous mixed density tumor matrix. Iodine enhancement is common and may be homogeneous or nonuniform. The MRI appearance is variable, but the tumor matrix is often isointense or hypointense on T1 images and isointense or hypointense with surrounding hyperintense edema on proton density and T2 images (Fig. 7-29). Gadolinium enhancement is common. After surgical biopsy or excision, combined chemotherapy and radiotherapy is the standard treatment for PNET.[36,38]

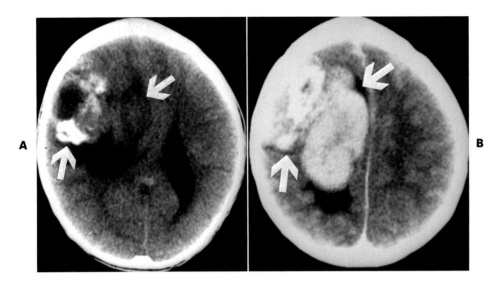

Fig. 7-28   Frontal cerebral PNET *(arrows)* demonstrated by precontrast **(A)** and postcontrast **(B)** CT as a mixed density, calcified, and markedly enhancing mass.

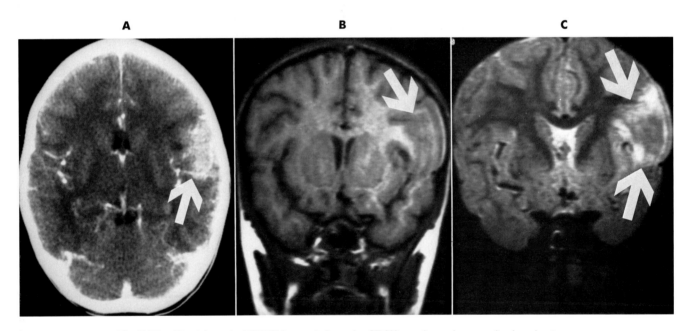

Fig. 7-29   Frontal cerebral PNET *(arrows)* shown by CT **(A)** as a hyperdense and enhancing tumor. **B,** On coronal T1 MRI the tumor is isointense to hypointense, whereas on coronal T2 MRI **(C)** the PNET shows central isointensity to hypointensity with surrounding hyperintensity.

MENINGEAL AND MELANOCYTIC TUMORS

The coverings, or meninges, of the CNS are divided into outer and inner layers.[67,68] The outer layer, the pachymeninges or dura mater, is a tough fibrous connective tissue sheath probably derived embryologically from prechordal plate mesenchyme and somatic segmented mesoderm. It forms a sac distinct from the vertebral column around the spinal cord and proximal nerve roots, fusing with the periosteum of the vertebrae at the intervertebral foramina and foramen magnum. In the cranial cavity the dura mater also serves as the periosteum of the inner surface of the bones forming the cranial cavity. Folds of the dura mater form the falx cerebri and tentorium cerebelli and provide conduits for the venous sinuses.

The inner layer, the leptomeninges, is composed of an outer arachnoid membrane and an inner pia mater. Together these form the boundaries of the subarachnoid space. The leptomeninges are in part derived embryologically from the neural crest and in part from the mesoderm. The pia mater closely invests the surface of the entire neuraxis and follows the contours of all of the sulci and fissures, as well as extending along the penetrating blood vessels. The arachnoid membrane loosely invests the inner surface of the dura and passes over the surface contours of the brain, forming local expansions of the subarachnoid space, the subarachnoid cisterns. The subarachnoid space, containing blood vessels and cerebrospinal fluid, is traversed by loose trabeculae of leptomeningeal connective tissue. Similar leptomeningeal tissue, more or less closely in communication with the subarachnoid space, forms the glomus and stroma of the choroid plexuses and a sheath around the larger penetrating blood vessels, the Virchow-Robin space. The arachnoid villi, or granulations, are local modifications of the leptomeninges along the tributary veins of the venous sinuses. These provide the mechanism of drainage of CSF from the subarachnoid space into the venous sinuses. The leptomeninges also contain a population of melanocytes, generally most numerous in dark-skinned individuals and at the base of the brain in structures such as the surfaces of the optic nerves and the medulla.

Primary neoplasms of the meninges are classified as meningiomas, meningeal sarcomatous tumors, and primary melanocytic tumors.[67,68] The meninges, particularly the leptomeninges, are most commonly involved secondarily by neoplastic processes such as tumor seeding, hematopoietic tumors, or tumors of adjacent structures, such as nerve root, pituitary, or pineal gland tumors. Other tumor types such as gliomas may rarely occur as primary meningeal tumors, presumedly originating in embryonic rests. These must be distinguished from subarachnoid seeding from primary intraparenchymal brain tumors.

The name *meningioma* is applied to the relatively common but histologically diverse soft tissue neoplasms arising in the meninges. Although occurring frequently in parafalcine locations, meningiomas may occur at any location within the cranial cavity and spinal canal or even arise as extracranial soft tissue masses.[67,68] Tumors arising

within the CNS parenchyma or in the ventricular system presumedly arise from the perivascular meningeal connective tissue sleeves or the meningeal core of the choroid plexus, respectively. Although more common in middle-aged adults, meningiomas may occur in children, frequently in the setting of an underlying disease such as neurofibromatosis or previous irradiation, and are more apt to behave in a malignant fashion.[16,55,66,67]

Meningiomas display a wide variety of histological appearances, including epithelial, mesenchymal, and secretory patterns, presumedly reflecting the multiple functions performed by normal arachnoidal cells (also called meningothelial cells or meningocytes).[67,68] Meningiomas are frequently calcified, often in the form of small sandlike granules (psammoma bodies) and may be highly vascular (Figs. 7-30 and 7-31). The histological subtypes have been traditionally grouped into the following categories: meningothelial or syncytial (emphasizing epithelial features), fibrous or fibroblastic (emphasizing mesenchymal features), transitional or mixed, psammomatous (heavily calcified), angiomatous (highly vascular), and papillary. Subcategories of meningiomas include those rich in lipid (lipoblastic or lipomatous meningiomas), mucopolysaccharide ground substances or other proteinaceous secretory materials (microcystic or secretory meningiomas), or macrophages (xanthomatous meningioma). Occasionally, meningiomas form bone, cartilage, or melanized cells. In addition, an angioblastic form has been recognized, although some if not all of this variant may be identical to the hemangiopericytomas seen in soft tissues elsewhere in the body.

Most of the histological variants have no particular prognostic significance and are designated simply as *meningioma NOS* in the proposed revision of the WHO classification, although some forms are more common in particular locations (for example, psammomatous meningioma occurring at the foramen magnum).[67] Both the angioblastic meningiomas and the papillary variants, however, have shown a tendency to more frequent and rapid recurrence and a greater propensity to form distant metastases, and are thus recognized as discrete WHO subtypes. In addition to the demonstration of CNS parenchymal invasion, the findings of increased mitotic activity, excessive pleomorphism, and necrosis have also been associated with more malignant clinical behavior and are used as criteria for the diagnosis of anaplastic meningioma.

Sarcomatous tumors of the meninges are rare but have developed in preexisting meningiomas and, less commonly, have arisen as primary malignant tumors.[67,68] In the former case the pathological features sometimes overlap with those of anaplastic meningioma and may develop over time in a meningioma with typical benign features in the initial stages. Primary malignant tumors are more common in children than in adults and have usually been reported in the setting of antecedent irradiation for a primary CNS or pericranial tumor.[16,55,66]

Meningeal sarcomas are generally massive circumscribed lesions, may contain areas of hemorrhage, necrosis,

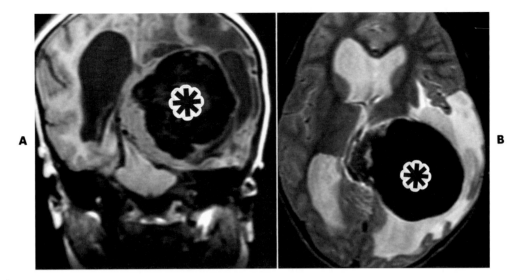

Fig. 7-30   Calcified cerebral meningioma *(asterisks)* shown by coronal T1 **(A)** and axial T2 **(B)** MRI as a huge isointense to hypointense tumor centered about the left trigone with surrounding T1 hypointense and T2 hyperintense edema.

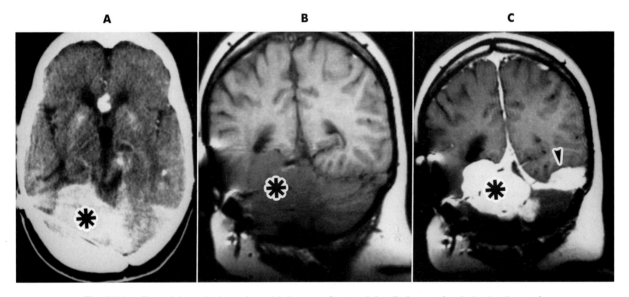

Fig. 7-31   Tentorial meningioma *(asterisks)* years after cranial radiotherapy for thalamic glioma. **A,** Contrast-enhanced CT shows marked iodine enhancement about the tentorium. Midline frontal, left thalamic, left temporal, and bilateral basal ganglia calcifications are also evident. Coronal T1 MRI images before **(B)** and after **(C)** gadolinium administration show isointense to hypointense tumor with marked enhancement. There are large supratentorial and infratentorial tumor components *(asterisks)* on the right with a smaller supratentorial component *(black arrowhead)* on the left and bilateral transverse sinus involvement.

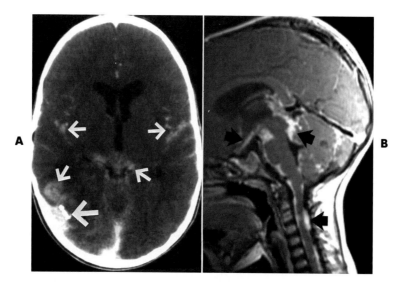

Fig. 7-32   Meningeal sarcomatosis shown by contrast-enhanced CT **(A)** as a calcified, enhancing right temporooccipital mass *(large white arrow)* with extensive intracranial enhancement *(small white arrows)*. **B,** Craniospinal MRI shows extensive gadolinium enhancement *(black arrows)* consistent with disseminated or multifocal tumor.

or cyst formation, and may disseminate in the subarachnoid space or form distant metastases (Fig. 7-32). Most are fibrosarcomas or poorly differentiated pleomorphic sarcomas with few characteristic features and are termed *meningeal sarcoma NOS* in the proposed revision.[67] Other variants of sarcoma with cartilaginous, myxoid, bony, or muscular components are named according to the predominant component. A diffuse form presenting as a widely disseminated subarachnoid sarcoma, *primary meningeal sarcomatosis,* is extremely rare but is most common in infants or children (Fig. 7-32).

In accordance with the embryological origin of melanin-producing cells in the neural crest, several tumors of presumed neural crest derivation, including some meningiomas and nerve sheath tumors, may exhibit the capacity to form melanin. Such tumors, referred to as *melanocytic meningiomas,* or *schwannomas,* are generally similar to their non–melanin producing counterparts.[67,68] The leptomeninges, however, normally contain a population of melanin-producing cells, the melanocytes. Such cells occasionally give rise to primary leptomeningeal melanocytic tumors analogous to melanocytic tumors arising in the skin or other tissues. *Malignant melanoma* is the most common form. It arises as a solitary meningeal nodule and shows rapid growth with diffuse spread in the subarachnoid spaces. The possibility that the leptomeningeal melanoma is a metastasis from a systemic primary may be difficult to exclude, particularly if the leptomeningeal tumor produces systemic metastases. Tumors with benign cytological features and lacking evidence of mitotic activity or rapid growth have been termed *melanocytomas* and may arise as solitary or multiple leptomeningeal or intraparenchymal

growths.[67] Such lesions are associated with pigmented cutaneous nevi or with neurocutaneous syndromes in a quarter of the cases (see Chapter 8).

Neuroimaging of meningioma often demonstrates a well-defined extracerebral or intraventricular mass with calcification and lytic or blastic bony involvement[5,19,27,73] (Figs. 7-30 and 7-31). The mass is usually isodense or hyperdense on CT. MRI usually demonstrates T1 isointensity to hypointensity and p/T2 isointensity to hyperintensity or occasional hypointensity (Figs. 7-30 and 7-31). Prominent iodine or gadolinium enhancement is common. Intrinsic punctuate, nodular, or linear low intensities may be seen with MRI and correlate with calcification or vascularity. A sharp interface with brain is often apparent by MRI and represents either CSF, edema, vascularization, or dural thickening. Meningeal sarcomatous tumors demonstrate a variety of findings including CT isodensity to hyperdensity and iodine enhancement plus T1 isointensity to hypointensity and p/T2 isointensity to hyperintensity or hypointensity and gadolinium enhancement by MRI (Fig. 7-32; see Posterior Fossa discussion). Cystic or necrotic components may appear with ring enhancement and edema. Melanin-containing tumors may be suspected by CT hyperdensity or by T1 hyperintensity and p/T2 hyperintensity or hypointensity on MRI depending on the concentration of melanin and the presence or absence of hemorrhage (see Posterior Fossa discussion). Sarcomas arising outside but secondarily involving the CNS are discussed and described in the section Parameningeal Tumors. Surgical excision is the primary mode of treatment for meningioma, whereas combined radiotherapy and chemotherapy is usually required for more malignant forms.[36,38]

TUMORS OF NERVE SHEATH CELLS

This group of tumors is discussed more fully in the section Posterior Fossa Tumors and also in Chapter 8, Neurocutaneous Syndromes.

MALIGNANT LYMPHOMAS

Although the CNS, unlike other systems, lacks a normal network of lymphatic channels and lymphoid structures and has traditionally been considered a site of immunological privilege, modern immunological techniques have increasingly demonstrated immunological components and functions in the CNS.[67,68] One particular normal cell component, the microglial cell, which colonizes the CNS during fetal development, is most likely a derivative of the mononuclear-phagocyte system analogous to the histiocyte in non-CNS tissue, although its function is not yet known.

Involvement of the CNS secondarily by lymphoid or other hematological malignancies is relatively common (see Metastatic Tumors). Primary CNS lymphoid malignancies, however, are rare, occur chiefly in the setting of an underlying congenital or acquired immunodeficiency disorder, and are most common in adults.* Although originally termed *reticulum cell sarcomas* or *microgliomas* and thought to represent the neoplastic counterpart of the microglial cell, primary malignant lymphomas of the CNS are now generally classified with the systemic non-Hodgkin's lymphomas (NHL) and, in common with the systemic forms of these neoplasms, can usually be demonstrated to express evidence of B-cell origin. Because of the different classification schemes for NHL in use worldwide, the WHO has recommended using local schemes to subdivide this group.[67]

Primary malignant lymphomas most commonly occur in the cerebrum and may be solitary or multifocal, circumscribed or infiltrative. Microscopic infiltration commonly follows the course of blood vessels and may mimic the infiltrative patterns of gliomas. Hemorrhage and necrosis may occur, further mimicking the appearance of malignant glial neoplasms. A characteristic feature is prominent perivascular proliferation of connective tissue (reticulin), that may sometimes be massive, thus the term *reticulum cell sarcoma*. Most lymphomas grow rapidly and diffusely and may spread into the subarachnoid space or, occasionally, form remote metastases. Most recur despite being radiosensitive. Common sites of involvement include the basal ganglia, corpus callosum, periventricular white matter, cerebellar vermis, and cerebral cortex. CT often demonstrates isodense or hyperdense lesions with moderate to marked homogeneous iodine enhancement.[5,19,40,48,72] Gyral or meningeal enhancement may also be seen. Rim or ring enhancement with central hypodensity (central necrotic tumor) may be seen especially in patients with AIDS or those who have received transplants and may be difficult to distinguish from abscess. Lymphoma may show T1 isointensity to hypointensity and p/T2 isointensity to hypointen-

sity with surrounding hyperintensity[5,19,72] (Fig. 7-33). Occasionally the lesions are primarily hypodense by CT with T1 hypointensity and p/T2 hyperintensity. Gadolinium enhancement may be homogeneous or heterogeneous, and there may be minimal or no mass effect and only mild edema.

TUMORS OF BLOOD VESSEL ORIGIN

Although tumors of blood vessel origin are made up of hemangioblastoma, hemangiopericytoma, and angiosarcoma according to the revised WHO classification,[67] these true neoplasms of blood vessel origin are exceedingly rare in childhood and are discussed primarily in the section Posterior Fossa Tumors. Cavernous angiomas are common vascular malformations (see Chapter 6) that may mimic vascular-origin tumors and intratumoral hemorrhage. This is particularly a problem when the angioma causes acute or subacute hemorrhage with surrounding edema.[34,51,57]

GERM CELL, MALFORMATIVE, AND NEUROENDOCRINE-ORIGIN TUMORS

Since most germ cell, malformative, and neuroendocrine-origin tumors occur along the midline about the third ventricle and within the posterior fossa, detailed discussions and illustrations are presented in respective sections.

LOCAL EXTENSION FROM REGIONAL TUMORS

The CNS and its meningeal coverings and the PNS reside in direct contact or in proximity to virtually all body structures, representing derivatives of all three germ cell layers, from skin to bone to gastrointestinal tract. Although natural barriers are provided by the pachymeninges and other connective tissue coverings, these barriers may be broached in various ways depending on the biology of the neoplasm. Neoplasms arising in any of these structures may extend directly to involve components of either the PNS or the CNS and may produce damage by compression or by invasion. Tumors involving the CNS, for example, may arise from the bones of the skull or vertebral column or may enter the CNS via the neural or vascular foramina. Tumors involving the PNS constitute virtually all known neoplasms.[67] These are discussed in the section on Parameningeal Tumors and in Chapter 10, Acquired Abnormalities of the Spine and Spinal Neuraxis.

METASTATIC TUMORS

In addition to involvement by direct extension the CNS and PNS may be involved by distant metastasis. These may arise from neoplasms originating within the CNS or PNS or from neoplasms originating primarily in other tissues.[67,68] As discussed in other sections, some primary CNS neoplasms, especially PNETs, malignant gliomas, and germ cell tumors, show a propensity to disseminate in the subarachnoid space. These may secondarily invade the CNS at these distant sites where their characteristics are generally similar to those at the site of origin.

Most metastatic neoplasms arising from non-CNS pri-

*References 16, 31, 32, 37, 62, 64, 67, 68.

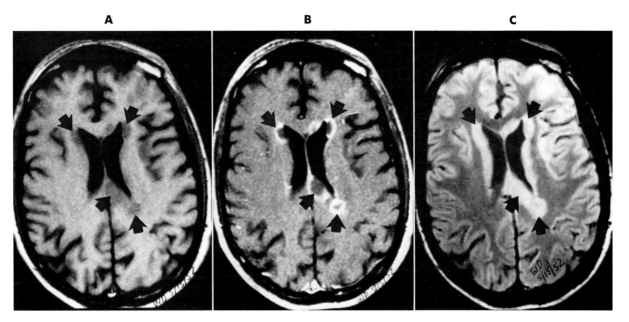

Fig. 7-33 Cerebral lymphoma *(arrows)* in AIDS. **A,** Axial T1 MRI shows multiple low intensity nodular lesions including involvement of the corpus callosum. **B,** Gadolinium T1 axial MRI shows ring enhancement. Some of the lesions are isointense to hyperintense, whereas others are isointense to hypointense on axial p MRI **(C).** (Courtesy J. Suojanen, M.D., New England Deaconess Hospital, Boston.)

mary tumors are blood borne, although the subarachnoid space provides another mechanism for further spread of tumors reaching the CNS originally by direct extension. Other than CNS involvement by systemic neoplasia such as leukemia, histiocytosis, or neuroblastoma, hematogenous metastases from a distant primary tumor is less frequent in childhood than in adulthood.[16,67,68] The primary neoplasm is usually a sarcoma, commonly osteosarcoma or rhabdomyosarcoma. With improved treatment of Wilms' tumor, CNS metastases are now exceedingly rare. CT or MRI may demonstrate single or multiple masses (Fig. 7-34), often enhancing, but with variable edema.[5,19]

Leukemia

In childhood leukemia, as with any CNS malignancy, it is important to distinguish CNS involvement from treatment effects.[38] Although leptomeningeal leukemic infiltration is common (acute lymphoblastic forms), brain infiltration via perivascular (Virchow-Robin) spaces is unusual. Meningeal leukemia is infrequently demonstrated by CT or MRI. Ventricular and subarachnoid space dilatation may be seen, but meningeal enhancement or meningeal-based masses are rare. Leukemic masses (chloroma) may be encountered more often with acute myeloblastic leukemia[44,52,79] (Figs. 7-35 and 7-36). Leukemic masses are hypercellular and often appear similar to lymphoma, including CT isodensity to hyperdensity, T1 isointensity to hypointensity, and p/T2 isointensity to hypointensity or occasional hyperintensity.[5,19] Marked iodine or gadolinium enhancement is expected. CNS disease in leukemia may be related to

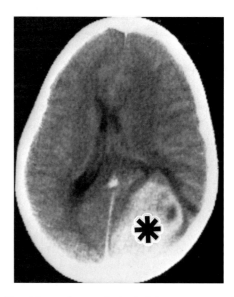

Fig. 7-34 Metastatic cerebral rhabdomyosarcoma *(asterisk)* shown by CT as an isodense to hyperdense enhancing mass with surrounding low density edema.

infarction, hemorrhage, infection, or complications and sequelae of chemotherapy or radiotherapy.[36] Perivascular or intravascular leukemic involvement with occlusion may produce edema, infarction, or hemorrhage. Hemorrhage may also result from thrombocytopenia. Cerebral venous or dural sinus thrombosis with hemorrhagic infarction may

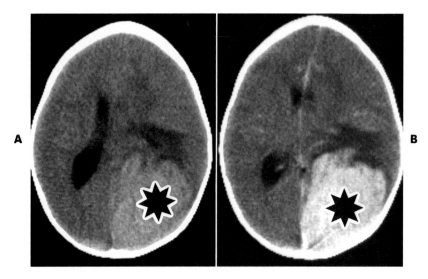

Fig. 7-35   Cerebral chloroma *(star)* shown by precontrast **(A)** and postcontrast **(B)** CT as an isodense to hyperdense enhancing mass with adjacent low density edema.

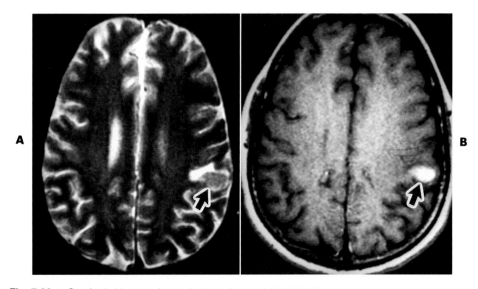

Fig. 7-36   Cerebral chloroma *(arrows)* shown by axial T2 MRI **(A)** as an isointense to hypointense mass with surrounding hyperintensity. Marked gadolinium enhancement is demonstrated on the axial T1 MRI **(B)**. (Courtesy M. Mantello, M.D., Boston.)

also occur, particularly as a complication of L-asparaginase therapy (see Chapter 6).

Histiocytosis

Histiocytosis (Langerhans' cell) is a reticuloendothelial disorder of unknown origin with tissue infiltration by reticulum cells, histiocytes, plasma cells, and leukocytes. The involvement may be isolated (eosinophilic granuloma) or associated with systemic involvement (malignant histiocytosis). Intracranial involvement is usually associated with systemic disease, and the findings may include hydroceph-

alus, demyelination, and single or multiple masses involving the optic and hypothalamic region (diabetes insipidus) or, rarely, the cerebellum or spinal cord.[5,13,19] Similar to other hypercellular neoplasms, histiocytosis often appears isodense to hyperdense by CT and enhances with iodine. These are T1 isointense to hypointense and enhance with gadolinium, and are p/T2 isohypointense often with surrounding hyperintensity (see Third Ventricular and Parameningeal sections). After tissue confirmation or tumor excision, radiotherapy, chemotherapy, or both are standard treatment for this pseudoneoplastic process.[38]

UNCLASSIFIED TUMORS

Despite the use of routine and novel methods of tissue analysis using light microscopy, electron microscopy, immunohistochemistry, cytogenetics, and other techniques, a small number of tumors still remain unclassified, whether through limitations of sampling or tissue preservation or because of the unique manifestations of neoplasia.[67] Whereas some tumors can be eventually grouped with comparable reported cases into newly defined groups, such as the recently described desmoplastic ganglioglioma of infancy, others remain elusive and merit a descriptive category while awaiting further definition.

REFERENCES
Cerebral hemispheric tumors

1. Altman N: MR and CT of gangliocytoma, *AJNR* 9:917, 1988.
2. Altman N, Fitz C, Chuang S, et al: Radiology of primitive neuroectodermal tumors in children, *AJNR* 6:15, 1985.
3. Ambrosino M, Hernanzschulman M, Genieser N, et al: Brain tumors in infants less than a year of age, *Pediatr Radiol* 19:1:6, 1988.
4. Armstrong E, Harwood-Nash D, Fitz C, et al: CT of neuroblastomas and ganglioneuromas in children, *AJNR* 3:401, 1982.
5. Barkovich A: *Pediatric neuroimaging,* New York, 1990, Raven.
6. Barnes P, Lester P, Yamanashi, et al: MR imaging in childhood intracranial masses, *Magn Res Imaging* 4:41, 1986.
7. Becker L: An appraisal of the WHO classification of tumors of the CNS, *Cancer* 56:1858, 1985.
8. Berger M, Kincaid J, Ojemann G, et al: Brain mapping techniques to maximize resection, safety, and seizure control in children with brain tumors, *Neurosurgery* 25:786, 1989.
9. Bird C, Drayer B, Medina M, et al: Gd-DTPA enhanced MR imaging in pediatric patients after brain tumor resection, *Radiology* 169:123, 1988.
10. Brooks B, King D, El Gammal T, et al: MR imaging in intractable complex partial seizures, *AJNR* 11:93, 1990.
11. Burger P: Malignant astrocytic neoplasm: classification, pathology, anatomy, and response to therapy, *Semin Oncol* 13:16, 1986.
12. Burke JW, Podrasky AE, Bradley WG Jr: Meninges: benign postoperative enhancement on MR images, *Radiology* 174:1:99, 1990.
13. Castel J, Diard F, Chateil J, et al: Value of CT in histiocytosis X of the base of the skull in children, *Ann Radiol* 31:3:151, 1988.
14. Castillo M, Davis P, Takei Y, et al: Intracranial ganglioglioma: MR and CT, *AJNR* 11:109, 1990.
15. Coates T, Hinshaw D, Peckman N, et al: Pediatric choroid plexus neoplasms: MR, CT, and pathology, *Radiology* 173:81, 1989.
16. Cohen M, Duffner P: Tumors of the brain and spinal cord, In Swaiman K: *Pediatric neurology,* St Louis, 1989, Mosby–Year Book.
17. Constine L, Konski A, Ekholm S, et al: Adverse effects of brain irradiation correlated with MR and CT, *Int J Radiat Oncol Biol Phys* 13:88, 1987.
18. Davis D, Kelly P, Marsh W, et al: Computer-assisted stereotactic biopsy of intracranial lesions in pediatric patients, *Pediatr Neurosci* 14:31, 1988.
19. Davis P: Tumors of the brain, In Cohen M, Edwards M, editors: *MR imaging of children,* Philadelphia, 1990, BC Decker.
20. Davis P, Wichman R, Takei Y, et al: Primary cerebral neuroblastoma, *AJNR* 11:115, 1990.
21. Dean B, Drayer B, Bird C, et al: Gliomas: classification with MRI, *Radiology* 174:411, 1990.
22. Destian S, Sze G, Krol G, et al: MR imaging of hemorrhagic intracranial neoplasms, *AJNR* 9:115, 1988.
23. Dooms G, Hect S, Brant-Zawadski M, et al: Brain radiation lesions: MR imaging, *Radiology* 158:149, 1986.
24. Dorne H, O'Gorman A, Melanson D: CT of intracranial gangliogliomas, *AJNR* 7:281, 1986.
25. Earnest F, Kelly P, Scheithauer B, et al: Cerebral astrocytomas, histopathologic correlation of MR and CT contrast enhancement with stereotactic biopsy, *Radiology* 166:823, 1988.

26. Ellenbogen R, Winston K, Kupsky W: Tumors of the choroid plexus in children, *Neurosurgery* 25:327, 1989.
27. Elster A, Challa V, Gilbert T, et al: Meningiomas: MR, *Radiology* 170:857, 1989.
28. Elster A, DiPersio DA: Cranial postoperative site: assessment with contrast-enhanced MR imaging, *Radiology* 174:1:93, 1990.
29. Elster A, Moody D, Ball M, et al: Is Gd-DTPA required for routine cranial MR imaging? *Radiology* 173:231, 1989.
30. Elster A, Rieser G: Gd-DTPA enhanced cranial MR imaging in children: initial experience and recommendations, *AJNR* 10:1027, 1989.
31. Epstein L, DiCarlo F, Joshi V, et al: Primary lymphoma of the CNS in children with AIDS, *Pediatrics* 82:355, 1988.
32. Federle M: A radiologist looks at AIDS, *Radiology* 166:553, 1988.
33. Figeroa R, el Gammal T, Brooks B, et al: MR in primitive neuroectodermal tumors, *J Comput Assist Tomogr* 13:773, 1989.
34. Gomori JM, Grossman RI, Goldberg HI, et al: Occult cerebral vascular malformations: high-field MR imaging, *Radiology* 158:707, 1986.
35. Halbach V, Higashida RT, Hieshima GB, et al: Venography and venous pressure monitoring in dural sinus meningiomas, *AJNR* 10:6:1209, 1989.
36. Halperin E, Kun L, Constine L, Tarbell N: *Pediatric radiation oncology,* New York, 1989, Raven.
37. Haney P, Yale-Loehr A, Nussbaum A, et al: Imaging of infants and children with AIDS, *AJR* 152:1033, 1989.
38. Heideman R, Packer R, Albright L, et al: Tumors of the central nervous system. In Pizzo P, Poplack D, editors: *Pediatric oncology,* Philadelphia, 1989, JB Lippincott.
39. Heinz E, Heinz T, Radtke R, et al: Efficacy of MR vs. CT in epilepsy, *AJNR* 9:1123, 1988.
40. Jack C, O'Neill B, Banks P, Reese D: CNS lymphoma: histologic types and CT appearance, *Radiology* 167:211, 1988.
41. Jack C, Sharbrough F, Marsh W: MR imaging for quantitative evaluation of resection for temporal lobe epilepsy, *Radiology* 169:463, 1988.
42. Jelinek J, Smirniotopoulos J, Parisi J, et al: Lateral ventricular neoplasms of the brain, *AJNR* 11:567, 1990.
43. Johnson P, Hunt S, Drayer B: Human cerebral gliomas: correlation of postmortem MR imaging and neuropathologic findings, *Radiology* 170:211, 1989.
44. Kao S, Yuh W, Sato Y, et al: Intracranial granulocytic sarcoma (chloroma): MR findings, *J Comput Assist Tomogr* 11:938, 1987.
45. Kelly P, Daumas-Duport C, Kispent D, et al: Imaging-based stereotaxic serial biopsies in untreated intracranial glial neoplasms, *J Neurosurg* 66:865, 1987.
46. Krol G, Galicich J, Arbit E, et al: Preoperative localization of intracranial lesions on MR, *Am J Neuroradiol* 9:513, 1988.
47. Latchaw R, L'Heureux P, Young G, et al: Neuroblastoma as CNS disease, *AJNR* 3:623, 1982.
48. Lee Y, Bruner J, Van Tassel P, et al: Primary CNS lymphoma: CT and pathologic correlation, *AJNR* 7:599, 1986.
49. Lee Y, Van Tassel P: Intracranial oligodendrogliomas, *AJR* 152:361, 1989.
50. Lee Y, Van Tassel P, Bruner J, et al: Juvenile pilocystic astrocytomas: CT and MR, *AJNR* 10:363, 1989.
51. Lemme-Plaghos L, Kucharczyk W, Brant-Zawadzki M, et al: MRI of angiographically occult vascular malformations, *AJR* 146:1223, 1986.
52. Leonard K, Mamourian A: MR of intracranial chloromas, *AJNR* 10:567, 1989.
53. Loeffler J, Rossitch E, Siddon R, et al: Stereotactic radiosurgery in treatment of intracranial malformations and tumors in children, *Pediatrics* 85:774, 1990.
54. Menkes J: *Textbook of child neurology,* ed 3, Philadelphia, 1985, Lea & Febiger.
55. Moss S, Roskwald G, Chou S, et al: Radiation-induced meningiomas in pediatric patients, *Neurosurgery* 22:758, 1988.
56. Naidich T, Quencer R, editors: *Clinical neurosonography,* New York, 1987, Springer-Verlag.
57. New PFJ, Ojemann RG, Davis KR, et al: MR and CT of occult vascular malformations of the brain, *AJNR* 7:771, 1986.
58. Packer R, Sutton L, Atkins T, et al: Cognitive function in children receiving whole-brain radiotherapy and chemotherapy, *J Neurosurg* 70:707, 1989.

59. Pederson H, Gjerris F, Klinken L: Malignancy criteria in CT of primary supratentorial tumors in infancy and childhood, *Neuroradiology* 31:24, 1989.
60. Powers T, Partain C, Kessler R, et al: CNS lesions in pediatric patients: Gd-DTPA enhanced MR imaging, *Radiology* 169:723, 1988.
61. Prados M, Levin V: Malignant supratentorial gliomas of childhood, *Pediatr Neurosci* 13:144, 1987.
62. Price D, Inglese C, Jacobs J, et al: Pediatric AIDS: neuroradiologic and neurodevelopmental findings, *Pediatr Radiol* 18:445, 1988.
63. Radkowski M, Naidich T, Tomita T, et al: Neonatal brain tumors: CT and MR, *J Comput Assist Tomogr* 12:10, 1988.
64. Ramsey R, Geremia G: CNS complications of AIDS: CT and MR findings, *AJR* 151:449, 1988.
65. Rippe DJ, Boyko OB, Friedman HS, et al: Gd-DTPA enhanced MR imaging of leptomeningeal spread of intracranial CNS tumor in children, *AJNR* 11:329, 1990.
66. Ron E, Modan B, Boice J, et al: Tumors of the brain and nervous system after radiotherapy in childhood, *N Engl J Med* 319:1033, 1988.
67. Rorke L, Gilles F, Davis R, et al: Revision of the WHO classification of brain tumors for childhood, *Cancer* 56:1869, 1985.
68. Russell D, Rubenstein L: *Pathology of tumors of the nervous system,* ed 4, Baltimore, 1977, Williams & Wilkins.
69. Sage M: Blood-brain barrier: phenomenon of increasing importance to the imaging clinician, *AJR* 138:887, 1982.
70. Schad L, Boesecke R, Schlegal W, et al: Three-dimensional image correlation of CT, MR, and PET in radiotherapy treatment planning of brain tumors, *J Comput Assist Tomogr* 11:948, 1987.
71. Schmitt H, Wowra B, Sturm V: The stereotactic approach to focal lesions in the deep brain of children and adolescents, *Brain Dev* 10:305, 1988.
72. Schwaighofer B, Hesselink J, Press G, et al: Primary intracranial lymphoma: MR, *AJNR* 10:725, 1989.
73. Spagnoli M, Goldberg H, Grossman R, et al: Intracranial meningiomas: MR imaging, *Radiology* 161:369, 1986.
74. Spoto G, Press G, Hesselink J, et al: Intracranial ependymoma and subependymoma, *AJNR* 11:83, 1990.
75. Storrs B: Stereotactic procedures in children. In McLaurin R, Schut L, Venes J, et al, editors: *Pediatric neurosurgery,* ed 2, Philadelphia, 1987, WB Saunders.
76. Sze G, Krol G, Olsen W, et al: Hemorrhagic neoplasms: MR mimics of occult vascular malformation, *AJR* 149:1223, 1987.
77. Sze G, Soletsky S, Bronen R, et al: MR imaging of the cranial meninges, *AJNR* 10:965, 1989.
78. Triulzi F, Franceschi M, Fazio F, et al: Nonrefractory temporal lobe epilepsy: 1.5 T MR imaging, *Radiology* 166:181, 1988.
79. Wang AM, Lin JCT, Power TC, et al: Chloroma of cerebellum, tentorium, and occipital bone in acute myelogenous leukemia, *Neuroradiology* 29:590, 1987.
80. Wechslerjentzsch K, Witt J, Fitz C, et al: Unrespectable gliomas in children—tumor volume response to radiation therapy, *Radiology* 169:237, 1988.
81. Zagzag D, Goldenberg M, Brem S: Angiogenesis and blood-brain barrier breakdown modulate CT contrast enhancement: an experimental study in a rabbit brain tumor model, *AJNR* 10:529, 1989.
82. Zhang J, Levesque MF, Wilson CL, et al: Multimodality imaging of brain structures for stereotactic surgery, *Radiology* 175:435, 1990.

Tumors about the third ventricle

Tumors about the third ventricle (see box on p. 235) may be subdivided into perisellar and anterior third ventricular tumors, pineal region and posterior third ventricular tumors, and paraventricular (for example, thalamic), intraventricular, and interventricular tumors.[37,38,46] Symptoms and signs may arise as a result of increased intracranial pressure from obstructive hydrocephalus. Neuroendocrine presentations with anterior pituitary-hypothalamic involvement include hypopituitarism (for example, growth retardation, delayed puberty), or, rarely, hyperpituitarism (for example, gigantism, galactorrhea, hypogonadism). Hypothalamic and neurohypophyseal dysfunction may be manifested as precocious puberty, diencephalic syndrome, or diabetes insipidus.[1,7,9]

Involvement of the optic pathway results in impaired visual acuity and visual field defects and is common in neurofibromatosis.[13] Ocular movement and pupillary abnormalities may be present including cranial neuropathy (III to VI), Horner's syndrome, Parinaud's syndrome, or nystagmus.[9] Common neoplastic processes include gliomas, germ cell neoplasms, and malformative tumors.[37,38] Less common or infrequent processes include pituitary, neuronal, pineal cell, vascular-origin, lymphomatous, or metastatic tumors. Nonneoplastic tumors often requiring differentiation are arachnoid cyst, sphenoidal encephalocele, the rare circle of Willis or vein of Galen aneurysm, granuloma (for example, tuberculous, fungal, sarcoid), arachnoiditis, or infundibulohypophysitis. Neoplasms and other processes of parameningeal origin (skull base, sinus, orbit) may invade or extend to involve this region.[41,45]

NEUROEPITHELIAL TUMORS
Glial tumors

Of the neuroepithelial tumors, *gliomas* constitute the largest group of neoplasms occurring about the third ventricle (see box on p. 235) and may arise from the optic pathways, hypothalamus, thalamus, midbrain, or walls of the third ventricle.[37,38] The optic pathway and hypothalamus are the most common sites of origin. The pilocytic cell subtype of *astrocytoma* characteristically occurs during childhood, often with slow infiltrative growth, and is more commonly solid than cystic in this region.[23] Other astrocytic subtypes or mixed subtypes commonly occur in this region also. Ependymoma, oligodendroglioma, and choroid plexus tumor[39] are somewhat unusual in this region, although mixed glial neoplasia is often encountered.[37] Imaging cannot reliably distinguish one tumor type from another, and there is significant overlap in imaging features for lower-grade versus higher-grade glial neoplasms. The subependymal giant cell tumor of tuberous sclerosis often demonstrates astrocytic and neuronal differentiation, is commonly calcified, and is usually situated near the foramen of Monro, producing asymmetrical obstructive hydrocephalus (see Chapter 8).

Neoplasms arising from the optic pathway constitute one of the common perisellar tumors of childhood.[13,32,37] Exclusively intraorbital lesions include hamartomas, nerve sheath hypertrophy or hyperplasia, or low-grade astrocytomas. Tumors rising from the chiasm and optic tracts may range from hamartomas or low-grade astrocytomas to anaplastic astrocytomas. Optic pathway tumors are commonly associated with neurofibromatosis 1 (see Chapter 8) and may be asymptomatic when discovered by routine screening.[13,32] An exclusively intraorbital optic glioma

TUMORS ABOUT THE THIRD VENTRICLE

ANTERIOR THIRD VENTRICULAR (PERISELLAR)

1. Glial tumors (IA)*
   a. Astrocytic (optic, hypothalamic)
   b. Other gliomas or mixed gliomas

2. Malformative tumors (VII)
   a. Craniopharyngioma
   b. Rathke's cleft cyst
   c. Cyst NOS (not otherwise specified)
   d. Lipoma
   e. Dermoid-epidermoid cyst
   f. Hamartoma

3. Germ cell tumors (VI)
   a. Germinoma
   b. Teratoma
   c. Other

4. Tumors of neuroendocrine origin (VIII)
   a. Pituitary adenoma

5. Meningeal tumors (II)

6. Metastatic tumors (X)

7. Neuronal tumors (IB)
   a. Ganglioglioma

8. Lymphoma (IV)

9. Parameningeal tumors (IX)

POSTERIOR THIRD VENTRICULAR (PINEAL REGION)

1. Germ cell tumors (VI)
   a. Germinoma
   b. Teratoma
   c. Other

2. Pineal cell tumors (ID)
   a. Pineoblastoma (PNET — IC)
   b. Pineocytoma

3. Glial tumors (IA)
   a. Astrocytic
   b. Other gliomas

POSTERIOR THIRD VENTRICULAR—Cont'd

4. Malformative tumors (VII)
   a. Cyst NOS (not otherwise specified)
   b. Lipoma
   c. Hamartoma

5. Neuronal tumors (IB)
   a. Ganglioglioma

6. Meningeal tumors (II)
   a. Meningioma

7. Metastatic (X)

8. Lymphoma (IV)

9. Blood-vessel origin tumors (V)

THIRD PARAVENTRICULAR/INTRAVENTRICULAR

1. Glial tumors (IA)
   a. Astrocytic
   b. Choroid plexus tumors
   c. Other, mixed gliomas (for example, giant cell tumor)

2. Germ cell tumors (VI)
   a. Germinoma
   b. Teratoma
   c. Other

3. Malformative tumors (VII)
   a. dermoid/epidermoid cyst
   b. colloid cyst
   c. cyst NOS (not otherwise specified)
   d. hamartoma (tuberous sclerosis, neurofibromatosis)

4. Neuronal tumors (IB)
   a. Ganglioglioma

5. Pineal cell tumors (ID)

6. Metastatic tumors (X)

7. PNET (IC)

8. Lymphoma (IV)

9. Blood-vessel origin tumors (V)

*Parenthetical data following each tumor type are designations referring to the outline of the revision of the WHO classification, as presented in the box on p. 205.

rarely occurs. More often, there is intraorbital, intracanalicular, and intracranial optic nerve involvement. Glial neoplasms arising primarily within the hypothalamus also range from low-grade astrocytomas to more anaplastic forms. When only a large intracranial suprasellar mass is demonstrated, it may be difficult to distinguish a chiasmatic glioma from a hypothalamic glioma. Not only may it be difficult to distinguish hypothalamic glioma from optic chiasm glioma without other optic pathway involvement, but also it may be difficult to distinguish it from germinoma without pineal region involvement, or distinguish it from the rare hypothalamic hamartoma.

Neuroimaging of optic glioma may reveal optic nerve or chiasm expansion (Figs. 7-37 and 7-38) with extension along the optic nerves anteriorly or the optic tracts posteriorly, occasionally to the level of the lateral genicu-late bodies and rarely along the optic radiations.[1,7,32] With hypothalamic glioma, the mass or expansion is centered behind the chiasm and above or behind the infundibulum (Fig. 7-39). The tumor is usually isodense or low density by CT, isointense or low intensity by T1 MRI and isointense to hyperintense by p/T2 MRI[1,7] (Fig. 7-40). Calcification, cyst, hemorrhage, or tumor hyperdensity is unusual when compared with craniopharyngioma (calcification, cyst) or germinoma (tumor hyperdensity, hemorrhage). Enhancement by iodine or gadolinium is frequently but not invariably seen and may be homogeneous or irregular. If a nonenhancing suprasellar mass is of small dimension and confined to the hypothalamus, particularly along the tuber cinereum, a hamartoma should be suspected, especially if the manifestation is precocious puberty.[2,4,35]

Other sites of neuroepithelial or glial tumor origin or

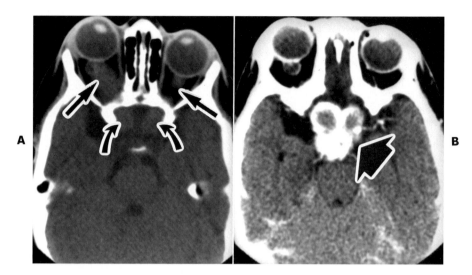

Fig. 7-37   Optic glioma demonstrated by precontrast **(A)** and postcontrast **(B)** CT with bilateral intraorbital (**A,** *straight black arrows*), intracanalicular, and intracranial (**A,** *curved black arrows*) optic nerve expansions. Marked iodine enhancement of the chiasmatic tumor is also apparent (**B,** *large black arrowhead*).

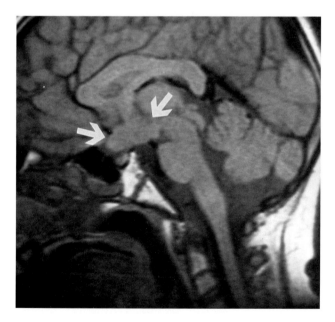

Fig. 7-38   Optic-hypothalamic glioma in NF 1 demonstrated by sagittal T1 MRI as an isointense suprasellar mass *(arrows)* involving the optic and hypothalamic structures.

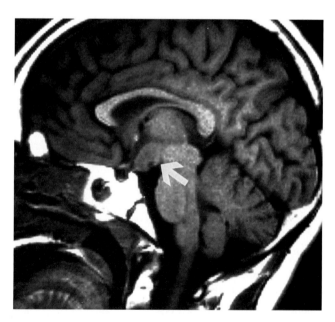

Fig. 7-39   Hypothalamic astrocytoma *(arrow)* with gelastic seizures shown by sagittal T1 MRI as an isointense to hypointense mass that is high intensity on axial p/T2 MRI.

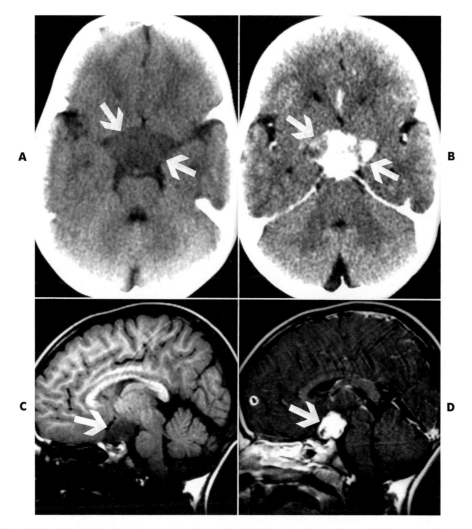

Fig. 7-40   Hypothalamic astrocytoma *(arrows)* with diencephalic syndrome. Precontrast **(A)** and postcontrast **(B)** CT images show isodense to hypodense enhancing suprasellar mass. Sagittal T1 images before **(C)** and after **(D)** gadolinium injection show hypointense enhancing tumor involving the chiasm, hypothalamus, and third ventricle with intact posterior pituitary bright spot. The tumor is high intensity on axial p/T2 MRI.

predominant involvement about the third ventricle include the thalamus, the midbrain, the walls of the third ventricle, and the foramina of Monro. The tumor may be circumscribed (for example, a tectal glioma or the giant cell tumor of tuberous sclerosis). In other cases the tumor may be infiltrative with poor margination, anatomical distortion, and extension across the midline (for example, thalamic astrocytoma). The CT density, MRI intensity, and enhancement characteristics are variable and similar to glial tumors at other sites whether low grade, anaplastic, or of mixed histology (Figs. 7-41 to 7-45). The range of findings includes signal homogeneity or heterogeneity and uniform or irregular enhancement (nodular or ringlike) with calcification, cystic or necrotic areas, hemorrhage, or edema.[1,7] Some of the latter features are seen particularly with higher-grade tumors (anaplastic glioma, glioblastoma).

Neuronal tumors

Neuronal tumors of the CNS including gangliocytoma, ganglioglioma, and their anaplastic forms may also occur about the third ventricle. Although showing a tendency for cyst formation and calcification as discussed in the previous section, these are often difficult to differentiate from glial tumors in this region (see Cerebral Hemispheric and Posterior Fossa sections).

Primary pineal cell tumors

The pineal gland or epiphysis is formed from an evagination of the dorsal surface of the embryonic neural tube at the junction of the mesencephalon and diencephalon.[27,37,38] The mature gland consists primarily of parenchymal cells (pinealocytes), which are specialized neurosecretory cells with characteristic clubbed argyrophilic

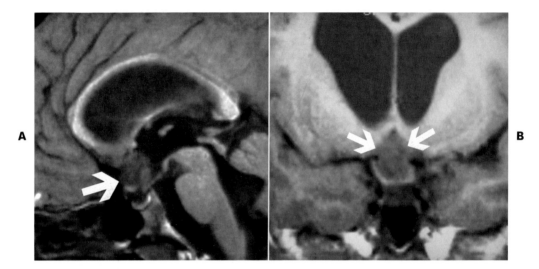

Fig. 7-41   Anterior third ventricular mixed oligodendroglioma-astrocytoma *(arrows)* shown by sagittal **(A)** and coronal **(B)** T1 MRI as a suprachiasmatic, third ventricular isointense mass that is isointense to hyperintense on axial proton density and T2 MRI.

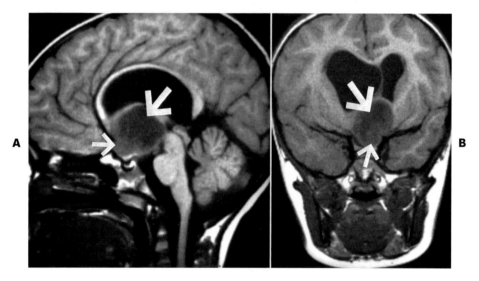

Fig. 7-42   Third ventricular astrocytoma shown by sagittal **(A)** and coronal **(B)** T1 MRI as a large suprachiasmatic and suprahypothalamic intraventricular mass with isointense solid tumor component *(small arrows)* and hypointense liquified or cystic component *(large arrows)*.

A   B   C

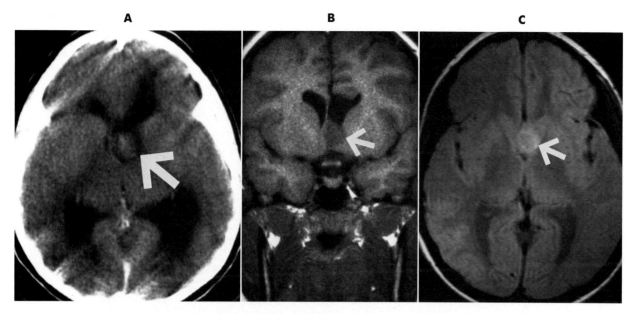

Fig. 7-43   Foramen of Monro astrocytoma *(arrows)* shown by CT **(A)** as an isodense mass at the left foramen of Monro producing asymmetrical hydrocephalus. Coronal T1 MRI **(B)** demonstrates an isointense to hypointense mass that is isointense to hyperintense on p/T2 MRI **(C)**.

processes. Pinealocytes transiently resemble photoreceptor cells during embryonic development, express the retinal S-antigen, synthesize and secrete melatonin, and may contain melanin pigment. Other components of the normal pineal gland include a stroma of blood vessels, fibrillary astrocytes, and an innervation of sympathetic nerve fibers. The ependyma-lined pineal recess of the third ventricle extends into the base of the gland, which frequently becomes calcified in later life.

Tumors of the pineal gland are rare and include a variety of types.[37,38] Germ cell tumors (see subsequent discussion), presumedly derived from germ cell rests, account for the majority of neoplasms and were referred to previously as *pinealomas,* a now obsolete term that did not distinguish germ cell neoplasms from neoplasms of pinealocytes. Neoplasms composed of cells resembling pinealocytes are divided into well-differentiated forms (pineocytoma), more common in adults, and poorly differentiated forms (pineo-blastoma), more common in children. A variety of other neoplasms has been reported including gliomas and tumors of other tissue types such as meningiomas, melanomas, or nonneoplastic cysts. These tumors are discussed under their own headings elsewhere. The proximity of the gland to the midbrain, to the third ventricular outflow and cerebral aqueduct, and to the meninges and deep cerebral veins accounts for some of the clinical manifestations of pineal tumors.[9] This location also facilitates the spread of high-grade pineal neoplasms into the ventricular system or subarachnoid space.

PINEOCYTOMAS. Pineocytomas have been reported more frequently in older adults than in children and, in contrast to pineoblastomas, have shown no sex predilection. In addition to resembling normal pinealocytes, pineocytoma cells may show evidence of either neuronal or astrocytic differentiation or both, and some tumors express retinal S-antigen or melatonin.[37,38] Pineocytomas are generally circumscribed and may be calcified. However, tumors lacking evidence of neuronal differentiation, that is, showing only pinealocytic features or pinealocytic and astrocytic features without neuronal features, resemble pineoblastomas in growth rate and malignant potential and may metastasize in the cerebrospinal fluid pathways.[37,38]

PINEOBLASTOMAS. Most pineoblastomas occur in the first decade and are more common in males. The association of pineoblastoma with bilateral retinoblastoma has been recognized (trilateral retinoblastoma), and an association with medulloblastoma has also been suggested. Because of the high cellularity and largely undifferentiated appearance, these tumors resemble medulloblastomas and PNETs occurring in other parts of the CNS. As a result the proposed revision of the WHO classification[37] classifies pineoblasto-mas with PNETs. Pineoblastomas are considered to be highly malignant neoplasms with a propensity to disseminate in the cerebrospinal fluid pathways. Neuroimaging of pineoblastoma often reveals a large lobulated pineal region mass with calcification [1,5,7,11,43] (Figs. 7-46 and 7-47). By CT the tumor matrix is often isodense to hyperdense, whereas by MRI it is isointense to hypointense on T1

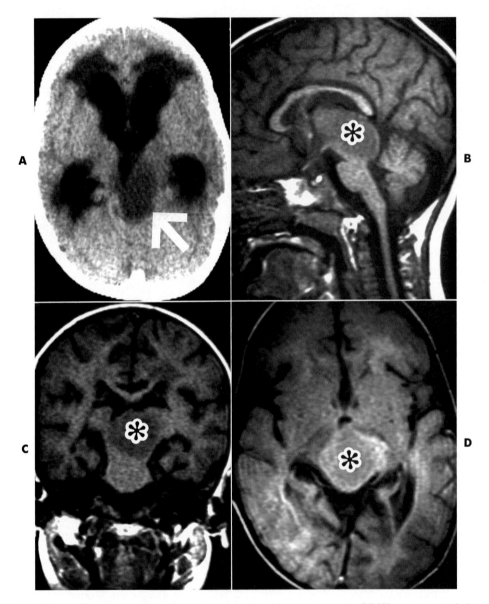

Fig. 7-44   Thalamic-mesencephalic astrocytoma in infancy as shown by CT **(A)** as an eccentric low density thalamic and midbrain mass (arrow) producing hydrocephalus with periventricular edema. Sagittal **(B)** and coronal **(C)** T1 MRI show the isointense to hypointense thalamic and midbrain tumor *(asterisks)* with aqueductal occlusion. The tumor is isointense to hyperintense on axial proton density **(D)** and T2 MRI.

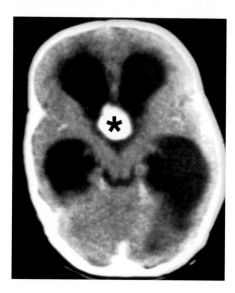

Fig. 7-45 Third ventricular choroid plexus papilloma *(asterisk)* shown by CT as a hyperdense enhancing tumor at the junction of the dilated anterosuperior third ventricle and dilated foramina of Monro and producing hydrocephalus. (Courtesy C. Humphrey, M.D., Lewiston, Maine.)

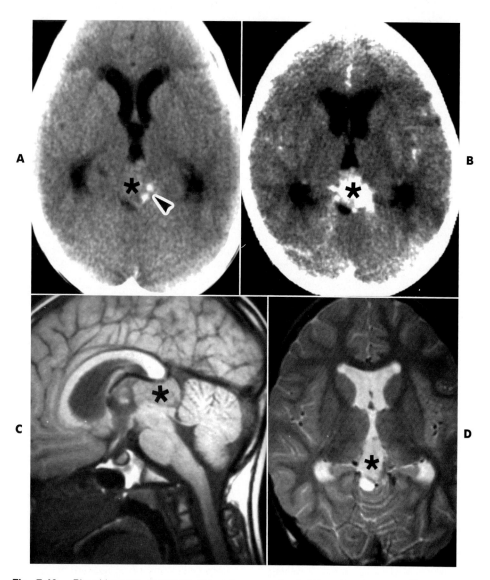

Fig. 7-46 Pineoblastoma *(asterisk)* shown by precontrast **(A)** and postcontrast **(B)** CT as an isodense to hyperdense enhancing pineal region mass with calcification *(black arrowhead)* plus hydrocephalus. **C,** Sagittal T1 MRI shows the tumor as an isointense mass compressing the tectum and occluding the aqueduct. **D,** The tumor is isointense to hyperintense on T2 MRI.

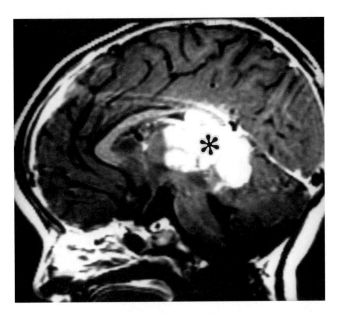

Fig. 7-47   Pineoblastoma *(asterisk)* shown by sagittal T1 MRI as a huge gadolinium-enhancing pineal region tumor with aqueductal occlusion and hydrocephalus.

images and isointense to hypointense or hyperintense on p/T2 images. Marked enhancement by iodine and gadolinium is common. There may be extensive invasion and CSF seeding, which is usually better demonstrated with gadolinium-enhanced MRI. The neuroimaging findings in pineocytoma, however, are often similar to those in pineoblastoma both of which may be difficult to distinguish from germ cell tumors.*

Regarding diagnosis and treatment of neuroepithelial tumors about the third ventricle, the clinical presentations (for example, visual loss, neurofibromatosis) and imaging findings (for example, optic pathway involvement) may be sufficiently characteristic to distinguish optic glioma from other tumors in the suprasellar region. Biopsy may be required, although excision is usually impossible. Optic and hypothalamic gliomas are therefore treated primarily with radiotherapy in progressive cases.[32] Partial excision may be possible for glial, neuronal, and other neoplasms about the foramina of Monro or within the third ventricle, but is usually not possible for thalamic or thalamomesencephalic tumors. Again, radiotherapy is an important modality for tumor control in progressive cases.[14] Ventricular shunting of associated hydrocephalus is usually necessary especially in cases in which only biopsy or partial resection is possible. As mentioned in the previous section, combined chemotherapy and radiotherapy is the treatment choice after biopsy or excision of PNET in this region. Treatment strategies for pineal region tumors are presented in the section on germ cell tumors. MRI is the preferred modality for follow-up in all of these cases.[1,7]

---

*References 1, 5, 7, 11, 31, 43.

MENINGEAL AND MELANOCYTIC TUMORS

Meningioma, meningeal sarcomas, and melanocytic tumors are rare in childhood.[37] These are more fully presented in the Cerebral Hemispheric and Posterior Fossa Tumor sections as well as in Chapter 8. Melanin-containing hamartomas may occur with neurofibromatosis 1. These are of high intensity on T1 and p/T2 MRI and appear within the basal ganglia and deep capsular structures.[13,29] These may be a source of confusion regarding tumor when there are clinical or other imaging findings relative to the optic pathways (see Chapter 8).

NERVE SHEATH CELL TUMORS

Neurilemmoma and neurofibroma are rarely if ever encountered about the third ventricle. These are more fully presented in the Posterior Fossa Tumor section of this chapter and in Chapter 8.

MALIGNANT LYMPHOMA

Central nervous system lymphoma may be encountered in childhood with parameningeal, meningeal, or brain involvement as presented in the previous section.

TUMORS OF BLOOD VESSEL ORIGIN

Hemangioblastoma, hemangiopericytoma, and angiosarcoma are very rare tumors encountered in childhood. The tumors of this category are more fully presented in the Posterior Fossa Tumor section.

GERM CELL TUMORS

Rubenstein and Russell[38] have classified pineal region tumors (see box on p. 235) according to germ cell origin, pineal cell origin, glial cell origin, neuronal origin, and others. Germ cell tumors of the CNS, a subset of extragonadal germ cell tumors, occur most frequently in the pineal and suprasellar regions or other midline locations. These tumors of the CNS clinically and pathologically resemble germ cell tumors arising outside the CNS and are classified along schemes adopted for germ cell tumors arising in the testis or ovary.[37,38] Arising in the embryonic yolk sac, primordial germ cells migrate widely throughout the early embryo and persist in sites such as the mediastinum and diencephaloepiphyseal region, where they may play a role in development or maturation of these structures. Germ cell tumors in the CNS presumedly arise from neoplastic transformation of such cells. Although the mechanism of transformation is not known, the high incidence of pineal region tumors in the second decade and in males suggests a neuroendocrine influence.

The WHO classification of germ cell tumors recognizes the categories of germinoma, embryonal carcinoma, choriocarcinoma, endodermal sinus tumor (also sometimes referred to as yolk sac carcinoma), teratomas, and mixed germ cell tumors composed of any combination of the previous categories.[37,38] By definition all of the germ cell tumors are malignant with the capacity for rapid and invasive growth and distant spread. This includes teratomas

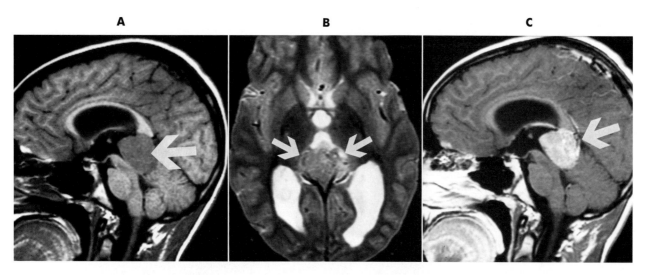

Fig. 7-48   Pineal germinoma *(arrows)* shown by sagittal T1 MRI **(A)** as an isointense pineal region mass compressing the tectum and occluding the aqueduct. **B,** The tumor is isointense to hypointense on axial T2 MRI. **C,** Marked gadolinium enhancement is demonstrated by postinjection sagittal T1 MRI.

containing any of these elements or areas of frank carcinoma or sarcoma. Other forms of teratoma are either benign or of uncertain malignant potential.

Germinomas

Originally termed *pinealoma* when manifested as a pineal region tumor and *ectopic pinealoma* when manifested in the anterior third ventricle or hypothalamus, the CNS germinoma is now thought to be identical to its gonadal counterparts, the ovarian dysgerminoma and the testicular seminoma.[37,38] Germinomas are the most common variety of intracranial germ cell tumor and are also the most common tumor arising in the pineal region.[9] Males predominate in cases of pineal region germinomas, but neither gender predominates in cases of suprasellar tumors. Intracranial germinomas may be circumscribed or ill defined, contain extensive calcification, infiltrate adjacent structures, disseminate in the CSF pathways, or form extraneural metastases. The tumors consist of two cell populations, the neoplastic germ cells, and reactive mononuclear cells. The neoplastic germinoma cells typically contain placental alkaline phosphatase, a useful immunohistochemical marker, but usually do not reveal alphafetoprotein (AFP) or human chorionic gonadotropin (HCG). Occasionally, elevated levels of HCG are present in the CSF. Although classified as malignant tumors, pure germinomas are generally highly radiosensitive.

Other forms of pure malignant germ cell tumor are rare and occur as pineal, sellar, suprasellar, or parasellar tumors. All three types are highly malignant tumors that grow rapidly and display metastatic behavior.[5,19,20,28] Embryonal carcinomas consist of primitive epithelium resembling primitive embryonic tissues and expressing cytokeratin and vimentin intermediate filament proteins. Endodermal sinus tumors contain epithelial structures resembling embryonic yolk sac epithelium and characteristically producing AFP, which can be demonstrated in tumor cells as well as in CSF or serum. Choriocarcinomas resemble placental tissues with the formation of cytotrophoblastic and syncytiotrophoblastic elements. These show a pronounced tendency to hemorrhage, and characteristically produce HCG, which can be demonstrated, along with other placental markers, in syncytiotrophoblastic elements as well as in CSF and serum.[37,38]

Neuroimaging demonstrates a midline or paramedian pineal region, hypothalamic, bifocal, or third periventricular mass.[1,7] Often the mass is associated with abnormal pineal calcification. The tumor is occasionally hemorrhagic but rarely cystic (see Fig. 7-51). CT often demonstrates an isodense to hyperdense and enhancing tumor matrix, with MRI showing isointensity to hypointensity and gadolinium enhancement on T1 images with isointensity to hypointensity or occasional hyperintensity on p/T2 images* (Figs. 7-48 to 7-50).

Occasionally the tumors are primarily of low intensity on T2 MRI with surrounding high intensity edema. The T2 hypointensity may correlate with the CT hyperdensity appearance often seen with hypercellular neoplasms (low intracellular free water content) such as germinomas and primitive neuroectodermal tumors. The surrounding high intensity often correlates with edema. Other causes for T2 MRI hypointensity in these tumors include calcification, hemorrhage, or hypervascularity (Fig. 7-51). With hypothalamic involvement producing diabetes insipidus, the normal posterior pituitary bright spot is absent[15] (Figs. 7-49 and 7-50).

Teratomas

Teratomas are defined as neoplasms composed of a mixture of differentiated tissues representing derivatives of

*References 1, 5, 7, 11, 19, 43.

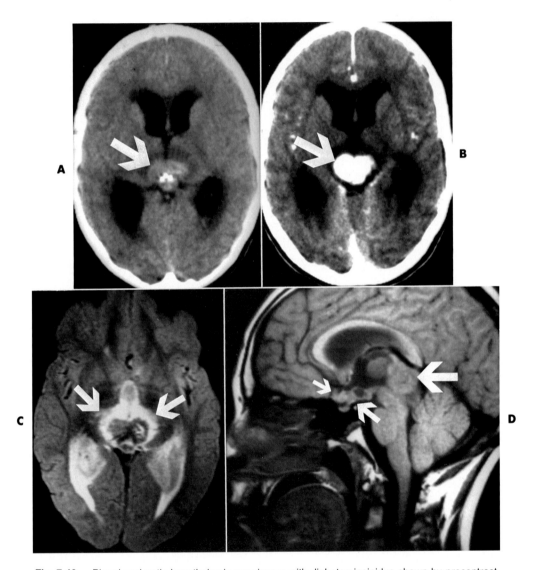

Fig. 7-49   Pineal and optic-hypothalamic germinoma with diabetes insipidus shown by precontrast **(A)** and postcontrast **(B)** CT *(arrow)* as an isodense to hyperdense enhancing pineal region mass with calcification and hydrocephalus. **C,** Axial T2 MRI shows an isointense to hypointense tumor *(arrows)* with surrounding hyperintensity. **D,** Sagittal T1 MRI shows the pineal region mass *(large arrow)* and additional nodular involvement of the chiasm and hypothalamus *(small arrows)* with absent posterior pituitary bright spot.

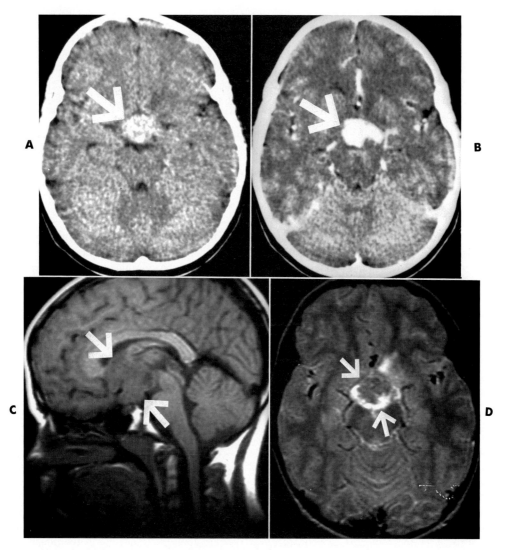

Fig. 7-50   Suprasellar germinoma with diabetes insipidus *(arrows)* shown by precontrast **(A)** and postcontrast **(B)** CT as a large hyperdense enhancing suprasellar mass. **C,** Sagittal T1 MRI shows a large isointense tumor engulfing the chiasm, hypothalamus, and anterior third ventricle. The posterior pituitary bright spot is absent. **D,** On the axial T2 MRI the tumor is isointense to hypointense with surrounding hyperintensity.

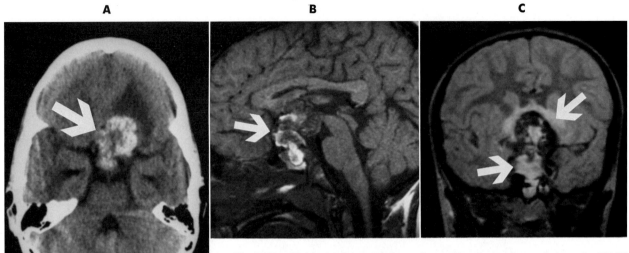

Fig. 7-51   Hemorrhagic suprasellar embryonal carcinoma *(arrows)* shown by CT **(A)** as a hyperdense tumor with adjacent low density edema. **B,** Sagittal T1 MRI shows the large intrasellar-suprasellar isointense to hypointense tumor with hemorrhagic high intensities (methemoglobin). **C,** Coronal p/T2 MRI shows internal hemorrhagic high and low intensities (methemoglobin and deoxyhemoglobin) with surrounding high intensity edema.

all three embryonic germinal layers.[37,38] Although relatively common in the sacrococcygeal region, intracranial or spinal cord teratomas are rare. These tend to occur chiefly in younger males in the pineal region, suprasellar region, pituitary fossa, or fourth ventricle. Teratomas are usually circumscribed, often cystic masses and may contain calcifications, bone, cartilage, teeth, and adipose tissue. Occasionally there is a tendency to spontaneous hemorrhage. Teratomas are divided into mature teratomas or immature teratomas depending on whether the tissue components resemble mature adult tissues or immature embryonic tissues. In CNS teratomas the immature tissues are frequently neuroectodermal and are more commonly encountered in fourth ventricle tumors. Mature teratomas are slow growing and generally considered benign, particularly if complete excision is possible. Immature teratomas may behave in a benign or malignant fashion, with abundant embryonic tissues suggesting the capacity for more rapid growth and metastasis. Teratomas containing other germ cell tumor types or areas of carcinoma or sarcoma, sometimes referred to as teratocarcinomas, are considered malignant and generally behave commensurately with their worst components.[37] Neuroimaging of teratoma usually reveals heterogeneous CT densities or MRI intensities within a lobulated mass including fat, calcification, ossification, and cartilage[1,5,7,43] (Figs. 7-52 and 7-53). Enhancement may be evident especially in the more malignant forms.

Other germ cell tumors

Germ cell tumor combinations constitute a substantial percentage of CNS germ cell neoplasms (for example, embryonal carcinoma with endodermal sinus tumor). These are classified as mixed germ cell tumors with a listing of the individual components.[37] Although germinomas and teratomas may occur in pure form more commonly than the other varieties, the combination of teratoma and germinoma is relatively frequent. Clinical behavior and prognosis depend on the worst component present. Elevated levels of markers such as AFP or HCG in CSF or serum may be a clue to the presence of endodermal sinus tumor or choriocarcinoma components when found in a patient with apparent germinoma, teratoma, or embryonal carcinoma.

Germ cell tumors are to be distinguished from glial neoplasms arising from the optic chiasm, hypothalamus, thalamus, or midbrain, as well as from pineal region or periventricular neuronal tumors (ganglioglioma). These should also be distinguished from malformative tumors (for example, craniopharyngioma), histiocytosis, or seeding (for example, medulloblastoma). Current management of germ cell tumors, or pineal region tumors in general, usually calls for biopsy confirmation and tumor excision if possible, especially for teratomas.[9] Germinomas are highly radiosensitive with good prognosis and often also responsive to chemotherapy. The more malignant germ cell tumors (embryonal carcinoma, choriocarcinoma, endodermal sinus tumor, immature teratoma, and teratocarcinoma) usually require a combination of chemotherapy and radiotherapy and have a much poorer prognosis. Ventricular shunting of associated hydrocephalus is often required using filtration devices to prevent seeding of the peritoneum. Added chemotherapy may be important in preventing or eradicating extraneural spread, that is, ventricular shunt seeding and hematogeneous metastasis. Craniospinal MRI with gadolinium enhancement is important for detecting CSF seeding to decide whether additional spinal neuraxis radiotherapy is necessary. MRI is recommended as the primary follow-up modality for this category of tumors.[1,7]

A   B   C

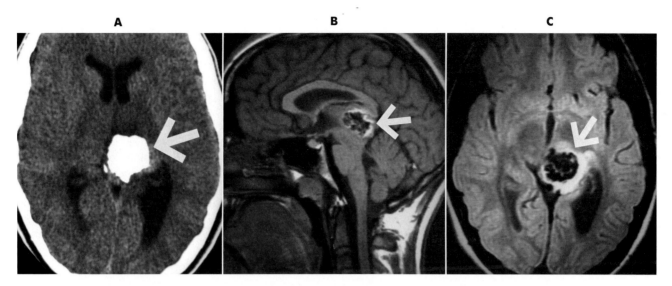

Fig. 7-52   Parapineal mature teratoma *(arrows)* shown by CT **(A)** as a nonspecific left paramedian pineal region calcific high density. Sagittal T1 MRI **(B)** and axial p MRI **(C)** show internal cortical and medullary ossific low and high intensities with an isointense to hyperintense cartilaginous rim.

A   B   C

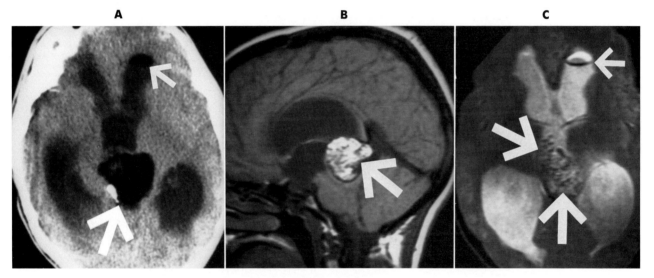

Fig. 7-53   Pineal region teratoma with undifferentiated elements shown by axial CT **(A)** as a fatty pineal region low density with calcification *(large arrow)* producing hydrocephalus and associated with left frontal horn fat-CSF level *(small arrow)*. **B,** Sagittal T1 MRI shows the fatty high intensity pineal region tumor (arrow). **C,** Axial T2 MRI shows the isointense to hypointense fatty pineal region mass *(large arrows)* and the left frontal horn fat-CSF level with chemical shift artifact *(small arrow)*.

MALFORMATIVE TUMORS

The category of malformative tumors includes a variety of space-occupying lesions, both neoplastic and nonneoplastic, whose common feature is their apparent origin in some abnormality of tissue development.[37,38] A number of lesions in this category are nonneuroepithelial and are often cystic tumors composed of tissues foreign to the CNS. In this category are the neoplastic but benign craniopharyngiomas, a variety of generally nonneoplastic cysts with characteristic clinical and pathological features, and nonneoplastic masses of adipose tissue (lipomas). The remaining lesions are the neoplastic granular cell tumors, also referred to as hypothalamic choristomas, and the hamartomas, which are nonneoplastic masses composed of mature elements normal to the area, that is, neuroepithelial or neural crest derivatives, but lack normal organization. Because of their presumed origin from migrating embryonic germ cells, the germ cell neoplasms could also logically be placed in this category, as could the vascular malformations, but these entities are discussed elsewhere.

Craniopharyngioma

Craniopharyngioma is a benign but aggressive neoplasm arising in the suprasellar or intrasellar regions and occurring most frequently in children or adolescents. Generally thought to arise from remnants of Rathke's pouch, the tumor is composed of characteristic squamous epithelium, referred to as adamantinomatous because of its resemblance to the neoplastic epithelium constituting the adamantinoma of the jaw.[37,38] Craniopharyngiomas may be solid or, more characteristically, cystic tumors, and the cysts are typically filled with a cholesterol-rich fluid grossly resembling motor oil. The tumors frequently calcify; formation of metaplastic

bone is also common. Although histologically benign, craniopharyngiomas tend to compress, envelop, or infiltrate adjacent structures and produce a florid reactive gliosis when involving brain. As a result, surgical extirpation is difficult and recurrence is likely. The pathological features of some craniopharyngiomas are difficult to distinguish from those of suprasellar epidermoid cysts.

Neuroimaging demonstrates a mass of variable size with a cystic component and calcification* (Figs. 7-54 to 7-57). The tumor matrix or solid component may be isodense or hypodense on CT and T1 isointense to hypointense with p/T2 isointensity to hyperintensity on MRI. Iodine and gadolinium enhancement of the solid

---

*References 1, 7, 16, 18, 24, 34.

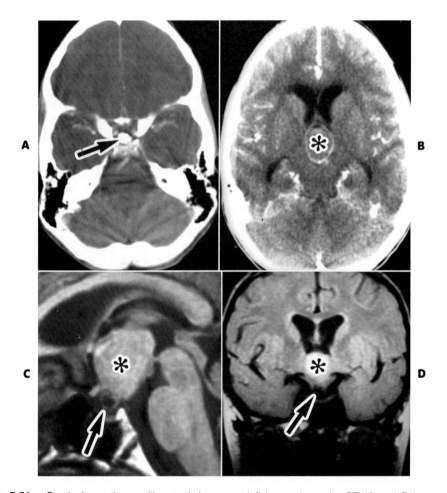

Fig. 7-54   Craniopharyngioma with growth hormone deficiency shown by CT (**A** and **B**) as an isodense to hypodense suprasellar tumor *(asterisk)* with intrasellar calcification *(arrow)*, rim enhancement, and hydrocephalus. **C,** Sagittal T1 MRI shows isointense to hyperintense proteinaceous cyst *(asterisk)* with hypointense calcification *(arrow)*. **D,** The cystic component *(asterisk)* is shown as hyperintense on coronal proton density image, whereas the calcification *(arrow)* remains low intensity.

tumor or cyst wall is commonly seen (Figs. 7-54 and 7-55). The calcified, ossified, or keratinized components are usually CT hyperdense and often MRI hypointense. The CT and MRI character of the cyst depends on content (Figs. 7-54 to 7-58). The contents may be primarily low density by CT (cholesterol or CSF-like fluid) or isodense to hyperdense (proteinaceous fluid, hemorrhage, keratin, calcium). By MRI the cyst is commonly of high intensity on all sequences as related to aqueous cholesterol, hemorrhage (methemoglobin), or proteinaceous fluid. MRI hypointensity of the cyst may indicate a predominance of keratin, calcium, or iron. Occasionally, small CSF-like cystic densities or intensities are seen within or around the tumor that may

represent arachnoidal encystment. Craniopharyngioma is to be differentiated primarily from a cystic, calcified glioma or a teratoma.

Rathke's cleft cyst

Rathke's pouch is an embryonic upward growth of ectoderm from the primitive oral cavity (stomodeum), which is the precursor of the anterior and intermediate lobe of the pituitary as well as the pars tuberalis. Persistence of the intrasellar extremity of Rathke's pouch occasionally results in formation of an epithelium-lined Rathke's cleft cyst. The cyst is usually located between the pars distalis and the pars nervosa of the pituitary and, if large, may lead

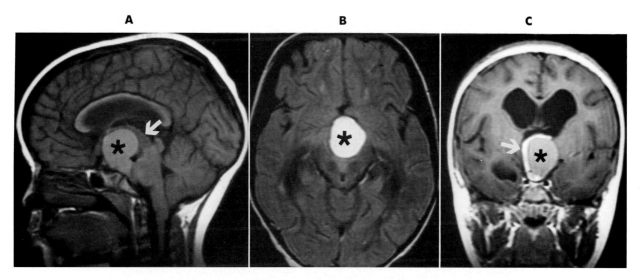

Fig. 7-55 Craniopharyngioma with cholesterol cyst *(asterisk)* demonstrated by sagittal T1 **(A)** and axial proton density **(B)** MRI as a large high intensity suprasellar mass. **C,** The solid laminar portion of the tumor *(arrow)* enhances with gadolinium on coronal T1 MRI.

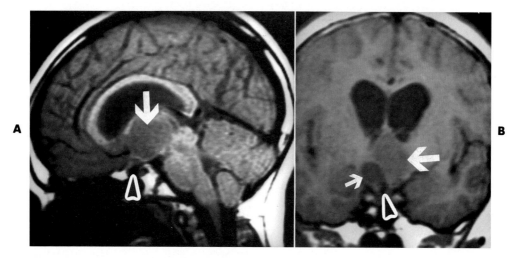

Fig. 7-56 Craniopharyngioma with intra–third ventricular component shown by sagittal **(A)** and coronal **(B)** T1 MRI as a large isointense to hypointense suprachiasmatic solid and cystic tumor *(large arrow)* filling the third ventricle. Associated suprasellar CSF-intensity cyst *(small arrow)* and hypointense calcification *(arrowhead)* are also shown.

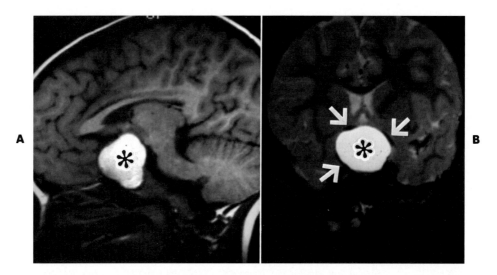

Fig. 7-57   Cystic intrasellar-suprasellar craniopharyngioma with cholesterol content and mural calcifications. The cyst is demonstrated as marked hyperintensity *(asterisk)* on sagittal T1 **(A)** and coronal T2 **(B)** MRI, whereas the mural calcifications are low intensity on all sequences (arrows).

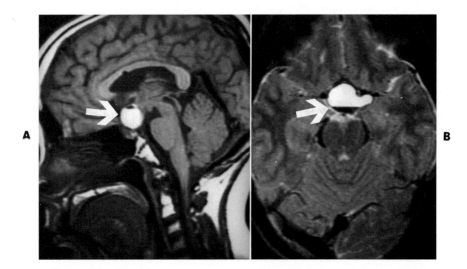

Fig. 7-58   Craniopharyngioma with hemorrhagic cyst (arrows) after surgery and radiotherapy. Sagittal T1 MRI **(A)** shows high intensity suprasellar mass, whereas axial T2 MRI **(B)** shows high intensity over low intensity fluid level consistent with hemorrhage.

to compression of the pituitary or adjacent structures. Although usually intrasellar and lined by cuboidal or columnar mucus-secreting epithelium, Rathke's cleft cysts may occur in the suprasellar region, undergo squamous metaplasia or hemorrhage, and overlap pathologically with craniopharyngiomas. Neuroimaging usually demonstrates an intrasellar or suprasellar cystic mass whose CT and MRI signal characteristics vary with cyst content[1,7,22,30] (Fig. 7-59). Serous fluid may appear isodense to hypodense by CT and follow CSF intensities on MRI. Mucoid or cholesterol cysts may appear of high intensity throughout the MRI sequences. More complex cysts with prominent cellular desquamation may appear CT hyperdense and MR hypointense or may show heterogeneous signal characteristics with abnormal enhancement. Calcification is rare. Differential considerations include craniopharyngioma, arachnoid cyst, pituitary cyst, and the rare cystic pituitary adenoma.

Colloid cysts

Although of probable neuroepithelial derivation, the tissue origin of the third ventricular colloid cyst, an

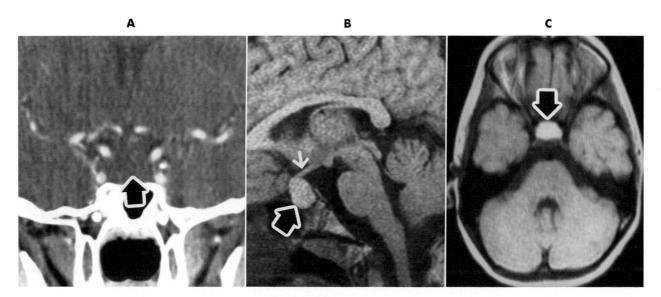

Fig. 7-59   Rathke's cyst *(black arrow)* shown by coronal CT **(A)** as an isodense nonenhancing intrasellar-suprasellar mass that is high intensity on sagittal **(B)** T1 MRI and high intensity on axial p **(C)** MRI. Notice the relationship of the cyst dome to the anterior optic pathways (white arrow).

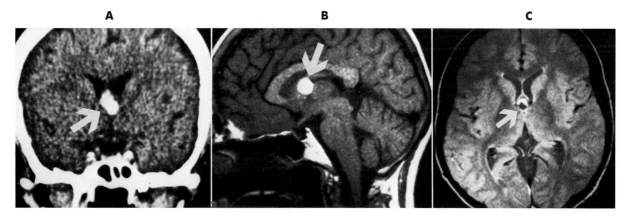

Fig. 7-60   Colloid cyst *(white arrow)* shown by direct coronal CT **(A)** as a nodular high density of the anterosuperior third ventricle. The cyst is high intensity on sagittal T1 MRI **(B)** and mixed high and low intensity on axial proton density MRI **(C)**. (Courtesy J. Suojanen, M.D., New England Deaconess Hospital, Boston.)

epithelium-lined cyst with a fibrous wall and proteinaceous content, has not yet been established.[37,38] Although some cysts are discovered as incidental findings in adults, the location of the cysts in the wall or roof of the third ventricle at the foramen of Monro may lead to obstruction of the foramen and acute hydrocephalus. Occasionally the colloid cyst may hemorrhage. CT and MRI findings vary with cyst content, which may include secretory and breakdown products of the epithelial lining of the cyst wall including mucin, lipid, cholesterol, CSF, hemorrhage, hemosiderin, and trace paramagnetic metals (magnesium, copper, and the

like).[1,7,26,40] The cysts are more commonly of high density and nonenhancing by CT but occasionally may appear isodense to hypodense. By MRI the lesions may be of low or high intensity on T1 and p/T2 images, again depending on the dominant elements within the cyst (Fig. 7-60).

Other cysts

Other cysts arise from a variety of neuroepithelial or meningeal components and in a variety of locations in and around the CNS. Neuroepithelial cysts may occur within the ventricles, in the CNS parenchyma, or in the subarachnoid

A   B   C

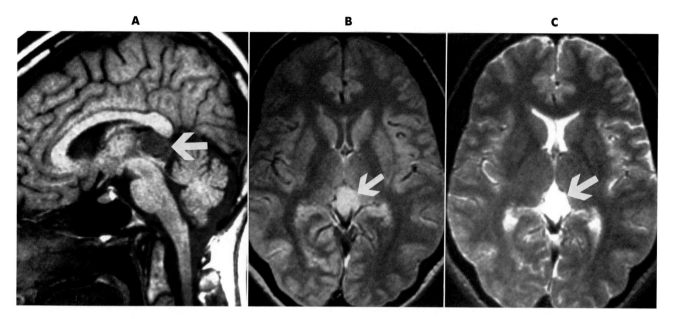

Fig. 7-61   Pineal cyst *(arrows)* shown by sagittal T1 MRI **(A)** as a hypointense pineal mass deforming the adjacent tectum. The cyst is hyperintense on axial p **(B)** and T2 **(C)** MRI.

space. These are lined by a monolayer of columnar or cuboidal, often ciliated cells resembling ependyma or choroid plexus.[37,38] Glial cysts generally lack a recognizable epithelial lining and consist of a variably thick wall of fibrillary glial tissue. Neuroepithelial and glial cysts presumedly develop from rests of normal ependymal, choroidal, or glial tissue. Some glial cysts may actually represent the residuum of burned out or involuted glial neoplasms. Arachnoid cysts, lined by flattened arachnoid cells and collagen, may arise from loculations of the leptomeninges following previous inflammation or from defects in meningeal development. All cysts act as slowly expanding masses that compress and indent surrounding structures. Nonneoplastic cysts must be differentiated from cysts arising in neoplasms.

Arachnoid cysts often occur suprasellar[47] or about the quadrigeminal plate region and are more fully discussed in Chapter 3. Ependymal and choroid plexus cysts occur intraventricularly. Pineal cysts are neuroglial-lined cysts representing vestigial remnants of pineal cavities after diverticulation of the posterior third ventricular roof.[27] Others may form after pineal parenchymal necrosis. The cysts are usually of low density by CT and difficult to detect and separate from CSF within the confluence of cisterns about the quadrigeminal plate. By MRI the cysts may be T1 isointense to hypointense, commonly isointense to hyperintense on proton density images, and markedly hyperintense on T2 images, probably related to proteinaceous fluid content[1,7,27] (Fig. 7-61). These are often incidental. There may be associated tectal deformity. Occasionally it is difficult to distinguish a pineal cyst from an arachnoid cyst of the quadrigeminal cistern, but aqueductal stenosis with

hydrocephalus is rarely associated. Cysts lined by epithelium resembling either columnar mucus-secreting gastrointestinal epithelium or pseudostratified ciliated respiratory epithelium are called, respectively, enterogenous or bronchial cysts.[37] These are rarely found in the region of the sella or posterior fossa. More commonly they are encountered paraspinally or intraspinally as part of the neurenteric continuum, as presented in Chapter 10.

Lipomas

Lipomas occur as localized proliferations of adipose tissue alone or as a dominant component of a mesenchymal hamartoma, the latter often consisting also of muscle, fibrous tissue, and vascular elements.[37,38] The common intracranial locations are hypothalamic, the quadrigeminal plate region, and pericallosal. These are rarely symptomatic themselves but may be associated with developmental brain malformations (for example, callosal dysgenesis), or seizure disorders (for example, partial complex or gelastic seizures associated with hypothalamic lesions). Lipomas probably result from faulty inclusion of the mesoderm during neural tube closure with subsequent induction to form fat. Lipomas may blend with the underlying CNS tissue and frequently invest nerve roots and blood vessels, making resection difficult. Neuroimaging reveals a midline or paramedian fatty low-intensity by CT, and occasionally shows calcification. MRI shows characteristic findings for fat including T1 and p high intensity, T2 low intensity, and chemical shift artifact[1,3,7,44] (Figs. 7-62 and 7-63). A hypothalamic or infundibular lipoma is distinguished from ectopic posterior pituitary by absence of a normal posterior pituitary bright spot in the latter (Figs. 7-63 and 7-64).

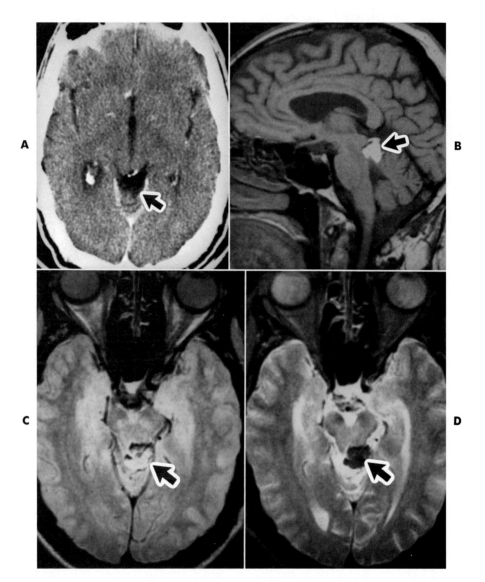

Fig. 7-62   Quadrigeminal plate lipoma *(arrows)* shown by axial CT **(A)** as cisternal fatty low density deforming the tectum. The lipoma is typically high intensity on sagittal T1 **(B)** and axial p **(C)** MRI with hypointensity on the axial T2 **(D)** MRI. The chemical shift artifact is most pronounced on the axial p image **(C)**.

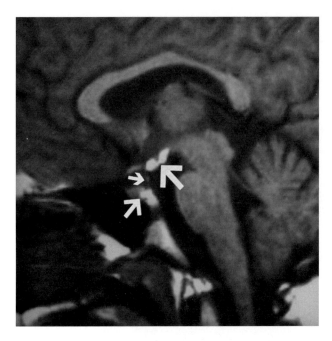

Fig. 7-63   Hypothalamic lipoma *(large arrow)* shown by sagittal T1 MRI as a bilobar high intensity. A normal posterior pituitary bright spot is apparent *(medium-sized arrow)*. There may be a small lipoma *(small arrow)* of the pituitary stalk.

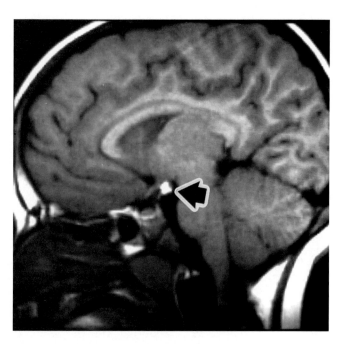

Fig. 7-64   Ectopic posterior pituitary in a child with hypopituitarism but no diabetes insipidus. Sagittal T1 MRI demonstrates hypothalamic nodular high intensity *(arrow)* with lack of a posterior pituitary bright spot. (Also see Chapter 2.)

Granular cell tumor

On the basis of its predilection for the neurohypophysis and resemblance to the choristoma of the infundibulum, the rare but distinctive *granular cell tumor* has been postulated to be a benign neoplasm of neurohypophyseal origin and has also been referred to as an infundibuloma.[6,37,38] The tumors, however, have been described in other CNS locations including the spinal cord. These are identical in morphological and immunocytochemical features to the granular cell tumors, also known as granular cell myoblastomas, of the peripheral nervous system, which are thought to be of Schwannian origin.

Hamartomas

Hamartomas are masses of mature nonneoplastic tissue of varying growth potential native to the particular site but disorganized.[37,38] Because of the importance of cell migration in the formation of the CNS, processes interfering with normal development may cause aberrant or arrested migration. Foci of ectopic gray matter or glial tissue in the CNS or leptomeninges are most frequently associated with other malformations and are appropriately designated as heterotopias or dysplasias. Although many do not produce mass effect, these may enter into the differential diagnosis of other masses.[25,29] In some instances a hamartoma may provide the focus in which a neoplasm such as a ganglioglioma or meningeal glioma subsequently arises. Hamartomas may be composed of disorganized mature neurons (neuronal hamartoma), disorganized glial elements with thickened blood vessels (glial hamartoma), or disorganized

neuronal and glial elements (neuronoglial hamartoma).[37] Meningioangioneurinomatosis is a rare condition consisting of local proliferation of arachnoid cells, vessels, and Schwann cells. It is often associated with other features of neuroectodermal dysplasia and may occur at any level of the CNS. Ectopic masses of neural, glial, or meningeal tissue may develop in juxtacranial or extracranial locations as well and may give rise to hamartomatous lesions such as a nasal glioma. Such developmental lesions may account for the origin of primary neuroepithelial or meningeal neoplasms outside the CNS.

The best known and most commonly symptomatic hamartomatous condition of childhood is hypothalamic hamartoma or hamartoma of the tuber cinereum.[2,4] This may be classically associated with precocious puberty, partial complex seizures (gelastic type), or neurofibromatosis. Neuroimaging reveals an isodense or low density suprasellar mass of variable size by CT, whereas MRI often reveals the mass as T1 isointense, p isointense to hyperintense, and T2 hyperintense[1,2,4,7] (Fig. 7-65). Abnormal iodine or gadolinium enhancement is usually absent. The lesion is occasionally detected only with MRI but may be obscured on T2 images by surrounding high-intensity CSF. Differential considerations include hypothalamic glioma or ganglioglioma.

Epidermoid and dermoid cysts

Dermoid and epidermoid tumors tend to be cystic and probably result from inclusion of epithelial elements at the time of neural tube closure in early embryonic develop-

A   B   C

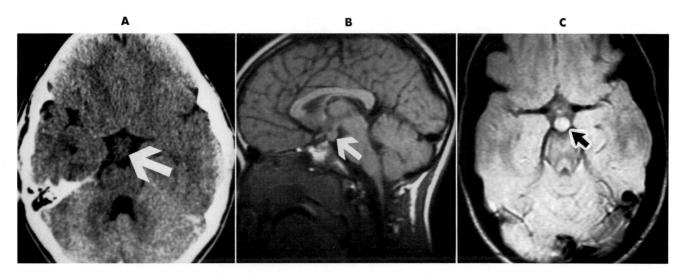

Fig. 7-65   Hamartoma of the tuber cinereum *(arrows)* with precocious puberty. **A,** Axial CT shows a nodular posterior suprasellar, nonenhancing isodensity. **B,** Sagittal T1 MRI demonstrates the isointense nodule with central hypointensity. **C,** Axial proton density MRI shows the high intensity nodule with more central hyperintensity. The hamartoma stands out against the low intensity suprasellar CSF on the proton density image **(C).**

ment.[3,37,38] *Epidermoid cysts* are of ectodermal origin and lined with keratinizing stratified squamous epithelium. These often contain desquamated cellular debris and cholesterol, the latter as a breakdown product of keratin. The contents are often brittle, white, and pearllike (pearly tumors or cholesteatomas). A slowly expanding mass results from progressive exfoliation of ketatinized cholesterol-rich material into the interior of the cyst. Rupture of the cyst contents into the subarachnoid spaces or ventricles may lead to chemical or granulomatous meningitis. Rarely is there neoplastic transformation into squamous carcinoma. These tumors tend to occur off-midline in the cerebellopontine angle, parasellar region, or cranial diploe. The calvarial site might actually be the most common location of epidermoid cysts in childhood.

Dermoids are also of ectodermal origin. Additional elements are derived from skin appendages including hair, sebaceous glands, and sweat glands. In addition to the desquamated debris of squamous epithelial cells, keratin, and cholesterol, the breakdown products of hair combined with sweat and sebaceous gland secretions produce an oily lipidlike mixture. Occasionally these also contain calcification, bone, cartilage, or, rarely, teeth, thus raising the question of a link with true teratomas. Dermoids usually occur in a median location, more commonly in the posterior fossa or spinal canal, and may communicate with the skin via a dermal sinus tract through a bony defect. Occasionally these arise about the third ventricle or frontally. Dermoids also expand by accumulation of exfoliated contents and may also rupture producing a chemical or granulomatous meningitis.

Neuroimaging may classically demonstrate a midline discrete suprasellar or third periventricular lesion in the case of a dermoid cyst, or a paramedian, parasellar lesion extending into the available spaces of the middle, anterior, or posterior cranial fossa in the case of an epidermoid cyst[1,3,7,17] (Fig. 7-66). Epidermoids are described as following CSF densities and intensities on CT and MRI respectively. Dermoid cysts are believed to more often contain calcification, occasionally as a formed element (for example, tooth) and more often contain fatlike densities and intensities. Iodine or gadolinium contrast enhancement and edema are unusual unless there is an inflammatory reaction or a complicating infection such as a dermoid with abscess (Fig. 7-67). Rarely these tumors may be predominantly of high density on CT and of low intensity on MRI because of the high keratin content relative to cholesterol or water. Due to the slow growth rate, soft consistency, and a tendency to extend into available spaces (especially epidermoids), hydrocephalus is infrequent except for very large or intraventricular tumors. It may be impossible at times to distinguish dermoid from epidermoid, or either from teratoma (see Figs. 7-52 and 7-66). In fact, epidermoids occurring in children, as contrasted with those occurring in adults, are often discrete, midline or paramedian, often contain identifiable fatlike intensities, and therefore are more difficult to distinguish from dermoids (Fig. 7-66). Cyst rupture may result in chemical arachnoiditis and granulomatous foreign body reaction with meningitis and hydrocephalus. Occasionally, intraventricular lipid-CSF levels may be seen or lipid particles in the subarachnoid spaces (see Fig. 7-53).

The treatment of malformative tumors is primarily surgical. Cellular proliferation and desquamation result in solid or cystic expansions containing liquid or semiliquid breakdown products. Excision and containment of cyst

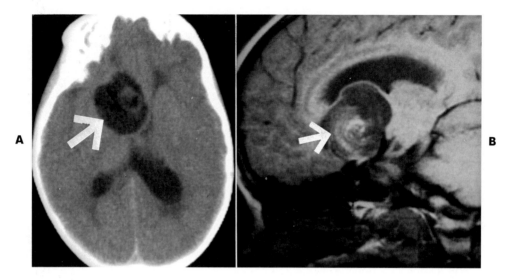

Fig. 7-66   Right suprachiasmatic epidermoid *(arrows)* shown by axial CT **(A)** as a low density, nonenhancing mass with an eccentric isodense nodule. **B,** Sagittal T1 MRI shows the low intensity mass above and lateral to the optic chiasm with fatlike high intensity nodules and swirls.

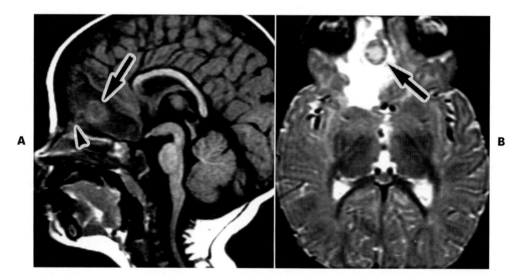

Fig. 7-67   Abscessed frontal dermoid cyst *(arrow)* shown by sagittal T1 MRI **(A)** as a low intensity mass with an isointense ring, isointense dermal sinus *(arrow head)* extending from the nasion, and surrounding low intensity edema. **B,** Axial T2 image shows the hyperintense mass with isointense to hypointense ring and surrounding high intensity edema.

content is difficult in this anatomically sensitive region, and removal is often incomplete. Staged resections or reoperation may be necessary in case of extensive or recurring tumors. Regional radiotherapy is an important addition, particularly in the management of residual or recurrent craniopharyngioma.

TUMORS OF NEUROENDOCRINE ORIGIN

Tumors of neuroendocrine origin include pituitary adenoma, pituitary carcinoma, and the rare paraganglioma.[37] As a derivative of Rathke's pouch epithelium, the anterior pituitary gland or adenohypophysis may give rise to benign or malignant epithelial neoplasms, which are termed *pituitary adenomas* or *carcinomas,* respectively. These may express any of the hormones secreted by the normal adenohypophysis. Pituitary adenomas are currently divided into hormonally active and inactive groups, with active tumors making up about three quarters of the total. These are more common in adults than in children, with particular age and gender incidence varying with the particular hormonal type or tumor.[10,37,38]

Clinical manifestations of pituitary adenomas take three forms: overproduction of hormone by the tumor, underproduction of other pituitary hormones due to compression or destruction of the remaining gland, and direct effects of the intrasellar or suprasellar mass on surrounding structures and on intracranial pressure. The most common hormonally active tumors secrete or make prolactin, growth hormone, or adrenocorticotropic hormone. Mixed secretory tumors constitute at least 10% of pituitary adenomas and are manifested in varying combinations, generally in accordance with the familial interrelationships of the various hormones. Hormonally inactive adenomas (null-cell adenomas) may fail to make hormone, make inadequate amounts of hormone to cause clinical symptoms, or make defective hormone. Many of the prolactin- or ACTH-secreting tumors are microadenomas, measuring less than 1 cm in diameter. Growth hormone–secreting tumors, tumors secreting both prolactin and growth hormone, and the null-cell adenomas are frequently large and may infiltrate adjacent structures. Local growth and infiltration may cause erosion of the surrounding sphenoid bone leading to expansion of the sella turcica and encroachment on the cavernous sinuses. Suprasellar extension can result in compression of the optic chiasm, hypothalamus, and frontal lobes.

Most pituitary tumors have benign cytological features, although focal infiltration of tissues may occur. In rare instances tumors show the cytological features of epithelial cell malignancy, generally associated with more extensive invasion of surrounding structures, rapid growth, and the formation of subarachnoid or distant extraneural metastases. Such malignant pituitary adenomas or pituitary carcinomas are usually hormonally inactive.

Neuroimaging may show an isodense or low density (occasionally high density) intrasellar or intrasellar and suprasellar mass with parasellar extension on CT. Calcification and cyst formation are unusual. Occasionally, intratumoral hemorrhage may be evident before or after chemical treatment. MRI often shows isointensity to hypointensity on T1 images with p/T2 hyperintensity or occasional hypointensity, depending on the tumor matrix*

---

*References 1, 7, 8, 21, 23, 42.

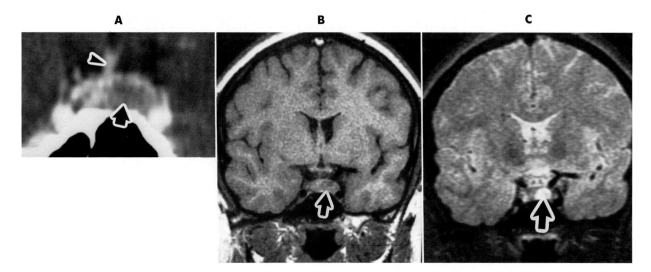

Fig. 7-68   Prolactin-secreting pituitary microadenoma *(arrows)* shown by direct coronal contrast-enhanced CT **(A)** as a hypodense area within the enhancing pituitary gland with upward convexity of the gland and contralateral tilting of the enhancing stalk *(arrowhead).* Coronal T1 MRI **(B)** shows the adenoma as hypointense, whereas the coronal T2 MRI **(C)** demonstrates hyperintensity.

(Figs. 7-68 and 7-69). Intratumoral hemorrhage may appear T1 hyperintense with T2 hypointensity or hyperintensity (Fig. 7-70). Iodine or gadolinium enhancement is more common with macroadenomas than with microadenomas. Treatment options include medical therapy (for example, bromocriptine), surgical excision (transsphenoidal or craniotomy), and localized radiotherapy. An extremely rare case of pituitary-hypothalamic paraganglioma is shown in Fig. 7-71.

LOCAL EXTENSIONS FROM REGIONAL TUMORS

Local extensions from regional tumors are discussed in the Parameningeal Tumor section.

METASTATIC TUMORS

Metastatic tumors are discussed primarily in the Cerebral Hemispheric Tumor section. The third ventricular structures are commonly involved with tumor seeding and histiocytosis, especially in the suprasellar region[12] (Fig. 7-72).

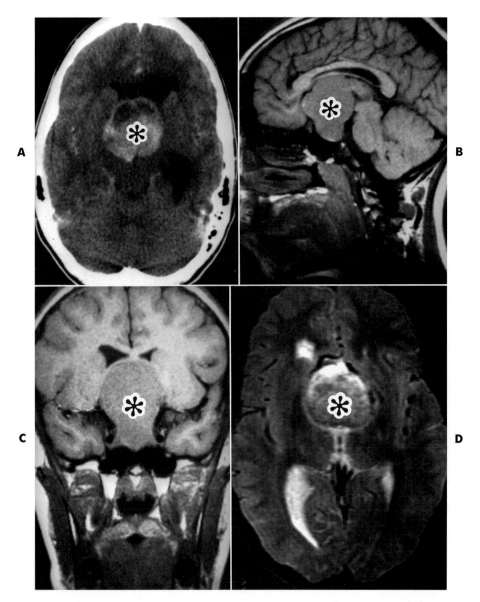

Fig. 7-69   Prolactin-secreting pituitary macroadenoma *(asterisks)* shown by CT **(A)** as a large isodense to hyperdense and enhancing intrasellar-suprasellar mass with cystic changes and hydrocephalus. Sagittal **(B)** and coronal **(C)** T1 MRI show the isointense intrasellar and suprasellar components with sellar expansion, loss of the pituitary-hypothalamic and optic landmarks, and obliteration of the third ventricle. **D,** Axial T2 MRI demonstrates the isointense to hypointense character of tumor matrix with associated cyst and edema hyperintensities.

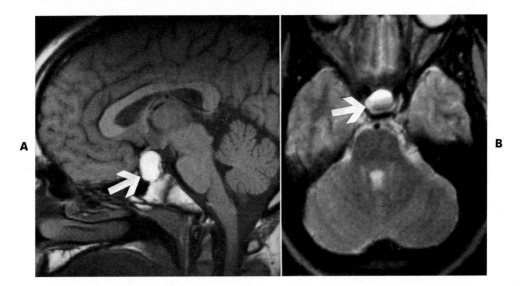

Fig. 7-70   Cystic and hemorrhagic pituitary adenoma (*arrow*) shown by sagittal T1 MRI **(A)** as a hyperintense intrasellar-suprasellar mass extending to the optic chiasm. **B,** Axial T2 MRI shows the tumor with hyperintense over hypointense fluid level consistent with hemorrhage.

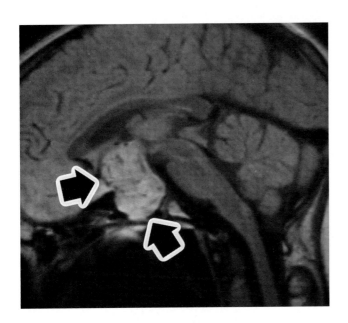

Fig. 7-71   Rare pituitary-hypothalamic paraganglioma (*arrows*) shown by sagittal proton density MRI as a large intrasellar-suprasellar high intensity mass containing linear vascular flow signal voids.

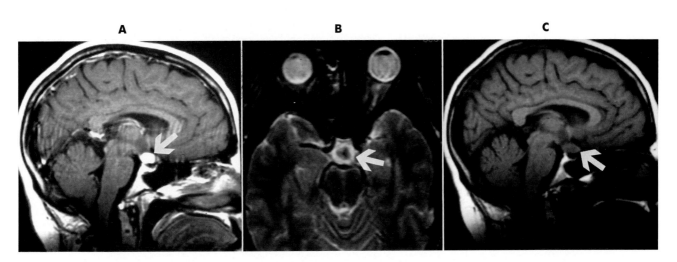

Fig. 7-72   Malignant histiocytosis (arrows) with hypothalamic involvement shown by sagittal T1 MRI **(A)** as an isointense to hypointense mass that is hypointense with peripheral hyperintensity on axial T2 MRI **(B)** and enhances with gadolinium on sagittal T1 MRI **(C)**.

REFERENCES
Tumors about the third ventricle

1. Barkovich A: *Pediatric neuroimaging,* New York, 1990, Raven.
2. Barral V, Brunelle F, Brauner R, et al: MRI of hypothalamic hamartomas in children, *Pediatr Radiol* 18:449, 1988.
3. Beltinger C, Saule H: Imaging of lipoma of the corpus callosum and intracranial dermoids in the Goldenbar syndrome, *Pediatr Radiol* 18:72, 1988.
4. Burton E, Ball W, Crone K, et al: Hamartoma of the tuber cinereum, *AJNR* 10:497, 1989.
5. Chang T, Teng M, Gno W, et al: CT of pineal tumors and intracranial germ cell tumors, *AJNR* 10:1039, 1989.
6. Cone L, Srinivasan M, Romanul FCA: Granular cell tumor (choristoma) of the neurohypophysis: two cases and a review of the literature, *AJNR* 11:403, 1990.
7. Davis P: Tumors of the brain. In Cohen M, Edwards M, editors: *MR imaging of children,* Philadelphia, 1990, BC Decker.
8. Davis P, Hoffman J, Malko J, et al: Gd-DTPA and MR imaging of pituitary adenoma, *AJNR* 8:817, 1987.
9. Edwards M, Hudgins R, Wilson C, et al: Pineal region tumors in children, *J Neurosurg* 68:689, 1988.
10. Elster AD, Chen MYM, Williams DW III, et al: Pituitary gland: MR imaging of physiologic hypertrophy in adolescence, *Radiology* 174:681, 1990.
11. Ganti S, Hilal S, Stein B, et al: CT of pineal region tumors, *AJNR* 7:97, 1986.
12. Graif M, Pennock J: MR imaging of histiocytosis X in the CNS, *AJNR* 7:21, 1986.
13. Gray J, Swaiman K: Brain tumors in children with neurofibromatosis: CT and MR imaging, *Pediatr Neurol* 3:335, 1987.
14. Grigsby PW, Thomas PRM, Schwartz HG, et al: Irradiation of primary thalamic and brainstem tumors in a pediatric population: a 33-year experience, *Cancer* 60:2901, 1987.
15. Gudinchet F, Brunelle F, Barth M, et al: MR imaging of the posterior hypophysis in children, *AJNR* 10:511, 1989.
16. Hillman TH, Peyster RG, Hoover ED, et al: Infrasellar craniopharyngioma: CT and MR studies, *J Comput Assist Tomogr* 12:702, 1988.
17. Horowitz BL, Chari MV, James R, et al: MR of intracranial epidermoid tumors: correlation of in vivo imaging with in vitro^{13}C spectroscopy, *AJNR* 11:299, 1990.
18. Hurst RW, McIlhenhy J, Park TS, Thomas WO: Neonatal craniopharyngioma: CT and ultrasonographic features, *J Comput Assist Tomogr* 12:858, 1988.
19. Kilgore D, Strother C, Starshak R, et al: Pineal germinoma: MR imaging, *Radiology* 158:435, 1986.
20. Komatsu Y, Narushima K, Kobayashi E, et al: CT and MR of germinoma in the basal ganglia, *AJNR* 10:S9, 1989.
21. Kucharczyk W, Davis D, Kelly W, et al: Pituitary adenomas: MR imaging, *Radiology* 161:761, 1986.
22. Kucharczyk W, Peck W, Kelly W, et al: Rathke cleft cysts: CT and MR, *Radiology* 165:491, 1987.
23. Lee Y, Van Tassel P, Bruner J, et al: Juvenile pilocystic astrocytomas: CT and MR, *AJNR* 10:363, 1989.
24. Linden CN, Martinez CR, Gonzalvo AA, et al: Intrinsic third ventricle craniopharyngioma: CT and MR findings, *J Comput Assist Tomogr* 13:362, 1989.
25. Lis S, Lampropoulos C, Sarwar M: Quadrigeminal plate hamartoma, *AJNR* 10:S56, 1989.
26. Maeder P, Holtas S, Babibuyuk L, et al: Colloid cysts of the third ventricle, *AJNR* 11:575, 1990.
27. Mamourian A, Towfighi J: Pineal cysts: MR imaging, *AJNR* 7:1081, 1986.
28. Matthews VP, Broome DR, Smith RR, et al: Neuroimaging of disseminated germ cell neoplasms, *AJNR* 11:319, 1990.
29. Mirowitz SA, Sartor K, Gado M: High-intensity basal ganglia lesions on T1-weighted MR images in neurofibromatosis, *AJNR* 10:159, 1989.
30. Mize W, Ball WS Jr, Towbin RB, et al: Atypical CT and MR appearance of a Rathke cleft cyst, *AJNR* 10:S83, 1989.
31. Nakagawa H, Iwasaki S, Kichikawa K, et al: MR imaging of pineocytoma: report of two cases, *AJNR* 11:185, 1990.
32. Pierce S, Barnes P, Loeffler J, et al: Definitive radiation therapy in the management of symptomatic optic glioma, *Cancer* 65:45, 1990.
33. Pojunas K, Daniels D, Williams A, et al: MR imaging of prolactin-secreting microadenomas, *AJNR* 7:209, 1986.
34. Pusey E, Kortman K, Flannigan B, et al: MR of craniopharyngiomas, *AJNR* 8:439, 1987.
35. Reith K, Comite F, Dwyer A, et al: CT of cerebral abnormalities in precocious puberty, *AJNR* 8:283, 1987.
36. Rice JF, Eggers DM: Basal transsphenoidal encephalocele: MR findings, *AJNR* 10:S79, 1989.
37. Rorke L, Gilles F, Davis R, et al: Revision of the WHO classification of brain tumors for childhood, *Cancer* 56:1869, 1985.
38. Russell D, Rubenstein L: *Pathology of tumors of the nervous system,* ed 4, Baltimore, 1977, Williams & Wilkins.
39. Schellhas K, Siebert R, Heithoff K, et al: Congenital choroid plexus papilloma of the third ventricle, real-time sonography, and MR imaging, *AJNR* 9:797, 1988.
40. Scotti G, Scialfa G, Colombo N, et al: MR in colloid cysts of the third ventricle, *AJNR* 8:370, 1987.
41. Som P, Dillon W, Sze G, et al: Benign and malignant sinonasal lesions with intracranial extension: MR imaging, *Radiology* 172:763, 1989.
42. Steiner E, Imhof H, Krosp E: Gd-DTPA–enhanced MR imaging of pituitary adenomas, *Radiographics* 9:587, 1989.
43. Tien R, Barkovich A, Edwards M: MR imaging of pineal tumors, *AJNR* 11:557, 1990.
44. Truwit C, Williams RG, Armstrong EA, et al: MR imaging of choroid plexus lipomas, *AJNR* 11:202, 1990.
45. Vogl T, Dresel S, Bilanink L, et al: Tumors of the nasopharynx and adjacent areas: MR imaging with Gd-DTPA, *AJNR* 11:187, 1990.
46. Waggenspack G, Guinto F: MR and CT masses of the anterior superior third ventricle, *AJR* 152:609, 1989.
47. Woodruff W, Heinz E, Djang W, et al: Hyperprolactinemia with suprasellar cystic lesions, *AJNR* 8:113, 1987.

Posterior fossa tumors

Posterior fossa tumors often manifest as increased intracranial pressure due to obstructive hydrocephalus at the level of the fourth ventricle and aqueduct. Often there are cerebellar signs such as ataxia and nystagmus. Brain stem involvement may reveal bilateral cranial nerve and pyramidal tract signs, whereas cerebellopontine angle lesions may produce unilateral cranial nerve palsies, such as sensorineural hearing loss or facial palsy. Meningeal involvement often results in a stiff neck or head tilt. Common posterior fossa neoplasms (see box on p. 261) of childhood are medulloblastoma, cerebellar astrocytoma, and brain stem glioma.[22,23] Less frequent tumors include ependymoma, dermoid or epidermoid, nerve sheath cell tumors, and choroid plexus neoplasms. Neuronal, meningeal, lymphomatous, blood vessel origin, germ cell, and metastatic tumors are rare in this location. Nonneoplastic tumors are common in this compartment, especially in infancy, and include the Dandy-Walker spectrum of retrocerebellar cysts, arachnoid cyst, encysted fourth ventricle, and the pseudotumor effect of Chiari II malformation. Parameningeal processes that may encroach on the posterior fossa are those arising from the skull base, petrous temporal bone, or suboccipital soft tissues and include sarcoma, chordoma, neuroblastoma, PNET, histiocytosis, paraganglioma,[19,28] mastoiditis, cellulitis, abscess, or cholesteatoma.

POSTERIOR FOSSA TUMORS

1. **Glial tumors (IA)***
   a. Astrocytoma (cerebellar, brain stem)
   b. Ependymoma
   c. Choroid plexus tumors
   d. Mixed gliomas

2. **PNET (IC)**
   a. Medulloblastoma

3. **Malformative tumors (VII)**
   a. Dermoid-epidermoid
   b. Cyst NOS (not otherwise specified)
   c. Hamartoma (gangliocytoma)

4. **Germ cell tumors (VI)**
   a. Teratoma

5. **Neuronal (IB)**
   a. Ganglioglioma
   b. Gangliocytoma

6. **Nerve sheath cell tumors (III)**
   a. Neurilemmoma

7. **Parameningeal tumors (IX)**

8. **Tumors of meningeal origin (II)**
   a. Meningioma
   b. Meningeal sarcoma
   c. Melanocytic tumors

9. **Lymphoma (IV)**

10. **Metastatic (X)**

11. **Blood-vessel origin tumors (V)**
    a. Hemangioblastoma

*Parenthetical data following each tumor type are designations referring to the outline of the revision of the WHO classification, as presented in the box on p. 205.

NEUROEPITHELIAL NEOPLASMS

The largest group of neoplasms arising within the posterior fossa are gliomas, the commonest of which are astrocytomas followed by mixed gliomas, ependymomas, choroid plexus tumors, and, rarely, glioblastomas.[22,23]

Cerebellar astrocytoma

Cerebellar astrocytoma is one of the two most common posterior fossa neoplasms of childhood, with medulloblastoma (PNET) being the other. Of the histological subtypes of astrocytoma, the pilocytic pattern is by far the most common[17] followed by the fibrillary, mixed (astrocytoma-ependymoma, astrocytoma-oligodendroglioma, and so on) and infrequent anaplastic forms. The vast majority of astrocytomas (pilocytic or fibrillary) tend to be slow growing, sharply demarcated, and well differentiated. These are usually noninvasive and nonmetastasizing, although tissue structure and function are widely variable. These have the best prognosis for any CNS neoplasm of childhood and usually require only surgical excision.

Cerebellar astrocytoma may arise within the vermis, hemisphere, or occupy a paramedian position. Infrequently the astrocytoma may be centered about the cerebellopontine angle or middle cerebeller peduncle. Those actually arising from the pontocerebellar junction are more appropriately classified as brain stem gliomas.[5] The same may be true for those arising from or involving the cerebellomedullary junction (inferior cerebellar peduncle) or the cerebellomesencephalic junction (superior cerebellar peduncle). Macrocysts or microcysts tend to form. The tumor may appear grossly cystic or grossly solid, although both forms contain numerous microcysts. The macrocyst content may be quite variable depending primarily on the protein concentration of the cyst fluid. The classic gross pathological description is that of a cerebellar mass consisting of a large cyst with a solid mural tumor nodule. In actuality, there is a broad spectrum ranging from an entirely microcystic but solid-appearing tumor to a macrocyst containing solid tumor nodules or laminar wall tumor, or an entirely noncystic or solid tumor.[22,23] Virtually all of these tumors produce hydrocephalus by compression or displacement of the fourth ventricle or aqueduct.

Neuroimaging of cerebellar astrocytoma demonstrates a midline, paramedian, or unilateral cerebellar mass of variable density or intensity characteristics depending on the predominance or combination of cystic and solid components and the nature of the cyst content[1,4,17] (Figs. 7-73 to 7-75). The classic appearance is that of a large cystic mass with an eccentric mural tumor nodule or nodules. By CT the cystic or microcystic component is commonly of low density, whereas a more solid tumor appears isodense (Fig. 7-75). The low density cystic component may display attenuation values at or higher than that of CSF depending on the protein content. Iodine enhancement of the nodular component is also characteristic (Fig. 7-75). Occasionally there may be a large, relatively uniform low density mass without abnormal enhancement that may be difficult to distinguish from a developmental cystic malformation, although the attenuation values are usually higher than CSF values. Infrequently the tumor appears as a uniform isodense or an irregular mixed density mass with either homogeneous or inhomogeneous enhancement. When a cerebellar astrocytoma occurs in the midline, differentiation from medulloblastoma or ependymoma may be difficult. However, cerebellar astrocytoma rarely demonstrates tumor hyperdensity, hemorrhage, or calcification on precontrast studies. The pattern of iodine enhancement may also be quite variable, including diffuse or focal, nodular or rimlike, homogeneous or irregular (Fig. 7-75). There has been no reliable correlation between enhancement and histology or grade of malignancy. Furthermore, enhancement may be seen within solid as well as microcystic portions of the tumor. The rimlike enhancement along the cyst margin does not invariably indicate cerebellar infiltration by tumor.

By MRI the macrocystic component may follow CSF

A   B   C

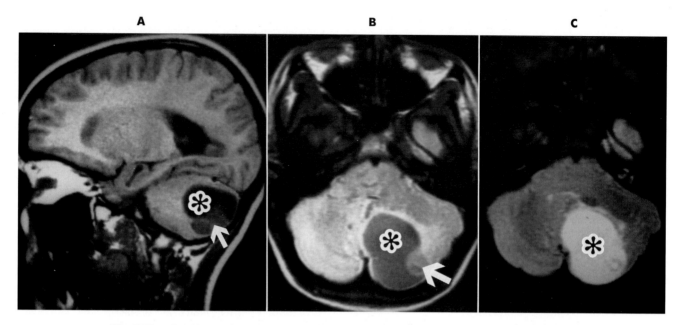

Fig. 7-73   Cerebellar astrocytoma best shown by sagittal T1 **(A)** plus axial proton density **(B)** MRI with low intensity macrocystic component *(astericks)* and isointense microcystic-solid components *(arrows)*. The solid component is obscured by high intensity cyst content on axial T2 **(C)** image. High intensity rim effect on the p **(B)** and T2 **(C)** images is consistent with edema.

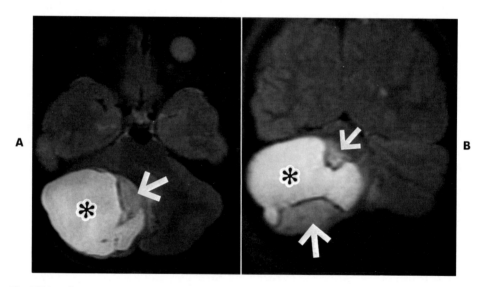

Fig. 7-74   Cerebellar astrocytoma best shown by axial **(A)** and coronal **(B)** T2 MRI with isointense microcystic-solid components *(arrows)* and hyperintense macrocystic fluid content *(asterisks)*. The components were not readily separated on sagittal T1 or axial p images.

intensities throughout the sequences or display intensity patterns characteristic of proteinaceous fluid[1,4] (Figs. 7-73 and 7-74). The microcytic component is commonly of low intensity on T1 MRI and isointense to hyperintense on proton density and T2 MRI images. The nodular or laminar solid component is commonly T1 isointense and isointense to hyperintense on proton density and T2 images, although tumor nodule hypointensity has also been observed. The signal variability of the tumor components accounts for the complexity of the MRI patterns, so all parameters (T1, p, T2) are necessary for achieving the optimal contrast between cystic versus solid tumor components, as well as differentiating tumor from adjacent brain. The distinction is important, since the more solid or microcystic components may be obscured by the macrocyst contents on one sequence but separated on others (Figs. 7-73 and 7-74). Gadolinium may also be helpful, although the enhancement patterns are quite variable and similar to those described

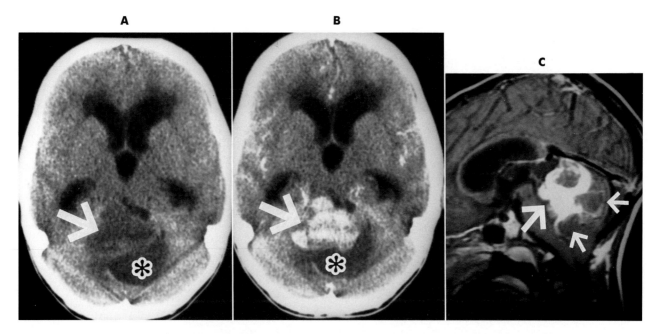

Fig. 7-75   Midline cerebellar astrocytoma shown by CT (**A** and **B**) with isodense enhancing nodules *(arrows)* and low density cystic areas *(asterisks)* plus hydrocephalus with periventricular edema. **C,** Sagittal T1 image after injection shows the vermain mass with high intensity nodular and ringlike gadolinium enhancement. The mass compresses the fourth ventricle, and there is aqueductal kinking with tonsillar herniation.

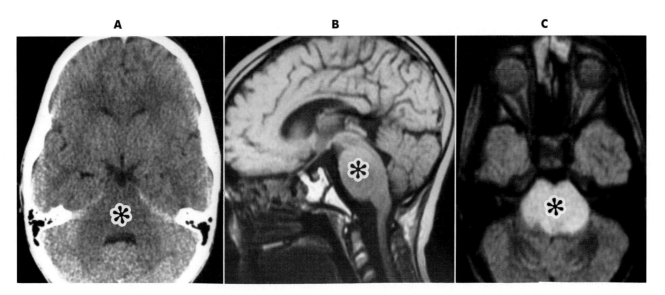

Fig. 7-76   Brain stem glioma shown by CT (**A**) as an isodense to hypodense pontine expansion *(asterisk)* with obliteration of the cisterns about the pons and flattening of the fourth ventricle. Sagittal T1 (**B**) and axial p (**C**) MRI shows T1 isointense to hypointese and p hyperintense pontine expansion *(asterisks)* extending into the midbrain above and the medulla below.

previously for iodine enhancement with CT. Since surgery is the primary and often exclusive mode of treatment, if the tumor is judged to be completely excised and benign, then CT may be used for routine follow-up. For suspected recurrence, however, intravenous iodine enhancement may be required along with density measurements of the surgical defect to detect increased protein content especially if the cyst wall is left in place. Recurrent tumors, particularly those involving the brain stem, are best evaluated with MRI.

Brain stem tumors

Brain stem tumors are overwhelmingly gliomas and most often astrocytomas of varying subtypes and histological variation including heterogeneous or mixed grades of malignancy.[5,22,23] The range of histology includes pilocytic, anaplastic, and glioblastomatous forms, occasionally mixed glioma, and neuronal tumors. Brain stem neoplasia may commonly arise in the pons with diffuse infiltration caudally involving the medulla, or rostrally into the midbrain (Fig. 7-76). Symptomatic hydrocephalus is un-

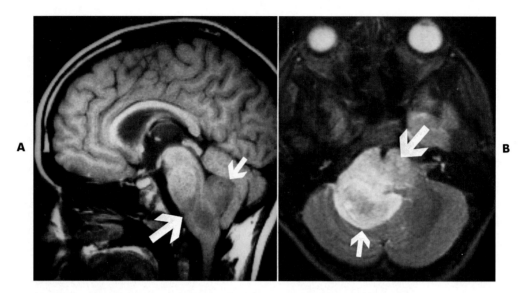

Fig. 7-77   Brain stem glioma shown by sagittal T1 **(A)** and axial T2 **(B)** MRI as a pontomedullary expansion *(large arrow)* with dorsal exophytic *(small arrow)* and right cerebellopontine angle components that are T1 isointense to hypointense and T2 isointense to hyperintense.

usual until late in the disease course. There may be symmetrical growth with circumferential expansion. Asymmetrical growth may produce exophytic extension ventrally into the prepontine cisterns, ventrolaterally into the cerebellopontine angle, dorsally into the fourth ventricle, or dorsolaterally into the middle cerebellar peduncle and cerebellum (Figs. 7-77 and 7-82). Occasionally the tumor appears confined to the pons, midbrain (for example, tectum), or medulla (Figs. 7-76, 7-78, and 7-79). Combined midbrain-thalamic or cervico-medullary involvement is often seen in childhood also (Figs. 7-79 to 7-81). Epstein[5,6] has devised an anatomical classification of brain stem tumors based on combined clinical and neuroradiological findings with relevance to treatment and prognosis. The categories include diffuse, focal, cystic, and cervicomedullary types. Although location and character never ensure histological or biological specificity, tendencies do exist.

Focal tectal, midbrain-thalamic, and cervicomedullary tumors may be of lower grade with a relatively better prognosis. By location the segmental pontine or diffuse brain stem tumors often have a poorer prognosis. These may be low grade, anaplastic, or glioblastomatous in nature. Cystic pontine glial tumors (Figs. 7-81 and 7-82) may be of relatively benign histology (for example, pilocytic) similar to that of cerebellar astrocytoma. Often, however, the cystic or necrotic tumors are higher grade (for example, glioblastoma). Surgery with biopsy, partial excision, or cyst decompression may be considered for cystic tumors, exophytic neoplasms, and especially for cervicomedullary tumors.[5,6] Radiotherapy, or chemotherapy and radiotherapy,[5] is considered the proper approach for treating pontine and diffuse neoplasms. Radiotherapy may be an important adjunct for operable but incompletely resected or recurrent tumors, such as those at the cervicomedullary junction.

Tectal or quadrigeminal plate tumors may be relatively benign in behavior, occurring as low-grade gliomas, hamartomas, or, occasionally, gliosis.[18,24] Most often these produce obstructive hydrocephalus and are more readily detected by MRI than CT (Fig. 7-78). These isolated expansions may be followed by MRI after ventricular shunting. Radiotherapy is reserved for those tumors demonstrating definite growth or those associated with more specific neurological symptoms or signs (for example, visual). Thalamomesencephalic tumors may be confirmed by stereotactic biopsy. Treatment primarily consists of radiotherapy, especially for the higher-grade glial tumors.

Neuroimaging findings in brain stem tumors depend on the level and extent of brain stem involvement.[1,4,11,15] There is usually symmetrical or asymmetrical expansion of the brain stem with compression or obliteration of adjacent cisterns, the fourth ventricle, or the aqueduct. By CT the expansion may be isodense or of low density, whereas MRI often demonstrates T1 isointensity to hypointensity with p/T2 isointensity to hyperintensity (Figs. 7-76 to 7-82). Enhancement with iodine or gadolinium is variable and may be diffuse, nodular, or ringlike along the margins of a cyst or about an area of necrosis (Fig. 7-82). CT almost always detects pontine, diffuse, and combined midbrain-thalamic expansions. Tectal tumors (except for hydrocephalus) and cervicomedullary tumors may be readily depicted only with MRI (Figs. 7-78 and 7-79). Furthermore, MRI more accurately and precisely defines the extent of involvement, which is often underestimated by CT. Of further impor-

A   B   C

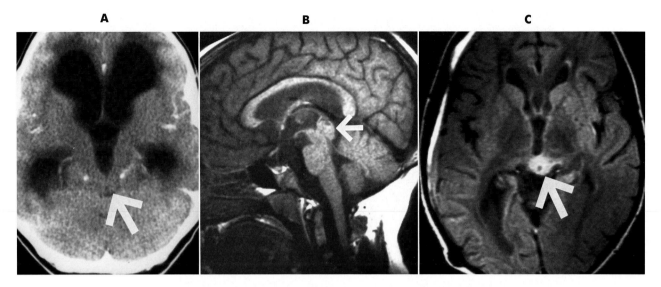

Fig. 7-78   Tectal glioma with aqueductal stenosis and hydrocephalus. **A,** CT shows severe third and lateral ventricular dilatation with periventricular edema and questionable tectal mass *(arrow)*. Sagittal T1 **(B)** and axial p **(C)** MRI demonstrate the tectal expansion *(arrow)* that is T1 isointense to hypointense and p/T2 isointense to hyperintense with aqueductal occlusion.

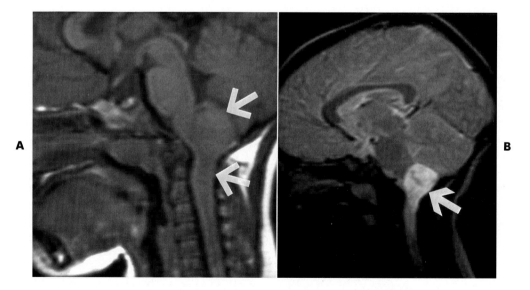

A   B

Fig. 7-79   Cervicomedullary low grade astrocytoma *(arrows)* shown by sagittal T1 MRI **(A)** as an isointense to hypointense expansion of the medulla and upper cord with filling of the cisterna magna. The tumor is isohyperintense on sagittal p images and hyperintense on sagittal T2 images (B).

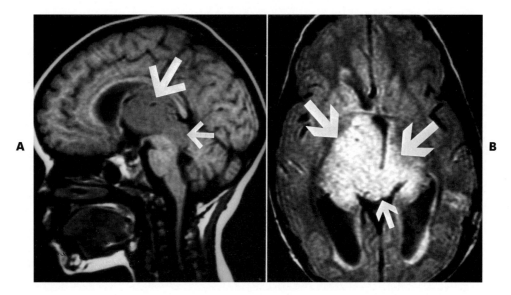

Fig. 7-80   Midbrain and bilateral thalamic low grade astrocytoma shown by sagittal T1 MRI **(A)** as an isointense expansion of the tectum *(small arrows)* and thalami *(large arrows)* with hydrocephalus. **B,** Axial proton density MRI shows the mass to be isointense to hyperintense.

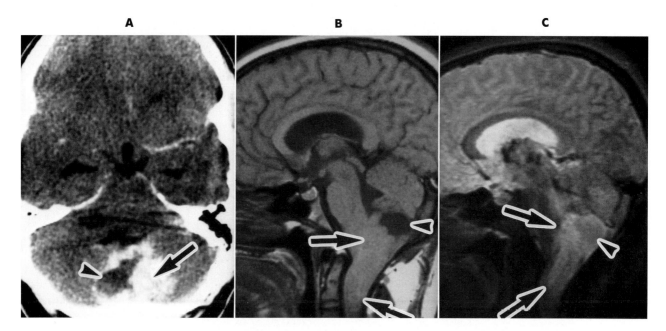

Fig. 7-81   Cervicomedullary anaplastic astrocytoma shown by CT **(A)** as a cystic *(arrowheads)* and enhancing *(arrows)* tumor of the lower posterior fossa. **B,** Sagittal T1 MRI shows isointense to hypointense eccentric cervicomedullary expansion *(arrows)* with exophytic cisterna magna component and cyst *(arrowhead).* The tumor is isointense to hyperintense on sagittal p and T2 **(C)** MRI.

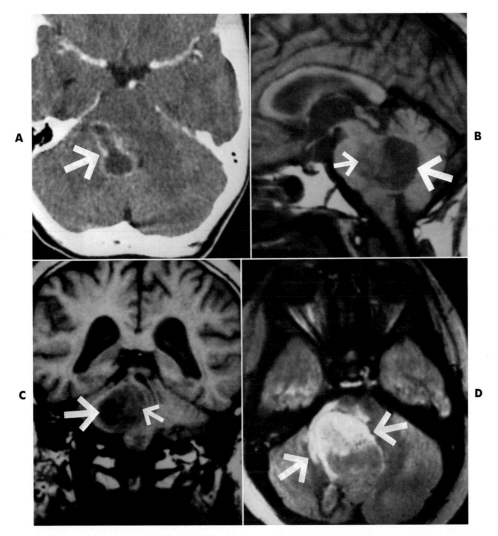

Fig. 7-82   Brain stem glioblastoma centered about the middle cerebellar peduncle shown by CT **(A)** as a low density lesion with margin enhancement *(arrow)*. Sagittal **(B)** and coronal **(C)** T1 MRI and axial p MRI **(D)** show a pontocerebellar and right cerebellopontine angle mass with isointense nodular components *(small arrows)* and cystic necrotic component *(large arrows)* that is T1 hypointense and p/T2 hyperintense. Biopsy tract is present in **D.**

tance, MRI may provide improved specificity for nonneoplastic lesions of the brain stem including infarction, encephalitis, demyelination (multiple lesions), or vascular malformation. For these reasons MRI is recommended as the primary modality for diagnosis, treatment planning, and follow-up of brain stem glioma.[1,4]

Ependymal tumors

Ependymomas are uncommon tumors of the posterior fossa in childhood (after medulloblastoma, cerebellar astrocytoma, and brain stem glioma). Ependymomas contain cells or structures resembling (1) the epithelial lining cells of the ventricular system and central canal, (2) astrocyte-like derivatives that form the subependymal glial layer, and (3) ventricular lining cells with vascular or pial foot processes (tanycytes) found in some parts of the CNS.[22,23] Ependymal tumors thus show considerable histological diversity, depending on which pattern predominates, and may be difficult to distinguish from astrocytomas (even expressing GFAP) or oligodendrogliomas. Although the traditional histological divisions into cellular, epithelial, and fibrillary types convey little prognostic significance, the rare papillary subtype is considered to be more aggressive. The myxopapillary ependymoma, distinguished by papillary architecture and the presence of a myxoid stroma, is uncommon in children and occurs almost exclusively in the filum terminale of the caudal spinal canal, which it resembles.[22,23] The subependymoma (subependymal glomerate astrocyte), probably derived from the subependymal astrocytes, is discussed with the mixed gliomas in the Cerebral Tumor section.

Most ependymomas grow in or adjacent to the ventricular system, although extraventricular and even subarachnoid or extra-CNS tumors occur and presumedly arise from ependymal rests. Tumors are usually strikingly circumscribed and may contain areas of calcification, thrombosis or hemorrhage, focal necrosis, or vascular hyperplasia, and even dysplastic cartilage or bone. Anaplastic cellular features and prominent mitotic activity along with increasingly prominent vascular hyperplasia and necrosis distinguish anaplastic ependymoma. These occur most frequently in the lateral ventricles of children. The term *ependymoblastoma,* used in some series as a synonym for anaplastic or malignant ependymoma, is best reserved for a variant of primitive neuroectodermal tumor (PNET) showing primitive ependymal differentiation. The soft and papillary tumors arising in the fourth ventricle enlarge and then occlude the chamber resulting in obstructive hydrocephalus. Often there is extension through the outlet foramina into the cisterna magna, cisterns about the brain stem, cerebellopontine angle, and through the foramen magnum into the upper cervical canal about the cord. Frequently there is adherence to or invasion of the cerebellum and brain stem, as well as encasement of vertebrobasilar and cranial nerve structures. Seeding occurs primarily with the anaplastic forms.

Heterogeneity is characteristic of ependymomas on neuroimaging and reflects a mixture of solid tumor, cyst, necrosis, edema, calcification, or hemorrhage[1,4,26] (Figs. 7-83 and 7-84). The tumor is often eccentrically placed within the posterior fossa. It may be small and confined to the fourth ventricle with early hydrocephalus, or large and extensive with obliteration of posterior fossa landmarks. By CT the tumor is usually of mixed density, often with calcification, but with variable and usually nonuniform iodine enhancement (Fig. 7-83). Similar heterogeneity is often demonstrated by MRI with mixed intensities throughout the pulse sequences. Usually the tumor is predominantly isointense to hypointense on T1 images, and p/T2 isointense to hyperintense with variable and nonuniform gadolinium enhancement (Figs. 7-83 and 7-84). The heterogeneous signal characteristics and calcification may only occasionally assist in differentiation from cerebellar astrocytoma or medulloblastoma. Complete surgical resection is often not possible, and residual tumor as demonstrated by neuroimaging is often the most important prognostic factor along with age (children less than 2 years of age rarely survive). Radiotherapy and chemotherapy may be important adjuncts. The associated hydrocephalus often requires shunting.

Choroid plexus tumors, mixed gliomas, and neuronal tumors

Choroid plexus tumors include papilloma and carcinoma and are primarily discussed and illustrated in the Cerebral Hemispheric Tumors section. However, these tumors may occasionally arise within the posterior fossa, usually within the fourth ventricle or infrequently within the cerebellopontine angle[1,4,22,23] (Fig. 7-85). *Mixed gliomas* most commonly occur in the cerebrum in childhood but may occasionally be encountered in the cerebellum or brain stem, as discussed earlier.[22,23] *Neuronal tumors* (gangliocytoma and ganglioglioma) are relatively rare in the posterior fossa in childhood[3,22,23] and are more completely discussed and illustrated in the Cerebral Hemispheric Tumor section. A classic type of gangliocytoma may be confined to the cerebellum as a malformative or dysplastic gangliocytoma (Lhermitt-Duclos) and presents as a mass often in late childhood[1,4,25] (Fig. 7-86). Ganglioglioma may rarely occur within the posterior fossa, involving the cerebellum, brain stem, or both[1,3,4] (Fig. 7-87).

PNETs and medulloblastomas

Neoplasms in the primitive neuroectodermal category (PNET) are among the most common and controversial tumors of childhood. Again, for consistency of definition, the term *PNET* has been used as a generic name for otherwise unclassifiable neoplasms resembling primitive neuroectodermal tissue.[7,22,23] In view of the disproportionately high frequency of PNET in the cerebellum the designation *medulloblastoma* has been retained for the usual cerebellar tumor. Cerebellar medulloblastoma, in many series, is the most common posterior fossa tumor of childhood.[12,23] There is a tendency for CNS seeding, although systemic metastases are rare (bone, lymph nodes, lung). Medulloepithelioma is another rare type of PNET in infancy and childhood that may arise within the brain stem or cerebellum.

Medulloblastoma in the vast majority of cases arises in the midline from the cerebellar vermis and grows into the fourth ventricle. The tumor often infiltrates or adheres to surrounding cerebellar vermian and paramedian hemispheric structures. Occasionally there is direct involvement of the brain stem. Often there is spread through contiguous CSF spaces to surfaces of the cerebellum, brain stem, cord, cranial nerves, and meninges. In fact, medulloblastoma is the most common childhood tumor producing intracranial and intraspinal seeding. In fact, seeding may be present initially. The tumor may contain areas of necrosis or cysts, but hemorrhage or calcification is unusual. Rarely in older children, medulloblastoma may arise from the cerebellar hemisphere according to the external granular cell migration theory. Otherwise, this rapidly growing tumor tends to occur in younger children (under 8 years of age) usually with a short duration of symptoms because of hydrocephalus from early invasion of the fourth ventricle.

Neuroimaging of medulloblastoma demonstrates a midline or, occasionally, paramedian tumor with distortion, displacement, dilatation, or obliteration of the fourth ventricle.[1,4] By CT the tumor is commonly isodense to hyperdense, whereas MRI shows T1 isointensity to hypointensity, proton density isointensity to hyperintensity, and T2 isointensity to hyperintensity or occasional T2 hypoin-

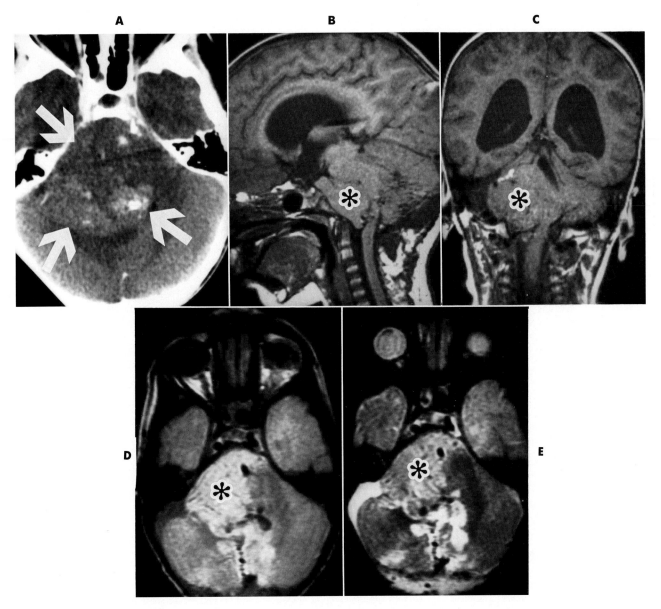

Fig. 7-83   Ependymoma shown by preoperative CT **(A)** as a mixed density, nonuniform enhancing, and poorly defined tumor *(arrows)* with calcific high densities. Postoperative sagittal **(B)** and coronal **(C)** T1 MRI plus axial p **(D)** and T2 **(E)** MRI show large residual tumor *(asterisk)* ventral and dorsal to the brain stem with extension into the right CP angle. The tumor is T1 isointense and p/T2 hyperintense with intermixed hypointensities. (From Healey E, et al: *Neurosurgery* 28:666, 1991.)

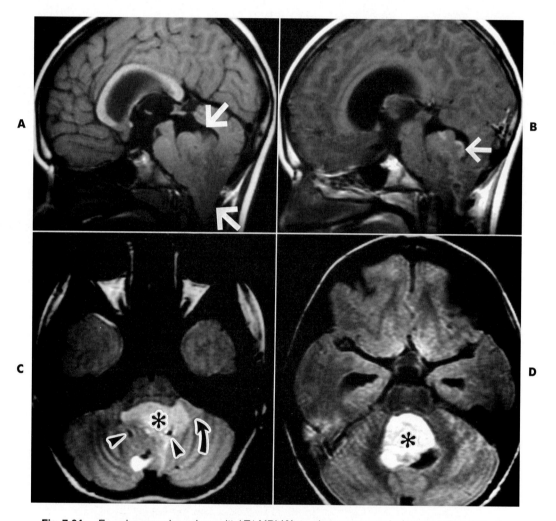

Fig. 7-84 Ependymoma shown by sagittal T1 MRI **(A)** as a heterogeneous isointense to hypointense tumor *(arrows)* extending from within the fourth ventricle along and compressing the dorsal brain stem into the upper cervical canal. **B,** Minimal gadolinium enhancement is present (arrow) on postinjection T1 MRI. **C** and **D,** Axial proton density MRI show the tumor *(asterisks)* as high intensity with extension into the left CP angle *(curved arrow).* Calcific hypointensities *(arrowheads)* are also evident.

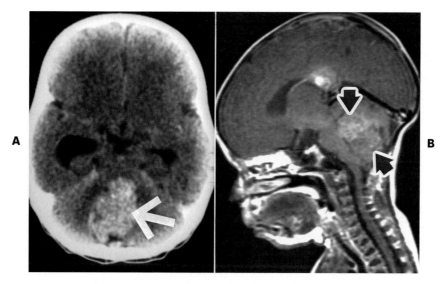

Fig. 7-85 Choroid plexus carcinoma of the fourth ventricle *(arrows)* shown by CT **(A)** as a high density enhancing midline posterior fossa tumor with calcification and hydrocephalus. **B,** Sagittal T1 MRI after injection demonstrates gadolinium enhancement.

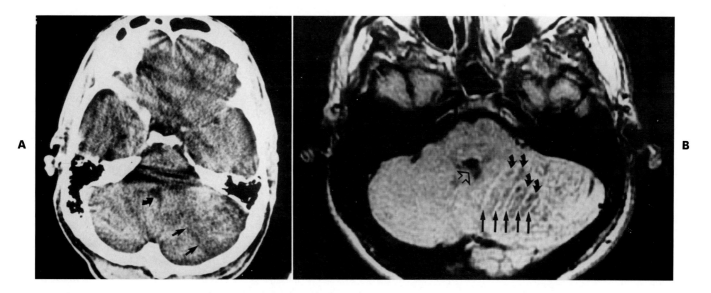

Fig. 7-86 Cerebellar gangliocytoma of Lhermitte-Duclos. **A,** CT shows a mixed density nonenhancing cerebellar mass *(arrows)* displacing the fourth ventricle *(curved arrow).* **B,** Axial T1 MRI shows alternating gray matter isointensities *(curved arrows)* and white matter hyperintensities *(straight arrows)* consistent with dysplastic folia and disordered myelination. The fourth ventricle is displaced *(open arrowhead).* (Courtesy of J. Suojanen, M.D., New England Deaconess Hospital, Boston.)

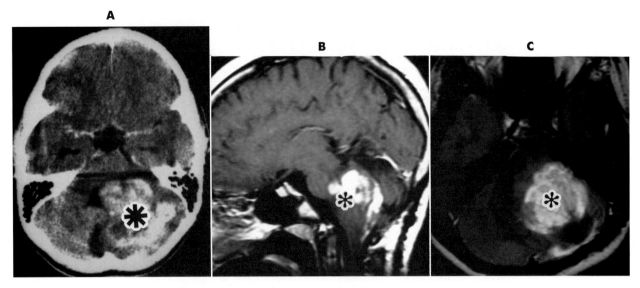

Fig. 7-87   Posterior fossa ganglioglioma shown by CT **(A)** as an isodense and low density enhancing tumor *(asterisk)* involving the cerebellum, brain stem, and fourth ventricle. **B** and **C** demonstrate a Gadolinium-enhancing tumor *(asterisks)* on sagittal T1 **(B)** that is isointense to hyperintense *(asterisk)* on axial p image **(C)** .

tensity with surrounding high intensity edema (Figs. 7-88, 7-90, and 7-94). There is almost always marked iodine or gadolinium enhancement, which is often uniform in character (Figs. 7-88 and 7-90). The tumor may be large and extensive, occasionally with enhancing intracranial dissemination apparent at initial presentation (Figs. 7-91 and 7-92). Heterogeneity may result from the presence of necrosis, cysts, calcification, hemorrhage, or lack of enhancement[1,4,21] (Figs. 7-88, 7-89, 7-93, and 7-94). The usual CT hyperdensity and occasional T2 MRI hypointensity correlates with the hypercellular nature of the tumor. Treatment consists of as complete a surgical excision as possible and shunting of hydrocephalus when necessary. Surgery is followed by preradiation chemotherapy and then craniospinal radiotherapy.[10,12] The presence or absence of spinal neuraxis seeding (Figs. 7-90 and 7-91) is established before chemotherapy and radiotherapy by way of gadolinium-enhanced total spinal MRI examination. This provides the indication and guide for higher dose radiotherapy of the spine. It is important not to confuse gadolinium-enhancing residual tumor or spread with operative intracranial or intraspinal hemorrhage (see Chapter 10).

MENINGEAL AND MELANOCYTIC TUMORS

Meningeal and melanocytic tumors are primarily discussed in the Cerebral Hemispheric Tumor section and in Chapter 8, and include meningioma, meningeal sarcomatous tumors (Fig. 7-95), and primary melanocytic tumors[22,23] (Fig. 7-96).

TUMORS OF NERVE SHEATH CELLS

Cranial and spinal nerve roots, their extensions as peripheral nerves, and the associated sensory and autonomic ganglia constitute the peripheral nervous system (PNS).[22,23] Every peripheral nerve consists of the axons traversing it, a population of nerve sheath cells closely associated with the neural elements, and various connective tissue coverings. Motor axons arise from cell bodies located in the motor nuclei within the CNS and derived from the neural tube, whereas sensory and peripheral autonomic fibers arise from nerve cells (ganglion cells) derived from the neural crest and located outside the CNS in the sensory ganglia. Nerve sheath cells, or Schwann cells, are also thought to originate embryologically from the neural crest. These invest the ganglion cells and both myelinated and unmyelinated axons, and subserve both structural and physiological functions. Schwann cells, analogous to the oligodendrocytes in the CNS, form and maintain the myelin sheath. The connective tissue coverings are divided into three layers. The *endoneurium* is a matrix of fibroblasts, collagen, and mucopolysaccharides which surround the individual axons and associated Schwann cells. The *perineurium* is a lamellated sheath of alternating collagen fibers and specialized cells of uncertain relationship to Schwann cells; it defines the individual peripheral nerve fiber bundles. The *epineurium* is an external sheath of fibroblasts and collagen blending with connective tissue.

Neoplasms of Schwann cells can occur at any point along the course of the peripheral nerve from the cranial or spinal

Text continued on p. 278.

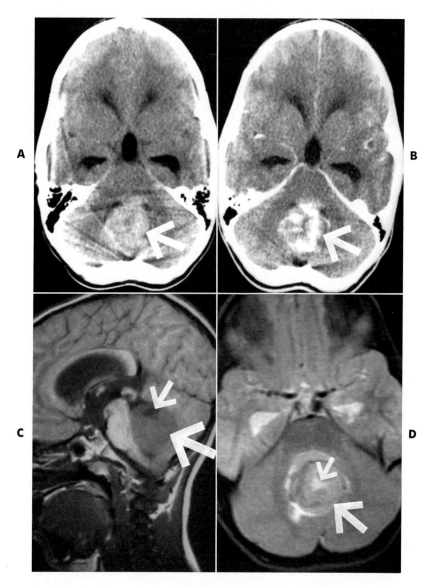

Fig. 7-88   Medulloblastoma demonstrated by CT (**A** and **B**) as a high density enhancing midline posterior fossa mass (arrows) with hydrocephalus. Sagittal T1 (**C**) and axial T2 (**D**) MRI show isointense to hypointense tumor *(large arrows)* with a T1 hypointense and T2 hyperintense cystic or necrotic area *(small arrows)*.

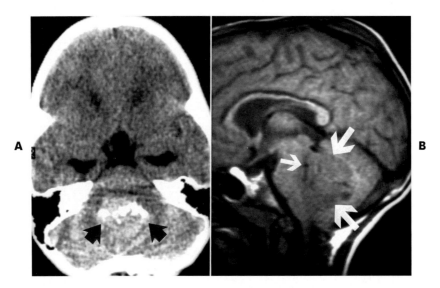

Fig. 7-89 Medulloblastoma shown by CT **(A)** as a high density tumor with nodular calcification *(arrows).* **B,** Sagittal T1 MRI demonstrates T1 isointense tumor *(large arrows)* with calcific low intensities *(small arrow).*

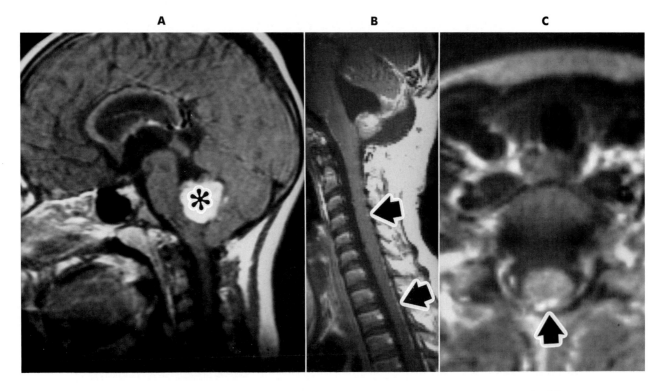

Fig. 7-90 Medulloblastoma with seeding shown as an isointense to hypointense mass on sagittal T1 MRI **(A)** with marked gadolinium enhancement *(asterisk).* Follow-up postoperative sagittal **(B)** and axial **(C)** T1 craniospinal MRI study shows gadolinium-enhancing operative site tumor and seeding with nodular cord implants *(arrows).*

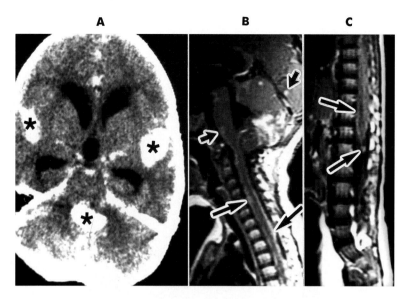

Fig. 7-91   Disseminated medulloblastoma at presentation shown by iodine-enhanced CT **(A)** as multiple-enhancing tumor sites including large midline cerebellar and bitemporal masses *(asterisks)*. **B** and **C,** Postoperative sagittal T1 craniospinal MRI show extensive laminar and nodular gadolinium enhancement at multiple brain and cord sites *(arrows)*.

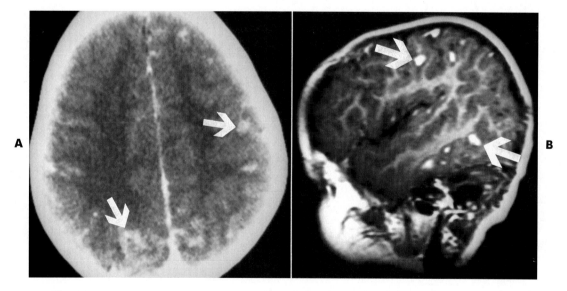

Fig. 7-92   Medulloblastoma with intracranial seeding *(arrows)* shown by CT **(A)** as multiple iodine-enhancing nodular areas. **B,** Parasagittal T1 MRI demonstrates multiple gadolinium-enhancing nodules.

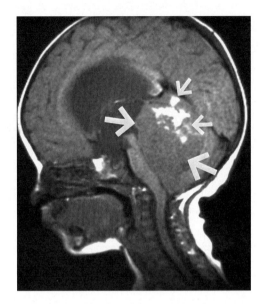

Fig. 7-93 Hemorrhagic medulloblastoma shown by sagittal T1 MRI as a huge isointense to hypointense tumor *(large arrows)* with hydrocephalus and high intensity areas consistent with hemorrhage *(small arrows)*.

A   **B**   **C**

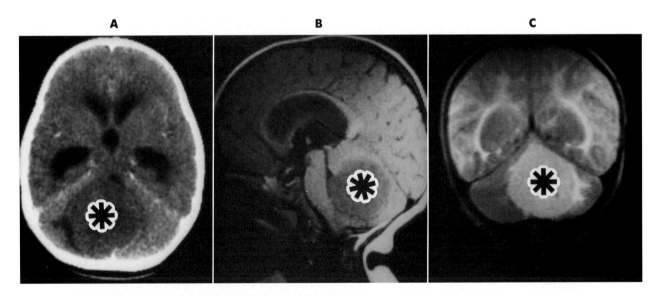

Fig. 7-94 Ganglioneuroblastoma (PNET) of the cerebellum shown by CT **(A)** as a large, low density, nonenhancing tumor *(asterisk)* with hydrocephalus. Sagittal T1 MRI **(B)** demonstrates isointensity to hypointensity, whereas coronal T2 MRI **(C)** demonstrates isointensity to hyperintensity

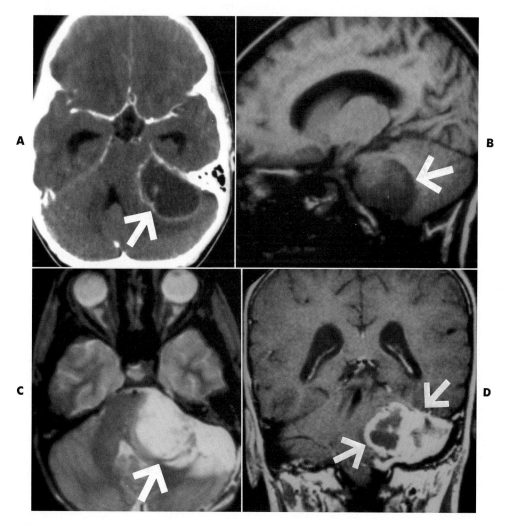

Fig. 7-95   Meningeal sarcoma shown by CT **(A)** as a low density, rim-enhancing left posterior fossa tumor (arrows) with broad-based interface along the petrous bone and tentorium. There is involvement of the cerebellum and pons. The tumor (arrows) is isointense to hypointense on sagittal T1 MRI **(B)** and hyperintense on axial p and T2 **(C)** MRI with marked, irregular enhancement on coronal T1 MRI **(D)** images.

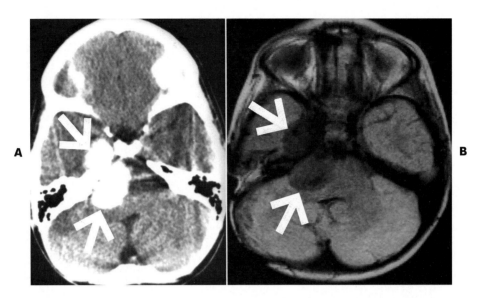

Fig. 7-96   Meningeal melanocytoma *(arrows)* shown by CT **(A)** as a high density enhancing right cerebellopontine angle and parasellar tumor. **B,** The tumor is hypointense on axial p/T2 MRI.

nerve root to the finest subcutaneous endings of the distal nerve twig. Although presumedly derived from the same or related cells, Schwann cell tumors are divided into two classes on the basis of growth pattern and behavior, schwannomas and neurofibromas. The schwannoma, or neurilemmoma, generally grows as a solid, generally rounded mass that compresses and displaces its nerve of origin. The neurofibroma grows infiltratively along its nerve of origin and thus tends to form a fusiform mass. Both types may occur as solitary or multiple lesions, although multiple lesions and certain clinicopathological presentations generally occur as manifestations of neurofibromatosis (see Chapter 8).

Schwannomas, also known as neurilemmomas because of their postulated origin from the perineurial connective tissue sheath, most commonly arise from cranial or spinal nerve roots, particularly the sensory roots, but are also occasionally found more distally in the PNS.[22,23] The most common intracranial schwannoma arises from the vestibular branch of cranial nerve VIII and is also referred to as an acoustic neurinoma.[9,13,20,30] More common in adults than in children, solitary schwannomas are generally incidental tumors, whereas multiple schwannomas are characteristic of neurofibromatosis. Whether associated with neurofibromatosis or not, most schwannomas grow as circumscribed or encapsulated, solid or cystic tumors that displace and compress rather than invade the nerve of origin. Microcystic degeneration, hemorrhage, calcification, and deposition of lipid (xanthomatous change) may occur. Schwannomas characteristically show two tissue patterns: (1) spindle cells arranged in bundles and palisades in a collagenous matrix (Antoni type A) and (2) polymorphic cells loosely arranged in a mucoid matrix (Antoni type B). Most schwannomas are

slowly growing tumors whose effects are caused by local mass effect. Evolution to anaplastic or malignant forms is rare.

Rare outside of the setting of neurofibromatosis, anaplastic or malignant neurilemmomas (schwannomas) almost always arise as de novo lesions rather than within preexisting benign schwannomas. These usually involve peripheral nerves rather than nerve roots. In contrast to benign schwannomas, malignant schwannomas tend to occur in younger adults and children. These show increased cellularity, pleomorphism, mitotic activity, and may contain areas of necrosis. The tumor may be circumscribed or infiltrate adjacent tissues. Local recurrence is common, but distant metastasis is generally a late development. Metaplastic change within the tumor with formation of osteoid, cartilage, striated muscle (malignant triton tumor), or other tissue types is relatively common. The difficulty in distinguishing high-grade malignant schwannomas from high-grade malignant neurofibromas has given rise to the proposed term *malignant peripheral nerve sheath tumor* to encompass the entire group.[22,23]

Although presumedly also arising from the Schwann cell, neurofibromas differ from schwannomas in growth pattern and histological appearance. These are encapsulated and less cellular lesions that grow infiltratively within the nerve of origin in a variably abundant collagenous or mucopolysaccharide matrix. Neurofibromas lack the characteristic Antoni type A and B patterns. Dermal neurofibromas may be single or multiple and are the most common manifestation of neurofibromatosis. Plexiform neurofibromas, so called because of the growth pattern of cylindrical enlargements along the course of the involved nerves, are characteristic of neurofibromatosis.[22,23] These

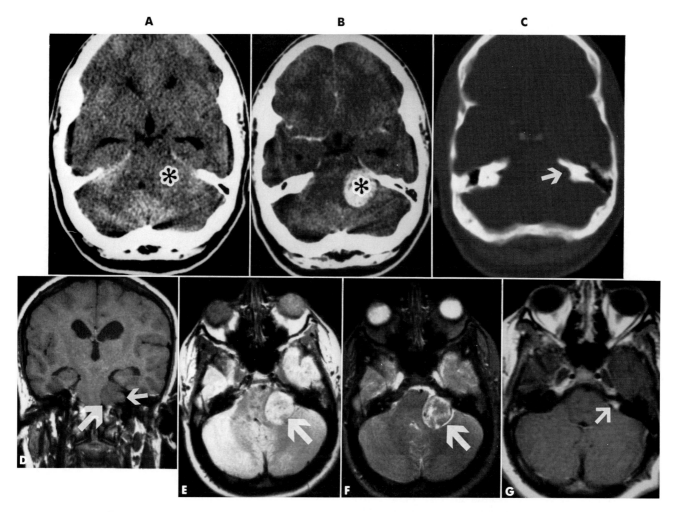

Fig. 7-97   Vestibular neurilemmoma demonstrated by CT **(A-C)** as an isodense **(A)** left cerebello-pontine angle mass *(asterisk)* that markedly enhances **(B)** and produces internal auditory canal (IAC) erosion and widening **(C,** *arrow)*. **D,** T1 coronal MRI shows an isointense tumor *(large arrow)* extending into and enlarging the IAC *(small arrow)*. The tumor (arrow) is isointense to hyperintense on axial p image **(E)** and is isointense to hypointense with internal and peripheral hyperintensities on axial T2 image **(F). G,** Postoperative axial T1 MRI shows residual enhancing IAC tumor *(arrow)*.

may involve singly or multiply any level of the peripheral nervous system from the spinal or cranial roots to the subcutaneous endings. Tumors arising from the proximal nerve roots in the intervertebral foramina may be compressed by the surrounding bone into the typical hourglass configuration (see Chapter 10). Unlike schwannomas, neurofibromas generally lack areas of cystic or xanthomatous degeneration and are not typically calcified.

Anaplastic neurofibromas arise almost exclusively from large peripheral nerves in the setting of neurofibromatosis and frequently in preexisting plexiform neurofibromas.[22,23] Previous radiation therapy may play a role in pathogenesis, but its contribution is difficult to separate from that of the underlying disorder. Although more common in adults, anaplastic neurofibromas occasionally occur in children. The higher-grade forms become indistinguishable from the anaplastic forms of schwannoma and may show similar metaplastic components.

In acoustic schwannomas or neurilemmomas neuroimaging reveals a unilateral, or, rarely, bilateral, intracanalicular, porus acousticus, or cerebellopontine angle mass usually of uniform density, intensity, and enhancement character[1,4,9,13,20] (Fig. 7-97). Rarely is there associated calcification, necrotic or cystic component, or hemorrhage. A characteristic finding is internal auditory canal or foraminal enlargement or erosion. Bilateral tumors are characteristic of neurofibromatosis 2 (see Chapter 8). CT demonstrates an isodense or low density mass, whereas MRI usually shows a T1 isointense to hypointense lesion that is isointense to hyperintense on proton density and T2 images (Fig. 7-97). Marked iodine or gadolinium enhancement occurs in most cases. Relatively sharp separation at the tumor-brain interface is usually seen with a CSF, vascular, dural, or capsular rim. Gadolinium enhancement is important for detecting smaller intracanalicular lesions de novo and for delineating residual tumor postoperatively (Fig. 7-97).

A   B   C

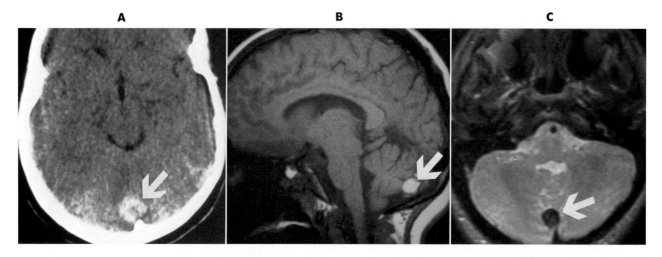

Fig. 7-98   Posterior fossa dermoid (arrows) in Goldenhar syndrome shown by CT **(A)** as a high density calcified nodule *(arrows)*. The dermoid has fatlike hyperintensities on T1 sagittal MRI **(B)** and is hypointense on both axial p and T2 **(C)** images.

MALIGNANT LYMPHOMA

Malignant lymphomas are presented primarily in the Cerebral Hemispheric Tumors section.

TUMORS OF BLOOD VESSEL ORIGIN

Compared with the nonneoplastic vascular malformative tumors (for example, cavernous angiomas), which may mimic true neoplasms clinically and radiologically and produce significant morbidity and mortality, true neoplasms of blood vessel origin are rare in the CNS. The WHO classification recognizes a separate category of vascular malformation. In its category Tumors of Blood Vessel Origin only the capillary hemangioblastoma and the monstrocellular sarcoma are included. In accordance with recent opinions as to the histogenesis of the monstrocellular sarcoma, the proposed revision of the WHO classification removes monstrocellular sarcoma to the category of Glial Tumors.[22] Along with the capillary hemangioblastoma, the subcategories of hemangiopericytoma and the extremely rare primary CNS angiosarcoma/neoplastic angioendotheliosis are included in the newer Blood Vessel Tumor category.[22] Inasmuch as tumors in both of these two new categories are extremely rare in children and raise unresolved questions of histogenesis, only the relatively common capillary hemangioblastoma is discussed.

The capillary hemangioblastoma is a distinctive benign neoplasm that arises most commonly in the paramedian regions of the cerebellum of young or middle-aged adults.[16,22,23] Most tumors are solitary, although multiple tumors and tumors in other locations are features of the autosomal dominant von Hippel–Lindau syndrome (see Chapter 8).[8] Capillary hemangioblastomas are usually grossly circumscribed and often cystic with the tumor itself forming a mural nodule within the cyst. The tumor consists of a meshwork of capillary-size blood vessels separated by a population of lipid-laden stromal cells of uncertain histogenesis. Hemorrhage into the tumor or cyst and reactive gliosis in the surrounding CNS parenchyma are common. Incompletely resected tumors may grow and invade brain. Second tumors, most frequently second primaries in patients with von Hippel–Lindau syndrome, may also appear. However, evolution into malignant forms does not appear to occur.

Hemangioblastomas are usually circumscribed, more often cystic than solid, and of similar appearance to cerebellar astrocytoma, that is, a cystic mass with a vascularized mural nodule[1,4,8,16] (see Chapter 8). Hemorrhage may occur, but calcification is very rare. CT may show an isodense to hypodense mass, whereas MRI demonstrates a CSF-intensity cyst or higher intensity cystic contents consistent with proteinaceous or hemorrhagic fluid. Marked iodine or gadolinium enhancement of the vascularized mural nodule or solid tumor is usually apparent, and there may be surrounding p/T2 hyperintense edema. Gadolinium-enhanced MRI may demonstrate small tumors not seen with iodine-enhanced CT. Surgery is the primary mode of therapy.

GERM CELL TUMORS

Germ cell tumors, except teratoma,[22,23] are extremely rare in the posterior fossa in childhood and are primarily discussed in the Tumors About the Third Ventricle section.

MALFORMATIVE TUMORS

Most malformative tumors occur about the third ventricle and are discussed in that section. However, a number of these are occasionally encountered in the posterior fossa including dermoid or epidermoid cyst, teratoma (also germ cell category), arachnoid cyst, and hamartoma (gangliocytoma). Epidermoids have been described as more commonly arising in the cisterns about the cerebellopontine angle, whereas dermoids more commonly arise in the

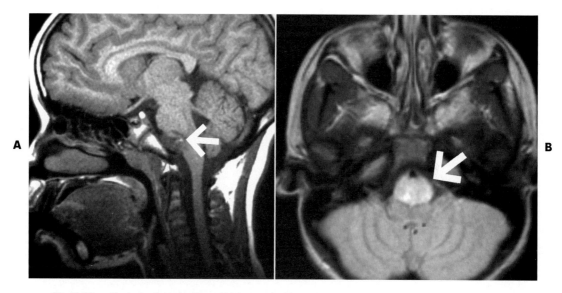

Fig. 7-99 Posterior fossa epidermoid *(arrows)* with recurrent aseptic meningitis shown by sagittal T1 MRI **(A)** as a hypointense tumor with nodular fatlike hyperintensities ventral to the medulla and pons. The epidermoid is hyperintense on both axial p **(B)** and T2 images.

midline related to the cerebellar vermis, within the fourth ventricle, or behind the cerebellum (Fig. 7-98). Epidermoids have been described as nonenhancing, CSF-like density or intensity masses rarely with fatty signal, whereas dermoids more often contain fatlike densities or intensities and calcification.[2,14,27,29] In our experience the classic adult appearance of an epidermoid is rarely seen. Epidermoids of childhood appear similar to dermoids and are more often discrete, midline or paramedian, and more often exhibit fatlike signals (Fig. 7-99). Epidermoid may not be readily distinguished from dermoid except for the presence of calcification or associated dermal sinus in the latter. Treatment is by way of surgical excision.

REFERENCES
Posterior fossa tumors

1. Barkovich A: *Pediatric neuroimaging,* New York, 1990, Raven.
2. Beltinger C, Saule H: Imaging of lipoma of the corpus callosum and intracranial dermoids in the Goldenbar syndrome, *Pediatr Radiol* 18:72, 1988.
3. Castillo M, Davis P, Takei Y, et al: Intracranial ganglioglioma: MR, CT, and clinical findings, *AJNR* 11:109, 1990.
4. Davis P: Tumors of the brain. In Cohen M, Edwards M, editors: *MR imaging of children,* Philadelphia, 1990, BC Decker.
5. Epstein F: A staging system for brainstem gliomas, *Cancer* 56:1804, 1985.
6. Epstein F, Wisoff J: Intrinsic brainstem tumors of childhood: surgical indications, *J Neuroncol* 6:309, 1988.
7. Figeroa R, el Gammal T, Brooks B, et al: MR in primitive neuroectodermal tumors, *J Comput Assist Tomogr* 13:773, 1989.
8. Filling-Katz M, Choyke P, Patronas N, et al: Von Hippel–Lindau disease: Gd-DTPA MR imaging, *J Comput Assist Tomogr* 13:743, 1989.
9. Hernanz-Schulman M, Welch K, Strand R, et al: Acoustic neuromas in children, *AJNR* 7:519, 1986.
10. Horowitz M, Kun L, Mulhern R, et al: Feasibility and efficacy of preirradiation chemotherapy for pediatric brain tumors, *Neurosurgery* 22:687, 1988.
11. Hueftle M, Han J, Kaufman B, et al: MR imaging of brainstem gliomas, *J Comput Assist Tomogr* 9:263, 1985.
12. Hughes EN, Shillito J, Sallan SE, et al: Medulloblastoma of the joint center for radiation therapy between 1968 and 1984: the influence of radiation dose on the patterns of failure and survival, *Cancer* 61:1992, 1988.
13. Kingsley D, Brooks G, Leung A, et al: Acoustic neuromas: MR imaging, *AJNR* 6:1, 1985.
14. Latock J, Kartush J, Kermink J, et al: Epidermoidomas of the CP angle and temporal bone: CT and MR, *Radiology* 157:361, 1985.
15. Lee B, Kneeland J, Walker R, et al: MR imaging of brainstem tumors, *AJNR* 6:159, 1985.
16. Lee S, Sanches J, Mark A, et al: Posterior fossa hemangioblastoma: MR imaging, *Radiology* 171:463, 1989.
17. Lee Y, Van Tassel P, Bruner J, et al: Juvenile pilocystic astrocytomas: CT and MR, *AJNR* 10:363, 1989.
18. Lis S, Lampropoulos C, Sarwar M: Quadrigeminal plate hamartoma, *AJNR* 10:S56, 1989.
19. Olsen W, Dillon W, Kelly W, et al: MR imaging of paragangliomas, *AJR* 148:201, 1987.
20. Press G, Hesselin K: MR imaging of CP angle and internal auditory canal lesions at 1.5 T, *AJNR* 9:241, 1988.
21. Rollins N, Mendelsohn D, Mulue A, et al: Recurrent medulloblastoma, Gd-DTPA MR imaging, *AJNR* 11:583, 1990.
22. Rorke L, Gilles F, Davis R, et al: Revision of the WHO classification of brain tumors for children, *Cancer* 56:1869, 1985.
23. Russell D, Rubenstein L: *Pathology of tumors of the nervous system,* ed 4, Baltimore, 1977, Williams & Wilkins.
24. Sherman J, Citrin C, Barkovich A, et al: MR imaging of the tectum, *AJNR* 8:59, 1987.
25. Smith RR, Grossman RI, Goldberg HI, et al: MR imaging of Lhermitte-Duclos disease: a case report, *AJNR* 10:187, 1989.
26. Spoto G, Press G, Hesselink J, et al: Intracranial ependymoma and subependymoma, *AJNR* 11:83, 1990.
27. Tampieri D, Melanson D, Ethier R: MR imaging of epidermoid cysts, *AJNR* 10:351, 1989.
28. Vogl T, Bruning R, Schedel H, et al: Paragangliomas of the jugular bulb and carotid body: MR imaging, *AJR* 153:583, 1989.
29. Yuh W, Barloon T, Jacoby C, et al: MR of fourth ventricular epidermoid tumors, *AJNR* 9:794, 1988.
30. Yuh W, Wright D, Barloon T, et al: MR imaging of primary tumors of trigeminal nerve and meckels cave, *AJNR* 9:665, 1988.

Parameningeal tumors

Parameningeal tumors (see box below) or tumorlike processes are those that arise outside, that is, extradural, but contiguous with the central nervous system. These may encroach on or invade the intracranial or intraspinal structures with or without producing specific neurological symptoms or signs. Such involvement often drastically changes therapeutic strategies and prognosis. Parameningeal tumors may arise from or involve the scalp, cranial vault, cranial base, sinuses or pharynx, orbits, petromastoid structures, or soft tissues of the face or neck* (see box on p. 283). Although invasive parameningeal processes are often malignant neoplasms, benign neoplasms or nonneoplastic processes (for example, inflammatory) may occasionally be aggressive. Dysplastic conditions may also be associated with bony defects or soft tissue masses and mimic neoplasm.

---

*References 1, 2, 5, 14, 22, 28, 31, 40, 48, 52, 55, 58, 63, 64, 74.

PATHOLOGICAL CLASSIFICATION OF PARAMENINGEAL TUMORS (IX)*

I. MESENCHYMAL

A. Osteochondral
   1. Chondrosarcoma
   2. Osteosarcoma
   3. Fibrosarcoma
   4. Ewing sarcoma
   5. Chondroma
   6. Osteochondroma
   7. Giant cell tumor
   8. Aneurysmal bone cyst
   9. Osteoma
B. Notochordal
   1. Chordoma
C. Lymphoma
D. Leukemia
E. Histiocytosis
F. Metastatic
G. Rhabdomyosarcoma
H. Fibroma/fibromatosis
I. Angiofibroma

II. CARCINOMA (RARE)

A. Oral cavity, pharynx
B. Sinus
C. Salivary gland
D. Thyroid

III. NEURAL

A. Neuroepithelial
   1. PNET
   2. Retinoblastoma
   3. Neuroblastoma
   4. Esthesioneuroblastoma
   5. Progonoma
B. Neural crest
   1. Neuroblastoma
   2. Ganglioneuroblastoma
   3. Ganglioneuroma
   4. Pheochromocytoma
   5. Paraganglioma
C. Nerve sheath
   1. Neurilemmoma
   2. Schwannoma
   3. Neurofibroma
   4. Plexiform neurofibroma

IV. MALFORMATIVE/DYSPLASTIC

A. Dermoid-epidermoid
B. Primary cholesteatoma
   1. Middle ear
C. Teratoma (germ cell tumor)
D. Lipoma
E. Coloboma
F. Vascular anomalies
   1. Hemangioma
   2. Vascular malformations
      a. Capillary
      b. Arterial
      c. Venous
      d. Lymphatic
      e. Combined (AVM)
G. Head/neck cysts
   1. Laryngocele
   2. Branchial cleft cyst
   3. Thyroglossal duct cyst
H. Cranioceles
I. Neurofibromatosis
J. Fibrous dysplasia

V. INFLAMMATORY

A. Lymphadenopathy-lymphadenitis
B. Cellulitis
C. Abscess
D. Granuloma
E. Parasitic infestation
F. Osteomyelitis
G. Sinusitis
   1. Polyps
   2. Cysts
   3. Mucocele
H. Orbital inflammation
   1. Cellulitis
   2. Abscess
   3. Pseudotumor
I. Otomastoid infection
   1. Otitis
   2. Mastoiditis
   3. Cholesteatoma
   4. Cholesterol granuloma

VI. POSTTRAUMA

A. Chronic hematoma (for example, sternomastoid)
B. Cephalohematoma
C. Growing fracture
D. CSF leak

*IX refers to the designation in the outline of the revision of the WHO classification, as presented in the box on p. 205.

The parameningeal neoplastic processes encountered in childhood include those of osseous, chondroid, or myeloid (reticuloendothelial) origin, other mesenchymal origin tumors, and those arising from notochordal remnants.[5,14,28] Other tumors of importance are those of neuroepithelial, neural crest, or nerve sheath origin, and those of neuroectodermal or mesodermal malformative origin.[53,54] The presence and nature of intracranial involvement are critical to patient management. With recent advances in craniofacial and skull base surgery, ablation may be possible without sacrificing function or cosmesis. In cases with intracranial involvement, surgery may serve primarily to establish the diagnosis and the extent of disease. Tumor debulking reduces the local tumor burden for subsequent chemotherapy and radiotherapy. Imaging often requires CT for bony involvement and calcification, and MRI for soft tissue components including neuroanatomy and vascularity.[31,63] Ultrasonography is often useful for screening of head and neck masses, that is, cystic versus solid, as well as for guiding needle aspiration or biopsy and for follow-up.

PARAMENINGEAL TUMORS AND THEIR DIFFERENTIAL DIAGNOSIS BY REGION

SKULL BASE

Neuroblastoma
Histiocytosis
Basal craniocele
Fibrous dysplasia
Chondrosarcoma
(Osteo) chondroma
Chondroma

CRANIAL VAULT

Cephalohematoma
Dermoid-epidermoid
Histiocytosis (for example, eosinophilic granuloma)
Neuroblastoma
Cranioceles
Hemangioma or other vascular anomaly
Fibrous dysplasia
Osteomyelitis
Growing fracture

SCALP

Cephalohematoma
Cellulitis
Abscess
Granuloma
Lipoma
Vascular anomalies (hemangioma, lymphatic, and so forth)
Dermoid cyst
Craniocele
Plexiform neurofibroma
Growing fracture
Fibroma/fibromatosis

ORBIT

Cellulitis, abscess, pseudotumor
Hematoma
Vascular anomalies (hemangioma, lymphatic, and so forth)
Retinoblastoma
Neuroblastoma
Histiocytosis
Dermoid-teratoma
Coloboma
Rhabdomyosarcoma
Neurofibromatosis (sphenoid dysphasia, buphthalmos)
Plexiform neurofibroma, optic glioma
Craniocele
Fibrous dysplasia
Leukemia, lymphoma

NASOSINUS-PHARYNX

Sinusitis (polyp, cyst, mucocele, granuloma)
CSF leak, hematoma, dehiscence
Neuroblastoma
Rhabdomyosarcoma
Angiofibroma
Fibrous dysplasia
Craniocele, heterotopia (nasal glioma), dermoid
Odontogenic tumors
Osteoma
Giant cell tumor
Histiocytosis, lymphoma, leukemia
Carcinoma, lymphoepithelioma

FACE AND NECK

Lymphadenitis
Cellulitis, abscess
Granuloma
Chronic hematoma (sternomastoid)
Vascular anomalies (hemangioma, lymphatic, and the like)
Congenital cysts (branchial cleft cyst, and the like)
Rhabdomyosarcoma
Lymphoma, leukemia
Neuroblastoma
Dermoid, teratoma, lipoma
Neurofibroma, paraganglioma
Fibroma/fibromatosis
Carcinoma (salivary, thyroid)

TEMPORAL BONE

Otitis, mastoiditis, cholesteatoma, cholesterol granuloma
CSF leak, hematoma, dehiscence
Neuroblastoma
Histiocytosis
Rhabdomyosarcoma
Primary cholesteatoma
Osteoma
Neurofibroma, paraganglioma
Fibrous dysplasia, osteopetrosis

MESENCHYMAL TUMORS

Osteochondral tumors may be benign or malignant and most often arise from the skull base. Probably the most common in this region in childhood is *chondrosarcoma*,[35,38] which is usually centered about the sphenoid or sphenooccipital synchondrosis (Fig. 7-100). *Chondroma* or osteochondroma[6] may also be encountered and associated with Ollier's disease (Fig. 7-101). There is usually slow growth but a tendency to malignant degeneration. *Osteosarcoma*[37] and *fibrosarcoma* are also rare but may arise after radiation therapy for other neoplasms in the region,[7] such as retinoblastoma (Fig. 7-102). Sarcomas are highly invasive tumors and may give rise to regional and distant lymphatic and hematogeneous metastases[72] (Fig. 7-103). *Chordoma*[8,32] is another rare but important tumor of childhood arising from intraosseous notochordal remnants of the skull base, and often centered about the synchondroses (Fig. 7-104). These are locally invasive tumors that destroy bone, although CSF seeding and systemic metastasis have been observed (Fig. 7-105). The chondroid variant of chordoma may be indistinguishable from chondrosarcoma. All of these tumors may have similar CT and MRI appearances.[5,14]

These are usually large solid tumors with variable bone destruction, calcified osteoid or chondroid matrix, and extradural soft tissue mass effect. There may be invasion of

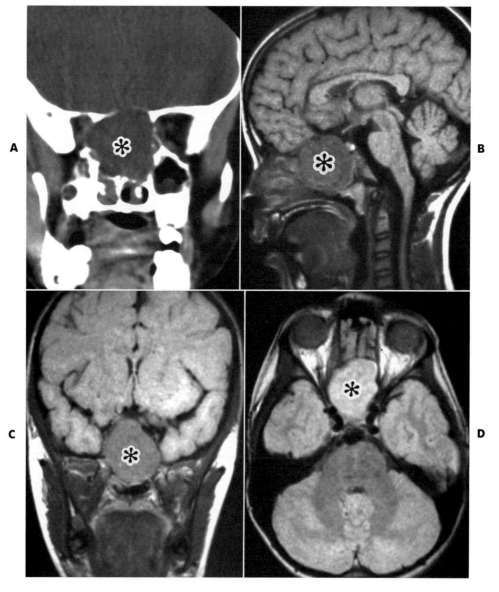

Fig. 7-100 Sphenoid chondrosarcoma *(asterisk)* shown by direct coronal CT **(A)** as an isodense expansion of the sphenoid sinus with bony thinning. The tumor is isointense to hypointense on sagittal **(B)** and coronal **(C)** T1 MRI and isointense to hyperintense on axial p/T2 MRI **(D)**.

adjacent brain structures along the planum sphenoidale, sella, or clivus. Often there is extension into the adjacent sinuses, nasopharynx, and other structures. CT may show an isodense to low density mass with high density calcific components or bony fragmentation along with variable iodine enhancement (Figs. 7-100, 7-101, 7-103 and 7-104). MRI reveals T1 isointensity to hypointensity and p/T2 isointensity to hyperintensity or hypointensity depending on mineral and tumor water content (Figs. 7-100, 7-101, 7-102, and 7-105). Nonspecific gadolinium enhancement may also occur. Occasionally, chondrosarcoma or chordoma may not contain identifiable calcification to allow differentiation from other soft tissue malignancies. Giant

cell tumor and aneurysmal bone cyst or other rare skull base tumors may also arise about the maxillomandibular complex, sinuses, or orbits and tend to expand rather than permeate bone.[5] These lesions may occur in combination and may contain blood elements with fluid levels. Sinus and calvarial osteomas are rarely symptomatic in childhood.

Other important mesenchymal tumors of childhood include rhabdomyosarcoma, fibroma or fibromatosis, and angiofibroma.[31] Rhabdomyosarcoma is the most common malignant soft tissue tumor of the head and neck region in childhood (Figs. 7-106 and 7-107) followed by lymphoma, other sarcoma, neuroblastoma, PNET, histiocytosis, and leukemia. Head and neck carcinomas (thyroid, salivary

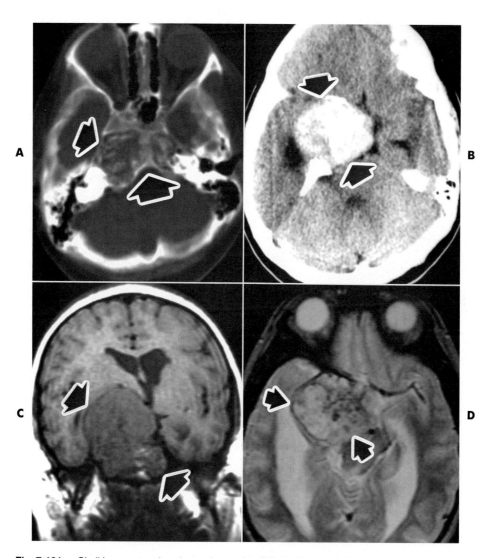

Fig. 7-101   Skull base osteochondroma (arrows) in Ollier's disease. **A,** Noncontrast CT shows mixed lytic and sclerotic expansion of the sphenoid body with chondroid matrix. **B,** Contrast CT shows high density enhancing suprasellar and right temporal mass. **C,** Coronal T1 MRI demonstrates the isointense to hypointense skull base mass with intracranial extension. **D,** On axial T2 MRI the mass is isointense to hyperintense with calcific hypointensities.

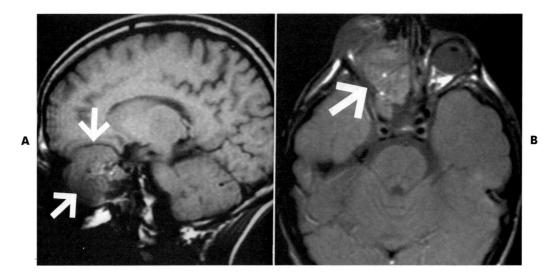

Fig. 7-102   Orbitoethmoid osteosarcoma *(arrows)* years after radiotherapy for bilateral familial retinoblastoma. Sagittal T1 MRI **(A)** demonstrates the isointense to hypointense tumor, which is isointense to hyperintense on axial p/T2 **(B)** images.

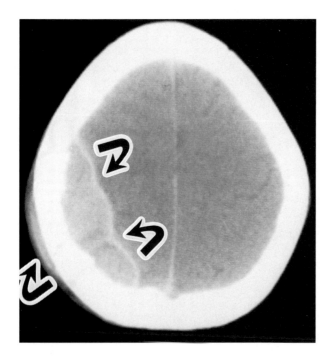

Fig. 7-103   Metastatic calvarial Ewing sarcoma *(curved arrows)* shown by CT as an isodense to hyperdense enhancing and bony destructive lesion of the parietal cranium with scalp and intracranial epidural involvement.

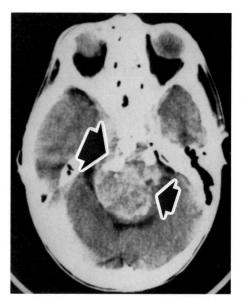

Fig. 7-104   Skull base chordoma *(arrows)* shown by CT as an isodense to hyperdense posterior fossa tumor with calcifications and enhancement.

A   B   C

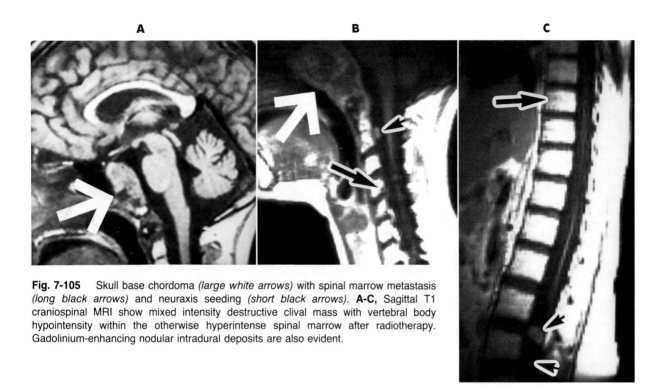

Fig. 7-105   Skull base chordoma *(large white arrows)* with spinal marrow metastasis *(long black arrows)* and neuraxis seeding *(short black arrows)*. **A-C,** Sagittal T1 craniospinal MRI show mixed intensity destructive clival mass with vertebral body hypointensity within the otherwise hyperintense spinal marrow after radiotherapy. Gadolinium-enhancing nodular intradural deposits are also evident.

A   B

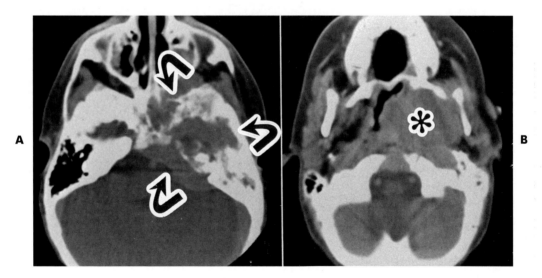

Fig. 7-106   **A** and **B,** infratemporal and skull base rhabdomyosarcoma shown by CT as an isodense, enhancing midline and left parapharyngeal tumor *(asterisk)* with middle cranial fossa and petrous temporal bony destruction and intracranial extension *(curved arrows)*.

A   B   C

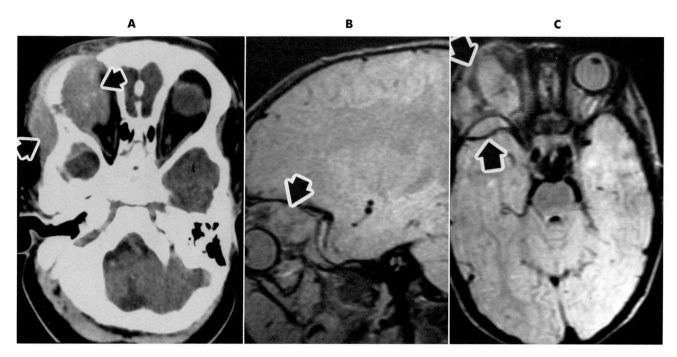

Fig. 7-107 Orbitocranial rhabdomyosarcoma *(arrows)* shown by contrast CT **(A)** as an isodense, calcified, and enhancing mass with bony destruction. Sagittal **(B)** and axial **(C)** p/T2 MRI show the isointense orbital tumor with intracranial extension.

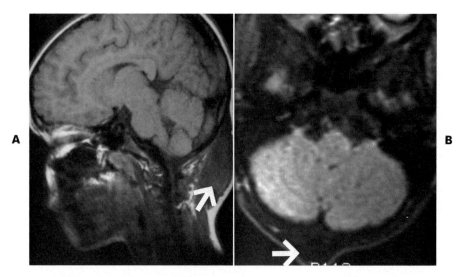

Fig. 7-108 Cervicooccipital subcutaneous benign fibroma *(arrow)* shown by sagittal T1 **(A)**, axial p, and axial T2 **(B)** MRI as a hypointense mass.

gland, sinus-pharynx, and so on) are quite rare.*

Rhabdomyosarcoma is an aggressive and invasive mesenchymal neoplasm, usually of the embryonal or alveolar subtype, and may arise within the sinus, pharynx, orbit, temporal bone, or neck.[31,34] Similar to other "small cell" or "round cell" malignancies of childhood as enumerated above, these hypercellular tumors often form large soft

tissue masses that infiltrate tissue planes and destroy bone in a permeative fashion, for example, orbit, sinus, or otomastoid[5,14,31,34] (Figs. 7-106 and 7-107). Regional and systemic metastasis may also occur. These often appear isodense to high density or occasionally low density by CT with frequent iodine enhancement. MRI may show nonspecific T1 isointensity to hypointensity and p/T2 isointensity to hypointensity or occasional hyperintensity depending on tumor water content (Fig. 7-107). The degree or character

*References 9, 61, 62, 65, 66, 68.

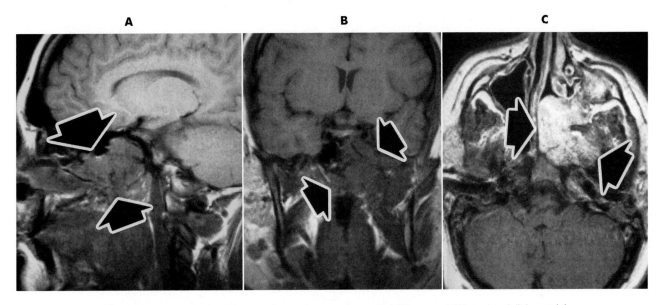

Fig. 7-109   Juvenile angiofibroma *(arrows)* shown by sagittal **(A)**, coronal **(B)**, and gadolinium-axial **(C)** T1 MRI as a large isointense to hypointense gadolinium-enhancing mass with vascular hypointensities.

of gadolinium enhancement is also variable and nonspecific.

Fibromas[5,14,31] are mesenchymal tumors that may be isolated and relatively benign in behavior, or aggressive, invasive, and malignant with extensive involvement, that is, fibromatosis or fibrosarcoma. CT and MRI may reveal isodensity to hypodensity and relative hypointensity throughout the sequences with minimal or no enhancement in lesions with a prominent fibrous component (Fig. 7-108). CT hypodensity and p/T2 MRI hyperintensity may be seen in lesions with higher water content, particularly the more malignant forms.

Juvenile *angiofibroma*[31] is a histologically benign but often aggressive and invasive fibrovascular tumor of adolescent males and arises from the posterolateral nasal cavity about the sphenopalatine foramen. These often extend further into the nasal cavity, nasopharynx, sinuses, or orbit. Occasionally there is intracranial extension. These are often large and highly vascular soft tissue masses causing recurrent epistaxis and nasal obstruction. By CT these are often isodense or low density masses showing marked iodine enhancement (Fig. 7-109). MRI commonly reveals T1 isointensity to hypointensity with p/T2 isointensity to hypointensity or hyperintensity (Fig. 7-109) depending on the combination of fibrous components (hypointensity), vascularity (flow signal voids or high intensity flow enhancement), and tumor water (occasionally cystic or edematous). Gadolinium enhancement is often marked. Angiography and preoperative embolization are important adjuncts to surgical resection.

Common reticuloendothelial or lymphoreticular para-

meningeal neoplasms in the pediatric age group include lymphoma, leukemia, and histiocytosis.[5,14,28,31,63] In some pediatric series *lymphomas*[20,26,31,36] are the commonest malignant solid tumor of the head and neck region, with non-Hodgkins's lymphoma being more common than Hodgkin's lymphoma. Hodgkin's disease frequently presents with cervical lymphadenopathy and usually spreads along contiguous nodal chains, whereas non-Hodgkin's lymphoma is often widespread initially with noncontiguous nodal spread. Also, lymphomas often occur in extranodal sites in children including the nasopharynx, adenotonsillar region, salivary glands, and sinuses. Head and neck lymphomas may be associated with childhood AIDS.[21,25,29,46] *Leukemia* may produce cervical lymphadenopathy in childhood and, rarely, leukemic tumors, that is, chloromas, the latter occurring especially with the myeloblastic forms.[31,70] These may be encountered intracranially or arise in the orbit, sinuses, pharynx, scalp, neck, or cranium (see Cerebral Hemispheric section).

Histiocytosis is a reticuloendothelial disorder of unknown origin that may be relatively isolated (for example, eosinophilic granuloma) or disseminated with visceral, cutaneous, and bony involvement (for example, malignant histiocytosis).[10,11,31,63] The condition is histologically characterized by tissue infiltration with reticulum cells, histiocytes, plasma cells, and leukocytes. Solitary or multiple soft tissue masses may be seen with lytic bony destruction involving the petromastoid, orbit, sinuses, cranial base, or cranial vault (Figs. 7-110 and 7-111). Intracranial involvement may also occur intradurally or extradurally with any of these lymphoreticular processes, as previously presented. CT

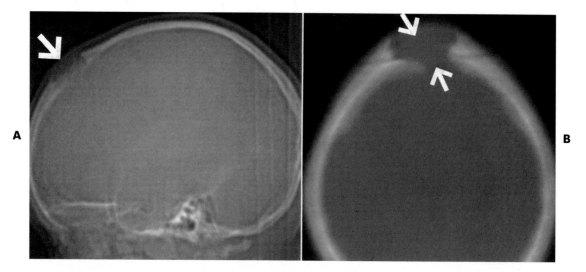

Fig. 7-110   Frontal calvarial histiocytosis (eosinophilic granuloma) shown by lateral scout projection **(A)** and axial CT **(B)** as a lytic diploic space mass *(arrow)* expanding and eroding into the inner and outer tables giving a beveled-edge appearance.

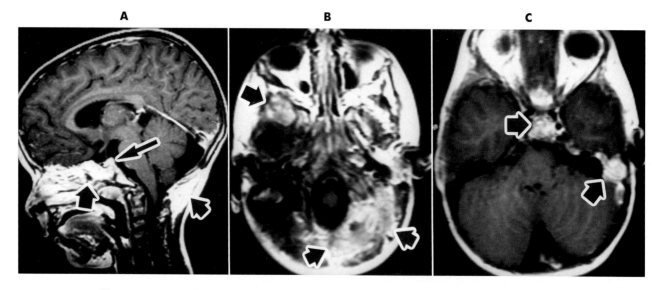

Fig. 7-111   Malignant histiocytosis with extensive skull base involvement *(arrows)*. Sagittal **(A)** and axial **(B** and **C)** T1 MRI show multiple, Gadolinium-enhancing and bone-destructive lesions including involvement of the sphenoid body, clivus, pituitary gland *(long black arrow)*, left petrous temporal bone, and occiput.

may often show isodense to high density masses in these hypercellular neoplasms, or occasional low density masses usually with prominent iodine enhancement. MRI often shows T1 isointensity to hypointensity with gadolinium enhancement and p/T2 isointensity to hypointensity or occasional hyperintensity[5,14] (Fig. 7-111). With involvement of the cranial base and vault, there may be focal or diffuse replacement of the marrow resulting in abnormal T1 isointensity to hypointensity. The absence of fatty T1 hyperintensity, particularly in the clivus, after 3 to 6 years of age, may be suspicious, since red to yellow marrow conversion has usually occurred by then. Other diagnostic considerations in the reticuloendothelial tumor category include the rare hematogenous metastasis from distant primaries.

NEURAL TUMORS

Neural tumors in the parameningeal category include neuroepithelial and neural crest origin tumors such as PNET, retinoblastoma, neuroblastoma, esthesioneuroblastoma, progonoma, and paraganglioma. Also included are the nerve sheath tumors, for example, schwannoma, neurofibroma, and plexiform neurofibroma.[53,54] *Neuroblastoma* is the most common of these solid tumors and may

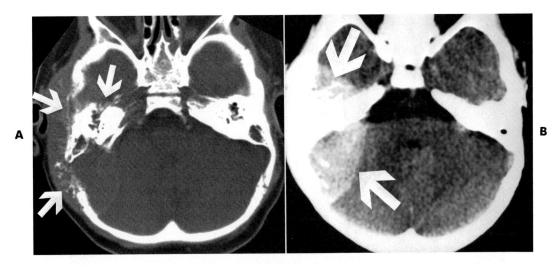

Fig. 7-112   **A** and **B,** Petrous temporal PNET *(arrows)* shown by CT as an isodense to hyperdense enhancing tumor with bony destruction and intracranial extension.

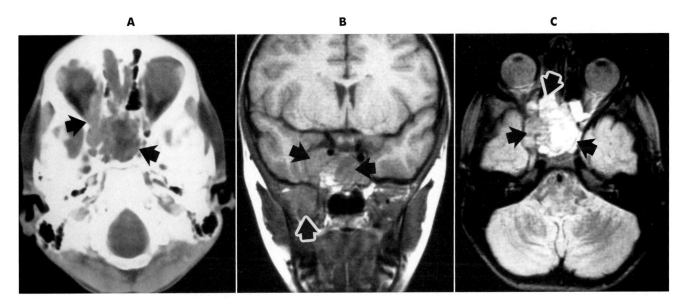

Fig. 7-113   Sphenoethmoidal and retromaxillary PNET *(black arrows)* shown by CT **(A)** as an isodense tumor with bone destruction. Coronal T1-MRI **(B)** shows the isointense-hypointense tumor, which is isointense to hyperintense on axial p/T2 MRI **(C)**. The tumor extends into the orbital apex and cavernous sinus.

arise or involve the skull base, cranial vault, scalp, orbit, sinuses, or temporal bone, or may present as a neck mass with cervical spinal involvement.[5,13,14,31,63] *Esthesioneuroblastoma* is a very rare variant that arises from the olfactory groove, often with extensive invasion of the adjacent skull, sinuses, orbit, and intracranial structures.[5,14] *Primitive neuroectodermal tumors* (PNETs) arising outside of the CNS are of similar location and gross appearance to neuroblastoma but usually lack any differentiated cellular elements.[5,14,31,53,63] *Progonomas* are rare retinal enlarge tumors often containing melanin that may arise from the cranial base or vault and invade adjacent brain.[5,28] Neuro-

blastoma, PNET, esthesioneuroblastoma, and progonoma have similar appearances by CT and MRI including soft tissue mass effect with permeative lytic bone destruction that is often calcified but infrequently cystic.[5,14,31,63] There may be single or multiple site involvement as part of disseminated or metastatic disease. CT and MRI may demonstrate isodensity to hyperdensity and isointensity to hypointensity, respectively, again related to tumor hypercellularity, along with prominent iodine or gadolinium enhancement[5,14] (Figs. 7-112 and 7-113). Again, significant tumor water may produce CT hypodensity and p/T2 MRI hyperintensity.

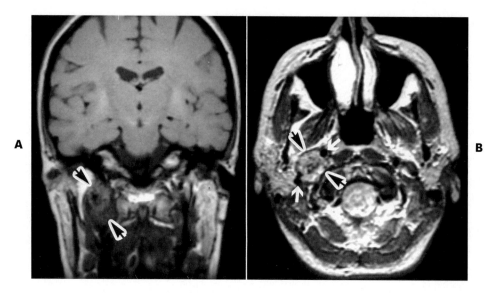

Fig. 7-114   Paraganglioma (glomus vagale) of the right neck *(black arrows)* shown by coronal T1 **(A)** and axial proton density **(B)** MRI as an isointense mass with internal vascular flow void signals. The mass is situated between the internal carotid arterial flow void anteriorly *(white arrows)* and the internal jugular venous flow void posteriorly *(white arrows)*. Gadolinium enhancement was also demonstrated. (Courtesy R. Schwartz, M.D., Brigham and Women's Hospital, Boston.)

From the point of view of taxonomy of *paraganglionic neoplasms*, the paraganglion system (neural crest origin) is a group of organs of the diffuse neuroendocrine system whose common feature is the storage and secretion of catecholamines.[53,54] This includes the adrenal medulla, groups of neuroendocrine cells associated with the sympathetic chain, and cell groups in other locations probably associated with parasympathetic nerves. Neoplasms of these structures include the pheochromocytomas, sympathetic paragangliomas, parasympathetic paragangliomas, and paragangliomas of uncertain origin. Pheochromocytomas usually arise in the adrenal medulla and secrete norepinephrine and epinephrine. The sympathetic paragangliomas arise from the sympathetic chain and sometimes secrete norepinephrine. The parasympathetic paragangliomas, also known as chemodectomas, arise from the carotid body, glomus jugular, glomus tympanicum, vagal body, or aortic body and generally secrete only small amounts of amines. The paragangliomas arise from uncertain cells of origin in the cauda equina, sella turcica, pineal region, or duodenum.

Most paragangliomas occur in adults, and clinical presentations depend on the anatomical location and functional status of the tumor. Important considerations are the possibilities of familial occurrence, association with various multiple endocrine neoplasia syndromes or neurofibromatosis, and the occurrence of bilateral or multiple tumors. Although most paragangliomas are histologically benign and grow slowly, with prognosis dependent on resectability and on the ability to control amine secretion, malignant forms sometimes develop. CT usually shows an isodense to hyperdense or low density soft tissue mass with bony erosion and marked iodine enhancement.[40] MRI may be characteristic by revealing T1 isointensity to low intensity with vascular signal voids plus p/T2 isointensity to hyperintensity with vascular flow voids or high intensity vascular flow enhancement[5,14,40,45,69] (Fig. 7-114). Gadolinium enhancement tends to be marked.

Nerve sheath tumors include schwannoma (neurilemmoma), neurofibroma, and plexiform neurofibroma, which are described in detail in the Posterior Fossa section and in Chapter 8. These tumors arise from peripheral cranial or somatic nerves (for example, vagus) within the neck, often as large, solid, or (rarely) cystic soft tissue masses. These tumors are usually isodense to hypodense by CT and show marked iodine enhancement. By MR these are often isointense to hypointense on T1 images, isointense to hyperintense on p/T2 images, and show gadolinium enhancement.[5,14] These may be large enough to erode bone, but calcification is unusual. Plexiform neurofibromas may be associated with underlying dysplastic defects in neurofibromatosis, as discussed later.

Retinoblastoma is the most common intraocular neoplasm of childhood.[4,48,53,54] It is often bilateral and occasionally familial. Leukocoria (white pupillary reflex)[30] and strabismus are the common clinical findings in this tumor of infancy and early childhood. Calcification occurs in greater than 90% of cases. CT usually reveals a high density intraocular mass with variable iodine enhancement[12,48] (Fig. 7-115). MRI demonstrates T1 isointensity to hypointensity relative to the vitreous with p/T2 isointensity to hypointensity and gadolinium enhancement.*

---

*References 5, 12, 14, 49, 57, 71.

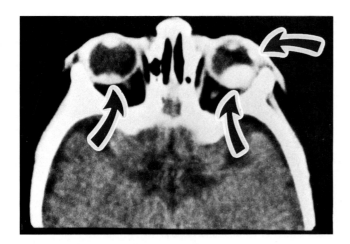

Fig. 7-115 Bilateral retinoblastoma *(arrows)* shown as intraocular calcified, enhancing high density nodular masses.

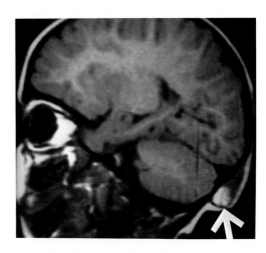

Fig. 7-116 Occipital subcutaneous dermoid cyst (arrow) without cranial or intracranial involvement. T1 sagittal MRI shows a high intensity mass with questionable fluid level. Other considerations include lipoma, sebaceous cyst, and lymphatic malformation.

Spread beyond the globe may occur by direct extension along the optic nerve, the perioptic subarachnoid space, or by lymphatic or hematogenous routes. Bilateral hereditary retinoblastoma may be associated with pineoblastoma, that is, trilateral retinoblastoma. Also, there is an increased susceptibility to radiation-induced malignancies, as well as second nonocular malignancies such as osteogenic sarcoma, fibrosarcoma, and rhabdomyosarcoma.

Other intraocular lesions included in the differential diagnosis of leukocoria,[30] intraocular calcification, or ocular hyperdensity by CT[33,47,48,50,57,71] include retinoma (benign variant of retinoblastoma), Coat's disease (retinal telangiectatic vascular anomaly with lipoprotein exudate), and persistent hyperplastic primary vitreous[41] (persisting embryonic hyaloid vascular system with vitreous hemorrhage, microphthalmia, and rare calcification). Also included are retrolental fibroplasia (retinopathy or prematurity with retinal detachment), chronic retinal detachment, and sclerosing endophthalmitis (larval granulomatous uveitis). Other considerations may include congenital cataract, coloboma, the rare retinal hemangioblastoma, and choroidal or retinal hemangioma with detachment.

BENIGN MALFORMATIVE TUMORS

Benign malformative and inflammatory processes make up the largest group of head and neck masses in childhood (greater than 80%).[31,63] Malformative lesions are commonly cystic, whereas malignant lesions are commonly solid. These include neuroectodermal[73] and mesodermal malformative lesions such as dermoid, epidermoid, teratoma, and lipoma. Also included are vascular anomalies (hemangioma and vascular malformations) as well as developmental cystic lesions of the neck such as laryngocele, branchial cleft cyst, and thyroglossal duct cyst. *Dermoids* or *epidermoids*, as discussed in previous sections, may also arise parameningeal (Figs. 7-116 and 7-117)

with or without intracranial connection (that is, sinus tract, bony defect, or compartment expansion). These may arise in the cranial vault, within the scalp, nasal or prenasal, intraorbitally (lacrimal fossa)[44] or in the middle ear (primary cholesteatoma). Dermoids of the nasofrontal region are to be differentiated primarily from encephaloceles and nasal "gliomas," that is, heterotopias. *Cystic teratomas* may also arise within the neck region. *Lipoma* may occur within the scalp, face, or neck (Fig. 7-118). *Coloboma* is a defect in closure of the fetal optic fissure (origin of the retina and optic nerve) and produces a malformed globe and optic nerve with an orbital cyst and microphthalmia[56] (Fig. 7-119).

Vascular anomalies include hemangiomas and vascular malformations.[24,43] The latter consist of capillary, arterial, venous, lymphatic (cystic hygroma), and combined malformations. These are often distinguished by clinical and imaging criteria, especially using spin echo (SE) MRI sequences with presaturation, and gradient echo (GE) sequences with gradient moment nulling. Vascular anomalies commonly arise or involve the scalp, cranial diploe, face, neck, orbit, nasosinus, and salivary glands (parotid). Hemangiomas are congenital tumors characterized histologically by endothelial proliferation. Parenchymal intensities are identified by MRI along with spin echo signal flow voids and gradient echo flow enhancement, which correlates with large arteries and veins in this "high flow" anomaly (Fig. 7-120). Parenchymal gadolinium enhancement is also demonstrated. Arteriovenous malformations are also "high flow" anomalies that exhibit SE vascular flow voids and GE flow enhancement but no parenchymal component. Lymphatic and venous malformations are "low flow" malformations (absence of SE vascular flow voids) consisting of cystic, septated, or cavernous channels (Fig. 7-121). Often there is a fibrofatty stroma. Phleboliths and gadolinium enhancement of the channels are typical of venous malfor-

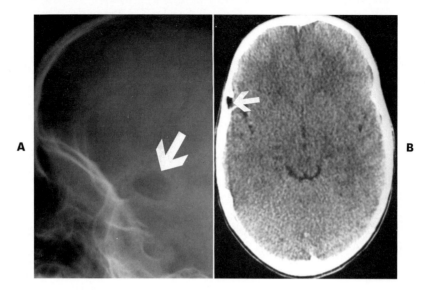

Fig. 7-117 Frontotemporal calvarial epidermoid (arrows) shown by lateral skull film **(A)** and axial CT **(B)** as a circumscribed lytic, diploic expansion with mildly sclerotic margins and CT fatty hypodensity with inner table breakthrough.

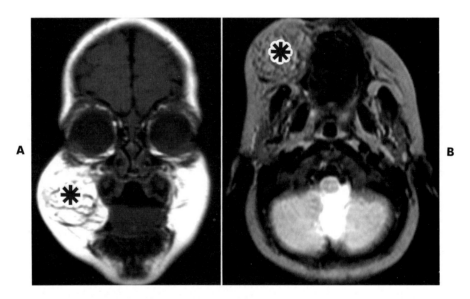

Fig. 7-118 Orbitofacial subcutaneous lipoma *(asterisk)* shown by coronal T1 **(A)** MRI as a septated high intensity mass that is isointense to hypointense on axial T2 MRI **(B).**

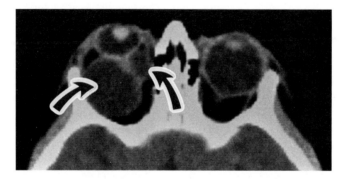

Fig. 7-119 Coloboma shown by CT as retroocular cystic masses *(arrows)* with microphthalmia.

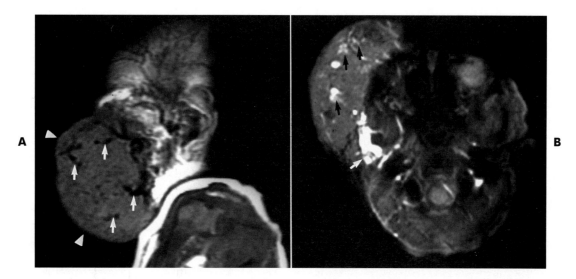

Fig. 7-120   Proliferating orbitofacial hemangioma that is T1 hypointense **(A)** (arrowheads) with internal vascular flow voids *(arrows)*, p/T2 hyperintense, and isointense **(B)** on axial gradient echo image with internal *(black arrows)* and peritumoral *(white arrow)* high intensity vascular flow enhancement.

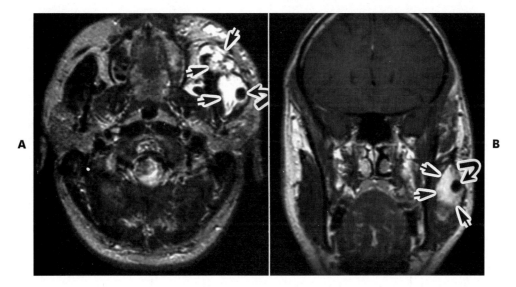

Fig. 7-121   Facial venous malformation *(straight arrows)* with phlebolith *(curved arrow)* shown by axial proton-density MRI **(A)** as a septated high intensity mass containing a hypointense phlebolith. **B,** Coronal T1 MRI shows marked gadolinium enhancement of the vascular spaces again with the hypointense phlebolith.

mations (Fig. 7-121). In lymphatic malformations, only the septae may show enhancement. Combined anomalies, such as a lymphaticovenous malformations, have features characteristic of their separate components. Involuting hemangiomas lacking vascular SE flow voids mimic the "low flow" malformations.

The *laryngocele* is a developmental appendicular sacculation of the laryngeal ventricle that is readily diagnosed by its air content and location within or adjacent to and communicating with the larynx.[31] The most common of the

branchial arch anomalies is the *branchial cleft cyst*, which arises after failure of cervical sinus obliteration (second branchial arch origin). These may occur anywhere from the tonsillar fossa to the supraclavicular region but are usually situated in the upper third of the neck anteromedial to the sternocleidomastoid muscle.[31] There may be an associated fistulous opening, and infection is common. Embryonic remnants of the thyroglossal duct may manifest as a cyst, sinus, or fistula. The mass is usually midline or paramedian occurring anywhere from the tongue base to the thyroid,

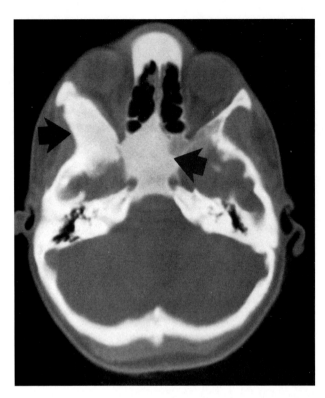

Fig. 7-122   Orbitocranial fibrous dysplasia *(arrows)* shown by axial CT with uniform ground-glass sclerotic thickening of the lateral orbital wall, sphenoid wing, and sphenoid body.

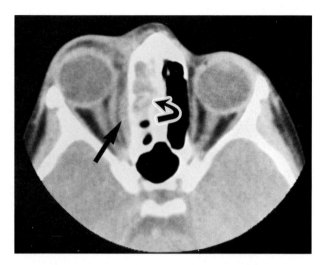

Fig. 7-123   Ethmoid sinusitis *(curved arrow)* and medial-orbital subperiosteal cellulitis *(straight arrow)* shown by axial CT without bone destruction or orbital fat involvement.

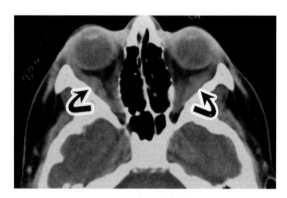

Fig. 7-124   Orbital inflammatory pseudotumor demonstrated by CT as bilateral nodular ocular muscular thickening (arrows).

often causing recurrent infection.[31] Ectopic thyroid should be ruled out. *Dysplastic conditions* that appear as masses or bone defects and are to be distinguished from parameningeal neoplastic conditions include cephaloceles especially those involving the orbit, sinus, nasopharynx, and skull base, or even the calvarial "-cele," which may present as a scalp mass.[18,31,39,51] Also, the dysplastic defects of neurofibromatosis may involve the sphenoorbital region including the sphenoid body or sphenoid wing, the petrooccipital structures, or the calvaria. These may be confused with neoplastic bony involvement particularly when associated with an overlying superficial plexiform neurofibroma[31,75] (see Chapter 3). Occasionally a *skeletal dysplasia* such as fibrous dysplasia may cause confusion. The characteristic "ground glass" sclerotic bony thickening is usually evident involving the orbit, sinuses (especially maxillary), facial bones, or skull base (Fig. 7-122). Calvarial fibrous dysplasia is usually lytic in appearance.

INFLAMMATORY TUMORS

Inflammatory processes are by far the commonest single cause of head and neck region "masses," especially cervical adenopathy, in childhood.[31,63] Often a trial of antibiotics serves to distinguish inflammatory masses from other developmental or neoplastic processes. Cranial base or calvarial *osteomyelitis* is exceedingly rare but may be

seen after penetrating trauma. *Scalp infections* (cellulitis, abscess, granuloma, parasitic) are quite common in childhood but are rarely complicated by bony or intracranial involvement. *Orbital cellulitis* or *abscess* is actually infrequent and more often is subperiosteal and associated with ethmoid sinusitis and preseptal periorbital cellulitis[27,48] (Fig. 7-123). *Orbital pseudotumor* is a lymphoid inflammatory process that often characteristically responds to steroids. It often has a rather typical CT or MR appearance including unilateral or bilateral uveoscleral thickening with enhancement, an enhancing retroocular mass, and extraocular muscle enlargement[3,19,27,48] (Fig. 7-124).

Sinusitis is commonly encountered in childhood and may be infectious (often unilateral) or allergic (usually symmetric).* Chronic sinusitis is characteristic of cystic fibrosis. The opacified paranasal sinus, which is smaller than normal, indicates hypoplasia. Inflammatory nasosinus lesions that may cause expansion include retention cysts,

---

*References 16, 17, 23, 31, 59, 60, 62, 76, 77.

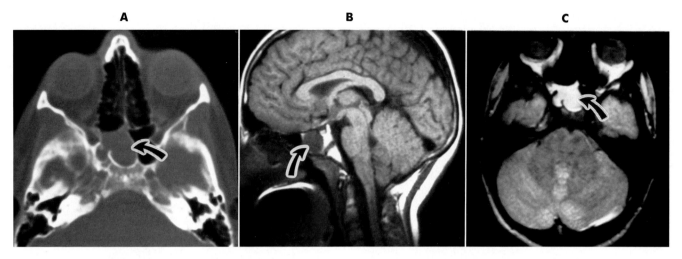

A   **B**   **C**

Fig. 7-125   Sphenoid mucocele *(arrows)* shown by CT **(A)** as an opacified and expanded sphenoid sinus. The mucocele is demonstrated by sagittal T1 MRI **(B)** as isointense to hypointense and by axial p MRI **(C)** as isointense to hyperintense.

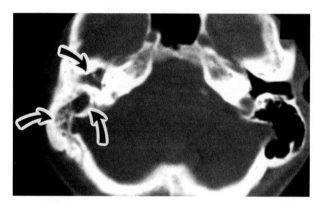

Fig. 7-126   Suppurative otomastoid infection (coalescent mastoiditis) shown by CT as an isodense opacified middle ear and mastoid with bony destruction *(arrows)*.

polyps (for example, cystic fibrosis or allergic), and mucoceles[15,67] (Fig. 7-125). Rarely a granulomatous process, such as aspergillosis, may secondarily invade the cranial contents.[76] Often this is associated with immunosuppression, (for example, after a transplant or with chemotherapy) or immunodeficiency, (for example, AIDS).[21,25,46] *Inflammatory diseases of the middle ear and mastoid* are also common in childhood.[63] Chronic, recurrent, or fulminant infections may occasionally destroy bone and secondarily involve the intracranial spaces. These may include cholesteatoma, cholesterol granuloma,[42] or coalescent mastoiditis with cellulitis or abscess (Fig. 7-126). Inflammatory processes of the neck are also very common and usually occur as adenopathy.[31] *Adenopathy* is often associated with other head or neck infections. Infrequently, cellulitis, abscess, granuloma, sialitis, or necrotic adenitis may occur. The latter may appear similar to an abscess, including a fluid center with rim enhancement.[31]

POSTTRAUMATIC TUMORS

Occasionally, posttraumatic lesions may be manifested as a mass and cause confusion. These include scalp, face, or neck hematomas, old calcified or ossified cephalohematomas in infancy, or growing fractures with subgaleal hygromas or leptomeningeal cysts. (see Chapter 6).[28,31]

REFERENCES
Parameningeal tumors

1. Armington WG, Harnsberger HR, Smoker WRK, et al: Normal and diseased acoustic pathway: evaluation with MR imaging, *Radiology* 167:509, 1988.
2. Arthur RJ, Brunelle F: Computerized tomography in the evaluation of expansile lesions arising from the skull vault in childhood—a report of five cases, *Pediatr Radiol* 18:294, 1988.
3. Atlas SW, Grossman RI, Savino PJ, et al: Surface-coil MR of orbital pseudotumor, *AJNR* 8:141, 1987.
4. Atlas SW, Kemp SS, Rorke L, et al: Hemorrhagic intracranial retinoblastoma metastases: MR pathology correlation, *J Comput Assist Tomogr* 1988:286, 1988.
5. Barkovich A: *Pediatric neuroimaging,* New York, 1990, Raven.
6. Beck DW, Dyste GN: Intracranial osteochondroma: MR and CT appearance, *AJNR* 10:S7, 1989.
7. Bronstein AD, Nyberg DA, Schwartz AN, et al: Soft tissue changes after head and neck radiation: CT findings, *AJNR* 10:171, 1989.
8. Brown RV, Sage MR, Brophy BP: CT and MR findings in patients with chordomas of the petrous apex, *AJNR* 11:121, 1990.
9. Casselman JW, Mancuso AA: Major salivary gland masses: comparison of MR imaging and CT, *Radiology* 165:183, 1987.
10. Castel J, Diard F, Chateil J, et al: Value of CT in histiocytosis X of the base of the skull in children, *Ann Radiol* 31:151, 1988.
11. Cunningham MJ, Curtis HD, Butkiewicz BL: Histiocytosis X of the temporal bone: CT findings, *J Comput Assist Tomogr* 12:70, 1988.
12. Danziger A, Price HI: CT findings in retinoblastoma, *AJR* 133:783, 1979.
13. David R, Lamki N, Fan S, et al: The many faces of neuroblastoma, *Radiographics* 9:859, 1989.
14. Davis P: Tumors of the brain. In Cohen M, Edwards M, editors: *MR imaging of children,* Philadelphia, 1990, BC Decker.
15. Dawson RC III, Horton JA: MR imaging of mucoceles of the sphenoid sinus, *AJNR* 10:613, 1989.

16. Digre K, Maxner C, Crawford S, et al: CT and MR findings in sphenoid sinus disease, *AJNR* 10:603, 1989.
17. Dillon WP, Som PM, Fullerton GD: Hypointense MR signal in chronically inspissated sinonasal secretions, *Radiology* 174:73, 1990.
18. Downey EF, Weinstein ZR: Unusual case of orbital encephalocele, *AJNR* 5:199, 1984.
19. Dresner SC, Rothfus WE, Slamovits TL, et al: Computed tomography of orbital myositis, *AJNR* 5:351, 1984.
20. Drossman SR, Schiff RG, Kronfeld GD, et al: Lymphoma of the mediastinum and neck: evaluation with Ga-67 imaging and CT correlation, *Radiology* 174:171, 1990.
21. Federle MP: A radiologist looks at AIDS: Imaging evaluation based on symptom complexes, *Radiology* 166:553, 1988.
22. Forbes GS, Earnest F IV, Waller RR: Computed tomography of orbital tumos, including late-generation scanning techniques, *Radiology* 142:387, 1982.
23. Glasier CM, Ascher DP, Williams KD: Incidental paranasal sinus abnormalities on CT of children: Clinical correlation, *AJNR* 7:681, 1986.
24. Graeb DA, Rootman J, Robertson WD, et al: Orbital lymphangiomas: clinical, radiologic, and pathologic characteristics, *Radiology* 175:417, 1990.
25. Haney PJ, Yale-Leohr AJ, Nussbaum AR, et al: Imaging of infants and children with AIDS, *AJR* 152:1033, 1989.
26. Harnsberger HR, Bragg DG, Osborn AG, et al: Non-Hodgkin's lymphoma of the head and neck: CT evaluation of nodal and extranodal sites, *AJNR* 8:673, 1987.
27. Harr DL, Quencer RM, Abrams GW, Computed tomography and ultrasound in the evaluation of orbital infection and pseudotumor, *Radiology* 142:395, 1982.
28. Harwood-Nash DC, Fitz CR: *Neuroradiology in infants and children,* St. Louis, 1976, Mosby–Year Book.
29. Holliday RA, Cohen WA, Schinella RA, et al: Benign lymphoepithelial parotid cysts and hyperplastic cervical adenopathy in AIDS-risk patients—a new CT appearance, *Radiology* 168:439, 1988.
30. Hopper KD, Katz NNK, Dorwart RH, et al: Childhood leukokoria: computed tomographic appearance and differential diagnosis with histopathologic correlation, *Radiographics* 5:377, 1985.
31. Humphrey C, Strand R, Barnes P: Imaging of the head and neck in childhood. In Healy G, editor: *Common problems in pediatric otolaryngology,* Chicago, 1990, Mosby–Year Book.
32. Krol G, Sze G, Arbit E: Intradural metastases of chordoma, *AJNR* 10:193, 1989.
33. Lallemand DP, Brasch RC, Char DH, et al: Orbital tumors in children: characterization by computed tomography, *Radiology* 151:85, 1984.
34. Latack JT, Hutchinson RJ, Heyn RM: Imaging of rhabdomyosarcomas of the head and neck, *AJNR* 8:353, 1987.
35. Lee Y, Van Tassel P: Craniofacial chondrosarcoma, *AJNR* 10:165, 1989.
36. Lee YY, Van Tassel P, Nauert C, et al: Lymphomas of the head and neck: CT findings at initial presentation, *AJNR* 8:665, 1987.
37. Lee YY, Van Tassel P, Nauert C, et al: Craniofacial osteosarcomas: plain film, CT, and MR findings in 46 cases, *AJNR* 9:379, 1988.
38. Lee YY, Van Tassel P, Raymond AK: Intracranial dural chondrosarcoma, *ANJR* 9:1189, 1988.
39. Levy RA, Wald SL, Aitken PA, et al: Bilateral intraorbital meningoencephaloceles and associated midline craniofacial anomalies: MR and three-dimensional CT imaging, *AJNR* 10:1272, 1989.
40. Lo WWM, Shelton C, Waluch V, et al: Intratemporal vascular tumors: detection with CT and MR imaging, *Radiology* 171:443, 1989.
41. Matee MF, Goldberg MF, Valvassori GE, Capek V: Computed tomography in the evaluation of patients with persistent hyperplastic primary vitreous (PHPV), *Radiology* 145:713, 1982.
42. Martin N, Sterkers O, Mompoint D, et al: Cholesterol granulomas of the middle ear cavities: MR imaging, *Radiology* 172:521, 1989.
43. Mulliken J, Glowacki J: Hemangiomas and vascular malformations in infants and children: a classification based on endothelial characteristics, *Plast Reconstr Surg* 69:412, 1982.
44. Nugent RA, Lapointe JS, Rootman J, et al: Orbital dermoids: features on CT, *Radiology* 165:475, 1987.
45. Olsen WL, Dillon WP, Kelly WM, et al: MR imaging of paragangliomas, *AJNR* 7:1039, 1986.
46. Olsen WL, Jeffrey RB Jr, Sooy CD, et al: Lesions of the head and neck in patients with AIDS: CT and MR findings, *AJNR* 9:693, 1988.
47. Peyster RG, Augsburger JJ, Shields JA, et al: Intraocular tumors: evaluation with MR imaging, *Radiology* 168:773, 1988.
48. Peyster RG, Hoover ED: *Computerized tomography in orbital disease and neuroophthalmology,* Chicago, 1984, Mosby–Year Book.
49. Price HI, Batnitzky S, Danziger A, et al: The neuroradiology of retinoblastoma, *Radiographics* 2:7, 1982.
50. Ramirez H, Blatt ES, Hibri NS: Computed tomographic identification of calcified optic nerve drusen, *Radiology* 148:137, 1983.
51. Rice JF, Eggers DM: Basal transsphenoidal encephalocele: MR findings, *AJNR* 10:S79, 1989.
52. Robinson JD, Crawford SC, Teresi LM, et al: Extracranial lesions of the head and heck: preliminary experience with Gd-DTPA–enhanced MR imaging, *Radiology* 172:165, 1989.
53. Rorke L, Gilles F, Davis R, et al: Revision of the WHO classification of brain tumors for children, *Cancer* 56:1869, 1985.
54. Russell D, Rubenstein L: *Pathology of tumors of the nervous system,* ed 4, Baltimore, 1977, William & Wilkins.
55. Schellhas KP: MR imaging of muscles of mastication, *AJNR* 10:829, 1989.
56. Simmons JD, LaMasters D, Char D: Computed tomography of ocular colobomas, *AJR* 141:1223, 1983.
57. Sobel DF, Kelly W, Kjos BO: MR imaging of orbital and ocular disease, *AJNR* 6:259, 1985.
58. Som PM, Braun IF, Shapiro MD, et al: Tumors of the parapharyngeal space and upper neck: MR imaging characteristics, *Radiology* 164:823, 1987.
59. Som PM, Dillon WP, Fullerton GD, et al: Chronically obstructed sinonasal secretions: observations on T1 and T2 shortening, *Radiology* 172:515, 1989.
60. Som PM, Dillon WP, Sze G, et al: Benign and malignant sinonasal lesions with intracranial extension: differentiation with MR imaging, *Radiology* 172:763, 1989.
61. Som PM, Sacher M, Stollman AL, et al: Common tumors of the parapharyngeal space: refined imaging diagnosis, *Radiology* 169:81, 1988.
62. Som PM, Shapiro MC, Biller HF, et al: Sinonasal tumors and inflammatory tissues: differentiation with MR imaging, *Radiology* 167:803, 1988.
63. Strand R, Humphrey C, Barnes P: Imaging of petrous temporal bone abnormalities in infancy and childhood. In Healy G, editor: *Common problems in pediatric otolaryngology,* Chicago, 1990, Mosby–Year Book.
64. Swartz JD: Current imaging approach to the temporal bone, *Radiology* 171:309, 1989.
65. Teresi LM, Lufkin RB, Vinuela F, et al: MR imaging of the nasopharynx and floor of the middle cranial fossa. Part I. Normal anatomy, *Radiology* 164:811, 1987.
66. Teresi LM, Lufkin RB, Wortham DG, et al: Parotid masses: MR imaging, *Radiology* 163:405, 1987.
67. Van Tassel P, Lee YY, Jing BS, et al: Mucoceles of the paranasal sinuses: MR imaging with CT correlation, *AJNR* 10:607, 1989.
68. Vogl T, Dresel S, Bilaniuk L, et al: Tumors of the nasopharynx and adjacent areas: MR imaging with Gd-DTPA, *AJNR* 11:187, 1990.
69. Vogl J, Bruning R, Schedel H, et al: Paragangliomas of the jugular bulb and carotid body: MR imaging, *AJNR* 10:823, 1989.
70. Wang AM, Lin JCT, Power TC, et al: Chloroma of cerebellum, tentorium, and occipital bone in acute myelogenous leukemia, *Neuroradiology* 29:590, 1987.
71. Wells RG, Sty JR, Gonnering RS: Imaging of the pediatric eye and orbit, *Radiographics* 9:1023, 1989.
72. West MS, Russell EJ, Breit R, et al: Calvarial and skull base metastases: comparison of nonenhanced and Gd-DTPA–enhanced MR images, *Radiology* 174:85, 1990.
73. Wismer GL, Wilkinson AH Jr, Goldstein JD: Cystic temporofacial brain heterotopia, *AJNR* 10:S32, 1989.
74. Zimmerman RA, Bilaniuk LT: Ocular MR imaging, *Radiology* 168:875, 1988.
75. Zimmerman RA, Bilaniuk LT, Metzger RA, et al: Computed tomography of orbital-facial neurofibromatosis, *Radiology* 146:113, 1983.
76. Zinreich SJ, Kennedy DW, Malat J, et al: Fungal sinusitis: diagnosis with CT and MR imaging, *Radiology* 169:439, 1988.
77. Zinreich SJ, Kennedy DW, Rosenbaum AE, et al: Paranasal sinuses: CT imaging requirements for endoscopic surgery, *Radiology* 163:769, 1987.

8 · Neurocutaneous Syndromes

Patrick D. Barnes
Bruce R. Korf

The neurocutaneous syndromes (see box at right) are a loosely defined group of conditions of neuroectodermal origin in which skin lesions coexist with prominent neurological abnormalities. Involvement of the skin and nervous system is about the only feature these disorders share; otherwise this is a heterogenous group that does not appear to share a common origin or development. By far the most common neurocutaneous syndromes of childhood, also referred to as phacomatoses (that is, birth marks), are neurofibromatosis and tuberous sclerosis. Less common syndromes include Sturge-Weber syndrome, von Hippel–Lindau disease, Klippel-Trenaunay-Weber syndrome, and ataxia-telangiectasia. Other rarer conditions are also listed in the box on p. 299. The involvement may not be limited to the central nervous system (CNS), peripheral nervous system (PNS), or to cutaneous manifestations. Lesions involving the eye, as well as tissues of mesodermal or endodermal origin, may occur. The lesions may be primarily dysplastic, neoplastic, or both. The syndromes associated with neoplasia include neurofibromatosis, tuberous sclerosis, von Hippel–Lindau disease, Gorlin's syndrome, ataxia-telangiectasia, and neurocutaneous melanosis. The syndromes associated primarily with vascular dysplasia are Sturge-Weber syndrome, Klippel-Trenaunay-Weber syndrome, ataxia-telangiectasia, and hereditary hemorrhagic telangiectasia.

Neurofibromatosis

At least two different forms of neurofibromatosis (NF) can often be distinguished clinically. Within a family, all affected individuals have the same type. The National

---

NEUROCUTANEOUS SYNDROMES

Common:	Neurofibromatosis
	Tuberous sclerosis
Less common:	Sturge-Weber Syndrome
	Klippel-Trenaunay-Weber syndrome
	von Hippel–Lindau syndrome
	Ataxia-telangiectasia
Rare:	Hereditary hemorrhagic telangiectasia (Osler-Rendu-Weber disease)
	Bannayan syndrome
	Epidermoid nevus syndrome
	Linear sebaceous nevus syndrome
	Hypomelanosis of Ito
	Incontinentia pigmenti
	Encephalocraniocutaneous lipomatosis
	Neurocutaneous melanosis
	Nevoid basal cell carcinoma syndrome (Gorlin's syndrome)
	Facial nevi with anomalous venous return and hydrocephalus

Institutes of Health Consensus Development Conference of 1987[8] has proposed the following classification based on two clinical categories: neurofibromatosis 1 (von Recklinghausen's neurofibromatosis or peripheral NF, that is, NF 1) and neurofibromatosis 2 (bilateral acoustic neurofibromatosis or central NF, that is, NF 2). NF 1 is considered to be present in an individual with two of the following criteria, provided that no other disease accounts for the findings:
1. At least six café-au-lait macules over 5 mm in greatest diameter if the individual is prepubertal, or six

macules over 15 mm. These are usually the first manifestations of NF in early childhood (95% of patients with NF 1 have at least one macule and 75% have six or more).

2. Based on historical grounds or physical examination, two or more neurofibromas of any type or one plexiform neurofibroma. Cutaneous neurofibromas usually begin to appear at puberty and increase in number with age.

3. Multiple axillary or inguinal freckles.

4. Sphenoid dysplasia or congenital long bone bowing or thinning with or without pseudoarthrosis.

5. Optic nerve glioma.

6. Two or more iris Lisch nodules. This hamartoma is specific for NF 1 and is present in 93% of affected patients over 6 years of age.

7. A first-degree relative (parent, sibling, or offspring) with NF 1 by the above criteria.

NF 1 constitutes greater than 90% of reported neurofibromatosis cases. It is inherited as an autosomal dominant trait with high penetrance and variable expression, and has a frequency of occurrence of 1/4000. Although an affected individual has a 50% chance of transmitting the condition to any offspring, it is not possible to predict severity for other family members. It has been estimated that 25% of individuals with NF 1 are "severely" afflicted with major neoplastic complications or dysplastic handicaps. Sporadic occurrences of new mutations occur in about 50% of patients and are associated with a very low recurrence rate for additional siblings. However, both parents of a child recently diagnosed with NF 1 must be thoroughly examined before declaring the child's condition a new mutation. Recent genetic linkage studies have revealed a gene locus for NF 1 on chromosome 17. Prenatal diagnosis is feasible for multigenerational families with NF 1.

NF 2 is considered to be present in an individual with either of the following: (1) CT or MRI evidence of bilateral internal auditory canal masses consistent with acoustic neuromas; or (2) a first-degree relative with NF 2 and one of the following: (a) CT or MRI evidence of a unilateral internal auditory canal mass consistent with acoustic neuroma, (b) a plexiform neurofibroma or two of the following: meningioma, glioma, or neurofibroma at any site, or (c) imaging evidence of an intracranial or spinal cord tumor. NF 2 is inherited as autosomal dominant with high penetrance and an occurrence frequency of 1/40,000. Most cases are familial, and genetic linkage has been established to chromosome 22; prenatal diagnosis is not yet available. The inevitable occurrence of bilateral acoustic neuroma usually presents in the second decade or later, usually with balance or hearing problems. Presenile posterior capsular cataracts characteristically occur in NF 2.

Neurofibromatosis (especially NF 1) is a disorder of multigerm-layer origin with dysplastic and neoplastic lesions primarily involving the neuroectodermal and mesodermal derivatives.[1,2,6,11,15] Commonly there are both dysplastic and neoplastic involvement of the CNS (neural tube origin) and PNS (neural crest origin), whereas the mesodermal involvement is exclusively dysplastic and primarily affects skeletal structures. In NF 2, only neoplasia involving both the CNS and PNS is seen. Clinical manifestations of CNS involvement occur commonly in patients with NF 1 and may or may not be directly related to specifically identifiable neuropathology. These include megalencephaly, other craniofacial dysmorphia, learning disabilities, seizures, neuroendocrine dysfunction (for example, precocious puberty, short stature, and, rarely, delayed puberty), intestinal motility disturbances, and migraine and tension headache syndromes. More specific or localizing neurological symptoms or signs may be indicators of identifiable disease processes. This may include visual impairment associated with buphthalmos or optic glioma, sensorineural hearing loss with acoustic neuroma (especially NF 2), or precocious puberty with a hypothalamic hamartoma or glioma. Other signs include increased pressure from hydrocephalus due to nontumor aqueductal stenosis or tumoral causes, cerebrovascular accidents associated with moyamoya syndrome, and neuropathy, radiculopathy, or myelopathy related to dural ectasia, neuroma, or cord glioma. Often CNS tumors such as optic glioma are discovered during asymptomatic screening. Cutaneous involvement produces cosmetic deformity and pruritus. Cutaneous or subcutaneous lesions occur much more frequently with NF 1 than with NF 2. Lesions other than café-au-lait spots, neuromas, and freckling include achromic nevi, xanthomas, angiomas, and lymphatic malformations. The neuromas may be simple schwannomas, neurofibromas, or plexiform neurofibromas. The cutaneous, subcutaneous, or deeper neuromas may involve the limbs, trunk, head and neck region, or intraspinal and paraspinal tissues. In addition to iris Lisch nodules, ocular manifestations may include buphthalmos (congenital glaucoma) or pulsating exophthalmos with palpebral or orbital plexiform neurofibroma and sphenoid dysplasia.

Clinical manifestations related to other mesodermal dysplasias or other non-CNS neoplasias include kyphoscoliosis, limb deformities, hypertension, pulmonary, gastrointestinal, or genitourinary dysfunction, and metabolic or endocrine disorders.[11,14,15] The kyphoscoliosis may be progressive and specific or nonspecific for NF 1. Overgrowth of any organ or tissue may occur, although the most common is that of limb overgrowth or focal gigantism. Limb deformities also commonly occur as a result of peripheral skeletal dysplasias including bowing, thinning, or pseudoarthroses (tibia, fibula, radius), bone cysts, fibrous dysplasia, and periosteal dysplasia with subperiosteal hemorrhage. Hypertension may be seen as related to renal artery stenosis, aortic coarctation, or pheochromocytoma. Congenital heart disease, including pulmonic or aortic stenosis and ventricular or atrial septal defect, has also been reported. Gastrointestinal hemorrhage or obstruction may occur related to neurofibromas, neurofibrosarcomas, or carcinoid tumor. Genitourinary abnormalities reported in neurofibromatosis include bladder neurofibromas or neurofibrosarcomas, Wilms' tumor (rarely), and genital enlargement. Respiratory symptoms may be related to pulmonary fibrosis or rare mediastinal tumors. Other reported endocrine and metabolic disorders in neurofibromatosis are osteomalacia, hyperparathyroidism, and multiple endocrine adenomatosis II. Other tumors reported include ganglioneuroma, xanthogranuloma, rhabdomyosarcoma, and leukemia.

NEUROIMAGING FINDINGS
Cranial and intracranial dysplastic abnormalities

The dysplasias of neurofibromatosis occurring at the cranial level may be either mesodermal or neuroectodermal in origin. Mesodermal dysplasias include defects of the sphenoid bone, calvarial defects, and other bony deformities.[2,6,9,11] The bony defects may be associated with overlying or adjacent plexiform neurofibromas or dural ectasia. The sphenoid dysplasia is usually unilateral with defective ossification and formation of the sphenoid wing (Figs. 8-1 and 8-2). The greater wing is involved more often than the lesser wing. The defect may be small and localized around the superior or inferior orbital fissure, or the optic foramen. Occasionally the defect is very large with total absence of the greater wing. The unossified greater wing (anterior wall of the middle cranial fossa and posterior wall of the orbit) often allows herniation of the temporal lobe and leptomeninges into the orbit, representing a sphenoid alar encephalocele or meningocele (dural ectasia). This may appear clinically as pulsating exophthalmos or anophthalmos. There may be an associated palpebral or intraorbital plexiform neurofibroma or buphthalmos (Figs. 8-1 and 8-2). Rarely the sphenoid dysplasia is in the midline with partial or complete absence of the sphenoid body, including partially absent sella, dorsum, or clivus and producing the appearance of an empty sella or transphenoidal encephalomeningocele (dural ectasia).

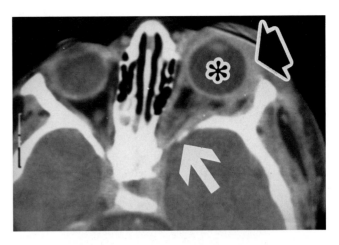

Fig. 8-1 Sphenoorbital dysplasia of NF 1 with palpebral plexiform neurofibroma. Contrast CT demonstrates the sphenoid wing defect *(white arrow)* and periorbital-intraorbital irregular and enhancing soft tissue masses *(black arrow)* along with buphthalmos *(asterisk).*

The dysplastic calvarial defects appear as rounded, oval, or irregular bone lucencies usually involving the lambdoid suture (left more often than right), often just posterior to the parietomastoid or occipitomastoid suture and often associated with deficient otomastoid pneumatization (Fig. 8-3). The defects rarely may be bilateral or multiple, and occasionally occur along the sagittal suture posteriorly. Overlying neurofibromatous tissue is less commonly associated, although large defects may be accompanied by an encephalomeningocele. Other reported defects include those involving the facial bones, dental structures, and petrous portion of the temporal bone. In one case a large

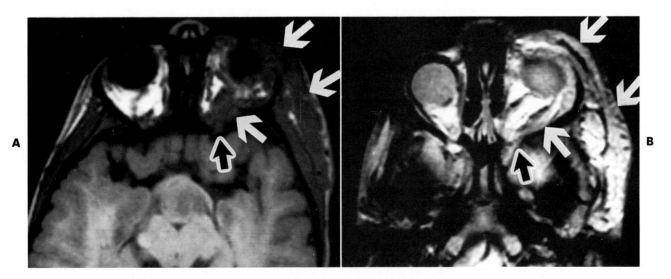

Fig. 8-2 Sphenoorbital dysplasia of NF 1 with palpebral plexiform neurofibroma. Axial T1 **(A)** and p/T2 **(B)** MRI demonstrate the sphenoid defect *(black arrows)* and periorbital-intraorbital irregular soft tissue tumor intensities *(white arrows).*

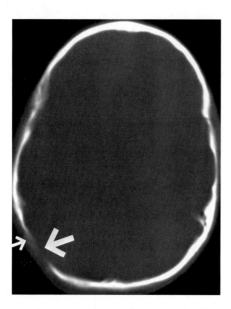

Fig. 8-3 Dysplastic parietooccipital cranial defect *(large arrow)* of NF 1 shown by CT as an irregular lytic bony defect adjacent to the lambdoidal suture *(small arrow)*.

petrooccipital skull base defect was associated with an adjacent scalp and facial plexiform neurofibroma in a child with nontumor sensorineural hearing loss on the same side (Fig. 8-4). Nontumor enlargement of the internal auditory canals has also been observed as a manifestation of dural ectasia with patulous or ectatic subarachnoid intrusions. Other, less common mesodermal dysplastic findings include dural and choroid plexus calcifications and vascular stenoses of the carotid and cerebral arterial structures.[3,6,20] Although the histogenesis of vascular neurofibromatosis remains unclear, the stenoses have been attributed to medial Schwann cell proliferation, secondary degenerative fibrosis, and intimal dysplasia. The reported vascular abnormalities include segmental or diffuse stenoses or ectasias of the carotid and cerebral arteries (Fig. 8-5) with or without basilar telangiectatic collaterals, that is, moyamoya syndrome (Figs. 8-6 and 8-7). The latter syndrome may be of multifactorial origin, having been observed in patients with neurofibromatosis who have had radiation therapy for optic pathway glioma.

The neural dysplasias of NF 1 occurring at the cranial level include buphthalmos, megalencephaly, neuroglial or neural crest migrational and proliferative malformations, and aqueductal stenosis.* Buphthalmos, or congenital

---

*References 1, 2, 4, 6, 12, 16, 18, 19.

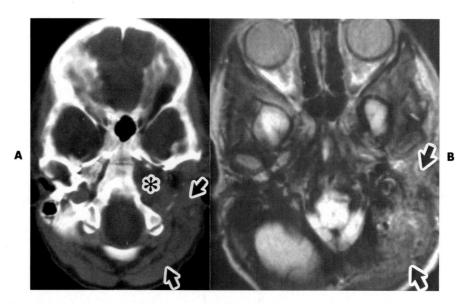

Fig. 8-4 Dysplastic petrooccipital defect *(asterisk)* of NF 1 shown by axial CT **(A)** with associated overlying plexiform neurofibroma *(black arrows)*, the latter shown better by axial proton density MRI **(B)**.

glaucoma, results from intraocular neurofibromatous involvement and resultant obstruction of aqueous outflow. If the process starts prenatally, enlargement of the globe results. Often there is associated palpebral or orbital plexiform neurofibroma or sphenoid dysplasia (Figs. 8-1 and 8-2). Other reported ocular dysplasias include anophthalmia and persistent hyperplastic primary vitreous. Megalencephaly represents an actual increase in brain volume not related to hydrocephalus but often associated with neuroglial histogenetic malformations. Rarely the "apparent" macrocephaly actually may represent increased soft tissues of the face and scalp related to neurofibromatous tissue or thickening of the cranial bones (macrocrania).

Probably the most common intracranial manifestation of NF 1, which may prove to be a major diagnostic criterion, is the "histogenetic foci" that are demonstrated only by MRI.[1,2,4,12,16] These are usually multifocal and appear as high intensity punctate, nodular, or occasionally confluent aggregates on proton density and T2 (p/T2) images (Figs. 8-8 and 8-9). Although often not identified on T1-weighted images, occasionally the abnormalities, particularly the globus pallidus foci, appear as hyperintense on T1-weighted images (Fig. 8-9). Gadolinium enhancement has not been observed. The intensity abnormalities on long TR sequences have been identified in the cerebellum, brain stem, spinal cord, basal ganglia, thalamus, deep capsular and

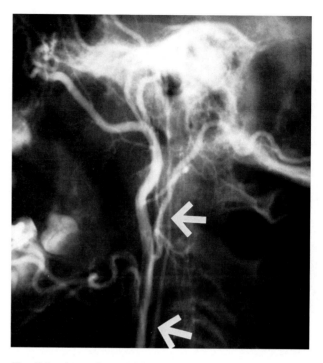

Fig. 8-5   Internal carotid hypoplasia of NF 1 shown by lateral common carotid angiogram as a thin column of intraluminal contrast *(arrows).*

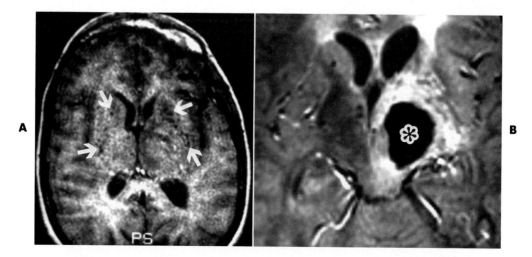

Fig. 8-6   Moyamoya in NF 1 after radiation therapy for optic glioma shown by axial T1 MRI **(A)** and axial p/T2 MRI **(B)** as deep ganglionic and capsular flow signal voids *(arrows)* plus left thalamic hemorrhage *(asterisk).*

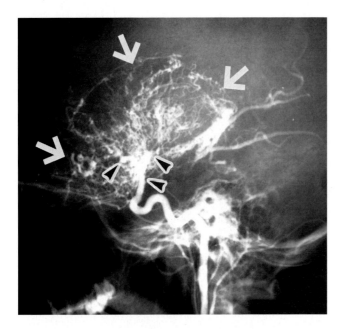

Fig. 8-7   Moyamoya in NF 1 shown by lateral carotid angiogram with supraclinoid internal carotid arterial stenosis *(arrowheads)* and extensive basilar telangiectatic collateralization *(arrows)*.

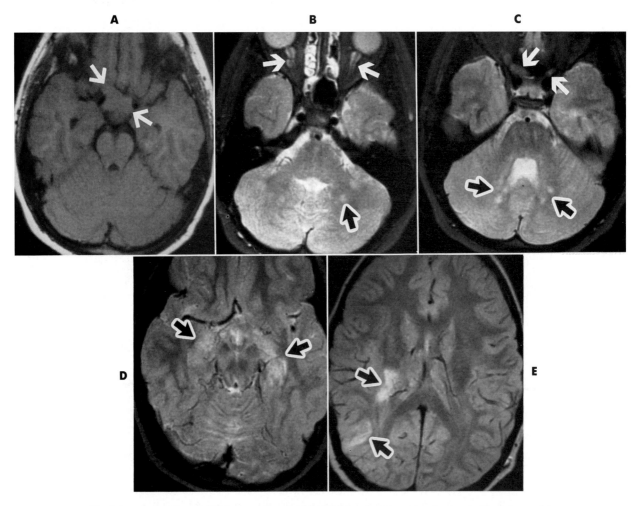

Fig. 8-8   Optic glioma in NF 1 shown by axial **(A)** T1 MRI as isointense involvement of the intracranial optic nerves, chiasm, and tracts *(arrows)*. **B-E,** Axial proton density and T2 MRI demonstrate the intraorbital and intracanalicular optic nerve involvement *(white arrows)* along with a number of high intensity areas, which are likely dysplastic *(black arrows)*.

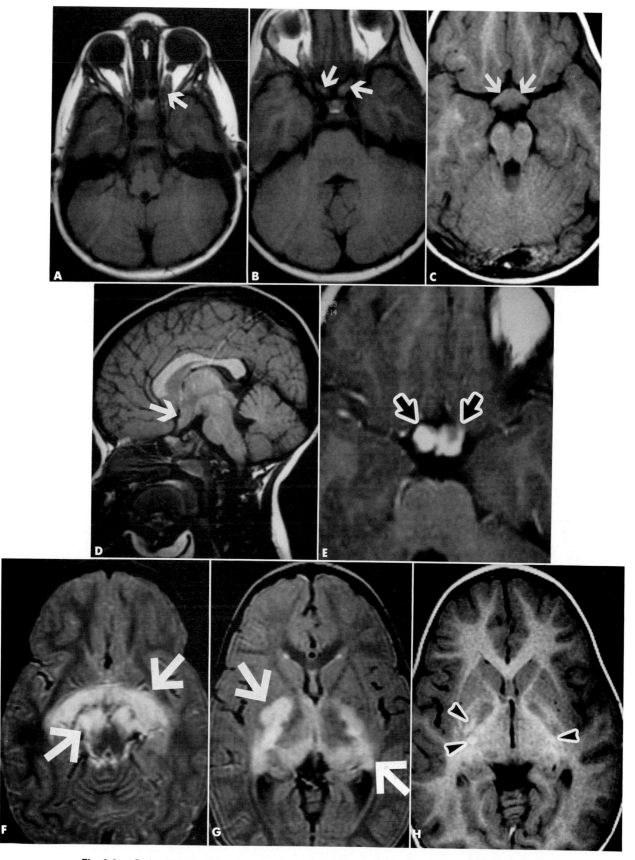

Fig. 8-9 Optic glioma in NF 1 shown by axial and sagittal T1 MRI **(A-E)** with involvement of the left intraorbital optic nerve *(A, arrow)*, both intracranial optic nerves *(B, arrows)*, the optic chiasm and tracts *(C* and **D,** *arrows)* with gadolinium enhancement only of the chiasmatic components **(E). F** and **G,** Axial proton density and T2 MRI show high intensity abnormalities along the optic tracts, basal ganglia, and capsular tracts *(arrows)*, which probably represent a combination of dysplastic and neoplastic involvement. **H,** Some of the globus pallidus and capsular foci are high intensity on axial T1 MRI *(arrowheads)*.

periventricular white matter, and corpus callosum. Histopathology in a few cases has revealed the well-known dysplastic findings of NF 1 including atypical glial cells and hamartomas of neural, glial, or meningoangiomatous nature. The T1 hyperintensity is thought to represent schwannosis, melanosis, or hypermyelination related to a neural crest migrational or proliferative disorder (Schwann cells and melanin pigment are of neural crest origin).[16] Other possibilities include absent or delayed myelination, since some of the T2-hyperintense foci may not be present on follow-up MRI and are often not seen in older patients with NF 1. The speculative potential that these foci are precursors for gliomatous degeneration or gliomatosis remains a concern because dysplastic glial tissue has been reported in areas of glial neoplasia in NF 1. The lack of mass effect and gadolinium enhancement may assist to differentiate dysplastic from neoplastic lesions. Confusion may persist, however, since the dysplastic intensity abnormalities are seen in the majority of patients with NF 1 and even more commonly in patients with NF 1 and optic glioma.[2]

Aqueductal stenosis may be nontumoral or associated with dysplastic or neoplastic periaqueductal or tectal deformities.[1,2,6] Tumoral aqueductal stenosis has been observed with subependymal hamartomas and gliomas (usually astrocytomas). The tumoral types may be detected and differentiated from the nontumoral types only with MRI (see Chapter 7). Follow-up MRI after ventricular shunting may demonstrate growth and provide the indication for more specific treatment, usually radiotherapy. Other reported histogenetic malformations in NF 1 include heterotopias, polymicrogyria, pachygyria, and hypothalamic hamartomas (see Chapters 3 and 7). The latter may be

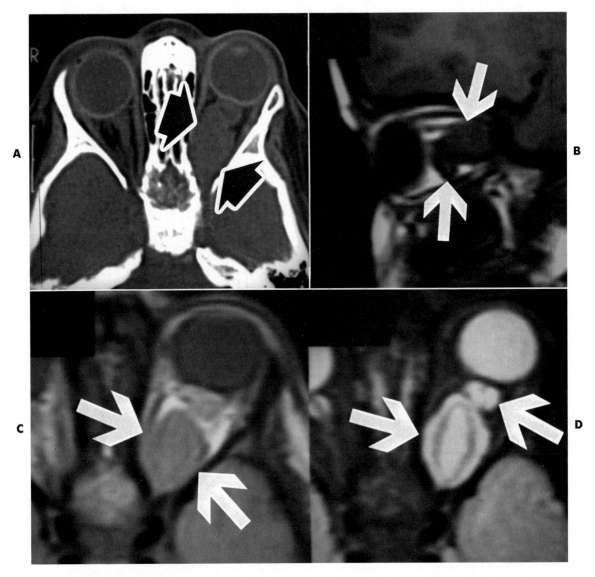

Fig. 8-10 Orbital optic glioma in NF 1 shown by CT **(A)** as an isodense lobulated tumor *(arrows)*. Sagittal T1 MRI **(B)** and axial proton density **(C)** and T2 **(D)** MRI show the irregular optic expansion confined to the orbit *(arrows)* and involving both nerve and nerve sheath (striate appearance, **D**).

associated with precocious puberty and indistinguishable from optic or hypothalamic glioma unless gadolinium enhancement or growth on serial follow-up is demonstrated to implicate glioma. The CT and MRI characteristics of hamartomas are more fully described in Chapter 7.

Cranial and intracranial neoplastic abnormalities

Glial neoplasia of the brain are characteristic of NF 1, whereas meningeal and nerve sheath tumors are distinctive of NF 2.[1,2,6,8,10] By far the commonest intracranial tumor in NF 1 is the optic pathway glioma, which usually occurs in the first two decades.[5,13,17] These are usually astrocytomas, often of the pilocytic type, and sometimes grow so slowly as to be considered hamartomatous rather than truly neoplastic. In fact, asymptomatic optic nerve thickening may be seen in up to 15% of patients with NF 1. (Fig.

8-10). Only a minority of the astrocytomas continue to grow, although some may become highly infiltrative and malignant. Lesions confined to the optic nerve (prechiasmatic) are amenable to resection and are associated with a better prognosis than are tumors involving the chiasm, tracts, or optic radiations beyond the lateral geniculate bodies (Figs. 8-8 and 8-9). The CT and MRI characteristics are more fully described in Chapter 7. Other neuroepithelial or glial neoplasms (most commonly astrocytomas) in neurofibromatosis include hypothalamic and third ventricular gliomas, cerebellar and brain stem glial tumors, and diffuse gliomas of the cerebral hemispheres, thalamus, or basal ganglia (Fig. 8-11). Rarely, fourth ventricular gliomas, ependymomas, glioblastomas, or retinoblastomas may be seen. More than one glioma may occur in the same patient simultaneously or over time. Unilateral acoustic

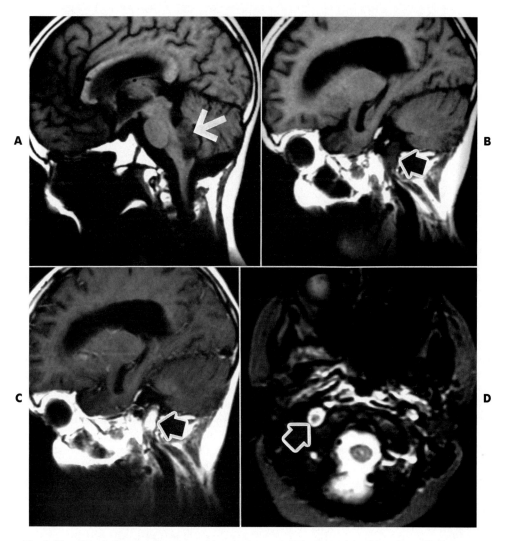

Fig. 8-11   Cerebellar astrocytoma and jugular foramen neurofibroma in NF 1 after radiotherapy for optic glioma. **A,** The fourth ventricular astrocytoma *(arrow)* is isointense to hypointense on mid-sagittal T1 MRI. **B** and **C,** The jugular foramen neurofibroma is demonstrated by parasagittal T1 MRI as an isointense to hypointense and gadolinium-enhancing mass *(arrows)* with central hypointensity and peripheral hyperintensity (arrows) on axial T2 MRI **(D).**

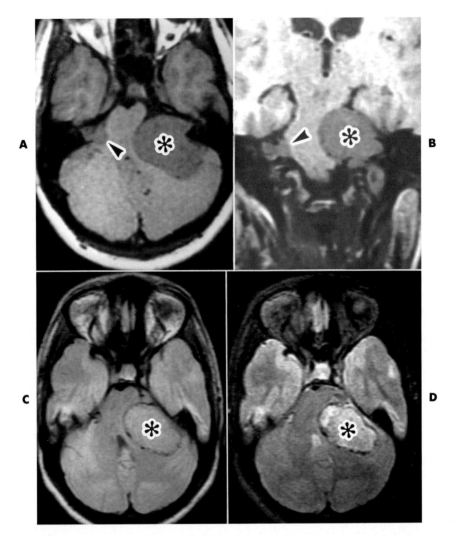

Fig. 8-12 Bilateral acoustic neuromas in NF 2 shown by MRI as bilateral large *(asterisk)* and small *(arrowhead)* isointense cerebellopontine angle and internal auditory canal masses on axial and coronal T1 images **(A** and **B).** The larger tumor *(asterisk)* is isointense to hyperintense on proton density **(C)** and T2 **(D)** images with a low intensity rim and compresses the brain stem.

neuroma rarely has been reported in NF 1. Craniofacial plexiform neurofibromas primarily occur in NF 1 and are often locally aggressive tumors that tend to extend centripetally along the involved nerve. Periorbital and intraorbital plexiform neurofibromata are often pervasive and may extend to involve the cavernous sinus. As mentioned before, often there is an association with sphenoid dysplasia and buphthalmos.

The common and characteristic intracranial neoplasia of NF 2 are neuromas (neurilemomas, schwannomas) and meningiomas. The meningeal and nerve sheath tumors occur earlier in life in patients with NF 2 than in those with sporadic occurrences. However, neuromas or meningiomas rarely are seen before puberty, even when associated with NF 2. Acoustic neuromas are more frequently encountered and are classically bilateral (Figs. 8-12 and 8-13). One or

more of cranial nerves III through XII may be involved, but the next most common in order are those of the fifth, ninth, and tenth (Fig. 8-11). Meningiomas may be single or multiple (including meningiomatosis) and are often associated with bilateral acoustic neuromas in NF 2 (Fig. 8-13). The meningiomas usually arise above the tentorium, often in a parasagittal or convexity extracerebral location, although lateral intraventricular tumors of choroid plexus origin with calcification are a classic occurrence in neurofibromatosis. The CT and MRI characteristics of neuromas and meningiomas are more fully described in Chapter 7.

Spinal dysplastic abnormalities

Spinal anomalies are primarily the result of mesodermal dysplasias involving bone and dura.[2,6,11] These are primarily, if not exclusively, associated with NF 1 (see also

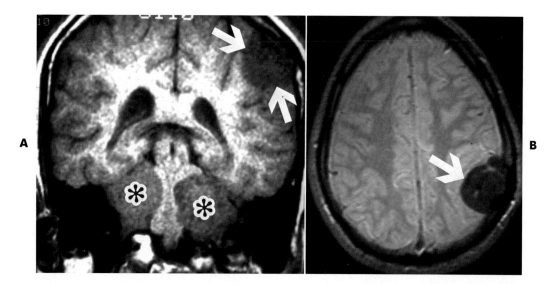

Fig. 8-13   Bilateral acoustic neuromas *(asterisks)* and cerebral convexity meningioma *(arrow)* in NF 2 shown by coronal T1 **(A)** and axial proton density **(B)** MRI. The cerebral convexity meningioma is hypointense on all sequences, which correlates with calcification on CT.

Chapter 9). The often characteristic bony deformities include cervical kyphosis, thoracic or lumbar kyphoscoliosis, vertebral scalloping and pencil-point deformities, hypoplasia of the pedicles, hypoplasia of the spinous or transverse processes, hyperplastic bony changes, and a twisted-ribbon or notched appearance of the ribs. Abnormal spinal curvature is probably the most common skeletal abnormality in NF 1, the majority occurring before age 15 years. Cervical kyphosis is highly suggestive of neurofibromatosis, especially when associated with vertebral scalloping, wedging, and apex erosion (Fig. 8-14). The kyphosis may be mild in younger patients and often progresses with age to a more severe deformity. Although the thoracic or lumbar scoliosis is often nonspecific in character, a more specific pattern may be seen, including an angular, short segment scoliosis involving five or fewer vertebral segments. This is characteristic for NF 1, particularly when associated with vertebral scalloping (Figs. 8-15 and 8-16). Associated kyphosis may be seen and is often a poor prognostic sign because of the tendency for progression and the poor response to treatment (see also Chapter 9).

Primary meningeal or dural dysplasia is often present and manifested as a widened dural sac (that is, dural ectasia) or dural diverticula (that is, meningocele). These may occur segmentally or diffusely. The meningoceles may extend through the intervertebral or sacral foramina as paraspinal, posterior mediastinal, or presacral masses (Figs. 8-17 to 8-19). Associated bony findings include a widened spinal canal, enlarged foramina, vertebral scalloping, and pedicle hypoplasia or thinning. The dural ectasia and diverticulae appear as low density spaces (comparable to cerebrospinal fluid [CSF]) by CT and are opacified with intrathecal water-soluble iodinated contrast material. On MRI these

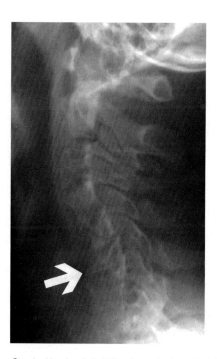

Fig. 8-14   Cervical kyphosis in NF 1 shown by lateral plain film with characteristic anterior vertebral deformity *(arrow).*

follow CSF intensities throughout the sequences (Figs. 8-17 to 8-19). The lesions of dural dysplasia should be distinguished from intraspinal or paraspinal neoplasia. Hydrosyringomyelia has also been reported as a dysplastic or degenerative feature of neurofibromatosis but is more often associated with neoplasm, as discussed in the next section.

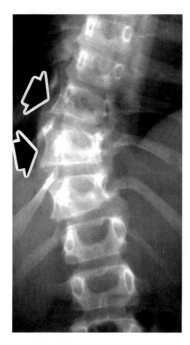

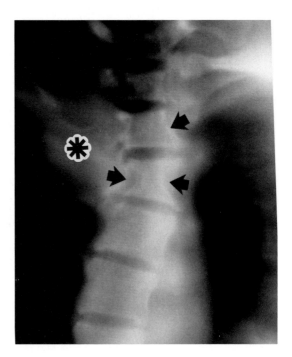

Fig. 8-15   Frontal plain film of the thoracic spine showing the dystrophic, short-segment kyphoscoliosis of NF 1 including vertebral and ribbon scalloping *(arrows)*.

Fig. 8-16   Frontal tomogram of upper thoracic spine in NF 1 showing characteristic vertebral scalloping *(arrows)* and paraspinal plexiform neurofibroma *(asterisk)*.

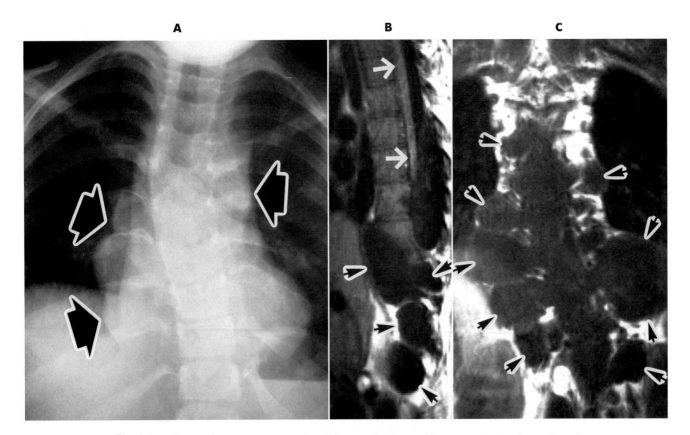

Fig. 8-17   Frontal thoracolumbar plain film **(A)** and MRI **(B** and **C)** in NF 1 with dural ectasia and multiple paraspinal meningoceles. **A,** Multiple paraspinal masses *(arrows)* are evident with scoliosis, canal widening, and rib deformities. **B** and **C,** Sagittal and coronal T1 MRI show the low intensity widening of the spinal canal with thinning of the spinal cord *(white arrows)* and multiple paraspinal CSF intensity meningoceles *(black arrows)* extending through the widened intervertebral foramina.

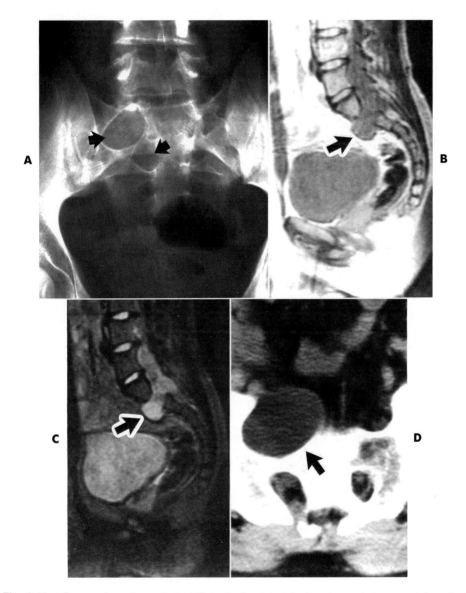

Fig. 8-18   Presacral meningocele in NF 1. **A,** Frontal plain film demonstrates sacral foraminal widening *(arrows)*. Sagittal proton density **(B)** and T2 **(C)** MRI plus CT **(D)** show the CSF intensity and CSF density extension *(arrows)* of the ectatic lumbosacral dural sac through the widened foramen.

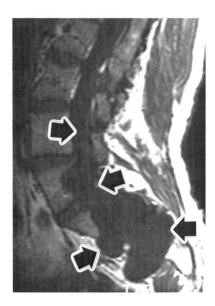

Fig. 8-19   Lumbosacral dural ectasia and multiple meningoceles in NF 1 shown by sagittal T1 MRI as CSF low intensity expansion of the central spinal canal *(top arrows)* and intervertebral foramina *(bottom arrows).*

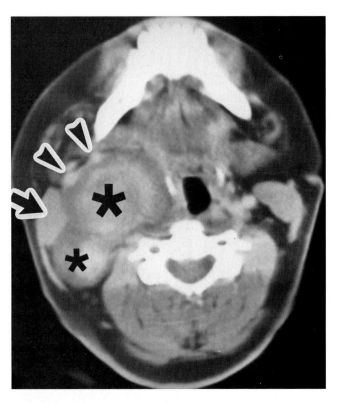

Fig. 8-20   Right neck neurofibroma in NF 1 shown by axial contrast CT as a bilobar isodense to hypodense and enhancing mass *(asterisk)* deep to the sternomastoid muscle *(arrow)* and displacing the carotid-jugular structures anterolaterally *(arrowheads).*

Spinal neoplastic abnormalities

Both simple neurofibromas and schwannomas occur in neurofibromatosis but may also be seen sporadically, particularly schwannomas.[2,6,7,11] The cutaneous simple and plexiform types of neurofibroma are characteristic of neurofibromatosis. Neurofibromas may be localized or diffuse, and may occur singly or at multiple levels. These consist of Schwann cells and fibroblasts with loosely arranged collagen fibers and mucoid material forming an intersecting pattern of wavy fascicles in which neuronal elements may be demonstrated. It is the more diffuse type, composed of tortuous cords, that is referred to as plexiform neurofibroma and is characteristic of neurofibromatosis. The occurrence of malignant schwannoma is also a recognized complication of neurofibromatosis. Neurilemoma (schwannoma, neurinoma) is a tumor composed of spindle-shaped cells considered to be Schwann cells. These are encapsulated or sometimes cystic tumors. Nerve fibers can usually be found stretched over the capsule but not within the tumor. Melanin pigmentation may be present in exceptional cases. Whereas neurilemomas are isointense to hypointense on T1 images, isointense to hyperintense on p/T2 images, and usually show uniform gadolinium enhancement, neurofibromas are more often isointense to hypointense on all sequences with a p/T2-hyperintense rim and nonuniform enhancement (Figs. 8-11 and 8-20 to 8-23). Plexiform neurofibromas are often T1 low intensity and p/T2 high intensity with irregular gadolinium enhancement (Fig. 8-24). By CT all of these tumors tend to be isodense to hypodense, and iodine enhancement is more often seen with schwannomas or neurilemomas than with simple neurofibromas or plexiform neurofibromas.

Paraspinal neuromas, especially neurofibromas, are characteristic of NF 1 and NF 2.[2,6,7] These may be seen as unilateral or bilateral, single or multilevel, discrete lesions of varying size or as diffuse, extensive plexiform tumors (Fig. 8-24). The tumors may involve or extend to involve the intraspinal, foraminal, or paraspinal structures as intradural, transdural (''dumbbell''), or extradural tumors producing spinal canal or foraminal enlargement (Figs. 8-24 and 8-25). Cord or nerve displacement or compression often leads to neurological symptoms and signs. Bilateral and multilevel tumors may be more characteristic of NF 2, especially in the absence of spinal bony or dural dysplasia. Spinal canal meningiomas are also more characteristic of NF 2, as are intramedullary cord tumors, especially ependymomas. Meningiomas may be single or multiple, occur intradural extramedullary, and displace or compress the cord. These are often the same intensity as the spinal cord on all sequences but are intensely enhanced with gadolinium. Ependymomas may be single (conus or filar), multiple, or diffusely involve the cord. Ependymomas and astrocytomas are usually indistinguishable and produce cord

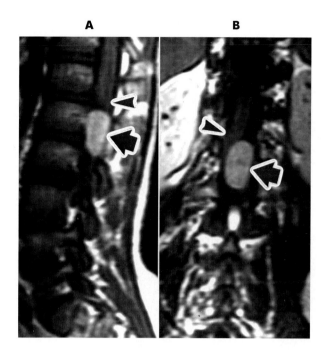

Fig. 8-21 Lumbar schwannoma in NF 1 demonstrated on sagittal **(A)** and coronal **(B)** T1 MRI as a gadolinium-enhancing intradural, extramedullary tumor *(arrow)* just caudal to the conus medullaris *(arrowhead)*.

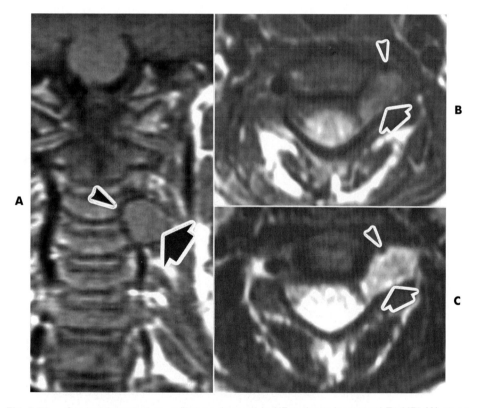

Fig. 8-22 Cervical foraminal neurofibroma *(arrows)* in NF 1 shown by coronal T1 MRI **(A)** as an isointense to hypointense tumor that is isointense on axial proton density MRI **(B)** and hyperintense on axial T2 MRI **(C)** with central hypointensity. There is displacement and narrowing of the left vertebral artery *(arrowheads)*.

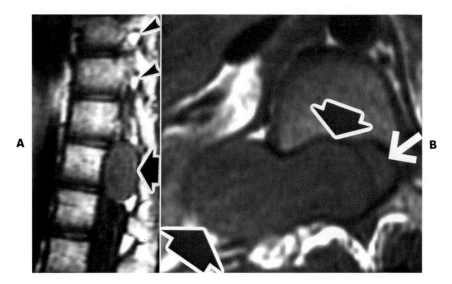

Fig. 8-23 Thoracolumbar schwannoma in NF 1. **A** and **B,** Sagittal and axial T1 MRI show the tumor as an isointense to hypointense mass with intraspinal, foraminal, and paraspinal components *(black arrows)*. There is obliteration of the epidural fat compared with the other intervertebral foramina *(arrowheads),* and the dural sac and cord are displaced and compressed *(white arrow).*

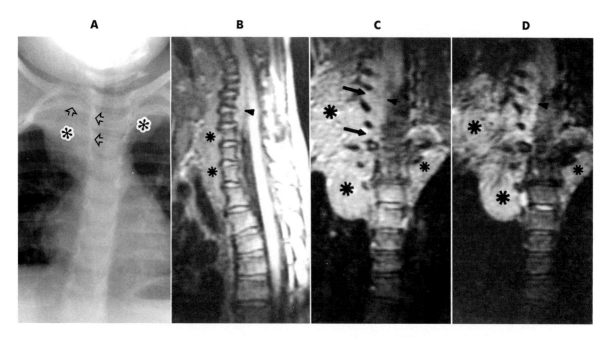

Fig. 8-24 Cervicothoracic paraspinal plexiform neurofibromata in NF 1 demonstrated by frontal plain film **(A)** as bilateral paraspinal (posterior mediastinal) masses *(asterisks)* with associated rib and vertebral scalloping plus pedicle thinning *(open arrows).* Sagittal **(B)** and coronal **(C)** proton density plus coronal T2 **(D)** MRI show isointense to hyperintense paravertebral masses *(asterisks)* with internal irregular low intensities. There is transforaminal *(arrow)* and intraspinal *(arrowhead)* extension.

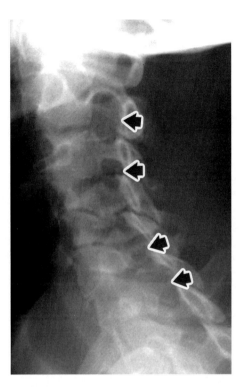

Fig. 8-25 Multiple enlarged intervertebral foramina *(arrows)* on oblique plain film of the cervical spine in NF 2 associated with multiple neurofibromata.

expansion with isointensity to low intensity on T1 images, isointensity to hyperintensity on p/T2 images, and frequent gadolinium enhancement. Cystic changes or hydrosyringomyelia commonly occurs with intramedullary tumors and occasionally may be seen with compressive extramedullary tumors. All of these tumors are more fully presented and illustrated in Chapter 10.

REFERENCES
Neurofibromatosis

1. Aoki S, Barkovich A, Nishimura K, et al: Neurofibromatosis types 1 and 2: cranial MR findings, *Radiology* 172:527, 1989.
2. Barkovich A: *Pediatric neuroimaging*, New York, 1990, Raven.
3. Beyer R, Paden P, Sobel D, et al: Moya-moya pattern of vascular occlusion after radiotherapy for glioma of the optic chiasm, *Neurology* 36:1173, 1986.
4. Bognanno J, Edwards M, Lee T, et al: Cranial MR imaging in neurofibromatosis, *AJNR* 9:461, 1988.
5. Brown E, Riccardi V, Mawad M, et al: MR imaging of optic pathways in neurofibromatosis, *AJNR* 8:1031, 1987.
6. Braffman B, Bilaniuk L, Zimmerman R: The CNS manifestation of the phakomatoses on MR, *Radiol Clin North Am* 26:773, 1988.
7. Burk D, Brunberg J, Kanal E, et al: Spinal and paraspinal neurofibromatosis: MR imaging, *Radiology* 162:797, 1987.
8. Conference Statement: Neurofibromatosis. NIH Consensus Development Conference, *Arch Neurol* 45:575, 1988.
9. Diebler C, Dulac O: *Pediatric neurology and neuroradiology,* New York, 1987, Springer-Verlag.
10. Gray J, Swaiman K: Brain tumors in children with neurofibromatosis: CT and MRI, *Pediatr Neurol* 3:335, 1987.
11. Holt J: Neurofibromatosis in children, *Am J Roentgenol* 130:615, 1978.
12. Hurst R, Newman S, Cail W: Multifocal intracranial MR abnormalities in neurofibromatosis, *AJNR* 9:293, 1988.
13. Jacoby C, Go R, Beren R: Cranial CT of neurofibromatosis, *AJR* 135:553, 1980.
14. Jones K: *Smith's recognizable patterns of human malformation,* Philadelphia, 1988, WB Saunders.
15. Klatte E, Franken E, Smith J: The radiographic spectrum in neurofibromatosis, *Semin Roentgenol* 11:17, 1976.
16. Mirowitz S, Sartor K, Gado M: High intensity basal ganglia lesions on T1-weighted MR images in neurofibromatosis, *AJNR* 10:1159, 1989.
17. Pomeranz S, Shelton J, Tobias J, et al: MR of visual pathways in neurofibromatosis, *AJNR* 8:831, 1987.
18. Reed D, Robertson W, Rootman J, et al: Plexiform neurofibromatosis of the orbit: CT evaluation, *AJNR* 7:259, 1986.
19. Rubenstein L: The malformative CNS lesions in central and peripheral forms of neurofibromatosis, *Ann NY Acad Sci* 486:14, 1986.
20. Tomsick T, Lukin R, Chambers A, et al: Neurofibromatosis and intracranial arterial occlusive disease, *Neuroradiology* 11:229, 1976.

Tuberous sclerosis

Tuberous sclerosis is a heredofamilial neurocutaneous syndrome or phacomatosis with multisystem involvement including neurological, cutaneous, ocular, renal, cardiac, pulmonary, and other organ manifestations.[2-4,6,7] The classic clinical triad is that of seizures, mental retardation, and adenoma sebaceum. It is inherited as an autosomal dominant trait with high penetrance and variable expression, but severity cannot be predicted. Approximately 60% to 80% of cases are sporadic and probably related to a new mutation. Careful examination of both parents is important, since subtle manifestations may be present in asymptomatic individuals. The most sensitive screening methods are complete skin examination and brain CT or MRI, although eye examination and renal or cardiac ultrasonography also may be necessary. The risk to future offspring from an affected parent is 50%, whereas the risk to offspring from unaffected parents is very low. Prenatal genetic screening is not yet available. A *definitive* diagnosis of tuberous sclerosis may be established when any one of the following are present: (1) cortical tubers or subependymal nodules (hamartomas), (2) multiple renal hamartomas (angiomyolipomas), (3) facial or truncal adenoma sebaceum or ungual fibroma (actually angiofibromas), or (4) giant cell tumors (neuroglial). In the absence of features required for definitive diagnosis, a *presumptive* diagnosis may be made with any two of the following: (1) hypopigmented macule (ash-leaf spot), (2) shagreen patch, (3) infantile spasms, (4) single retinal hamartoma (peridiscal astrocytic hamartoma), (5) multiple renal hamartomas or cysts, (6) cardiac rhabdomyoma, or (7) first-degree relative with tuberous sclerosis.

Over 90% of patients have skin lesions, nearly 90% have brain hamartomas demonstrated by CT, 50% have retinal hamartomas, and 50% to 80% have renal hamartomas as demonstrated by ultrasonography. The patient may be asymptomatic, mildly symptomatic, or disabled. Neurologically, many patients have seizures that may be generalized, partial, myoclonic, atypical absence, atonic, or infantile spasms. More than a third, and nearly all with seizure onset before 2 years of age, have some degree of mental retardation. There is no reliable correlation between the occurrence of seizures or mental retardation and the extent or severity of cutaneous or brain involvement. More focal neurological deficit or increased intracranial pressure due to hydrocephalus may indicate the presence of a large periventricular hamartoma or giant cell tumor. Renal angiomyolipomas and epithelial cysts are benign, multiple, bilateral, and usually asymptomatic, although hematuria, hypertension, pain, and renal failure have been reported. Cardiac rhabdomyomas may also be asymptomatic or produce blood flow obstruction, impaired myocardial function, or arrhythmia. Multiple pulmonary cysts or lymphangiomyomatosis may develop in adults and result in hemoptysis, pneumothorax, congestive heart failure, or pulmonary failure. Other manifestations include cranial, vertebral, or pelvic osteosclerosis, cysts of the small bones of the hand or foot, metatarsal periosteal reaction, gingival fibromas, enamel pits, hemangiomas and histiocytoid cellular features

of the spleen, hepatic hamartomas, and rare hamartomas of the mesentery, small bowel, pancreas, adrenal, or thyroid.

NEUROIMAGING FINDINGS

The essential neuropathological hallmark of tuberous sclerosis is hamartomatous lesions that occur subependymally, cortically, and subcortically.[1-3,5,8-12]

Subependymal nodules occur on the surface of the caudate nuclei, especially near the foramina of Monro, and are less commonly identified about the third or fourth ventricles or aqueduct. Calcification or iron deposition is common with increasing age. The nodules are composed of giant cells with neural or glial features plus vascular elements. The nodules may be the same density as brain on CT unless calcified. These are commonly isointense to hyperintense on T1 images and isointense to hypointense on

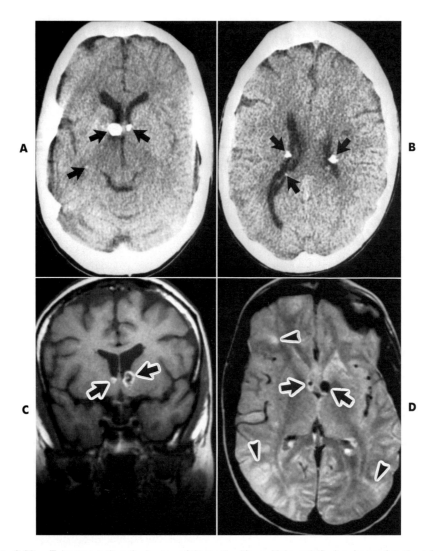

Fig. 8-26 Tuberous sclerosis in an adolescent with multiple calcified subependymal nodules demonstrated by CT **(A** and **B)** as multiple large and small high densities *(arrows).* **C,** Coronal T1 MRI demonstrates the nodules as isointense and hyperintense *(arrows).* **D,** Axial T2 MRI demonstrates the nodules as isointense or hypointense *(arrows).* Dysplastic cortical and subcortical high intensities *(arrowheads)* are also shown.

p/T2 images depending upon the mineral type and concentration (Fig. 8-26). Iodine or gadolinium enhancement is minimal or absent. The hyperintensity on T1 MRI may indicate a paramagnetic effect of calcium, associated iron, or other trace metals (Figs. 8-26 and 8-27). Although often better demonstrated with CT, calcifications may be detected by MRI (see Chapter 1). *Subependymal giant cell tumors* may develop from the nodules, obstruct the foramen of Monro, and cause hydrocephalus. The tumor is a periventricular, circumscribed, solid, or rarely cystic mass composed of giant cells with varying degrees of astrocytic and neuronal differentiation. These cells are often in a perivascular arrangement and are frequently calcified. As demonstrated by CT, these tumors are commonly large and calcified and enhance with iodine administration (Figs. 8-28 and 8-29). As opposed to the subependymal nodules, giant cell tumors appear on MRI as isointense or hypointense on T1 images, hyperintense on p/T2 images, and enhance with gadolinium (Figs. 8-28 and 8-29). Rarely, other neoplasms have been described in tuberous sclerosis, including malignant giant cell tumors, ependymomas, fibrillary astrocytomas, and gliomatosis. The ventriculomegaly commonly

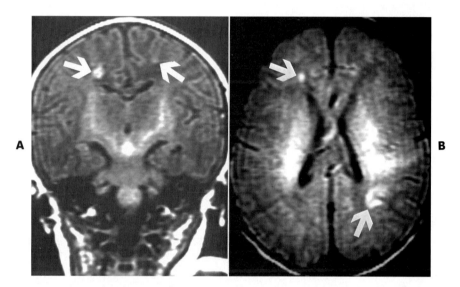

Fig. 8-27   Tuberous sclerosis in infancy with multiple dysplastic cerebral foci *(arrows)* shown as hyperintense on both T1 **(A)** and proton density **(B)** MRI.

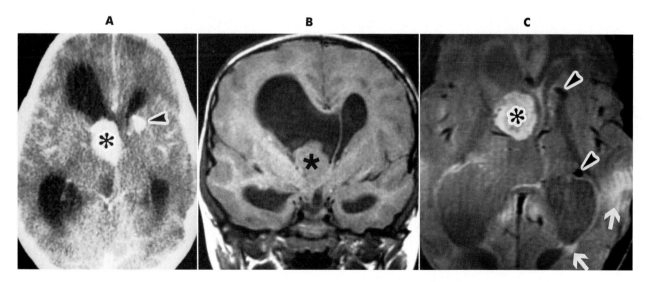

Fig. 8-28   Tuberous sclerosis with giant cell tumor. **A,** CT demonstrates a calcified, iodine-enhancing, high density periforaminal mass *(asterisk)* associated with hydrocephalus. Other calcified nodules are also demonstrated *(arrowheads)*. **B,** Coronal T1 MRI demonstrates the tumor as isointense *(asterisk)*. **C,** Axial T2 MRI demonstrates the tumor as hyperintense *(asterisk)*. Some of the calcified nodules appear low intensity *(arrowheads)*. Also shown are other T2 hyperintense periventricular, cortical, and subcortical dysplastic foci *(arrows)*.

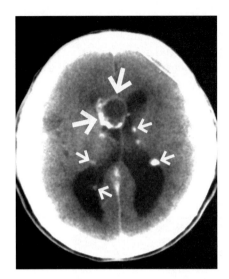

Fig. 8-29   Tuberous sclerosis with cystic giant cell tumor. CT demonstrates a periforaminal low density and calcified cystlike mass *(large arrows)* associated with other calcific high densities *(small arrows)* and hydrocephalus.

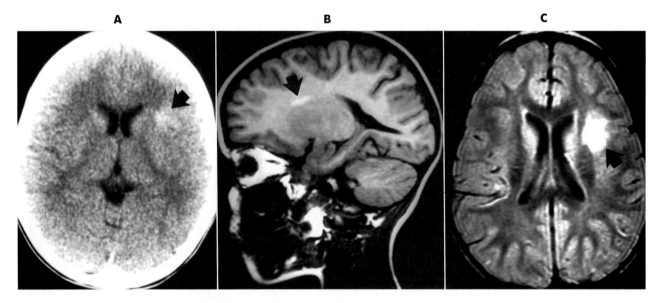

Fig. 8-30   Tuberous sclerosis with solitary tuber *(arrow)* shown by CT **(A)** as a focal high density. The tuber demonstrates hyperintensity on T1 **(B)** and p/T2 **(C)** MRI.

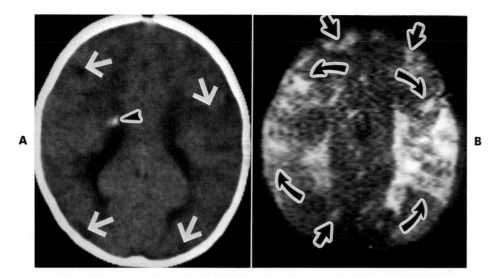

Fig. 8-31   Tuberous sclerosis in infancy with CT **(A)** showing multiple low intensity cerebral foci *(arrows).* Only a few calcific high densities are demonstrated *(arrowhead).* **B,** The corresponding dysplastic foci are demonstrated as high intensity *(straight and curved arrows)* on axial T2 MRI.

observed in tuberous sclerosis may be dysgenetic or atrophic rather than a representation of obstructive hydrocephalus.

Cortical tubers are sclerotic patches within a pachygyric-like cortex occurring more often frontally than occipitally and occurring infrequently in the cerebellum. There is involvement of cortical gyral gray and white matter with giant cells of both neural and glial character. Diminished and disordered myelination is common along with gliosis, but calcification is infrequent. There is disruption of the normal cortical lamination. Subcortically, heterotypic neurons and giant cells are demonstrated with gliosis and myelination defects in a radially oriented pattern extending from the subependymal regions to the cortex (disordered neuronal and glial migration). CT demonstrates the cortical and subcortical abnormalities as low density without abnormal enhancement or calcification early in life (see Fig. 8-31). With increasing age, the low density findings diminish or disappear and calcification appears. MRI demonstrates the lesions to be of low intensity on T1 images and high intensity on p/T2 images early in life (see Fig. 8-31). Again, with age the lesions become T1 isointense but maintain the p/T2 hyperintensity, which probably correlates with deficient myelin and gliosis (Figs. 8-26 and 8-28). The lesions may be few or many, and occasionally a solitary lesion presents with seizures in infancy, demonstrated as high density by CT and high intensity by p/T2 MRI (Fig. 8-30). Some of the lesions may appear cystlike, but neoplastic degeneration is rare.

REFERENCES
Tuberous sclerosis

1. Altman N, Purser R, Donovan Post M: Tuberous sclerosis: CT and MR imaging, *Radiology* 167:527, 1988.
2. Barkovich A: *Pediatric neuroimaging,* New York, 1990, Raven.
3. Braffman B, Bilaniuk L, Zimmerman R: The CNS manifestation of the phakomatoses on MR, *Radiol Clin North Am,* 26:773, 1988.
4. Diebler C, Dulac O: *Pediatric neurology and neuroradiology,* New York, 1987, Springer-Verlag.
5. Gardeur D, Palmieri A, Masholy R: CT in the phakomatoses, *Neuroradiology* 25:293, 1983.
6. Hanno R, Beck R: Tuberous sclerosis, *Neurol Clin* 5:351, 1987.
7. Jones K: *Smith's recognizable patterns of human malformation,* Philadelphia, 1988, WB Saunders.
8. Kingsley D, Kendall B, Fitz C: Tuberous sclerosis, *Neuroradiology* 28:38, 1986.
9. Lee B, Gawler J: Tuberous sclerosis: CT and conventional neuroradiology, *Radiology* 127:403, 1978.
10. Martin N, deBroucker T, Cambier J, et al: MRI of tuberous sclerosis, *Neuroradiology* 29:437, 1987.
11. McMurdo S, Moore S, Brant-Zawadzki M, et al: MR imaging of intracranial tuberous sclerosis, *AJNR* 8:77, 1987.
12. Nixon J, Houser O, Okazaki H: Cerebral tuberous sclerosis: MR imaging, *Radiology* 170:869, 1989.

Sturge-Weber syndrome

Sturge-Weber syndrome, or encephalotrigeminal angiomatosis, is a syndrome of facial port-wine stain in the distribution of the first division (V-1) of the trigeminal nerve together with ipsilateral leptomeningeal angiomatosis.[1,4,6,7,9] Seizures, mental retardation, and hemiplegia are common. Familial incidence is rare, and the majority of cases are sporadic. The facial capillary angioma of the dermis is usually unilateral, but bilateral involvement has been reported. The angioma usually involves the lid, forehead, and cheek, but there may be additional involvement of the trunk or limbs. Neurological symptoms and signs occur only, but not invariably, when the vascular malformation includes the V-1 territory. Visceral angiomatosis and an association with Klippel-Trenaunay-Weber syndrome has also been reported. Ipsilateral choroidal angioma is also frequent and may result in buphthalmos (congenital glaucoma). The pial angioma usually lies over the occipital lobe, with variable extension to the parietal and temporal lobes. Hemispheric or bilateral involvement is unusual. Seizures are present in greater than 90% of patients and may be partial or generalized. The seizures begin early in life and often become refractory to treatment. Homonymous hemianopsia, hemiplegia, hemisensory deficit, and mental retardation are also common. Subarachnoid or intracerebral hemorrhage is a rare occurrence. Neuropathological changes include pial venous angiomatosis, choroid plexus angiomas, arterial fibrosis, cortical and subcortical ischemic microangiopathy with necrosis, gliosis, demyelination, and progressive mineralization with both calcium and iron deposition.[1,4,6] Migrational anomalies with pachygyric-like changes have also been observed.[5] Hemiatrophy also results in craniocerebral asymmetry and occasional subdural hematomas.

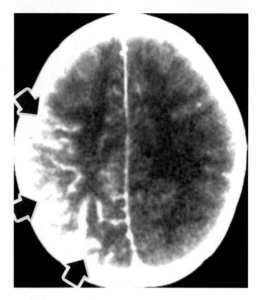

Fig. 8-32   Sturge-Weber syndrome and seizures in infancy with CT showing abnormal enhancement *(arrows)* without calcification.

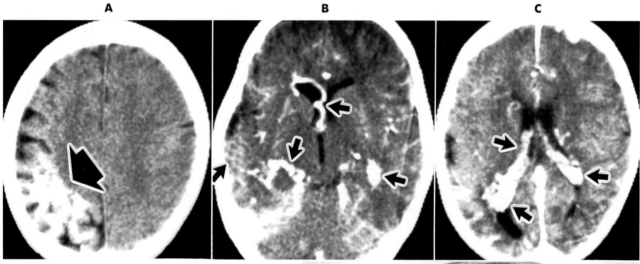

A   **B**   **C**

Fig. 8-33   Sturge-Weber syndrome in a juvenile with CT demonstration **(A-C)** of extensive calcification *(large arrow)*, atrophy, and abnormal cerebral and choroid plexus vascular enhancement *(small arrows)*. **D,** The venous phase of the lateral carotid angiogram shows anomalous cerebral venous structures *(arrows)*.

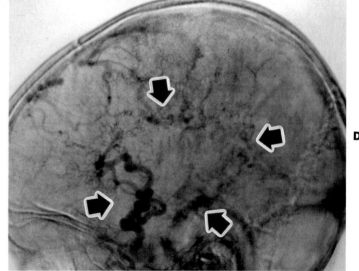

D

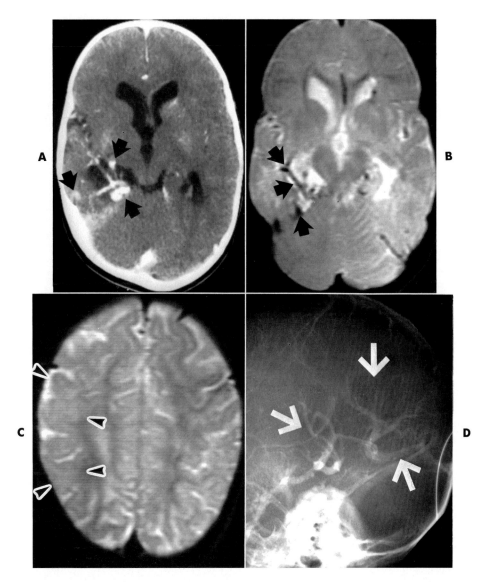

Fig. 8-34   Sturge-Weber syndrome. **A,** CT shows abnormal vascular enhancement *(arrows).* **B** and **C,** Axial T2 MRI show abnormal vascular flow voids *(arrows)* and pachygyric-like cortical morphology *(arrowheads).* **D,** The venous phase of the lateral carotid angiogram shows anomalous cerebral venous structures *(arrows).*

NEUROIMAGING FINDINGS

Neuroimaging findings include gyral calcification beginning in later infancy and progressing with age until the second or third decade.[1,3,4,6-8] It may often be confined to the occipital region or extend into the adjacent temporal and parietal areas (Figs. 8-32 and 8-33). Extensive hemispheric or bilateral calcification has been observed in some cases along with choroid plexus calcification. Iodine enhancement has been reported on CT, especially in early infancy and before the identification of mineralization (Figs. 8-32 and 8-33). The cortical and subcortical enhancement is probably related to impaired capillary permeability (blood-brain barrier breakdown) rather than subpial extension of the leptomeningeal angioma. As the calcification increases with age and atrophy, the iodine enhancement diminishes or may be obscured. Calcification is often better demonstrated by CT than by MRI except when acting as a paramagnetic element, when highly concentrated, when associated with iron, or when gradient echo techniques are used (see Chapter 1). The atrophy is readily demonstrated as ventricular and subarachnoid space dilatation on both CT and MRI, whereas gliosis and demyelination are better shown by MRI as high intensity abnormalities on p/T2 images. The pachygyric-like changes are also better demonstrated with MRI (Fig. 8-34). Prominent choroid plexus, deep midline, and subependymal periventricular vascular densities, intensities, or enhancement may be demonstrated by CT and MRI (Figs. 8-33 and 8-34). These correlate with angiographic findings of slow flow or nonopacification of the dysplastic or thrombosed superficial cortical veins with shunting and opacification of dilated medullary and deep veins.[2,10,11] Other vascular abnormalities (Figs. 8-33 and 8-34) include arterial, venous, or sinus thrombosis, often small cerebral arteries on the side of the pial malformation, numerous prominent veins and capillaries with dense angiographic staining in the involved lobe early in life, and, rarely, enlarged arterial feeders or other vascular malformations.

REFERENCES
Sturge-Weber syndrome

1. Barkovich A: *Pediatric neuroimaging*, New York, 1990, Raven.
2. Bentson J, Wilson G, Newton T: Cerebral venous drainage pattern of Sturge-Weber syndrome, *Radiology* 102:111, 1971.
3. Bilaniuk L, Zimmerman R, Hochman M, et al: MR of the Sturge-Weber syndrome, *AJNR* 8:945, 1987.
4. Braffman B, Bilaniuk L, Zimmerman R: The CNS manifestation of the phakomatoses on MR, *Radiol Clin North Am* 26:773, 1988.
5. Chamberlain M, Press G, Hesselink J: MR imaging and CT in Sturge-Weber syndrome, *AJNR* 10:491, 1989.
6. Diebler C, Dulac O: *Pediatric neurology and neuroradiology*, New York, 1987, Springer-Verlag.
7. Enrolras O, Riche M, Merland J: Facial port-wine stain and Sturge-Weber syndrome, *Pediatrics* 76:48, 1985.
8. Enzmann D, Hayward R, Norman D, et al: CT of Sturge-Weber disease, *Radiology* 122:721, 1977.
9. Jones K: *Smith's recognizable patterns of human malformation*, Philadelphia, 1988, WB Saunders.
10. Probst F: Vascular morphology and angiographic flow patterns in Sturge-Weber angiomatosis, *Neuroradiology* 20:73, 1980.
11. Stimac G, Soloman M, Newton T: CT and MR of angiomatous malformations of the choroid plexus in Sturge-Weber disease, *AJNR* 7:623, 1986.

Von Hippel–Lindau disease

Von Hippel–Lindau disease, or CNS angiomatosis, is of autosomal dominant inheritance with incomplete penetrance (linkage to chromosome 3) and consists classically of retinal, cerebellar, and visceral "angiomatosis."[1,2,4,7] In this syndrome angiomatosis refers to vascular neoplasia (hemangioblastoma) rather than to vascular malformations. The diagnosis may be confirmed in a patient with more than one hemangioblastoma of the CNS, one CNS hemangioblastoma plus visceral involvement, or one component of the disease and a positive family history. More specifically, the disease includes retinal, cerebellar, spinal cord, and, rarely, cerebral hemangioblastomas. Visceral lesions include renal carcinoma (multicentric or bilateral), pheochromocytomas, cysts of the kidney, liver, pancreas, spleen, adrenal glands, mesentery, omentum, and epididymis, as well as adenomas of the liver and epididymis. Occasionally, cutaneous or mucosal nevi may be seen. Retinal hemangioblastomas occur in the majority of patients and may be multiple and bilateral. Symptoms include visual impairment or eye pain related to the inflammatory and hemorrhagic components and the sequelae of retinal detachment, which

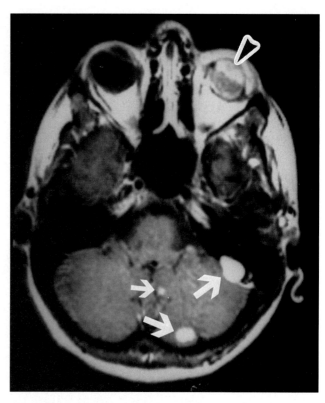

Fig. 8-35 Von Hippel–Lindau syndrome with axial T1 MRI showing high intensity, gadolinium-enhancing hemangioblastomas of the globe *(arrowhead)* and cerebellum *(arrows)*.

may obscure the primary abnormality. Cerebellar hemangioblastomas occur in one third to one half of cases and infrequently may be multiple. Hemangioblastomas are less commonly seen in the brain stem, especially in the medulla (area postrema), or spine, particularly the cervical or thoracic cord, and rarely involve the nerve roots or are located extradurally. Supratentorial hemangioblastomas are exceedingly rare. Neurological symptoms and signs include increased pressure, cerebellar dysfunction, subarachnoid hemorrhage, or myelopathy. Although retinal hemangioblastoma may appear in childhood, the CNS and other visceral lesions are usually not symptomatic until late in the second decade or adulthood. Asymptomatic or additional lesions may be demonstrated, however, with routine imaging screens.

NEUROIMAGING FINDINGS

Neuroimaging rarely directly demonstrates retinal hemangioblastomas as calcified, ossified, or enhancing lesions (Fig. 8-35). More often the complications associated with retinal detachment are observed (for example, hemorrhage). Cerebellar hemangioblastomas are classically subpial, hemispheric, and cystic, and may mimic a cystic astrocytoma.[1-6,8] The cystic component may be single or multiple and large, often obscuring the small vascularized mural nodule (Figs. 8-36 and 8-37). In less than half of the cases

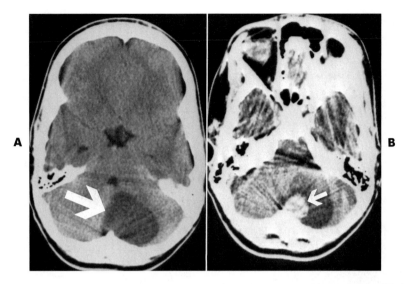

Fig. 8-36   Von Hippel–Lindau syndrome with cerebellar cystic hemangioblastoma. **A** and **B,** Axial CT scans show cerebellar low density cystic tumor *(A, arrow)* with nodular high density enhancement *(B, arrow).*

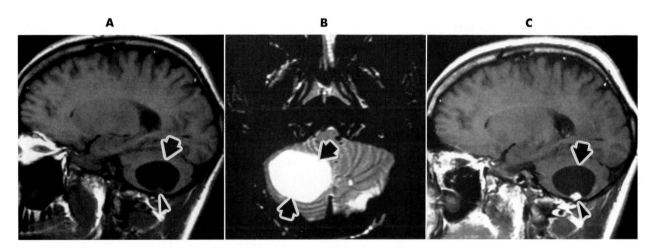

Fig. 8-37   Von Hippel–Lindau syndrome with recurrent cerebellar hemangioblastoma (same patient as in Fig. 8-36). There is a large cerebellar cyst *(arrows)* that is hypointense on sagittal T1 **(A)** and hyperintense on axial T2 **(B)** MRI obscuring the small nodular component *(arrowhead)* that markedly enhances with gadolinium on postinjection sagittal T1 MRI **(C).**

the tumor is entirely or predominantly solid. The solid form may occur as a very small nodule not detected by CT as readily as with MRI. The CT and MRI appearance of the cystic component varies with the cyst content. CSF-like, proteinaceous, or hemorrhagic density or intensity patterns may be seen. The nodule may be isodensity to low density relative to brain on CT, isointensity to low intensity on T1 MRI, and isointensity to hyperintensity on p/T2-MRI (Figs. 8-36 and 8-37). The nodular tumor or component may be readily demonstrated only with iodine or gadolinium enhancement (Figs. 8-35 and 8-37). Occasionally the

vascular components (feeding artery and draining vein) of the tumor nodule may be identified by MRI as tubular or pin-point flow voids or as flow enhancement. Cerebellar hemangioblastomas are rarely multiple but frequently recur after initial resection (Fig. 8-37). It is important to search for other CNS tumors (that is, brain stem, cord, cerebral), and gadolinium-enhanced MRI is the preferred method (Fig. 8-38). Gadolinium MRI is particularly important in screening of the cord, particularly to distinguish tumoral from nontumoral hydrosyringomyelia.

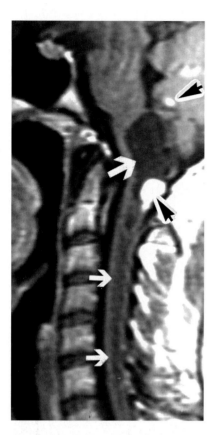

Fig. 8-38   Von Hippel–Lindau syndrome with cerebellar and cervicomedullary hemangioblastomas demonstrated by sagittal T1 MRI as a hypointense cystlike mass *(large white arrow)* with nodular gadolinium enhancement *(black arrows)* and hydrosyringomyelia *(small white arrows).*

REFERENCES
Von Hippel–Lindau disease
1. Barkovich A: *Pediatric neuroimaging,* New York, 1990, Raven.
2. Braffman B, Bilaniuk L, Zimmerman R: The CNS manifestation of the phakomatoses on MR, *Radiol Clin North Am* 26:773, 1988.
3. Coulam C, Brown L, Reese D: Hippel-Lindau syndrome, *Semin Roentgenol,* 11:61, 1976.
4. Diebler C, Dulac O: *Pediatric neurology and neuroradiology,* New York, 1987, Springer-Verlag.
5. Fill W, Lamiell J, Polk N: The radiographic manifestations of von Hippel–Lindau disease, *Radiology* 133:289, 1979.
6. Huson S, Harper P, Hourihan M, et al: Cerebellar hemangioblastoma and von Hippel–Lindau disease, *Brain* 109:1297, 1986.
7. Jones K: *Smith's recognizable patterns of human malformation,* Philadelphia, 1988, WB Saunders.
8. Sato Y, Wazir M, Smith W, et al: Hippel-Lindau disease: MR imaging, *Radiology* 166:241, 1988.

Other neurocutaneous syndromes

KLIPPEL-TRENAUNAY-WEBER SYNDROME

Klippel-Trenaunay-Weber syndrome (angioosteohypertrophy syndrome) is a sporadically occurring syndrome composed of capillary and cavernous malformations and varicosities that may occur unilaterally or bilaterally involv-ing the trunk or limbs.[2,9,14,20,34] Limb hypertrophy or hemihypertrophy is frequent. CNS vascular malformations (Fig. 8-39) may occur, including cerebral angiomas, spinal cord malformations, aplasia of the cervical internal carotid artery, and circle of Willis anomalies. Calcifications, microcephaly, and macrocephaly have been reported, as well as cerebral and cerebellar hemihypertrophy, scoliosis, and kyphosis. The disorder may be related to Sturge-Weber syndrome.

ATAXIA-TELANGIECTASIA

Ataxia-telangiectasia (Louis-Bar syndrome) is of autosomal recessive inheritance and includes facial and conjunctival (oculocutaneous) capillary telangiectasias, cerebellar atrophy (Chapter 4), and demyelination of the posterior columns and dorsal spinocerebellar tracts.[1,9,18,29,34] Progressive ataxia is characteristic along with choreoathetosis, mental retardation, apraxia, and hypotonia. Hemorrhage may occur as a result of cerebral telangiectasias. Cerebral infarction may occur secondary to embolization from pulmonary arteriovenous malformations (AVMs). Growth deficiency has also been reported. Cellular immunodeficiency with thymic and lymphoid hypoplasia is also characteristic, which predisposes the patient to recurrent infection and neoplasia, particularly lymphomas (Hodgkin's disease), but also leukemia and sarcomas.

HEREDITARY HEMORRHAGIC TELANGIECTASIA

Hereditary hemorrhagic telangiectasia (Osler-Rendu-Weber disease) is an autosomal dominant inherited disorder and includes cutaneous and mucous membrane telangiectasias.[9,19,30,34] Occasionally there is brain involvement including telangiectasias, AVMs, and aneurysms with subarachnoid or intracerebral hemorrhage and infarction. Cerebral abscess or infarction may result from embolization related to pulmonary vascular malformations. Seizures, hemiparesis, and visual and speech symptoms or signs may result.

BANNAYAN SYNDROME

Bannayan syndrome is a rare autosomal dominant inherited disorder with associated hemangiomas, lipomas, meningiomas, and macrocephaly.[19,34]

EPIDERMAL NEVUS SYNDROME

Epidermal nevus syndrome is a sporadic disorder characterized by linear epidermal nevi, skeletal anomalies, seizures, and developmental delay.[9,19,34] CNS involvement may include brain atrophy, porencephaly, hydrocephalus, white matter disease, calcifications, heterotopias, and lateral ventricular coarctation. Other lesions reported are gliomas, leptomeningeal hemangiomas, aneurysms, and kyphoscoliosis with cord compression.

LINEAR SEBACEOUS NEVUS SYNDROME

Linear sebaceous nevus syndrome is a sporadically occurring disorder with characteristic sebaceous nevus of Jadas-

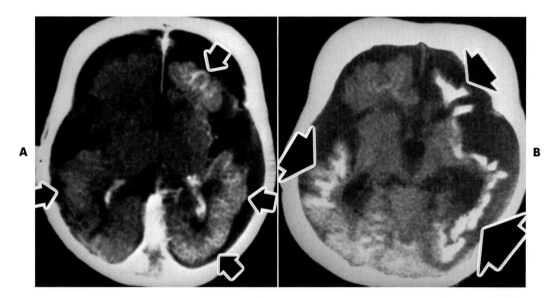

Fig. 8-39   Klippel-Trenaunay-Weber syndrome with Sturge-Weber features. **A** and **B**, Serial CTs show enhancing vascular malformations *(arrows)*, progressing to atrophy with calcifications (**B**, *arrowheads*).

sohn, which is a yellow plaque consisting of hyperkeratosis and hypertrophy of sebaceous glands.[3,5,19,21-24,34] The midline scalp or face location of the nevus is usually associated with neurological symptoms and signs including seizures, developmental delay, and mental retardation. The seizures may be partial or generalized and include infantile spasms and Lennox-Gestaut syndrome. Ocular manifestations are common, including microphthalmia and coloboma. Reported neuroimaging findings include hemimegalencephaly, hemiatrophy, hydrocephalus, choroid plexus papillomas, astrocytomas, and vascular malformations.

NEUROCUTANEOUS MELANOSIS

Neurocutaneous melanosis (Rokitansky-van Bogaert syndrome) is a syndrome composed of giant, pigmented, and occasionally hairy nevi in a truncal or capelike distribution. There is associated abnormal meningeal pigmentation and thickening (melanocytic proliferation) especially at the skull base but often also involving the cerebellum, brain stem, and basal ganglia.[*] The risk of malignant melanoma is in the range of 10% to 12%. The disorder probably represents an aberration of melanoblast origin and migration from the neural crest. Clinical manifestations include seizures, hydrocephalus, chronic meningitis, and cranial nerve palsy. Neurological involvement is more likely when pia-arachnoid melanosis is associated with head and scalp nevi. Neuroimaging may demonstrate hydrocephalus, hydrosyringomyelia, cisternal opacification, tumor masses, calcification, and enhancement.

NEVOID BASAL CELL CARCINOMA SYNDROME

Nevoid basal cell carcinoma syndrome (Gorlin's syndrome) is of autosomal dominant inheritance. The syndrome includes multiple nevoid basal cell lesions that are prone to carcinoma and involve the face, neck, arms, and trunk.[*] Odontogenic keratocysts characteristically involve the mandible or maxilla. Associated skeletal anomalies include absent ribs, scoliosis, kyphoscoliosis, craniocervical junction anomalies (for example, hypoplastic dens), cervical spondylolisthesis, and osteoporosis. A broad nasal bridge and frontoparietal bossing produce characteristic craniofacial dysmorphia. Other system anomalies reported include ocular malformations and brachydactyly. There may be calcification of the falx cerebri, falx cerebelli, or choroid plexus (Fig. 8-40). Agenesis of the corpus callosum, septum pellucidum cyst, hydrocephalus, and cerebellar atrophy have also been reported. There is a predisposition to tumors, including CNS tumors (Fig. 8-40) and especially medulloblastoma. Other reported tumors include meningioma, craniopharyngioma, fibrosarcoma, amelioblastoma, and coloboma. Mental retardation, seizures, and hydrocephalus are common neurological manifestations.

HYPOMELANOSIS OF ITO

Hypomelanosis of Ito possibly represents a chromosomal mosaicism and includes streaky patches of cutaneous hypopigmentation (incontinentia pigmenti achromians), skeletal malformations including scoliosis, kyphosis, syndactyly, cleft palate, and skull defects, and ocular abnormalities including strabismus, nystagmus, optic atrophy,

---

[*]References 7,9,12,13,17,19,34.

[*]References 6,9,10,15,16,19,26,34.

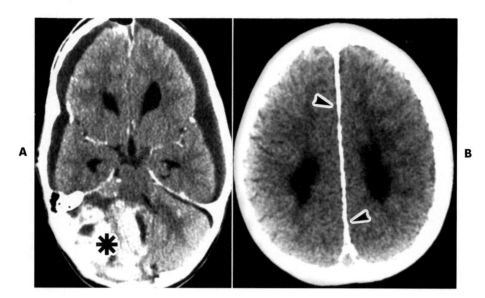

Fig. 8-40   Gorlin syndrome. **A** and **B,** CT scans demonstrate an irregular-enhancing posterior fossa medulloblastoma *(asterisk).* Bilateral subdural collections are also seen after shunting for hydrocephalus. Extensive dural calcification is seen along the falx *(arrowheads).*

coloboma, and microphthalmia.[8,9,19,31,34] Seizures, mental retardation, macrocephaly or microcephaly, and developmental delay are common. Neuroimaging has demonstrated asymmetrical cerebral atrophy, porencephaly, white matter degeneration, gliosis, and heterotopias.

INCONTINENTIA PIGMENTI

Incontinentia pigmenti (Bloch-Sulzberger syndrome) is an X-linked disorder with a characteristic skin rash beginning in infancy as truncal and limb erythematous and bullous lesions. These lesions rupture and become hyperkeratotic, evolving to streaks of hyperpigmentation.* Also there is abnormal dentition, alopecia, ocular anomalies (microphthalmia, optic nerve hypoplasia or atrophy), and skeletal anomalies including scoliosis. Seizures, mental retardation, microcephaly, and developmental delay are frequent. Recurrent meningitis and encephalitis have also been reported. Neuroimaging has demonstrated ischemic brain lesions including edema, gliotic white matter cavities, atrophy, porencephaly, microgyria, and microcephaly.

ENCEPHALOCRANIOCUTANEOUS LIPOMATOSIS

Encephalocraniocutaneous lipomatosis (Fishman's syndrome) is a syndrome that includes subcutaneous scalp and neck lipomas, intracranial and intraspinal lipomas, leptomeningeal lipogranulomatosis, facial papules, ocular choristomas, and unilateral parietal cranial vault and scalp thickening.[9,11,19,34] Ipsilateral cerebral abnormalities include microgyria, porencephaly, ventricular dilatation, cortical atrophy, cerebral and meningeal calcifications, and vascular malformations. Clinical manifestations include seizures and mental retardation.

*References 4,9,19,25,27,34

FACIAL NEVI WITH ANOMALOUS VENOUS RETURN AND HYDROCEPHALUS

Facial nevi with anomalous venous return and hydrocephalus is a disorder of similar embryogenesis to the Sturge-Weber syndrome. The port-wine nevus, however, primarily involves the lower face and neck, and hydrocephalus is the major manifestation rather than seizures or mental retardation.[9,28,32-34] There is associated hypoplasia of the distal lateral dural venous sinuses.

REFERENCES
Other neurocutaneous syndromes

1. Barkovich A: *Pediatric neuroimaging,* New York, 1990, Raven.
2. Baskerville P: The Klippel-Trenaunay syndrome: clinical, radiological, and hemodynamic features and management, *Br J Surg* 72:232, 1985.
3. Bianchine J: The nevus sebaceous of Jadassohn: a neurocutaneous syndrome and a potentially premalignant lesion, *Am J Dis Child* 120:223, 1970.
4. Carney R: Incontinenti pigmenti, *Arch Dermatol* 112:535, 1976.
5. Chalhub E, Volpe J, Gado M: Linear nevus sebaceous syndrome, *Neurology* 25:857, 1975.
6. Codish S, Kraszeski J, Pratt K: CNS developmental anomaly in basal cell nevus syndrome, *Neuropaediatric* 4:338, 1973.
7. Crisp E, Thompson J: Primary malignant melanomatosis of the meninges, *Arch Neurol* 38:528, 1981.
8. David T: Hypomelanosis of Ito: a neurocutaneous syndrome, *Arch Dis Child* 56:798, 1981.
9. Diebler C, Dulac O: *Pediatric neurology and neuroradiology,* New York, 1987, Springer-Verlag.
10. Ferrier P, Hinrichs W: Basal cell carcinoma syndrome, *Am J Dis Child* 113:538, 1967.
11. Fishman M, Chang C, Miller J: Encephalocraniocutaneous lipomatosis, *Pediatrics* 61:580, 1978.
12. Flodmark O, Fitz C, Harwood-Nash D, et al: Neuroradiologic findings in primary leptomeningeal melanoma, *Neuroradiology* 18:153, 1979.
13. Fox H: Neurocutaneous melanosis, *Arch Dis Child* 39:508, 1964.
14. Furukawa T: Sturge-Weber and Klippel-Trenaunay syndrome, *Arch Dermatol* 102:840, 1970.
15. Gorlin R: The multiple basal cell nevi syndrome, *Cancer* 18:89, 1965.

16. Hawkins J, Hoffman H, Becker L: Multiple nevoid basal cell carcinoma syndrome (Gorlin's syndrome), *J Neurosurg* 50:100, 1979.
17. Hoffman H, Freeman A: Primary malignant leptomeningeal melanoma in association with giant hairy nevus, *J Neurosurg* 26:62, 1967.
18. Hosking G: Ataxia-telangiectasia, *Dev Med Child Neurol* 24:77, 1982.
19. Jones K: *Smith's recognizable patterns of human malformation,* Philadelphia, 1988, WB Saunders.
20. Kuffer F: Klippel-Trenaunay syndrome, visceral angiomatosis, and thrombocytopenia, *J Pediatr Surg* 3:65, 1968.
21. Kurokawa T, Sasaki K, Honai T, et al: Linear nevus sebaceous syndrome, *Arch Neurol* 38:375, 1981.
22. Lansky L: Linear sebaceous nevus syndrome, *Am J Dis Child* 123:587, 1972.
23. Leonidas J, Wolpert S, Feingold M, et al: Radiological features of the linear sebaceous syndrome, *AJR* 132:277, 1979.
24. Levin S, Robinsen R, Aicardi J: CT in linear sebaceous naevus syndrome, *Neuroradiology* 26:469, 1984.
25. Morgan J: Incontinentia pigmenti, *Am J Dis Child* 122:294, 1971.
26. Murphy M, Tenser R: Nevoid basal cell carcinoma syndrome and epilepsy, *Ann Neurol* 11:372, 1982.
27. O'Doherty N, Norman R: Incontinentia pigmenti with cerebral malformation, *Dev Med Child Neurol* 10:168, 1968.
28. Orr C, Osher R, Savino P: The syndrome of facial nevi, anomalous cerebral venous return, and hydrocephalus, *Ann Neurol* 3:216, 1978.
29. Paller A: Ataxia-telangiectasia, *Neurol Clin* 5:447, 1987.
30. Schaumann B, Alter M: Cerebrovascular malformations in hereditary hemorrhagic telangiectasia, *Minn Med* 56:951, 1973.
31. Schwartz M, Esterly N, Fretzin D, et al: Hypomelanosis of Ito, *J Pediatr* 90:236, 1977.
32. Shapiro K, Shulman K: Facial nevi associated with anomalous venus return and hydrocephalus, *J Neurosurg* 45:20, 1976.
33. Stephan M: Macrocephaly in association with unusual cutaneous angiomatosis, *J Pediatr* 87:353, 1975.
34. Taybi H, Lachman R: *Radiology of syndromes, metabolic disorders, and skeletal dysplasias,* Chicago, 1990, Mosby–Year Book.

PART THREE

Spine Imaging

9 · Developmental Abnormalities of the Spine and Spinal Neuraxis

Patrick D. Barnes

Developmental aspects of the spine and spinal neuraxis

SPINAL COLUMN

Early in the embryonic period (the first 8 weeks after ovulation) the notochord serves as the developmental precursor (Fig. 9-1) for induction of the mesodermal germ layer, which gives rise to the mesenchymal elements forming the spinal column and paraspinal tissues, including bone, muscle, ligaments, disk, connective tissue, blood vessels, and meninges. The notochord also induces the neuroectoderm to form the neural tube, origin of the central nervous system, and the neural crest, origin of the peripheral nervous system.* The notochord also is respon-

___
*References 2, 15, 16, 18, 20, 25.

sible for serial segmental organization of mesodermal and neuroectodermal development, as well as final separation of neural tube derivatives (brain and spinal cord) from overlying ectodermal derivatives (skin), from surrounding mesodermal derivatives (spinal column, paraspinal muscles, dura, and so forth), and from underlying endodermal derivatives (respiratory, gastrointestinal, and genitourinary tracts and the coelomic cavities).

The notochordal process arises from the rostral primitive streak at the node of Henson, separating the dorsal amniotic cavity from the ventral yolk sac. The notochordal process in turn gives rise to the notochordal canal and then the notochordal plate. The primitive neurenteric canal, a remnant of the notochordal canal, allows direct communication between the yolk sac (endoderm) and amniotic cavity (Fig. 9-2). Persistence of the neurenteric canal with

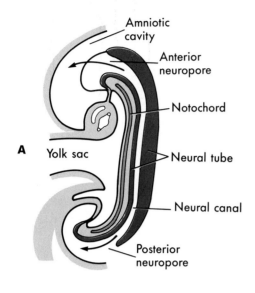

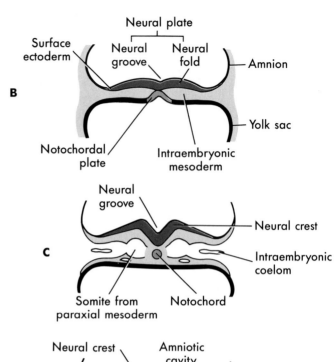

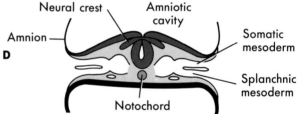

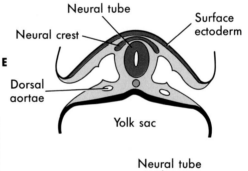

Fig. 9-1 Spinal column and spinal neuraxis development. **A,** Sagittal section of embryo at 24 days. **B-F,** Cross sections of the embryo from 18 to 28 days (see text). (Modified from Moore K: *The developing human,* ed 4, Philadelphia, 1988, WB Saunders.)

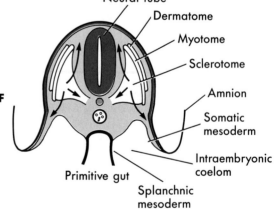

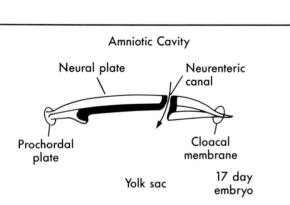

Fig. 9-2 The neurenteric canal. Midline sagittal section along the intercalated notochordal process at 17 days showing the amniotic cavity in communication with the yolk sac through the neurenteric canal at Henson's node. (Modified from French B: Abnormal development of the CNS. In McLaurin R, et al, editors: *Pediatric neurosurgery,* ed 2, Philadelphia, 1989, WB Saunders.)

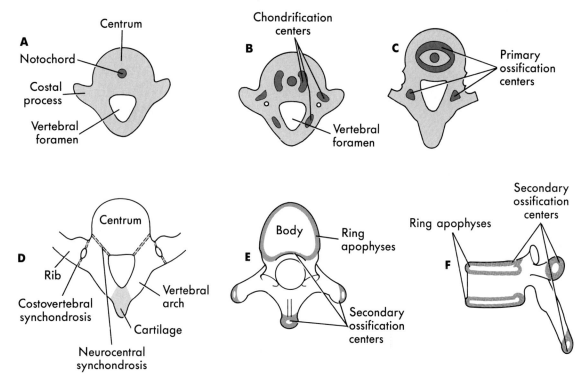

Fig. 9-3   Stages of vertebral development. **A,** Mesenchymal vertebra (approximately 5 weeks). **B,** Chondrification centers (approximately 6 weeks). **C,** Primary ossification centers (approximately 6 weeks). **D,** Thoracic vertebra at birth. **E** and **F,** Thoracic vertebra at puberty. (Modified from Moore K: *The developing human,* ed 4, Philadelphia, 1988, WB Saunders.)

abnormal endodermal-ectodermal adhesion in the presomite embryo (20 to 22 days) is the likely precursor for the range of malformations included in the neurenteric or split notochord spectrum.[15,20] The notochordal plate separates the endoderm ventrally from the neuroectoderm dorsally and becomes a solid rod of tissue, the notochord, which extends the entire length of the embryo from the level of the adenohypophysis to the tail by 22 days (Fig. 9-1). The persistence of notochordal remnants at sites along this path has been implicated in the pathogenesis of chordomas.[20]

The notochord separates from the ventral gut (yolk sac) and dorsal neural tube with migration of the intervening axial mesenchyme to form a longitudinal series of paired somites, or segments. The medial sclerotomes give rise to vertebral column elements (bone, cartilage, ligaments, disks, meninges), and the lateral myotomes give rise to the paraspinal muscles (Fig. 9-1).[18,20] This occurs at the same time that the neuroectoderm is directing segmental development of the neural tube to form the spinal cord and directing the neural crest to form the peripheral nerves and ganglia along dermatomes, all of which is integrated with the developing cardiovascular system. After neural tube closure and separation from the superficial ectoderm, the dorsal mesenchyme migrates around the neural tube to form the neural arches, meninges, and paraspinal muscles. The mesenchymal somites at each level proliferate dorsolater-

ally to surround the notochord (Fig. 9-1) and fuse to form the vertebral structures (bodies, neural arches, and disks) and ribs, with subsequent conversion to cartilage (chondrification) and then to bone (enchondral ossification).

Each vertebral segment develops separately (that is, segmentation) from the ones above and below. Failure of separation leads to segmentation anomalies, for example in Klippel-Feil syndrome, congenital scoliosis or kyphosis, and occipitalization of the atlas.[20] Starting at 4 weeks, each vertebral unit develops from three separate mesenchymal centers. The central portion, or centrum, of the vertebral body surrounds the notochord, and the two neural processes give rise to the dorsal body and neural arches. The latter extend dorsally to unite and enclose the neural tube (Fig. 9-3). Serial segmentation of the vertebral arches probably depends on development of the spinal ganglia as derived from the neural crest. Each mesenchymal vertebra becomes cartilaginous between 6 and 8 weeks, and then ossifies beginning at 9 weeks. Disorders of vertebral formation (for example, hemivertebra) also may lead to congenital scoliosis or kyphosis.

In the fetal period (after the first 6 to 8 weeks) chondrification of the mesenchymal vertebrae begins in each half of the body, with ossification of the cartilaginous centrum proceeding from thoracic to lumbar to cervical. Bone deposition takes place around preexisting vascular canals, giving a bipartite and coronal cleft appearance. The neural processes undergo subperiosteal (membranous) ossification, primarily in a rostrocaudal progression from cervical to thoracic to lumbosacral.[20,22]

In the postnatal period three separate centers of ossification are evident for each vertebral segment (Fig. 9-3), that is, the centrum and the paired neural processes. These are joined by the preossified cartilaginous neurocentral synchondroses.[20,22] Between 3 and 6 years of age the synchondroses ossify and unite the centrum and arch centers. The partially ossified vertebral centrae appear ovoid and of equal height to the disk spaces but are smaller than the corresponding spinal canal. The disk spaces actually represent disk tissue plus the nonossified portions of the adjacent bodies. Anterior and posterior vascular clefts are present within the ossified centra. With progressive ossification the bodies become more rectangular and of increased height. Anterosuperior and anteroinferior vertebral body indentations are apparent at about 5 years and represent exaggerations of the annular recesses for the cartilaginous ring apophyses. The latter begin ossification as small calcific foci between 6 and 9 years, form a complete ossified ring at about 12 years, and fuse to the body at maturity. Hyaline cartilage makes up the vertebral epiphyseal growth plate superiorly and inferiorly. Disorders of chondrification or ossification occurring about the weak points of vascular penetration of the ring and end-plate cartilage may provide the basis for Schmorl's nodes and Scheuermann's disease.

Spinous process ossification begins in the lumbosacral region in early infancy and proceeds cephalad, with completion in the cervical region in the second year after birth. Variations (that is, spina bifida benigna) are common, especially at the transitional segments, such as the lumbosacral, craniocervical, or cervicothoracic junctions.[11,20-22] Ossification of the posterior arch of the atlas may not occur until between 4 and 6 years, whereas that for the lumbosacral junction may not occur until between 7 and 10 years or may persist as a spina bifida variant. Bony union of the neurocentral synchondrosis begins in the cervical region at 3 years and progresses to the sacral level by 6 to 7 years.

The nucleus pulposus of the intervertebral disk is derived embryologically from notochordal and perichordal mesenchyme, whereas the annulus fibrosis and fibrocartilage originate from perichordal mesenchyme.[1,14,20,29] The nucleus at birth consists of mucoid substance, a product of notochordal degeneration, along with a few fibrocartilaginous elements. The nucleus is vascularized and 88% water at birth, becomes avascular at about 4 years, and is approximately 80% water at 12 years. The annulus has about 10% less water content than the nucleus. With age there is dorsal shift of the nucleus within the disk plus progressive fibrocartilaginous replacement of the mucoid substance and further loss of water (70% at 70 years). The changes in the vascularity of the disk space and in the nuclear matrix are often implicated, respectively, in the

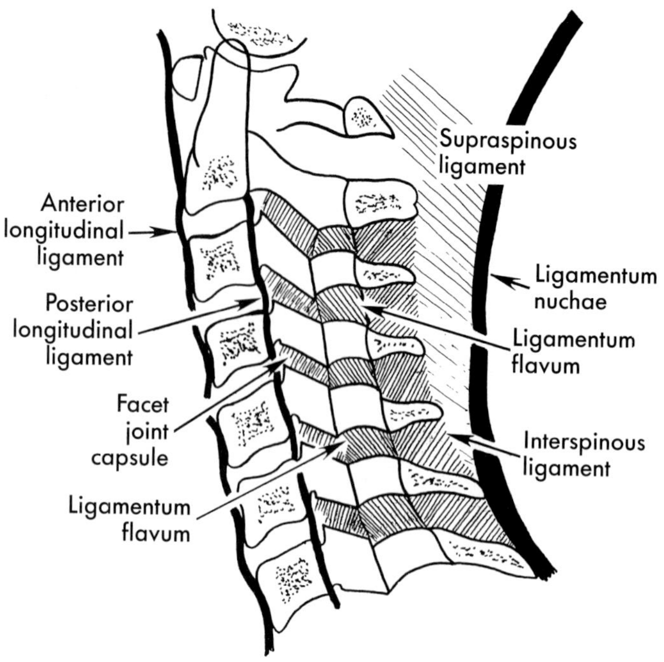

Fig. 9-4 Ligamentous structures of the cervical spine. (From Gerlock A, et al: *The cervical spine in trauma,* Philadelphia, 1978, WB Saunders.)

pathogenesis of diskitis/osteomyelitis, and disk herniation. The important ligamentous structures responsible for spinal stability include the anterior and posterior longitudinal ligaments continous with the annulus fibrosis, the facet joint capsular ligaments, the ligamentum flavum, and the interspinous and supraspinous ligaments (Fig. 9-4).

The thoracic and sacral curves are formed prenatally and are thus considered primary curvatures.[22] These persist postnatally until the child begins to assume an upright sitting or walking posture. As a result secondary lumbar and cervical curvatures form, although evidence also exists for prenatal formation of the latter.[22] The curves tend to straighten with recumbency in the infant and young child. The ossified bodies appear small in infancy compared with the adjacent disk spaces, spinal canal, and the fatty and venous epidural compartment. Early in life the craniospinal skeleton is composed primarily of incompletely ossified cartilage and red marrow.[7,9,19,25,27] In the spinal column this makes it difficult to separate the vertebral bodies and arches from adjacent ligamentous and disk structures on T1 images (see Fig. 9-14). With age there are relative increases in the fatty yellow marrow content that result in increased T1 intensity (see Fig. 9-15). This allows better separation of the cancellous or marrow portions of the bony column from the cortical portions and from the ligaments and disks, although chemical shift artifacts become more apparent. The red bone marrow contains 40% water, 20% protein, 40% fat, and is highly vascularized. Yellow bone marrow contains 15% water, 5% protein, 80% fat, and is much less vascularized.[25] Red to yellow bone marrow conversion

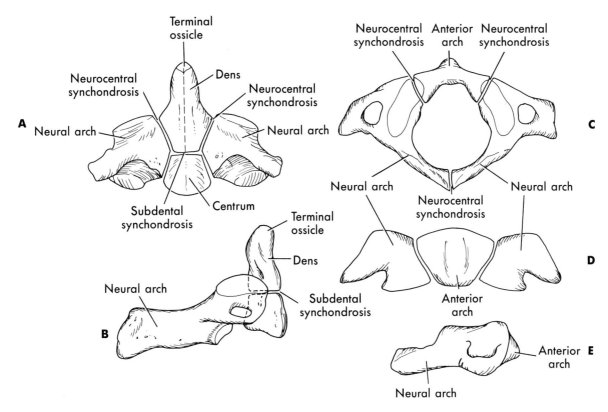

Fig. 9-5   Developmental components of the atlas and axis. **A,** Axis front view. **B,** Axis side view. **C,** Atlas top view. **D,** Atlas front view. **E,** Atlas side view. (From Gehweiler J, et al: *Radiology of vertebral trauma,* Philadelphia, 1980, WB Saunders.)

occurs with age and proceeds in an orderly, although not uniform, manner from the peripheral to the axial skeleton.[19,25] The adult pattern emerges primarily in the second decade and is complete by the twenty-fifth year. In the cranial base and vault of the infant (younger than 1 year of age), the bone marrow spaces usually appear T1 isointense to hypointense. Up to about 7 years a patchy T1 isointense to hypointense appearance occurs. From then until about 15 years a more uniform T1 hyperintense appearance is expected. The infant spinal marrow appears T1 isointense to hypointense (and T2 isointense) relative to muscle, whereas in the juvenile and adolescent, the spinal marrow often appears T1 isointense to hyperintense (and T2 isointense to hypointense) relative to muscle.[19] Diffuse isointensity to hypointensity on T1 images, particularly of the clivus and vertebral bodies, in the juvenile or adolescent may indicate bone marrow disease, that is, a hematopoietic disorder or a neoplastic process (see Chapter 10).

CRANIOCERVICAL JUNCTION

The craniocervical junction is embryologically, anatomically, and functionally a single unit with the primary purpose of providing support for and movement of the head upon the body (Figs. 9-5 to 9-10). The unit consists of the occipital bone, the atlas (C1) and the axis (C2), as well as the ligaments of the atlantooccipital and atlantoaxial articulations.* Rotation of the head primarily occurs at the atlantoaxial articulation, whereas flexion, extension, and lateral bending take place primarily at the atlantooccipital articulation. Components of the craniocervical junction are derivatives of the primitive mesenchyme of the last occipital sclerotome, or proatlas, and the first three cervical sclerotomes.[10,20,26] The skull base develops around the notochord, as does the spine, following the basic processes of segmentation, formation, chondrification, and then ossification. The cranial base is defined as the bony structure surrounding the foramen magnum and includes the basisphenoid and occipital bones[26] (Fig. 9-7). The occipital bone is composed of the basiocciput, the exocciput, and the occipital squamosa, which are separated from each other by cartilaginous synchondroses. The clivus is derived from the basiocciput. The lateral margins of the foramen magnum, the occipital condyles, and the hypoglossal canals develop from the paired exoccipital bones. The supraoccipital and interparietal calvaria arise from the squamosa. The basiocciput and exocciput undergo enchondral ossification; the squamosa undergoes membranous ossification, as does the remainder of the cranial vault. The sphenooccipital syn-

---

*References 3, 6, 10, 13, 23, 24, 26.

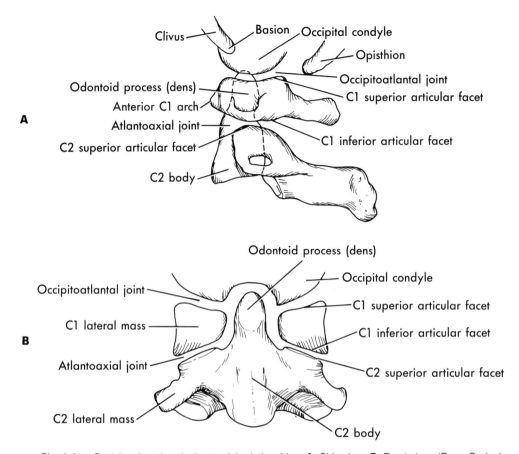

Fig. 9-6   Occipitoatlantal and atlantoaxial relationships. **A,** Side view. **B,** Front view. (From Gerlock A, et al: *The cervical spine in trauma,* Philadelphia, 1978, WB Saunders.)

chondrosis is an important landmark visible throughout childhood and ossifies between 16 and 20 years of age (Figs. 9-7 and 9-8).

The basioccipital and exoccipital portions of the occipital bone, their respective synchondroses, the lateral masses and posterior arch of the atlas, and the apex of the odontoid (ossiculum terminale) are derived from assimilation of the fourth occipital sclerotome, with contributions from the first and second cervical sclerotomes.[10] The anterior arch of the atlas arises as the only example of persistence of the embryonic vertebral hypochordal bow. The body of the odontoid originates from the first cervical sclerotome, and the body of the axis arises from the second and third cervical sclerotomes. Pathological processes occurring in this region may affect any or all of the components anatomically and functionally. Common disorders of segmentation, formation, assimilation, or enchondral ossification include, respectively, occipitalization of the atlas, odontoid hypoplasia with os odontoideum, and basilar impression.[10,23,26]

At birth, the occiput is ossified along with the lateral masses and posterior arch of the atlas. The anterior arch of the atlas may not be ossified at birth but is identifiable in most infants before 1 year. It unites with the lateral masses by 3 years.[10,20] The posterior arch centers ossify in the midline by 5 to 6 years. The body of the dens ossifies from two paramedian centers that are visible and fused at birth. Incomplete fusion is common as a sagittal lucent cleft visible until closure between 1 and 2 years. Subsequently it appears as a sagittally sclerotic line. The ossiculum terminale is the ossification center of the dens tip. It begins ossifying as early as 1 year, may also have a sagittally cleft appearance, and continues to ossify until approximately 3 years of age. The ossified dens tip unites with the body between 8 and 12 years and rarely persists as a normally separate ossicle.

The subdental synchondrosis is the cartilaginous growth plate between the body of the odontoid and the body of the axis and lies below the plane of the superior articular facets of the axis. The synchondrosis is normally a thin lucency at birth, which then ossifies with fusion of the dens body to the axis body between 4 and 6 years of age (Fig. 9-8). The cartilaginous neurocentral synchondroses between the ossified bodies, lateral masses, and posterior arches ossify with fusion by 6 years of age (Fig. 9-9). In early infancy, on open-mouth views, the lateral masses of the atlas often appear larger and laterally offset relative to the lateral masses of the axis. This pseudoJefferson fracture appear-

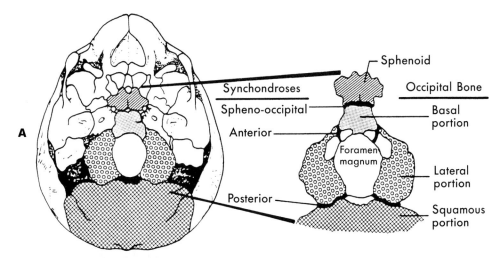

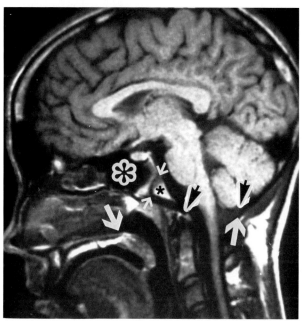

Fig. 9-7 Cranial base development and anatomy. **A,** The sphenoid and occipital bones plus synchondroses. **B,** Sagittal T1 MRI showing the pneumatized sphenoid body *(large asterisk),* sphenooccipital synchondrosis *(small white arrows),* clivus *(small asterisk),* and occipital squamosa *(large posterior white arrow).* McGregor's line extends from the hard palate *(anterior large white arrow)* to the occipital floor *(large posterior white arrow),* whereas McRae's line extends from the basion *(anterior black arrow)* to the opisthion *(posterior black arrow).* (Modified from Wald S, McLaurin R: Anomalies of the craniocervical junction. In McLaurin R, et al, editors: *Pediatric neurosurgery,* ed 2, Philadelphia, 1989, WB Saunders.)

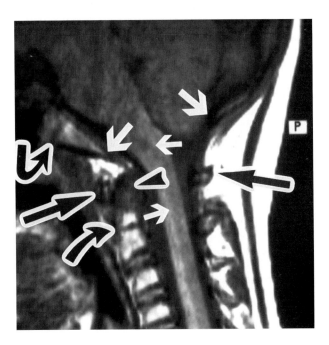

Fig. 9-8 Sagittal T1 MRI of the craniocervical junction and cervical spine showing the relationships of the basion *(anterior large white arrow),* dens *(black arrowhead),* anterior atlas arch *(anterior straight black arrow),* posterior atlas arch *(posterior straight black arrow),* opisthion *(posterior large white arrow),* subdental synchondrosis *(lower curved black arrow),* sphenooccipital synchondrosis *(upper curved black arrow),* medulla *(upper small white arrow),* and spinal cord *(lower small white arrow).*

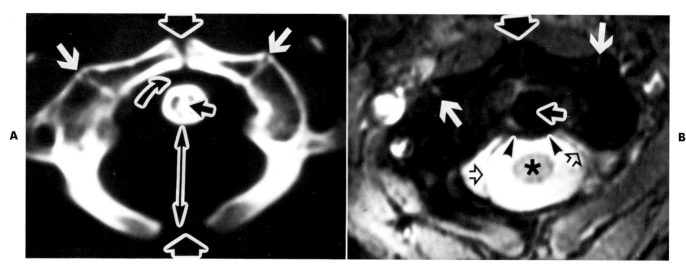

Fig. 9-9   Axial CT **(A)** and axial gradient echo MRI **(B)** at the level of the atlas and odontoid in a juvenile male showing the neurocentral synchondroses *(large white arrows)*, bifid anterior C1 arch *(large upper black arrow)*, preossified posterior arch junction *(large posterior black arrow)*, sclerotic sagittal fusion line of the dens *(small black arrow)*, transverse ligament *(black arrowheads)*, predental space *(curved black arrow)*, postdental dimension *(double black arrow)*. The dura *(outline black arrow)* and spinal cord *(asterisk)* stand out against the epidural venous and CSF high intensities **(B)**.

ance represents a normal variant and is related to the relatively faster growth of the atlas and skull base, which are of common embryologic origin, as compared with that of the axis, which is of similar origin and growth rate to the remainder of the cervical spine[24] (see Chapter 10).

The ligaments around the craniocervical junction (Fig. 9-10) are responsible for stabilizing the most unstable part of the axial skeleton.[6] The important intraspinal ligaments include the tectorial membrane, the apical ligament, the transverse and vertical portions of the cruciate ligament, the accessory atlantoaxial ligaments, and the alar ligaments. The tectorial membrane is a continuation of the posterior longitudinal ligament along the posterior dens to the clivus. The apical ligament extends from the dens tip to the clivus tip. The transverse cruciate ligament lies retrodentally and extends between the lateral masses of the atlas; the vertical cruciate ligament connects the dens body to the occiput. The paired accessory atlantoaxial ligaments attach the axis body to the lateral masses of C1. The paired alar ligaments extend from the dens apex to the inferomedial aspects of the occipital condyles. Important extraspinal ligaments are the anterior atlantooccipital ligament, which is continuous with the anterior longitudinal ligament, and the posterior atlantooccipital ligament, which is analogous to the ligamentum flavum. The apical and extraspinal ligaments primarily limit flexion and extension, whereas the alar ligaments limit lateral bending.

Although a number of landmarks may be used to assist in establishing normal or abnormal relationships at the craniocervical junction, there are two landmarks that are often the most practical (Fig. 9-7).[26] *McGregors's line* is drawn

from the posterior hard palate to the lowest point of the occiput. The dens tip is normally not more than 4.5 mm above this line, with greater than 7 mm being definitely abnormal. Although there is often wide variation, this may be the best landmark for screening, since it is readily identifiable and reproducible on lateral plain films. *McRae's line* defines the plane of the foramen magnum. The dens tip should always lie below this line. When the dens tip approaches this line, there is good correlation with symptomatology. Therefore this may be the most accurate guide in clinical assessment of craniocervical abnormalities.

In infants and young children the anterior atlas-dens interval (predental space) varies from 3 to 5 mm maximum in flexion, with approximately 2 mm excursion from extension to flexion (Figs. 9-6, 9-8, and 9-9). This interval represents a combination of incomplete ossification of the dens and normal peridental ligamentous laxity.[10,24] In adolescence and adulthood the interval is normally less than 3 mm. Primary stability of the atlantoaxial articulation is provided by the transverse cruciate ligament, and secondary stability is provided by the alar and apical odontoid ligaments. The critical dimension is the postdental space, that is, the distance from the posterior dens to the posterior arch of the atlas, or to the posterior margin of the foramen magnum, which normally is at least 15 mm in children and 19 mm in adults[10] (Figs. 9-6, 9-8, and 9-9). One may use the Steel rule of thirds regarding the area of the spinal canal at the C1 level (Fig. 9-9). The area is composed of one third dens, one third cord, and one third safe zone. The retrodental safe zone between the dens anteriorly and cord posteriorly approximates the transverse diameter of the dens

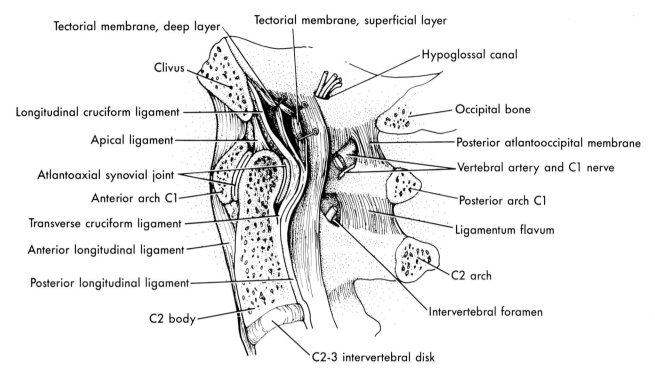

Fig. 9-10   Ligamentous structures of the craniocervical junction. (Modified from Gehweiler J, et al: *Radiology of vertebral trauma,* Philadelphia, 1980, WB Saunders.)

and is protected as a last resort by the alar and apical ligaments.[13] As a practical measure the ratios may be applied to the lateral or sagittal planes using the anteroposterior dens dimension (Fig. 9-8). The dens tip should align with the tip of the clivus, that is, the anterior margin of the foramen magnum (basion), in all positions (Figs. 9-6 and 9-8). The dens tip and clival tip should never be separated craniocaudally more than 1 cm. The posterior arch of the atlas and posterior margin of the foramen magnum (opisthion) should be aligned in flexion and extension.

Anterior placement (pseudosubluxation) of the bodies of C2 on C3, and C3 on C4, of 3 to 4 mm is commonly normal in the neutral to flexed position and often is accompanied by an apparently wide retropharyngeal space.[24] Normally, however, alignment of the posterior arches (spinolaminal junction lines) at C1, C2, and C3 is maintained even in flexion. The dural sac or spinal cord normally may be visualized on axial CT, especially in the higher cervical segments.[22] Often cervical lordosis is absent in the young child, with uneven angulation of the vertebral bodies. Also, the normal flexion curve is often lacking as compared with that in the adult cervical spine. In extension the anterior arch of the atlas commonly overrides the dens tip. Slight uniform pseudosubluxation of the bodies, or uniform rotation of the facets and spinous processes, over several cervical segments also may be seen normally. The interspinous distance at C1-C2 is normally wide, especially in flexion. All of these variations are seen primarily in infants

and young children up to approximately 8 to 10 years of age, at which time the craniocervical junction and cervical spine reach adult status developmentally.[10,24] Occasionally some of these variations persist into adolescence.

SPINAL NEURAXIS

As mentioned earlier the notochord is derived from the notochordal process at the cephalic end of the primitive streak at about the fifteenth day of gestation[2,15-17] (Fig. 9-1). The notochord dorsally induces the neural plate, which is contiguous with the overlying superficial ectoderm (neuroectoderm). The neural plate differentiates into the neural groove (with lateral neural folds) and the neural crest at 17 days. The neural folds close dorsally to form the neural tube, which becomes the neuroepithelial-lined central nervous system. The neural crest gives rise to the peripheral nervous system. The process of primary dorsal neural tube closure, that is, primary neurulation, is initiated near the craniocervical junction and proceeds cranially and caudally to separate the closing neural tube from the dorsal ectoderm (disjunction), from the surrounding mesoderm, and from the ventral endoderm (Fig. 9-1). The process extends rostrally to the lamina terminalis and closes the anterior neuropore to form the cephalic end of the neural tube (brain and cervicomedullary junction) at about 24 days' gestation. At the same time the process extends caudally to the upper lumbar level and closes the posterior neuropore to form the lower end of the primary neural tube

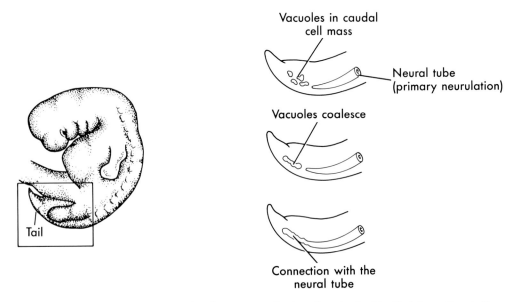

Vacuoles in caudal
cell mass

Neural tube
(primary neurulation)

Vacuoles coalesce

Connection with the
neural tube

Tail

Fig. 9-11   Caudal neural tube development-canalization. (see text). (Modified from French B: Abnormal development of the CNS. In McLaurin R, et al, editors: *Pediatric neurosurgery,* ed 2, Philadelphia, 1989, WB Saunders.)

(cervical, thoracic, and upper lumbar cord) at about 27 days.

Beyond the initial 4 or 5 weeks of gestation, as part of secondary neurulation, the primitive caudal cell mass in the embryonic tail fold is formed from fusion of the neuroepithelium with the caudal notochord[2,15] (Fig. 9-11). The caudal cell mass is the multipotential germ layer precursor for caudal neuroectodermal development (skin and caudal neural tube), caudal mesodermal development (lumbar and sacrococcygeal spinal column, dura, and paraspinal mesenchymal tissues), as well as caudal endodermal development (anorectal and urogenital structures). From 4 to 7 weeks the vacuoles and cells of the caudal cell mass coalesce (canalization) to form the neuroepithelial-lined caudal or secondary neural tube that joins with the primary neural tube above. From about 7 weeks on there is progressive reduction (retrogressive differentiation) of the cell mass and the caudal tube lumen to form the distal portion of the conus medullaris (normal termination of the spinal cord) and filum terminale. Also, there is simultaneous reduction or fusion of the caudal spinal column segments to form the coccyx and sacrum. The central canal of the spinal cord, terminal ventricle of the conus medullaris, and filum terminale are all neural tube vestiges. From the fetal period to the postnatal period and until about 2 years of age there is differentially more rapid longitudinal growth of the spinal column, so the conus undergoes relative ascent (Fig. 9-12) to eventually lie above the level of the L2-L3 interspace (conus tip usually at the L1-L2 or mid-L2 level).[12,16,18,28] There is an orderly segmental arrangement of the cauda equina nerve roots and anchoring of the conus medullaris by the filum terminale, which extends from the conus tip to the first coccygeal segment.

The closed neural tube develops into the central nervous system (CNS) (brain and cord); the adjacent neural crest develops into the peripheral nervous system (PNS)[18] (Fig. 9-13). The lumen of the neural tube becomes the ventricular system of the brain and central canal of the spinal cord. The neuroepithelial cells lining the neural tube give rise to all glial and neuronal elements (migration, proliferation, and differentiation), including the ependymal lining of the central canal and the white and gray matter of the cord proper.[4,5] The outer neural tube is enclosed by the primitive meninx (meninges), which is derived from the mesoderm and neural crest. The primitive meninx develops into the pia mater on the cord surface, and the arachnoid. Together these are referred to as the leptomeninges.[18] The outer meningeal layer is known as the dura mater. Within the subarachnoid space of the leptomeninges and central canal of the spinal cord, cerebrospinal fluid (CSF) is produced and circulated. The dura mater is the final barrier separating the CNS from the spinal and paraspinal mesenchymal tissues, as well as from the cutaneous elements dorsally and the visceral elements ventrally. The dural membrane and subarachnoid space extend caudally to terminate at about the S2 to S4 level.

The pial-lined cord terminates at the tip of the conus medullaris, whereas the pial-lined filum terminale extends caudally within the subarachnoid space and penetrates the dural sac termination near S2 to extend extradurally with a dural covering (Figs. 9-12, 9-14 to 9-16). The filum inserts upon the dorsal first coccygeal segment, often with a separate trunk extending dorsally to the skin surface as a dimple over the coccyx. The paired pial-lined anterior and posterior nerve roots emerge from the cord on each side and extend ventrolaterally within the subarachnoid space in the

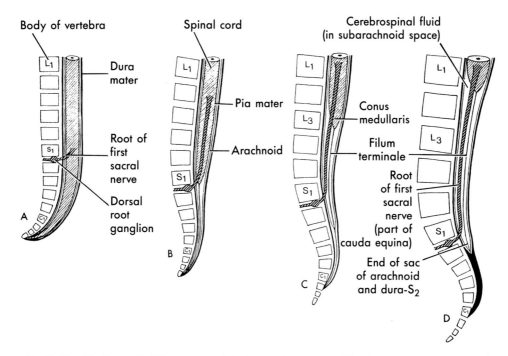

Fig. 9-12   The "ascent" of the conus medullaris at various stages of development. **A,** 8 weeks. **B,** 24 weeks. **C,** Newborn. **D,** 2 years to adulthood. (Modified from Moore K, *The developing human,* ed 4, Philadelphia, 1988, WB Saunders.)

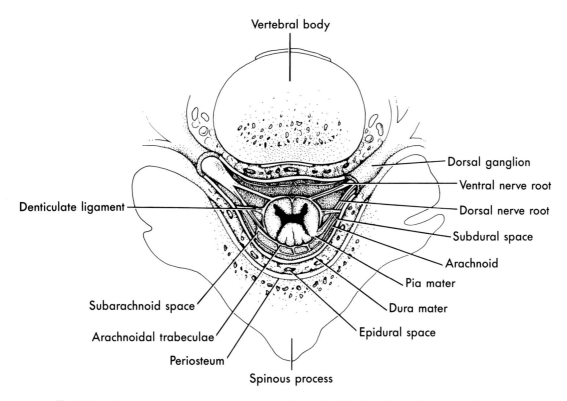

Fig. 9-13   The spinal cord, nerve roots, and meninges. (Modified from Gehweiler J, et al: *Radiology of vertebral trauma,* Philadelphia, 1980, WB Saunders.)

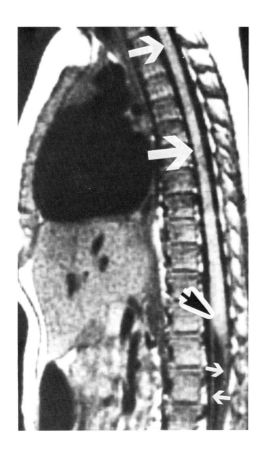

Fig. 9-14   Sagittal T1 MRI of the spine in an infant girl showing the immature spinal column and the difficulty of distinguishing disk spaces from vertebral bodies. Notice the cervical cord *(smaller white arrow)* and lumbar cord *(black arrow)* enlargements relative to the thinner thoracic cord *(larger white arrow)*. Anterior and posterior nerve roots *(very small white arrows)* of the cauda equina are seen in the lumbar region.

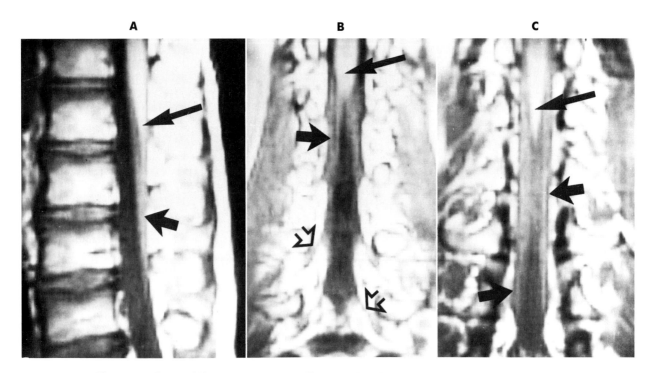

A   B   C

Fig. 9-15   Sagittal **(A)** and coronal **(B** and **C)** lumbar T1 MRI in a juvenile girl showing the conus medullaris *(long arrow)*, cauda equina nerve roots *(short arrows)*, and axillary nerve root sleeves *(open arrows)*. (From Barnes P, et al: *AJNR* 7:465, 1986).

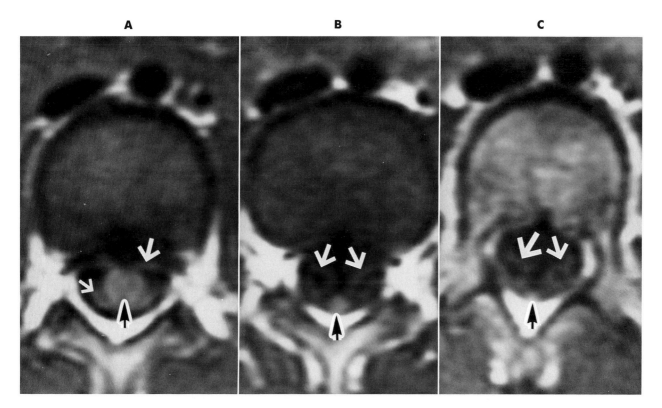

Fig. 9-16   Axial T1 MRI at the level of the caudal spinal cord **(A)**, conus medullaris tip **(B)**, and just below the conus **(C)** demonstrating the relationships of the cord *(black arrow,* **A** and **B)**, anterior nerve roots *(large white arrows)*, posterior nerve roots *(small white arrow)*, and the filum terminale *(black arrow,* **C)**.

direction of their respective intervertebral foramina. Beyond the dorsal root ganglia the nerve roots join to form the spinal nerves. The cauda equina nerve roots emerging from above the conus extend caudally and obliquely within the lumbosacral subarachnoid space to their respective intervertebral foramina according to the original levels of caudal neural tube formation before retrogressive differentiation and relative conus ascent.

Components of the PNS derived from the embryonic neural crest include the cranial, spinal, and visceral nerves plus the cranial, spinal, and autonomic ganglia, the paraganglia or chromaffin tissues (adrenal medulla, carotid body, and the like), and the Schwann cells and melanocytes.[18] Myelination of the nervous system begins in the fetus and continues into the postnatal period. Myelin is produced by Schwann cells and initially deposited in the distal portions of the PNS. The process continues proximally toward the spinal cord. Myelination of the spinal cord then proceeds in a caudocephalic direction within the white matter, the myelin produced by the oligodendrocytes, similar to the process taking place later in the brain. At term the PNS and spinal cord to the level of the brain stem are fully myelinated.[16,17]

The vast majority of developmental malformations of the spinal neuraxis (that is, myelodysplasias) result from disorders of neurulation and are referred to as dysraphic myelodysplasias. These disorders usually involve faulty closure of the neural tube or faulty dural separation (disjunction) of the neural tube from the integument, surrounding mesenchyme, or underlying viscera.[2]

The size and shape of the spinal canal, dural sac, and shape and position of the cord vary from level to level and also with age, although symmetry is normally maintained throughout[22,27] (Figs. 9-8, 9-9, 9-13 to 9-16). At the craniocervical junction the foramen magnum and dural sac are oval in the sagittal direction, whereas the cervicomedullary junction and upper cervical cord are round and centrally placed. In the cervical region in the first 6 postnatal months the dural sac and cord are round; in later infancy and childhood the cervical spinal canal, sac, and cord become more oval in the transverse dimension. The subarachnoid space and epidural space are small relative to the cross-sectional area of the cord in the cervical region. The lower cervical cord has a relatively pseudoexpanded appearance at the levels of origin of the brachial plexus roots. The thoracic spinal canal and sac are oval in childhood, with larger sagittal diameter, whereas the oval lumbar and sacral canal and sac are wider in the transverse dimension. The epidural space, which contains fat, venous elements, and extradural portions of the nerve roots, becomes wider in the thoracic and lumbosacral regions.

At the cervicothoracic junction and at the midthoracic

levels, the centrally placed spinal cord is smaller than it is in the cervical region, but it remains oval in the infant.[22] With normally increasing thoracic kyphosis, the spinal cord becomes more anteriorly positioned but remains midline. In the thoracic and upper lumbar spine the subarachnoid space is large relative to the cord. At the lower thoracic and upper lumbar level, the cord again appears enlarged at and just above the conus medullaris, the cone-shaped termination of the cord (Fig. 9-14). This is the level of origin of the large anterior and posterior nerve roots of the lumbar and sacral plexus and of the large anterior and posterior spinal arteries. Both the cervical and lumbar cord enlargements may be particularly striking in infancy, giving the false impression of expansion (Fig. 9-14).

In the older child and adolescent the transition from distal cord to conus medullaris is often more sharply defined than in the younger child or infant. Below the level of the conus the filum terminale and cauda equina nerve roots occupy the mid and posterior dural sac as a V-shaped formation on axial supine cross sections, the sacral roots arranged medially and the lumbar roots situated more laterally[8] (Figs. 9-15 and 9-16). The filum remains midline and dorsally positioned, with a diameter of less than 2 mm at the L5-S1 level. In the infant and young child the conus medullaris is centrally located within the dural sac. With normally increasing lordosis, the conus, filum, and caudae roots are often closely applied to the posterior dural sac. This may occasionally cause difficulty in separating the conus tip from adjacent caudae elements on sagittal MRI and give the false impression of a low-placed or tethered cord. This can usually be clarified with additional coronal or axial sections. The larger nerve roots within the subarachnoid space of the lumbar and cervical regions are often better visualized than at the thoracic levels. With age the entire central spinal canal becomes more triangular with the triangle apex posteriorly directed.[22]

REFERENCES
Developmental aspects of the spine and spinal neuraxis

1. Aguila LA, Piraino DW, Modic MT, et al: The intranuclear cleft of the intervertebral disk: magnetic resonance imaging, *Radiology* 155:155, 1985.
2. Barkovich A, Naidich T: Congenital anomalies of the spine. In Barkovich A: *Pediatric neuroimaging,* New York, 1990, Raven.
3. Calvy T, Segall H, Gilles F, et al: CT anatomy of the craniovertebral junction in infants and children, *AJNR* 8:489, 1987.
4. Curtin AJ, Chakeres DW, Bulas R, et al: MR imaging artifacts of the axial internal anatomy of the cervical spinal cord, *AJR* 152:835, 1989.
5. Czervionke LF, Daniels DL, Ho PSP, et al: The MR appearance of gray and white matter in the cervical spinal cord, *AJNR* 9:557, 1988.
6. Daniels, D, Williams A, Haughton V: CT of the articulations and ligaments at the occipitoatlantal region, *Radiology* 146:709, 1983.
7. Gilsanz V, Gibbens DT, Roe TF, et al: Vertebral bone density in children: effect of puberty, *Radiology* 166:847, 1988.
8. Grogan JP, Daniels DL, Williams AL, et al: The normal conus medullaris: CT criteria for recognition, *Radiology* 151:661, 1984.
9. Hajek PC, Baker LL, Goobar JE, et al: Focal fat deposition in axial bone marrow: MR characteristics, *Radiology* 162:245, 1987.
10. Harwood-Nash D: Anomalies of the craniovertebral junction, In Hoffman H, Epstin F, editors: *Disorders of the developing nervous system,* Boston, 1986, Blackwell.
11. Harwood-Nash D, Fitz C: *Neuroradiology in infants and children,* St Louis, 1976, Mosby–Year Book.
12. Hawass ND, El-Badawi MG, Fatani JA, et al: Myelographic study of the spinal cord ascent during fetal development, *AJNR* 8:691, 1987.
13. Hensinger R, Fielding J: The cervical spine. In Morrissy R, editor: *Lovell and Winter's pediatric orthopaedics,* ed 3, Philadelphia, 1990, JB Lippincott.
14. Ho PSP, Yu S, Sether LA, et al: Progressive and regressive changes in the nucleus pulposus. Part I, *Radiology* 169:87, 1988.
15. Lemire R, Siebert J, Warkany J: Normal development of the CNS. In McLaurin R, Schut L, Venes J, et al, editors: *Pediatric neurosurgery,* ed 2, Philadelphia, 1989, WB Saunders.
16. Lemire R, Warkany J: Embryology of the CNS: Part 1. IN Hoffman H, Epstein F, editors: *Disorders of the developing nervous system,* Boston, 1986, Blackwell.
17. Monajati A, Wayne WS, Rauschning W, et al: MR of the cauda equina, *AJNR* 8:893, 1987.
18. Moore K: *The developing human: clinically oriented embryology,* ed 4, Philadelphia, 1988, WB Saunders.
19. Moore S, Sebag G: Primary disorders of bone marrow. In Cohen M, Edwards M, editors: *MR imaging of children,* Philadelphia, 1990, BC Decker.
20. O'Rahilly R, Benson D: The development of the vertebral column. In Bradford D, Hensinger R, editors: *The pediatric spine,* New York, 1985, Theime.
21. Patel NP, Kumar R, Kinkhabwala M, et al: Radiology of lumbar vertebral pedicles: variants, anomalies, and pathologic conditions, *Radiographics* 7:101, 1987.
22. Petterson H, Harwood-Nash D: *CT and myelography of the spine and cord,* New York, 1982, Springer-Verlag.
23. Shapiro R, Robinson F: Anomalies of the craniovertebral border, *AJR* 127:281, 1976.
24. Swischuk L: *Emergency radiology of the acutely ill or injured child,* ed 2, Baltimore, 1986, Williams & Wilkins.
25. Vogler J, Murphy W: Bone marrow imaging: state of the art, *Radiology* 168:679, 1988.
26. Wald S, McLaurin R: Anomalies of the craniocervical junction. In McLaurin R, Schut L, Venes J, editors: *Pediatric neurosurgery,* ed 2, Philadelphia, 1989, WB Saunders.
27. Walker HS, Dietrich RB, Flannigan B, et al: Magnetic resonance imaging of the pediatric spine, *Radiographics* 7:1129, 1987.
28. Wilson DA, Prince JR: MR imaging determination of the location of the normal conus medullaris throughout childhood, *AJR* 152:1029, 1989.
29. Yu S, Haughton VM, Ho PSP, et al: Progressive and regressive changes in the nucleus pulposus. Part II, *Radiology* 169:93, 1988.

Dysraphic myelodysplasias

Approximately 2% of newborns have major congenital anomalies, nearly 60% of which involve the CNS. Dysraphic myelodysplasias are a spectrum of spinal neural tube malformations that as a group are among the most common of all CNS defects.* Early diagnosis and treatment are of critical importance to prevent progressive and irreversible neurological deficit.[6,56] *Spinal dysraphism* refers to the entire range of spinal column and neuraxis anomalies resulting from failure of primary or secondary neurulation.[21,31,33,50] The range includes defective midline closure and separation of neural, meningeal, bony, muscular, connective tissue, cutaneous, or visceral structures, with subsequent externalization or tethering of neural elements or persistence of neurenteric connections.

Spina bifida refers to defective vertebral or neural arch bony development and particularly to the characteristic

---

*References 1, 4, 7, 8, 12, 57.

```
PRIMARY NEURULATION DEFECTS

Craniorachischisis totalis
Myeloschisis
Myelocele
Myelomeningocele
Hemimyelocele
Chiari II malformation
Hydromyelia
```

```
SECONDARY NEURULATION DEFECTS

POSTERIOR DYSRAPHISMS
Lipomyelomeningocele
Dermal sinus
Tight filum terminale
Myelocystocele
Meningocele

ANTERIOR DYSRAPHISMS
Split notochord syndrome
Neurenteric cyst
Anterior meningocele
Diastematomyelia

CAUDAL DYSPLASIA SPECTRUM

DEVELOPMENTAL TUMORS
Lipoma
Dermoid-epidermoid
Teratoma
Hamartoma
Arachnoid cyst
Vascular anomalies
```

spinolaminal deformities.[4] *Spina bifida aperta* or *cystica* refers to the primary or combined (primary and secondary) neurulation defects that are overt or open dorsal myelodysplasias of exposed primitive neural tissue extending through the spina bifida (see box above). *Spina bifida occulta* refers to secondary neurulation defects which are the occult or skin-covered myelodysplasias (see box above, right).

CLINICAL MANIFESTATIONS

The presenting manifestations of dysraphic myelodysplasias may be considered in three categories: (1) direct observation of the superficial component of the dysraphic malformation, (2) associated developmental anomalies, or (3) neurological impairment resulting from the myelodysplasia.[*]

The first group comprises the most common of patient presentations and clinical findings, that is, dorsal cutaneous stigmata. This includes the flat or cystlike, non–skin covered dorsal midline lesions at birth (myelocele or myelomeningocele) as well as the skin-covered lesions that may be discovered at birth or later as dorsal midline subcutaneous lipomas, cutaneous hairy patches (hypertrichosis), hemangiomas, telangiectasias, hyperpigmentation (nevi), and skin dimples, tags, cysts, or sinus tracts. Also included in this category are patients with obvious spinal curvature abnormalities including scoliosis, kyphosis, torticollis, or Klippel-Feil deformity.

The second category includes patients who may have any of the manifestations in the first category but who primarily demonstrate developmental defects of other organ systems. This may include the VATERS association (*v*ertebral anomalies and ventricular septal defect, *a*nal atresia with or without fistula, *t*racheoesophageal fistula with *e*sophageal atresia, *r*adial dysplasias and renal anomalies, and *s*ingle umbilical artery), other anorectal or urogenital anomalies, and the caudal regression syndrome.

Within the third group are patients who may have any of the manifestations of the other two categories but who also initially display urologic, gastrointestinal, or musculoskeletal manifestations of neuropathic origin as related to cord tethering (traction) or compression with resulting neural ischemia.[55,56] The disorders include neurogenic bladder with incontinence, urinary retention, infection, reflux, or hydronephrosis. Anal sphincter dysfunction may occur with

constipation or encopresis. Gait disturbances often occur with limb paresis or atrophy, cavus foot deformity, and sensory or motor deficits.

Two clinical subcategories deserve further emphasis. The first concerns children who, after surgical repair of overt myelodysplasias at birth, subsequently develop one or more neurological syndromes related to associated CNS malformations or to sequelae of early surgical repair (these are discussed in the next section).[27,43] The second group includes children with developmental caudal endodermal syndromes (such as high imperforate anus, anal stenosis or atresia, omphalocele, and cloacal exstrophy) who also have lumbosacral dysgenesis and associated myelodysplasias further complicating the management of their anorectal and urogenital malformations.[13,63] In this group the myelodysplasias may include lipomyelomeningocele, myelocystocele, other tethering syndromes, presacral meningocele, or the caudal regression spectrum, each of which is discussed in upcoming sections.

IMAGING CONSIDERATIONS

Currently used modalities for imaging spinal dysraphism include radiography, ultrasonography, magnetic resonance, myelography, and computed tomography.[6-8,16,45-47] The plain film is the important initial test, since the majority exhibit findings that specifically implicate the dysraphic etiology. Furthermore, the spinal film serves as a guide to further, more definitive imaging. Radiographic findings may be those of congenital scoliosis or kyphosis (Fig. 9-17) including formation anomalies (such as butterfly vertebrae, hemivertebrae, or wedge vertebrae) or segmentation abnormalities (such as block vertebra, pedicle bar, or interlaminar fusion). These types of bony malformations may be associated with underlying myelodysplasia in 15% to 25%

---

[*]References 6, 23, 29, 31, 33, 35, 38, 55.

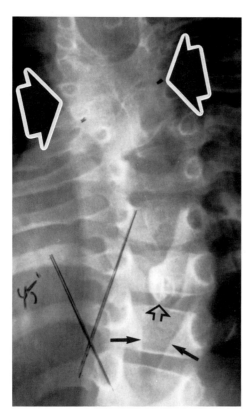

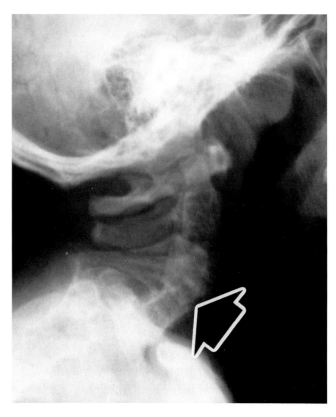

Fig. 9-17   Frontal plain film of thoracic congenital scoliosis with formation-segmentation anomalies *(large black arrows),* dysraphic spinolaminal defects *(small black arrows),* and ossified diastematomyelic peg *(open black arrow).* (From Barnes P: *Contemp Diagn Radiol* 13:1, 1990).

Fig. 9-18   Lateral cervical plain film of Klippel-Feil syndrome with segmentation (fusion) anomalies of the mid and lower cervical spine *(arrow).*

of cases, and usually those of the anterior dysraphic category within the neurenteric continuum or split notochord spectrum. These include diastematomyelia, neurenteric cyst, anterior meningocele, and split notochord syndrome. Klippel-Feil anomaly or syndrome is also included in this category (Fig. 9-18). The hallmark plain film findings of posterior dysraphism (Fig. 9-19) are related to defective spinolaminal development, including widening of the spinal canal with dural ectasia and eversion deformity of the laminae and spinous processes (that is, spina bifida). Associated myelodysplasia is present in more than 90% of cases, the vast majority occurring at the lumbar or lumbosacral level. In dysraphic myelodysplasias, associated scoliosis, kyphosis, or kyphoscoliosis may be congenital due to formation-segmentation anomalies as previously mentioned, or neuropathic due to cord tethering or compression with ischemia, hydromyelia, or myelomalacia (cord atrophy).

Ultrasonography (US) has become an effective modality for screening the fetus, young infant, or any patient with a spinal bony defect that provides an acoustic window (spina bifida, laminectomy).* US is particularly useful to docu-

*References 20, 34, 40, 42, 49, 53, 68.

ment normal conus level in infants with low-yield presentations (for example, sacral dimple only), or when there are equivocal plain film findings (Fig. 9-20). US also may be useful intraoperatively and for postoperative follow-up.

CT without CSF contrast enhancement may also be useful to detect bony dysraphic defects in questionable cases.[6,22] MRI is now the ideal modality for definitive spinal cord imaging in spinal dysraphism.[1,6,7,12,50] MRI is the first choice especially for higher-yield clinical presentations such as dorsal cutaneous stigmata with dysraphic plain film abnormalities, neurogenic bladder or bowel dysfunction, or limb deformity. Myelographic CT may no longer be necessary for assessing the subarachnoid space to delineate nerve root anatomy or filar thickening. Nonmyelographic CT may be helpful for bony canal morphology not clearly delineated by MRI or to confirm or further delineate calcific or bony elements, including ossific septation in diastematomyelia (see Fig. 9-51).

T1-weighted (short TR/short TE) MRI usually provides optimal visualization of anatomy starting with sagittal images for screening and localization.[6] Occasionally, additional coronal or axial T1 sections are needed to establish normal conus medullaris morphology and level by separating the conus tip from cauda equina nerve roots, especially

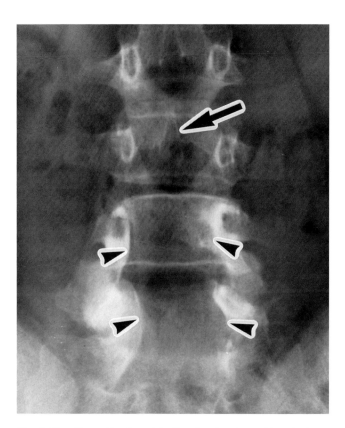

Fig. 9-19   Frontal lumbar plain film showing dysraphic spinolaminal defects *(arrowheads)* at L4, L5, and S1. The last intact neural arch (spinous process) is at L3 *(arrow)*. (From Barnes P: *Contemp Diagn Radiol* 13:1, 1990).

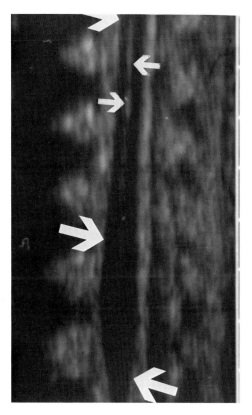

Fig. 9-20   Midsagittal sonogram of the lower back demonstrating the normally sonolucent spinal cord *(large arrows)* and conus medullaris *(bottom arrow)* with normal central echogenicity *(small arrows)*.

when exaggerated lumbar lordosis produces dorsal bowstringing of the conus-caudae elements (Fig. 9-16). Three planes are often required for complete evaluation of the myelodysplasia in anticipation of surgery. Additional axial sections are especially important for precise delineation of conus or placode and nerve root elements as related to bony and dural landmarks, as well as for associated mass lesions or septation in diastematomyelia (see Figs. 9-31 and 9-46). Two or more planes are often important for evaluating myelodysplasias complicated by severe spinal curvature deformity.

Occasionally, proton density (long TR/short TE) and T2 (long TR/long TE) images provide additional tissue characterization if needed to evaluate fatty, CSF, vascular, or mineralizing components. Axial T2 spin echo or T2/T2* gradient echo techniques provide myelography-like CSF enhancement that is particularly important in delineating diastematomyelic septation. Axial T1 or proton density/T2 sections may be necessary at the level of the dorsal cutaneous abnormality (for example, dimple) to evaluate for dermal sinus/stalk extent or communication and associated intraspinal dermoid or epidermoid cyst (see Fig. 9-34). T1 sagittal and coronal acquisitions may be needed for longitudinal screening of the remaining neuraxis for extent

of cord splitting in diastematomyelia or associated hydrosyringomyelia (see Figs. 9-23, 9-26, and 9-46). Thorough neuroimaging evaluation is important preoperatively, since newer microsurgical and electrophysiological monitoring techniques allow for safer, more precise, and more complete repair.

PRIMARY NEURULATION DEFECTS

Dysraphic myelodysplasias resulting from disorders of primary neurulation, that is, dorsal neural tube closure defects within the first 3 to 4 weeks of gestation,[4,6,20,29,65] are listed in the box on p. 345. In actuality, these may often represent combined primary and secondary neurulation disorders, since the myelodysplasias often occur or extend beyond the lower level of primary neural tube closure. Furthermore, it is logical to infer that faulty secondary closure may follow faulty primary closure. The most severe of the primary neural tube defects are craniorachischisis and myeloschisis. These result from complete failure of anterior and posterior neuropore closure in the former and failure of posterior neuropore closure in the latter. Long segments of open or externalized and exposed neural plaque (no meningeal or skin covering) are evident. These very rare malformations are incompatible with extrauterine life.

Myelocele and myelomeningocele

The most common defect of primary neurulation compatible with life is the myelocele or myelomeningocele, the classic "spina bifida" malformation[4,6] (Fig. 9-21). This is usually a more localized segment of incomplete neural tube closure at the lumbar, sacral, or, less frequently, thoracic level. The basic defect is a dorsally open neural tube; this plaque, referred to as the placode, is composed of primitive neural epithelium without meningeal, bony, or skin covering. Often there is a thin mesenchymal membranous covering. The primitive groove along the midline of the placode is continuous with the central canal of the spinal cord (closed neural tube) above which expresses CSF over the dorsal placode surface. The neural placode merges with the surrounding skin at its margins. The dorsal placode actually represents the everted, exposed interior of the neural tube, that is, the would-be ependymal-lined central canal. The ventral aspect is the intended pial-lined surface of the would-be spinal cord. Underlying the placode is the dural sac with the CSF-containing leptomeninges. The dural covering merges with the placode margins at the periphery along the placode-cutaneous interface.

Ventrolateral to the dural sac is the adipose- and venous-containing epidural space and in turn the often wide and flat vertebral bodies with everted dysplastic pedicles and laminae. The spinal canal is often large, the spinous processes are absent, and the paraspinal musculature markedly attenuated. The deformity may be further complicated by congenital or neuromuscular kyphoscoliosis (Fig. 9-22). The size of the dorsal myelocele or myelomeningocele (sac) at birth is usually related to the volume of ventrally collected CSF (Fig. 9-21). Most of the lesions are level with the skin surface, that is, myelocele, whereas others are elevated due to CSF expansion of the ventral dural sac, that is, myelomeningocele. Occasionally the placode appears disorganized due to intrauterine degeneration. The ventral pial-lined placode is composed of subpial gray and white matter with ventral nerve roots emerging ventromedially and the would-be dorsal nerve roots emerging ventrolaterally. The nerve roots traverse the ventral subarachnoid space often in a horizontal or even cephalad direction to reach their respective foramina.

Since the "surgical" neuroanatomy of the myelocele or myelomeningocele is predictable, neuroimaging is not ordinarily done before closure.[29] Early closure is critical to prevent infection and further neurological deterioration. Reconstruction and central suspension of the neural tube within the circumferentially closed and skin-covered dural sac have been recommended to minimize scarring and retethering of the neural elements. In hemimyelocele, or

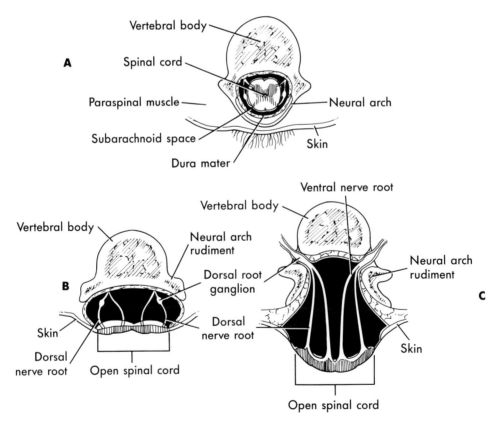

Fig. 9-21   Basic types of spinal bifida cystica. **A,** Normally neurulated cord within the intact dural sac and bony spinal canal. **B,** Myelocele with exposed, nonneurulated cord or placode through the defective dura, bony neural arches, and skin. **C,** myelomeningocele with distention of the ventral dural sac and elevation of the exposed placode.

hemimyelomeningocele, there is a myelocele or myelo-meningocele with associated diastematomyelia, that is, longitudinal splitting of the cord-placode into two hemicords or hemiplacodes.[4] There may be an intervening septum of bony or other tissue. The split may occur at, above, or below the myelocele or myelomeningocele. The lesion may involve one or both hemicords, and the involvement may occur at different levels, giving asymmetrical neurological findings.

Associated malformations of the CNS occur in some form or degree in every patient with spina bifida aperta and include Chiari II malformation, hydrocephalus, and hydromyelia[4,6,29,43,67] (Fig. 9-23). (Chiari II malformation and associated cerebral dysgenesis are discussed in detail in Chapter 3.) Obstructive hydrocephalus and hydromyelia related to Chiari II occur in most patients. Hydrocephalus, hydromyelia, or both may be present before surgical closure of the myelocele or myelomeningocele. Commonly the hydrocephalus or hydromyelia become evident only after surgical repair and closure of the CSF outlet (for example, terminal ventricle) at the level of the myelocele or myelomeningocele. Ventricular shunting is required in a high percentage of patients with ventriculomegaly, although the latter may primarily or additionally result from the cerebral dysgenesis associated with Chiari II malformation. Surgical diversion of the ventricular system for hydrocephalus often provides decompression of the hydromyelia. It is the early closure of the myelocele and the early manage-

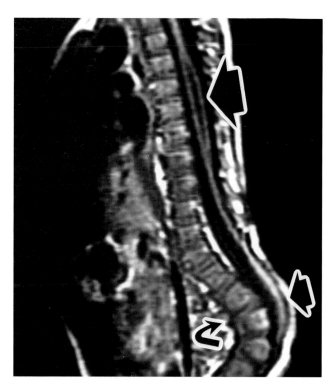

Fig. 9-22   Lumbar myelomeningocele after surgical repair with sagittal T1 MRI demonstration of lumbar kyphosis *(curved arrow)*, placode *(small arrow)*, and segmental thoracic hydromyelia *(large arrow)*.

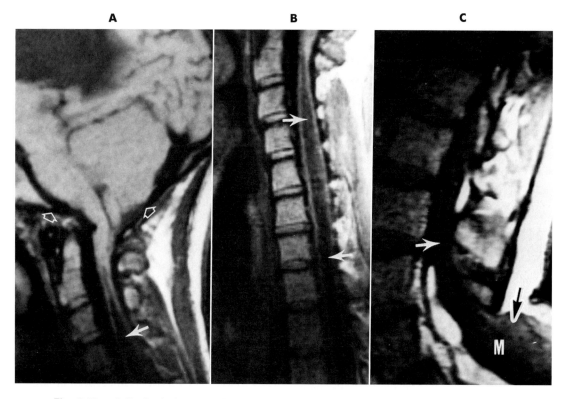

Fig. 9-23   A-C, Sagittal craniospinal T1 MRI in an adolescent male years after lumbosacral myelomeningocele repair with Chiari II malformation *(open arrows)*, hydrocephalus, and expanding hydromyelia *(white arrows)* extending to the level of the dorsal lumbosacral placode *(black arrow)* and meningocele *(M)*.

SEQUELAE OR COMPLICATIONS IN SPINA BIFIDA APERTA

Chiari II malformation
Hydromyelia-hydrobulbia
Hydrobulbia
Shunt malfunction
Encysted fourth ventricle
Brain stem/cervical cord compression
Intrinsic brain stem dysfunction
Hemimyelocele, hemimyelomeningocele
Developmental tumor
Cord ischemia (infarction, myelomalacia)
Progressive kyphoscoliosis
Scarring/retethering at operative site
Dural sac stenosis
Implant dermoid/epidermoid

---

ment of the hydrocephalus and hydromyelia, along with the prevention or early treatment of infection, that has allowed increased survival of these children.[43] The expected outcome of early intervention is therefore the stabilization of existing neurological deficits. Sequelae or complications may be encountered after initial repair, however, that produce changing or progressive neurological symptoms or signs. These are usually related to Chiari II malformation, cord ischemia, or prior surgical intervention[4,6,43] (see box above).

Neurological syndromes associated with the sequelae or complications of spina bifida aperta include increased intracranial pressure related to hydrocephalus or shunt malfunction. Also there may be brain stem, cerebellar, or cervical cord symptoms and signs related to fourth ventricular isolation, brain stem or upper cord compression, intrinsic brain stem dysfunction, or hydromyelia-hydrobulbia. Lower spinal cord level deficits or progressive neuromuscular scoliosis may result from hydromyelia, repair site scarring and retethering, operative site implant epidermoid, dural sac stenosis, cord ischemia with infarction or myelomalacia, previously unrecognized diastematomyelia (hemimyelocele, hemimyelomeningocele), compressive developmental mass (for example, lipoma), or tight filum terminale. Progressive kyphoscoliosis also may be congenital as related to formation-segmentation anomalies.

It is important to remember that any or all of the progressive symptoms or signs, especially those caused by expanding hydromyelia or hydrobulbia, may be directly or indirectly related to ventricular shunt malfunction.[43,54] Therefore cranial imaging is done first to check for changing ventricular size or fourth ventricular encystment. However, direct shunt system testing is indicated, since hydromyelia or other complications of malfunction may occasionally occur in the absence of increasing ventricular size. Fourth ventricular isolation occurs after lateral ventricular shunting, which results in secondary closure of the aqueduct.[4,6,43,67] With preexisting outlet fourth ventricular

obstruction from Chiari II malformation and continued CSF production by intraventricular choroid plexus, there is fourth ventricular expansion with subsequent brain stem compression. The enlarged or dilated fourth ventricle is readily diagnosed with CT (see Chapter 3). Preoperative MRI or intraoperative US may assist in catheter placement for decompression.

Brain stem compression, upper cervical cord compression, or both may occur as a result of foramen magnum or upper cervical canal impaction, upper cervical canal stenosis or constricting dural band, hydromyelia-hydrobulbia, or arachnoid cyst. Cervicooccipital surgical decompression may be necessary. More commonly, the brain stem dysfunction is related to intrinsic nuclear disorganization.[67] MRI readily demonstrates hydromyelia and hydrobulbia and serves as a preoperative guide. US may serve as an intraoperative guide for catheter placement and decompression. The hydromyelia may involve the entire cord length above the myelocele or myelomengingocele or may be confined to a short segment representing isolation of the central canal (Figs. 9-22 and 9-23).

Complications at the placode repair site include scarring of the cord or placode with retethering at the dorsal dural closure site.[4,6,43] Normally after surgery the cord-placode remains low-placed and dorsally or laterally contiguous with the dural surface at the repair site. CSF intensity should be evident surrounding the cord except at the repair site. The cord should follow an undulating course corresponding to the spinal curvatures rather than assuming an abnormally straightened course across the curves. Also, there should be no angulation or kinking of the cord-placode. An abnormally straightened course, angulation, kinking, or a direct cord interface with dural or extradural structures may suggest scarring with retethering.[14] However, the diagnosis of retethering, even with MRI, is often not possible. Retethering is a clinical diagnosis and MRI is primarily indicated to rule out other unexpected findings such as hydromyelia, developmental mass, and diastematomyelia. The absence of cord pulsation by real-time or Doppler ultrasonography or by cardiac-gated MRI has been proposed to support the diagnosis of cord retethering. The lack of positional change on sagittal MRI from supine to prone has also been suggested as a supportive sign.

Other potential complicating factors at the original repair site include dural sac stenosis and implant epidermoid.[4,6,43] Dural sac stenosis may be surgical and confined to the repair level as a localized constrictive deformity. Rarely, there may be preexisting localized or long segment spinal or dural sac stenosis. The implanted epidermoid produces neural compression and may be difficult to directly visualize by MRI except for mass effect, since these often have CSF-like intensity characteristics throughout the sequences (Fig. 9-24). Occasionally, fatty high intensity may be present on TI images. Cord ischemia with infarction, myelomalacia, or syrinx may produce a localized intramedullary water-intensity abnormality or focal cord narrowing. Myelomalacia may more appropriately refer to more extensive atrophy

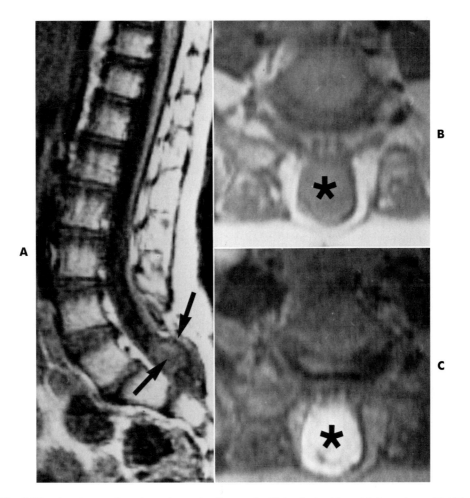

Fig. 9-24 Lumbosacral myelomeningocele after repair with implant epidermoid shown by sagittal T1 MRI **(A)** as an isointense to hypointense mass *(arrows)* at the level of the dorsal placode. **B** and **C,** The epidermoid *(asterisks)* is isointense to hypointense on axial p image **(B)** and isointense to hyperintense on axial T2 image **(C).**

or thinning of the cord over several segments. It may be difficult to differentiate myelomalacia from collapsed hydromyelia.

Hydrosyringomyelia

Hydromyelia is the specific term used for dilatation of the CSF-filled central canal of the spinal cord. *Syringomyelia* is the specific term used to denote cavitation (syrinx) within the cord. The one may not be readily distinguished from the other, however, since syrinx formation may occur secondary to hydromyelia, and syrinx may extend into and dilate the central canal producing secondary hydromyelia.* Therefore the term *hydrosyringomyelia* has been used for any or all of these situations. For the purposes of this discussion, however, *hydromyelia* designates developmental dilatation of the central canal, the so-called communicating type. This implies that the hydromyelic cord is in

continuity with the ventricular system via the obex and fourth ventricle, or is in continuity with the subarachnoid space through the terminal ventricle of the conus medullaris or the filum terminale. Hydromyelia is most commonly associated with Chiari malformations I, II, or III (Figs. 9-22, 9-23, and 9-25) as discussed in Chapter 3. *Syringomyelia,* or *hydrosyringomyelia,* may be the more useful term for describing those nondevelopmental causes including idiopathic, traumatic, degenerative, or neoplastic. In these situations the intramedullary CSF-filled space or spaces have been described as "noncommunicating" except secondarily by way of dissection into the central canal. Also, the fluid of the syrinx or hydrosyrinx may contain additional elements related to the pathological process, such as inflammatory or neoplastic cells, protein, hemorrhage, and so forth.

By far the most common category of hydromyelia or hydrosyringomyelia in childhood is the developmental category associated with Chiari malformations, spinal

*References 3, 10, 36, 48, 51, 61.

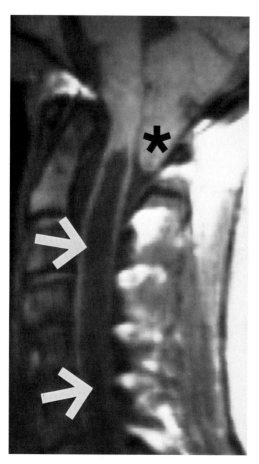

Fig. 9-25 Hydrosyringomyelia associated with Chiari I malformation shown by sagittal T1 MRI with low placed cerebellar tonsils *(asterisk)* and cervicomedullary junction relative to the foramen magnum. Marked intramedullary hypointensity and pulsatile CSF flow signal voids *(arrows)* are demonstrated along with cord expansion.

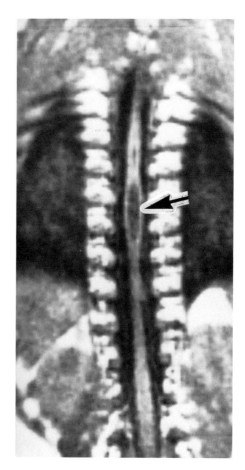

Fig. 9-26 Isolated central canal (hydromyelia) associated with lumbosacral tethered cord shown by coronal T1 MRI as a segmental low intensity cord expansion (arrows).

dysraphism, and craniocervical anomalies.[3,4,7] (Figs. 9-22, 9-23, and 9-26). Probably the most common acquired and nontraumatic cause is intramedullary neoplasm (see Chapter 10). The MRI appearance of hydrosyringomyelia is that of a short or long segment longitudinal intramedullary lesion of CSF intensity that may be thin, tubular, and difficult to distinguish from truncation artifact, or may be wide with sacculations or septations and expand the cord.[10,36,48] Accentuated CSF pulsations within may produce progressive T2 shortening and signal loss throughout the MRI sequences, especially if motion-compensating techniques are not used.[61] This phenomenon is most probably produced by transmitted vascular pulsations. Cord expansion and intramedullary signal void as seen on MRI may correlate with neurological findings indicating the need for decompression.[5,19] On follow-up after surgical intervention, decreased cord expansion and the absence of signal voids may further support clinical signs of response.[5,37,49] If no obvious developmental, traumatic, or inflammatory cause for hydromyelia or hydrosyringomyelia is evident in

childhood, then compressive or expanding neoplasm must be sought. MRI with gadolinium enhancement is the recommended imaging procedure.

Intramedullary gliosis and perimedullary arachnoiditis may be seen with hydrosyringomyelia from trauma or inflammation. The former may produce high intensities on proton density and T2-weighted MRI, whereas the latter may produce perimedullary loculation or nodular abnormality, both of which may mimic neoplasm. Gadolinium enhancement may occur occasionally and not allow differentiation from neoplasm. However, in the absence of trauma and because inflammatory or degenerative CNS processes are extremely rare causes of hydromyelia or hydrosyringomyelia in childhood, gadolinium enhancement becomes an important feature implicating neoplasm as the cause.

SECONDARY NEURULATION DEFECTS

Dysraphic myelodysplasias due to secondary neurulation defects are those occurring after or in spite of dorsal closure

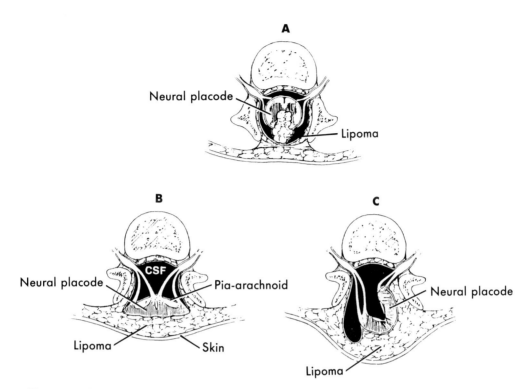

Fig. 9-27   Developmental types of lipomyeloschisis. **A,** Myelolipoma with incompletely neurulated cord and subpial lipoma into the dorsal cleft. **B,** Lipomyelocele with nonneurulated cord or placode continuous dorsally with the subcutaneous fat. **C,** Lipomyelomeningocele with rotated placode, nerve roots, and meningocele relative to the eccentric lipoma. (Modified from Barkovich A: *Pediatric neuroimaging,* New York, 1990, Raven.)

of the anterior and posterior neuropores. These usually result from defective caudal cell mass development (that is, disorders of canalization, retrogressive differentiation, and ascent) or persistence of primitive neurenteric connections.[4,6,7,12] Most are skin-covered malformations (occult dysraphisms) with underlying defects of bony, dural, and neural development, and usually with cord tethering. This category includes the subcategories of posterior dysraphism, anterior dysraphism (anomalies of the neurenteric continuum), the caudal dysplasia spectrum, and developmental tumors (see box on p. 345). Mixed forms containing components of each of the subcategories are often encountered in the same patient.

Lipomyelomeningocele

Lipomyelomeningoceles are probably the commonest of the occult dysraphic myelodysplasias.[4,7,12,14,41] These have also been referred to as lipomyeloschisis, lipomeningoceles, lipomyeloceles, myelolipomas, leptomyelolipomas, and lipomyelodysplasias (Figs. 9-27 to 9-33). There are almost always evident at birth as dorsal lumbosacral subcutaneous lipomas and often are without early neurological deficit. However, virtually all patients develop deficits over time. The basic malformation is similar to that of a myelocele or myelomeningocele, but with an additional lipoma and intact overlying skin. The speculated pathogenesis is that of premature disjunction, or premature separation, of the neural tube from the overlying ectoderm with interposition of mesenchyme before closure of the neural tube. There is subsequent induction of lipomatous tissue with invasion of the incompletely closed neural tube.[41] The caudal spinal cord almost always extends below the expected level for normal conus termination (above L2-3) into the lower lumbar or sacral levels.

At the level of the malformation the cord is usually nonneurulated as a dorsally open placode (plaque, groove, or cleft) that communicates with the central canal above and is adherent to the lipoma behind or below (Fig. 9-27). A dorsal dural defect of variable size is present with a bifid lumbar or sacral spinal canal through which the placode-

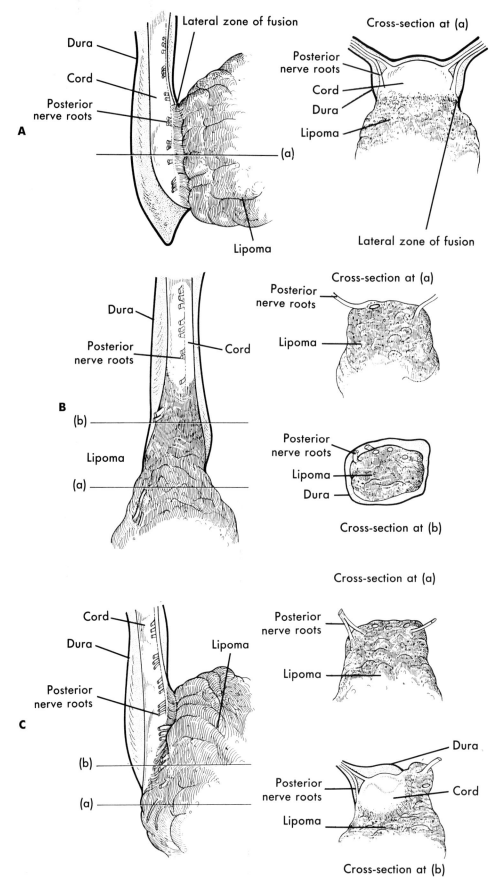

Fig. 9-28 Surgical classification of lipomyeloschisis. **A,** The dorsal lipoma. **B,** The caudal lipoma. **C,** The transitional lipoma. (Modified from Chapman P, Beyerl B: The tethered spinal cord. In Hoffman H, Epstein F, editors: *Disorders of the developing nervous system,* Boston, 1986, Blackwell.)

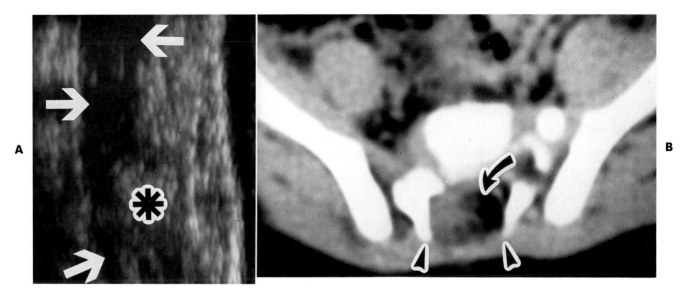

Fig. 9-29 Lumbosacral lipomyeloschisis shown by midsagittal sonogram **(A)** as an echogenic mass *(asterisk)* dorsally applied to the low-placed sonolucent cord-placode *(arrows)*. **B,** Axial CT demonstrates the fatty low intensity of the lipoma *(curved arrow)* and dysraphic bony defects *(arrowheads)*.

lipoma is widely or narrowly continuous with a dorsal subcutaneous lipoma. The lipomas may actually represent mesenchymal hamartomas, often containing multiple mesenchymal and neural elements including fibrous tissue, muscle, cartilage, bone, vascular tissue, epithelial cysts, and dysplastic or aberrant neuroglial tissue. Other theories speculate that the lipomas are malformations resulting from defective formation of the primitive meninges.[4] The lipoma is the primary tethering element, although a short thickened filum may contribute (see Fig. 9-31). Rarely is there an associated dermoid-epidermoid or diastematomyelia. The lipoma (Fig. 9-28) may be adherent to the cord-placode dorsally (dorsal lipoma), caudally (caudal lipoma), or combined (transitional lipoma). The lipoma may be localized or may extend rostrally into the central canal (intramedullary) or may extend dorsally and intradurally or extradurally. Occasionally with a caudal lipomyelomeningocele there may be only a small subcutaneous lipoma, or no lipoma, and instead there may be a cutaneous dimple (see Fig. 9-33). The meningocele manque variation refers to conus or placode attachment by a fibrous or neuroglial band to the dura dorsally with or without an intraspinal lipoma.[29]

As with the myelocele, the margins of the dorsally defective dura fuse circumferentially at the periphery of the placode-lipoma interface and enclose the ventrolateral leptomeninges and subarachnoid space (Figs. 9-27 and 9-28). Also, the dorsal and ventral nerve roots emerge ventrally and traverse the subarachnoid space to their respective foramina. The more laterally situated dorsal root entry zones of the cord-placode lie very near the line or zone of dorsal lipomatous attachment. The anatomy of the placode-lipoma-dural fusion zone and nerve roots is often

predictable, especially for the common dorsal lipoma variant (Fig. 9-28). For the caudal or transitional variants, however, nerve roots may traverse within the ventral or ventrolateral aspect of the lower portions of the lipoma (Figs. 9-28 and 9-30 to 9-33).

The term *lipomyelocele* has been used when the cord-placode-lipoma interface, that is, the *lipomyelo* component, lies entirely within the canal and without expansion of the ventral subarachnoid space (Figs. 9-27, 9-29, and 9-31). The term *lipomyelomeningocele* is applied when the subarachnoid space expands and the lipomyelo component extends to or beyond the posterior canal margin.[4] Often there is associated extension of the dural sac and subarachnoid space (meningocele) beyond the canal as a complex herniation into the dorsal subcutaneous tissues (Figs. 9-27 and 9-30). Also, there may be rotation of the lipomyelomeningocele with the rotated and herniated lipomyelo component eccentrically placed opposite the meningocele component (Figs. 9-27 and 9-32). This often places the cord-placode and nerve roots at the midline between the lipoma on one side and the subarachnoid space on the other in the direct path of the operative approach. The placode, in fact, may be further deformed or thinned by the herniating and intruding subarachnoid space, thus making it difficult to identify by MRI (Fig. 9-27).

Fibrovascular bands are almost always present at the superior and inferior margins of the dural defect at the levels of the first and last widely bifid neural arches.[4,41] These interlaminar bands, particularly at the upper margin, are also points for tethering and kinking of the cord-placode, which may result in ischemic injury. MRI in sagittal and axial planes is critical for surgical planning, particularly to

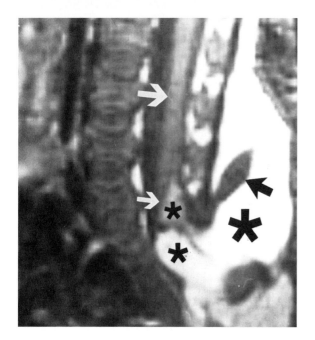

Fig. 9-30   Lumbosacral lipomyeloschisis shown by sagittal T1 MRI with low-placed cord-placode *(white arrows)*, intraspinal transitional lipomatous elements *(smaller asterisks)* in continuity with the subcutaneous fat *(large asterisks)* and the meningocele sac *(black arrow)*. (From Barnes P: *Neurol Clin North Am* 8:741, 1990.)

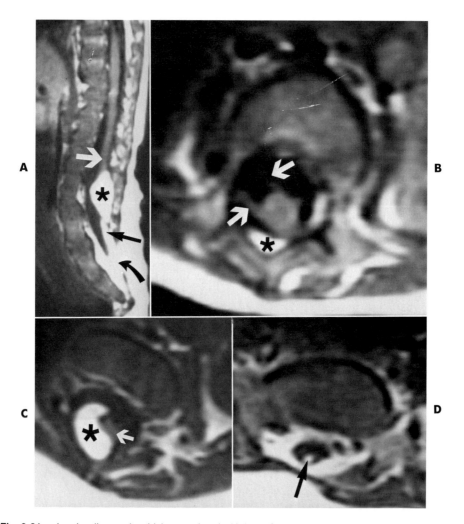

Fig. 9-31   Lumbar lipomyeloschisis associated with imperforate anus complex shown by sagittal **(A)** and axial **(B-D)** TI MRI including the low-placed cord *(white arrow, A, C)*, intraspinal transitional lipoma *(asterisk)*, fatty thickened filum *(straight black arrow)*, and continuity with the subcutaneous fat *(curved black arrow)*. Axial sections **(B** and **C)** best demonstrate the relationships of the cord *(white arrow, C)*, nerve roots *(white arrows, B)*, and lipoma *(asterisk)*.

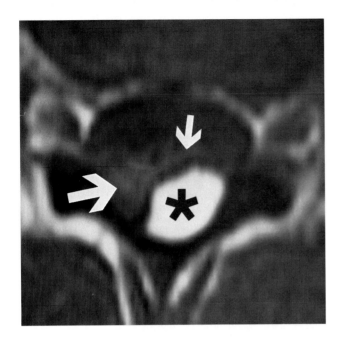

Fig. 9-32 Lumbar lipomyeloschisis demonstrated by axial T1 MRI with left-sided dorsolateral lipomatous component *(asterisk)* and right-sided rotated cord-placode *(large arrow)* and nerve roots *(small arrow)*.

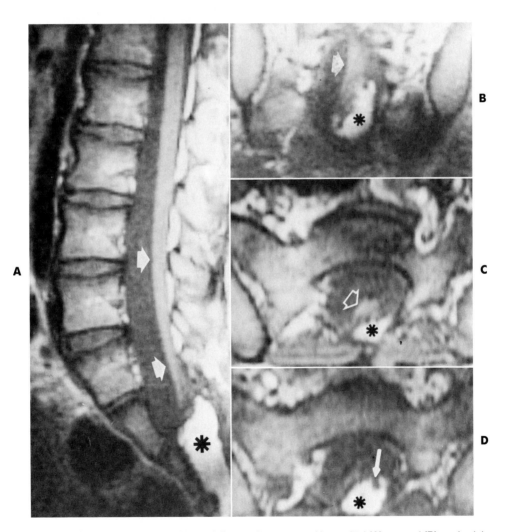

Fig. 9-33 Sacral dermal sinus with myelolipoma demonstrated by sagittal **(A)**, coronal **(B)**, and axial **(C** and **D)** T1 MRI as a low-placed, attenuated cord *(arrows)* with caudal lipomatous element *(asterisk)*.

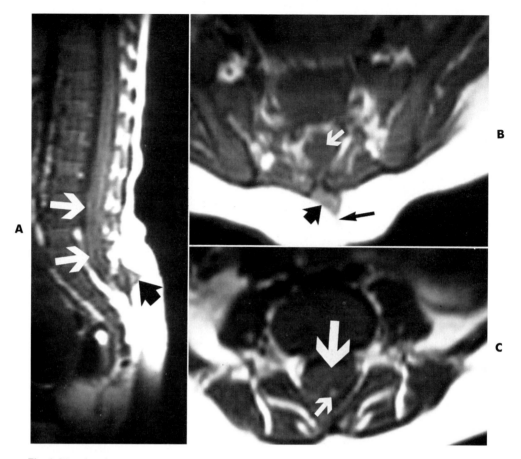

Fig. 9-34   Lumbosacral dermal sinus with dermoid cyst and abscess shown by sagittal **(A)** and axial **(B** and **C)** T1 MRI with low-placed cord and conus medullaris *(white arrows,* **A***)* and perimedullary thickening. **B,** The dorsal subcutaneous sinus *(thin black arrow)* and cyst *(black arrowhead)* communicate with the dural sac via spinolaminal defect. The abscessed intradural dermoid cyst is isointense to hypointense *(large arrow,* **C,** *small white arrow,* **B***).* **C,** Small, fatty-like high intensity *(small white arrow).*

delineate the important placode-lipoma-meningocele and nerve root relationships. Nonmyelographic CT may occasionally assist in identifying the important bony landmarks. The goal of surgery is to subtotally excise the extradural lipoma, release the placode-lipoma from its dural attachments, release other points of tethering, and close the dura to separate the neural elements and residual lipoma stump from the overlying skin and subcutaneous tissues.[29,31,38] Postoperative MRI should demonstrate this separation, although scarring with retethering of the placode-lipoma to the dura may not be directly diagnosed by MRI. In cases of neurologic deterioration after surgical repair, MRI may more importantly show other unsuspected sequelae or complications similar to those following the repair of myelocele or myelomeningocele, including changes of cord ischemia and hydromyelia. Other sequelae or complications may include CSF leak with pseudomeningocele deformity, neural injury, and multiple tethering sites.

Dermal sinuses

Dermal sinuses are epithelial tracts, stalks, or fistulas that extend from the skin surface into the deeper tissues.* These malformations are more often single than multiple and probably result from delayed and incomplete separation of the dorsally closing neural tube from the overlying cutaneous ectoderm during disjunction.[4] The tract or fistula may end in the subcutaneous tissues or a bony neural arch, or it may extend deeper between the spinous processes, along a spinous groove, or through a bifid spine to end with tenting of the dura (Fig. 9-34). The dural-penetrating sinus may communicate with the subarachnoid space and be a source of CSF leakage or may insert upon a low-placed conus medullaris, thickened filum, nerve root, or localized dorsal fibrous thickening on the cord (Fig. 9-35). Often the tract or stalk may terminate in a dermoid cyst, epidermoid cyst, or

*References 4, 6, 7, 29, 31, 38.

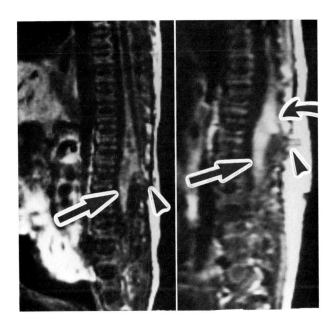

Fig. 9-35   Lumbar dermal sinus with cord tethering shown by sagittal T1 MRI. The dorsal dermal sinus *(arrowhead)* extends intraspinally and inserts into a localized dorsal thickening *(curved arrow)* of the low-placed conus medullaris *(straight arrows).*

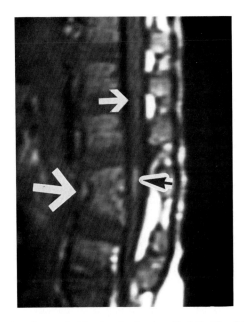

Fig. 9-36   Congenital lumbar kyphosis with fatty filar thickening (filar lipoma) and borderline low-placed conus medullaris demonstrated by sagittal T1 MRI. The conus termination *(small white arrow)* is near L2-3. There is an L4-5 block vertebra with kyphosis *(large white arrow).* There is high intensity fatty thickening of the filum *(black arrow).*

lipoma (Fig. 9-33). The blind-ending sinus contains dermis and hair follicles, as well as sweat and sebaceous glands. The sinus associated with a deeper dermoid or epidermoid cyst is lined by stratified squamous epithelium. The dermoid, epidermoid, or lipoma is usually intradural in location and encapsulated by reactive glial and fibrovascular tissue. The mass may be the termination of a thickened filum or low-placed conus medullaris, or adherent to nerve roots (Figs. 9-33 and 9-34). There may be compression of the cord or nerve roots. Rarely the dermoid or epidermoid may arise in a intramedullary location and produce cord expansion.

The majority of dermal sinuses are found dorsally at the lumbosacral level and less often at the occipital, thoracic, or sacrococcygeal levels. Ventral dermal sinuses are very rare. The sinus tract or fistula follows a segmental distribution originating at the skin level as a midline or paramedian dimple or ostium, and it courses cephalad toward the conus tip to the level determined by fetal conus ascent. Other cutaneous stigmata may be present including patchy pigmentation, hairy nevus, or angioma. Complications of dermal sinuses other than those associated with compression or tethering include multilevel sinuses with or without associated tumors, chemical meningitis due to discharge of tumor contents, and infection resulting in epidural, intradural, or intramedullary suppuration (Fig. 9-34). The cutaneous-lined dermal sinus courses within a collagenous enclosure and commonly appears as low intensity lesions on all MRI sequences and as high density on CT (Figs. 9-34 and

9-35). The entire length of the sinus may be difficult to delineate because of the oblique course of the sinus relative to the plane of section. Associated lipoma is identified as high intensity on T1 and p images and low intensity on T2 images (Fig. 9-33). A dermoid cyst may only occasionally be differentiated from an epidermoid cyst (Fig. 9-34) by fattylike content, calcium, or formed elements (for example, a tooth). Otherwise, the dermoid-epidermoid may be of similar intensity to CSF or cord on all MRI sequences, making it difficult to identify in the absence of mass effect (Figs. 9-24 and 9-34). More extensive or diffuse mass effect and enhancement may be seen with an infected dermal sinus and cyst and related to abscess and arachnoiditis (Fig. 9-34).

Tight filum terminale syndrome

The tight filum terminale syndrome, also known as the tethered cord syndrome, refers to low position of the conus medullaris (below the L2-3 level) associated with a short, thickened filum (greater than 2 mm at the L5 or S1 level).* The malformation probably results from incomplete or defective retrogressive differentiation with failure of involution of the caudal neural tube, or from failure of lengthening of the filum during involution of the caudal neural tube and relative conus ascension.[4] The filar thickening is usually fibrous but may often be fatty (filar lipoma), fibrofatty (fibrolipoma), or, less often, cystic

---

*References 4, 6, 9, 12, 21, 31, 56.

A   B   C

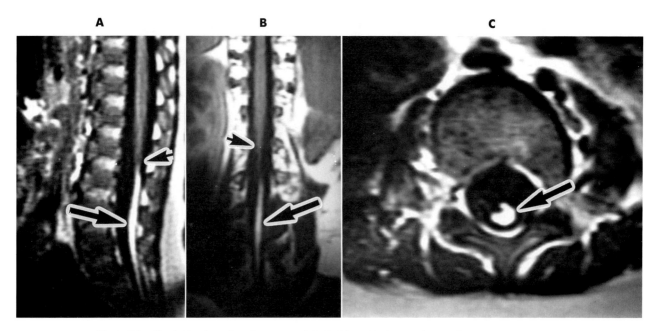

Fig. 9-37   Borderline low-placed conus medullaris *(short black arrow)* with diffuse filar lipoma *(long black arrow)* shown by sagittal **(A)**, coronal **(B)**, and axial **(C)** T1 MRI as marked hyperintense fatty thickening along the entire filum *(black arrow, **C**)*.

(Figs. 9-36 and 9-37). Also, the thickened filum may insert into a caudal malformative tumor such as a lipoma, dermoid, or epidermoid. The thickening may involve the intradural filum, extradural filum, or both.

The filum and elongated or attenuated cord may be tightly applied dorsally along the lumbar lordosis and be difficult to delineate with sagittal or coronal MRI. Axial sections may then be required. Often there is a widened sac (dural ectasia) and scoliosis. Infrequently the cord extends to the caudal point of tethering and terminates directly (absent filum) into a small lipoma or dermoid (Fig. 9-33). Occasionally, there is filar thickening with a normal conus level, including filar lipoma or fibrolipoma as an otherwise incidental finding. Filar thickening is commonly associated with other overt or occult myelodysplasias including myelomeningocele, lipomyelomeningocele, diastematomyelia, and dermal sinus.

Rarely a borderline low conus (L2-3 or L3) is demonstrated by sagittal MRI without obvious filar thickening or other cause of tethering. Axial T1-weighted sections from the conus tip to the sacral levels should then be obtained to demonstrate the focal thickening, which usually occurs distally (L5-S1). This technique may be preferred to axial T2-weighted spin echo or T2/T2★ gradient echo sections. Rarely will myelographic CT be needed to clarify the MRI findings. Occasionally, additional findings that may assist in differentiating the tethered from the nontethered low conus may be present on sagittal T1 MRI. The loss of the normally sharp transition from the tubular cord to the cone configuration of the conus medullaris gives the appearance of an elongated or attenuated caudal cord segment. Another finding may be that of a caudal intramedullary "water" intensity lesion, which may represent infarction, myeloma-

lacia, or hydrosyrinx, or it may represent a local dilatation of the central canal or terminal ventricle (hydromyelia). The absence of cord pulsation on ultrasonography or cardiac-gated MRI is a questionably helpful sign. The absence of a tethering lesion by neuroimaging in a patient with progressive neurological impairment and low position of the conus should not defer further clinical or imaging evaluation nor defer consideration for surgery.

Myelocystocele

Myelocystocele is a very rare anomaly and probably a variant of myelomeningocele in which the hydromyelic cord-placode and accompanying leptomeninges herniate through a bifid canal.[4,14,63,64] These occur most frequently at the lumbosacral level (Fig. 9-38) and classically may be associated with other caudal malformations including lumbosacral spinal anomalies with anorectal and urogenital malformations (for example, cloacal exstrophy).[13,63] Rarely are these encountered at higher spinal levels (Fig. 9-39). The terminal myelocystocele (Fig. 9-38) consists of a dilated central canal (hydromyelia) and dilated terminal ventricle of the conus-placode continuous with a large dorsal, ependymal-lined cyst within or adjacent to the meningocele sac, the latter continuous with the subarachnoid space. The cyst of the myelocystocele is usually larger and is located posteroinferior or occasionally superior to the meningocele sac. A lipomatous component may be present, that is, a lipomyelocystocele.

Meningocele

Meningoceles are uncommon saccular dural protrusions extending beyond the confines of the spinal canal and containing CSF-filled arachnoid but no neural elements.[4,6]

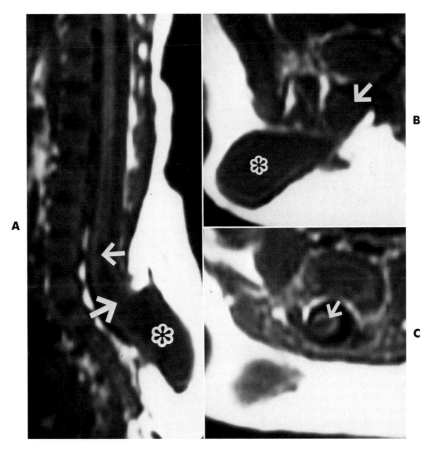

Fig. 9-38   Lumbosacral terminal myelocystocele shown by sagittal **(A)** and axial **(B** and **C)** T1 MRI with hydromyelia *(small arrows,* **A, C** *)* and cystic dilatation of the terminal ventricle *(large arrow,* **A, B***)* and the meningocele sac *(asterisks).*

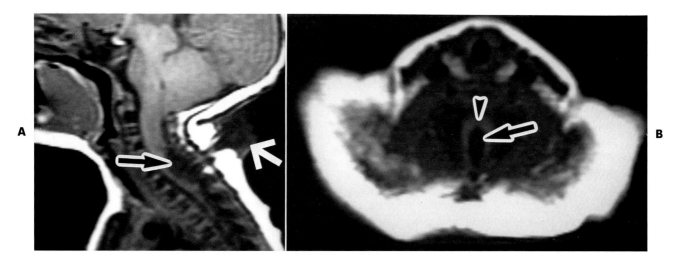

Fig. 9-39   Cervical myelocystocele shown by sagittal **(A)** and axial **(B)** T1 MRI with segmental cystic dilatation of the central canal *(black arrows)* extending from the nonneurulated cord-placode *(arrowhead)* through the dysraphic spinal canal and subcutaneous fatty tissues into the dorsal meningocele *(white arrow).*

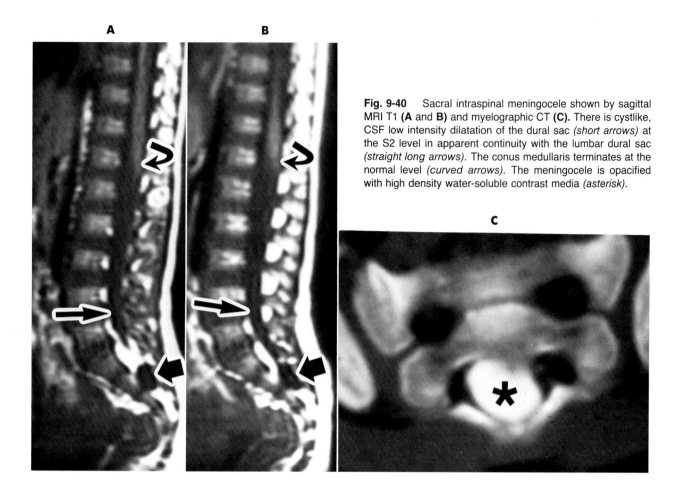

A   B

Fig. 9-40   Sacral intraspinal meningocele shown by sagittal MRI T1 **(A** and **B)** and myelographic CT **(C).** There is cystlike, CSF low intensity dilatation of the dural sac *(short arrows)* at the S2 level in apparent continuity with the lumbar dural sac *(straight long arrows).* The conus medullaris terminates at the normal level *(curved arrows).* The meningocele is opacified with high density water-soluble contrast media *(asterisk).*

C

The meningeal herniation may traverse a small or large bony defect, such as a spina bifida, or protrude through an enlarged existing opening such as an intervertebral or sacral foramen. Meningoceles may occur at the craniocervical junction, or at the cervical, thoracic, lumbar, sacral, or, rarely, the coccygeal level. The meningoceles may protrude dorsally, ventrally, or laterally and are rarely multiple. Intraspinal meningoceles have been described (Fig. 9-40), as well as meningoceles extending along the axillary sleeves of nerve roots (Tarlov's cyst). At the cervicooccipital level, the dorsal meningocele may be associated with Chiari malformation (see Chapter 3). The dorsal lumbar and dorsal or anterior sacral meningoceles may be associated with other myelodysplasias, including low-placed conus with thickened filum (posterior dysraphism).

The very rare anterior meningocele occurring above the sacral level may be considered an anomaly in the neurenteric spectrum (see Fig. 9-44) and is associated with vertebral body defects (anterior dysraphism). Anterior sacral or presacral meningoceles are associated with anterior dysraphic sacral or sacrococcygeal bony anomalies and may occur as isolated malformations or in association with anorectal and urogenital anomalies in the caudal dysplasia spectrum.[4,6,13,63] The meningocele may be manifested as a retrorectal mass with urinary, rectal, menstrual, or pain symptoms. Commonly there is a wide sacral intraspinal

dural sac (dural ectasia) communicating via a wide or narrow neck through the sacral defect with a simple or loculated presacral meningocele. Sacral nerve roots may be adherent to the sac wall or neck. Associated sacral bony anomalies include hemihypoplasia with a sickle configuration, absent coccygeal and lower sacral segments, and dorsal sacral dysraphic defects (Fig. 9-41).

Presacral meningoceles extending through a large sacral foramen and associated with a large sacral canal are characteristic of the dural ectasia of neurofibromatosis, as discussed in Chapter 8. Lateral thoracic or lumbar meningoceles extending through enlarged intervertebral foramina are also associated with dural ectasia and occur in neurofibromatosis but may be seen in Marfan's syndrome or be idiopathic. Occasionally, local or diffuse CSF-filled expansions occur intraspinally with widening of the spinal canal and thinning of the pedicles. These have been referred to as intraspinal meningoceles and may represent localized dural ectasia, cystic dilatation of the leptomeninges herniating through a dural defect, or arachnoid cysts (Fig. 9-40). Dural ectasia occurs with spinal dysraphism, neurofibromatosis, Marfan's syndrome, Ehlers-Danlos syndrome, or may be idiopathic (Fig. 9-42). Other entities included in the plain film differential diagnosis of spinal canal widening and pedicle thinning are hydrosyringomyelia and intraspinal neoplasm.

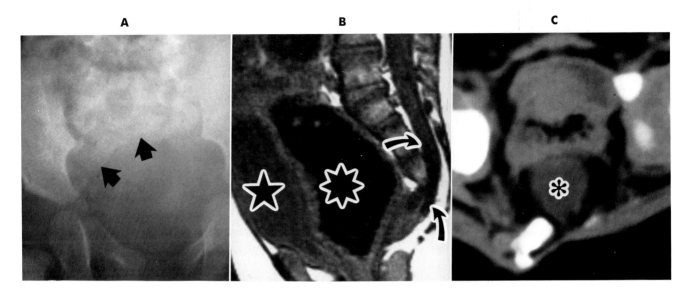

Fig. 9-41   Presacral meningocele associated with imperforate anus complex and sacral dysplasia. **A,** Frontal plain film shows sickle-shaped, hypoplastic sacrum *(arrows)*. **B,** Sagittal T1 MRI shows the CSF hypointense meningocele *(lower curved arrow)* continuous with the ectatic lumbar dural sac *(upper curved arrow)* and extending into the posterior pelvis. There is marked bladder *(star)* and bowel *(asterisk)* dilatation. **(C),** Axial CT image shows the CSF density presacral meningocele *(asterisk)*.

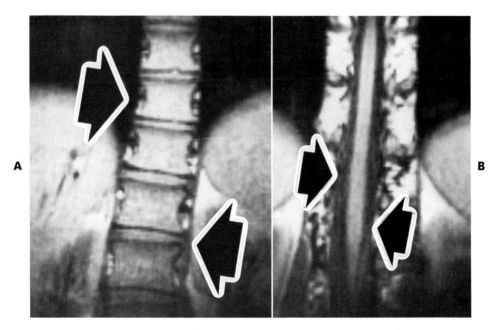

Fig. 9-42   Dural ectasia with idiopathic thoracolumbar scoliosis shown by coronal T1 MRI. **A,** There is rightward curvature deformity with canal widening but questionable pedicle thinning *(arrows)*. **B,** The spinal cord is normal, but there is dural sac widening *(arrows)*.

NEURENTERIC CONTINUUM DEFECTS

The most common CNS malformations of the neurenteric continuum include diastematomyelia, neurenteric cyst, and anterior meningocele.[4,6] These are all part of a spectrum of anomalies that may also be included in the split notochord spectrum. The basic developmental defect is probably persistence of the embryonal adhesion between the endoderm and ectoderm that produces splitting or deviation of the notochord.[4,14] This in turn results in variable persistence of the connections or communications between the ventral gut and dorsal integument via the intervening and notochordally induced mesenchyme (spinal column) and neural tube (spinal cord). These may also be designated as anterior dysraphic or ventral neural tube closure anomalies that occur in spite of dorsal neural tube closure. However, associated dorsal neural tube and skin involvement may occur. In fact it is this author's speculation that other dorsal neural tube anomalies not directly involving the primitive placode, such as dorsal meningoceles and dermal sinuses, may more appropriately belong in this category. Common to CNS involvement for all of the malformations of this spectrum are vertebral formation-segmentation anomalies (that is, anterior dysraphism) such as hemivertebrae, butterfly vertebrae, block vertebrae, pedicle or interlaminar fusion, and canal widening. The presentation may be that of congenital scoliosis or kyphosis or Klippel-Feil syndrome. Neural arch or spinolaminal defects (that is, posterior dysraphism) may also be present.

Split notochord syndrome

Any of the CNS anomalies in the neurenteric continuum may occur in isolation or in association with other neural or extraneural anomalies, including the rare split notochord syndrome.[4,6,14] This syndrome more specifically refers to a very rare spectrum of malformations resulting from complete or partial failure of obliteration of the primitive neurenteric connections, whether or not associated with spinal CNS involvement. At the one extreme there is total failure of neurenteric involution with visceral fistulization, usually of midgut or enteric origin. The fistula extends through the abdomen or thorax, through the deformed spinal column, meninges, and spinal cord to the dorsal skin surface. This rare anomaly has been designated the *dorsal enteric fistula*. Even rarer is the associated dorsal bowel herniation with open or membrane-covered dorsal cutaneous ostium expressing meconium or feces. More commonly, partial obliteration along the visceral or enteric side of the continuum may give rise to endodermally derived foregut, midgut, or hindgut diverticulae, duplications, cysts, sinuses, or cords. This may result in any number of thoracic, abdominal, or, rarely, pelvic masses involving foregut derivatives (pharyngeal, laryngotracheal, bronchopulmonary, esophagogastric, duodenal, hepatic, pancreatic, or biliary), midgut derivatives (small intestine to transverse colon), or hindgut derivatives (transverse colon to the anal canal, urogenital sinus, and cloaca). Because of visceral migration and rotation, the intraabdominal enteric end of the malformation may extend through the diaphragm in continuity with a mediastinal component, which in turn is continuous with a cervical or thoracic spinal component. These anomalies may include the dorsal enteric sinus, dorsal enteric diverticulum or duplication, and the dorsal enterogenous cyst.[4,14]

Neurenteric cyst and anterior meningocele

Partial persistence of the neural end of the neurenteric continuum may give rise to characteristic vertebral anomalies as outlined above, as well as meningoceles, diastematomyelia, and arachnoid or neuroglial cysts. Often, visceral elements are present in cystic malformations of the neural end of the spectrum, such as respiratory or intestinal epithelial-lined intraspinal neurenteric cysts.[24,30,44] Clinical presentations may include pulmonary or gastrointestinal symptoms or signs (for example, respiratory distress or intestinal obstruction), spinal curvature deformity, or spinal level neurological involvement. Involvement of the visceral end of the neurenteric spectrum may be accompanied by involvement of the neural end and vice versa. Therefore discovery at one side of the continuum may prompt a search for involvement at the other.

CNS involvement in neurenteric cyst almost always is indicated by plain film demonstration of spinal column anomalies.[24,30,44] In addition to those anomalies listed above, close scrutiny may reveal a midline bony ostium or tunnel-like defect at the center of a butterfly vertebra representing a remnant of the primitive neurenteric canal of Kovalevsky. There may or may not be an associated posterior mediastinal or abdominal mass as a separate or contiguous component. The cyst may be located prevertebrally, intraspinally, or dorsal extraspinally (Figs. 9-43; see also Figs. 9-45 and 9-60). The intraspinal cyst may expand the canal and lie ventral, lateral, or dorsal to the cord, within the cord, or both (Figs. 9-43, 9-45, and 9-60). The cysts usually occur in the lower cervical or upper thoracic region and, rarely, at the lumbar or sacral levels. When there is a tandem extraspinal-intraspinal cyst combination, an intercommunication or interconnection as a sinus or stalk may be apparent extending through the bony spinal defect (Fig. 9-45). The cyst content may be primarily serous and difficult to separate from surrounding CSF on all MRI sequences. Mucoid or hemorrhagic cyst content may give T1 hyperintensity as well as p/T2 hyperintensity. Meningoceles are discussed in a previous section. Occasionally, an anterior meningocele may be difficult to differentiate from a neurenteric cyst containing serous fluid. With a meningocele the cord and nerve roots are often deviated *toward* the opening of the meningocele (Fig. 9-44), whereas with a neurenteric cyst the neural elements are usually displaced *away* from the lesion.

Diastematomyelia

Diastematomyelia designates sagittal division, splitting, or clefting of the spinal cord.[4,6,14,28,32] There is a female preponderance, and the majority (70% to 80%) occur in the

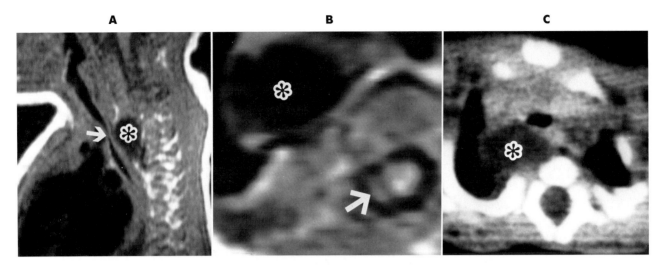

Fig. 9-43   Cervicothoracic neurenteric cyst shown by sagittal **(A)** and axial **(B)** T1 MRI and by CT **(C)**. A CSF density and CSF intensity cyst *(asterisks)* is present in the posterosuperior mediastinum associated with cervicothoracic junction vertebral anomalies and producing tracheal airway obstruction *(arrow,* **A** *). An isointense to hyperintense intraspinal component (arrow,* **B** *)* is demonstrated adjacent to the cord.

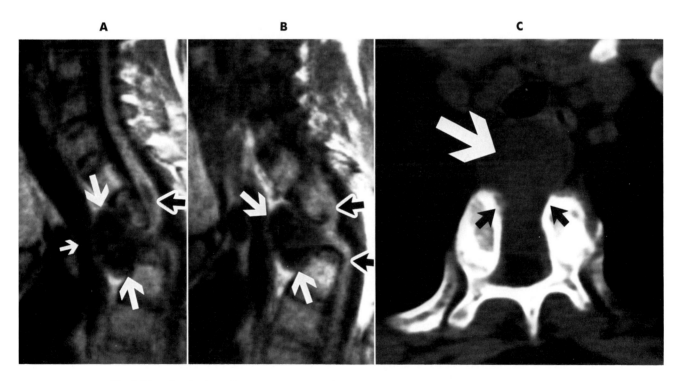

Fig. 9-44   Cervicothoracic anterior meningocele shown by sagittal T1 MRI **(A, B)** and axial CT **(C)**. The CSF intensity and CSF density meningocele *(large white arrows,* **A-C** *)* is continuous with the ectatic spinal dural sac and extends anteriorly through the vertebral defect *(black arrows,* **C** *)* into the posterosuperior mediastinum with impression on the tracheal airway *(small white arrow,* **A** *)*. The cord and nerve roots *(black arrows,* **A, B** *)* are deviated into the mouth of the meningocele, and there is a small syrinx *(black arrow,* **A)**.

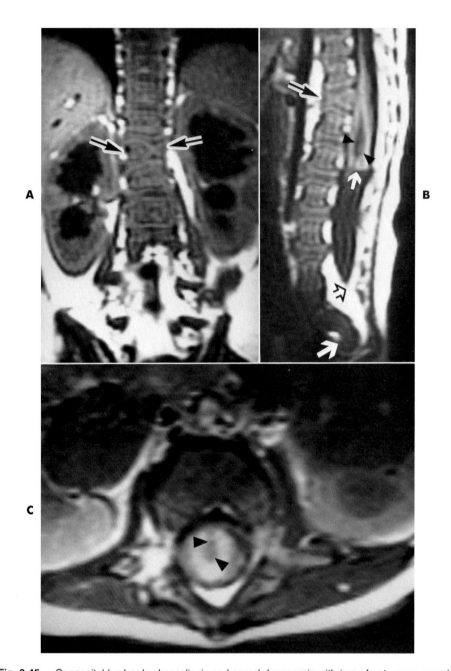

Fig. 9-45   Congenital lumbar kyphoscoliosis and sacral dysgenesis with imperforate anus complex shown by coronal **(A)**, sagittal **(B)**, and axial **(C)** T1 MRI. Lumbar hemivertebral and wedge vertebral anomalies *(large black arrow)* are present with shortened sacrum *(large white arrow)*, dural sac stenosis *(open black arrow)*, and blunted, dysplastic caudal cord *(small white arrow)*. There is low intensity, intramedullary cystlike expansion *(black arrowhead)* with an anterior cord cleft at a slightly higher level related to the vertebral anomaly. This may represent an intramedullary neurenteric spectrum cyst. Also there is bilateral hydronephrosis.

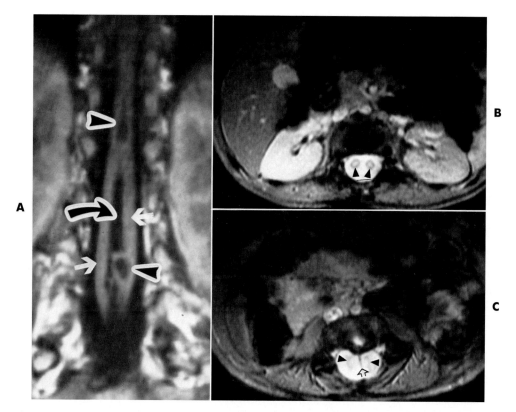

Fig. 9-46   Lumbar septate diastematomyelia with syringohydromyelia. **A,** Coronal T1 MRI demonstrates the intermedullary split (*curved black arrow*), the two hemicords (*white arrows*), and the syringohydromyelia (*black arrowheads*). The septum is somewhat apparent. **B** and **C,** Axial T2★ gradient echo MRI showing the hemicords with high intensity syringohydromyelia in each (*arrowheads*). The low intensity septum (*open arrow*) stands out against the high intensity CSF **(C).**

lumbar or thoracolumbar region. They occur less often in the thoracic region, and rarely in the cervical region or at multiple levels. The split may extend through the full thickness of the cord or partially as a deep fissure or cleft (Figs. 9-46 to 9-51). Commonly the complete split becomes a partial split at the cranial and caudal ends in transition to the whole cord. The diastematomyelia may divide the cord into symmetrical or asymmetrical hemicords, each usually with one dorsal and one ventral nerve root[39,58] (Fig. 9-47). This is to be distinguished from the very rare diplomyelia, or duplication of the cord, in which there are two separate whole cords, each with a complete set of nerve roots.

In diastematomyelia there may or may not be a septum extending through the split.[39,58] In about half of the cases the hemicords are contained together entirely within a single ectatic dural enclosure continuous with that for the whole cord above and below the split (Fig. 9-49). An intermedullary septum is rarely present. In other cases the hemicords are each contained within separate dural enclosures with septation of the interdural or meningeal space (Figs. 9-46 to 9-48, and 9-51). Above and below, the separate dural sacs are reconstituted as a single dural sac at or just before the point where the hemicords reunite to form the whole cord.

The septum, which is usually single, may be composed of one or a combination mesenchymal or neural elements, including cortical or medullary bone, cartilage, fibrous tissue, vascular structures (epidural venous), or neuroglial tissue (Figs. 9-46 to 9-48, and 9-51). The more common bony peg or spur may be a partial or complete bridge between the posterior margin of the vertebral body and the anterior aspect of the neural arch. There may be an associated cartilaginous synchondrosis or fibrous pseudoarthrosis. Fibrous or neuroglial bands (meningocele manque variation) may be present in either the septate or nonseptate types.

The hemicords usually reunite above and below the split.[39,58] Rarely is there extended splitting caudally that results in symmetrical or asymmetrical division of the conus and filum, and symmetrical or asymmetrical distribution of the filum and caudae equina nerve roots (Fig. 9-51). Hydromyelia is occasionally present extending into the hemicords[59] (Figs. 9-46 and 9-47). Low termination of the conus medullaris is present in the majority of cases. In septate diastematomyelia the spur or band lies at the lower end of the split. Other septae must be sought for or ruled out, however, especially when one is present at a site other

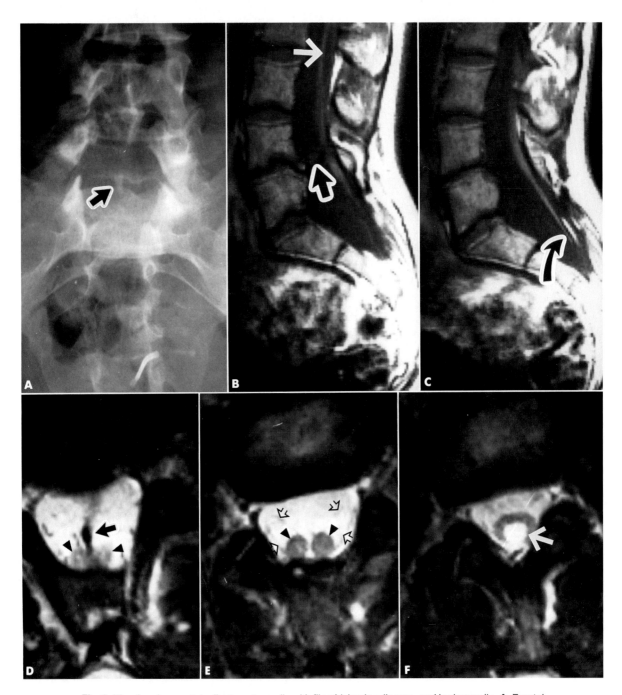

Fig. 9-47   Lumbar septate diastematomyelia with filar thickening, lipoma, and hydromyelia. **A,** Frontal plain film shows L5-S1 dysraphism and ossified septum *(arrow).* **B** and **C,** Sagittal T1 MRI demonstrating the cortical bony septum or peg *(black arrow),* the hydromyelia *(white arrow),* and the thickened filum *(curved arrow)* with adjacent lipoma. **D-F,** Axial T2 MRI scans demonstrate to better advantage the septum *(black arrow,* **D** *),* hemicords *(arrowheads),* nerve roots *(open black arrows),* and the hydromyelia *(white arrow).*

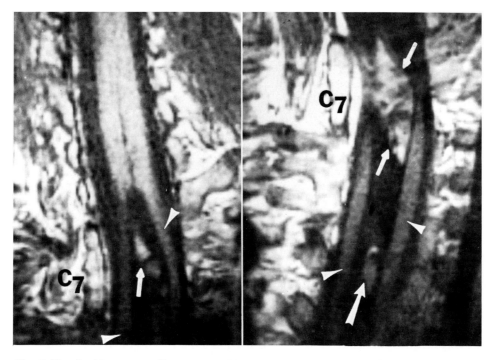

Fig. 9-48   Double septate diastematomyelia in Klippel-Feil syndrome with congenital thoracic scoliosis. Coronal T1 MRI shows the high intensity medullary bony upper and lower septae *(arrows)* within the intermedullary split plus the hemicords *(arrowheads).* (From Barnes P: *Contemp Diagn Radiol* 13:1, 1990).

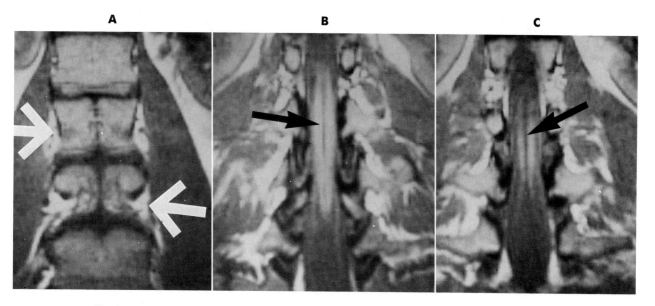

Fig. 9-49   Nonseptate lumbar diastematomyelia with tethered cord due to tight filum. Coronal T1 MRI shows butterfly vertebral deformities *(white arrows)* and nonseptate sagittal splitting of the cord *(black arrows).*

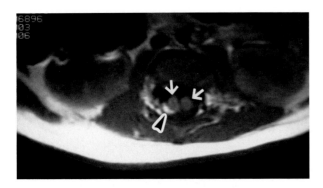

Fig. 9-50 Lumbar diastematomyelia with axial T1 MRI showing the hemicords *(arrows)* and associated lipoma *(arrowhead)*.

tion defects (hemimyelocele), as discussed earlier, or with other secondary neurulation defects. In fact, nonseptate diastematomyelia itself is usually incidental to other, more clinically important myelodysplasias such as lipomyelomeningocele, and tight filum terminale.[58]

Important aspects of neuroimaging include the often characteristic plain film findings, the necessity for thorough MRI evaluation for surgical planning, and the complementary role of CT.[4,6,14,60,66] Radiographic findings that may be suggestive of and often localize the level of septate diastematomyelia include formation-segmentation anomalies, as previously described. Occasionally there is direct plain film visualization of the ossific peg or spur (Fig. 9-47; see also Fig. 9-17).[28] Multiplanar MRI is required to provide complete delineation regarding the nature and extent of cord splitting, level of conus termination, presence or absence of septation, multilevel splitting, multiple septations, other tethering lesions as previously outlined, and associated hydromyelia.

Axial images are particularly important for delineating the split and septation, especially in rotated or tilted complexes associated with scoliosis or kyphosis. CSF-

than the caudal end of the split (Fig. 9-48). The septum is usually the source of cord tethering in septate diastematomyelia, but additional tethering may result from associated filar thickening, developmental tumor, or tethering nerve roots. Diastematomyelia may occur with primary neurula-

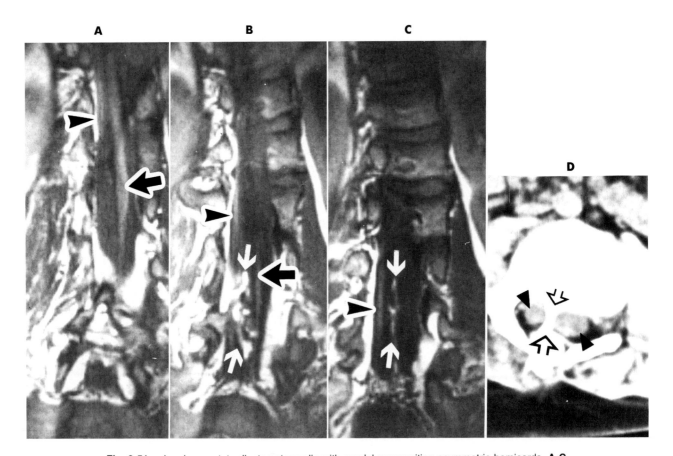

Fig. 9-51 Lumbar septate diastematomyelia with caudal nonreuniting asymmetric hemicords. **A-C,** Coronal T1 MRI showing the smaller right *(black arrowheads)* and larger left *(black arrows)* hemicords extending caudally beyond the split conus medullaris *(black arrow, **A**)* as asymmetrical cauda equina nerve root trunks. The cortical and the medullary bony septum is seen as mixed high and low intensities *(white arrows)* and confirmed by axial CT **(D)** as a high density partition *(open arrows)* separating the hemicords and their dural tubes *(arrowheads)*.

enhanced MRI techniques are often necessary to delineate the septal tissue. If the septum contains elements other than the fatty high intensity marrow of medullary bone, the septum may not be distinguished from low intensity CSF on T1-weighted images (Figs. 9-46 and 9-47). Cortical bony, cartilaginous, fibrous, vascular, or neuroglial elements may only be identified as low intensity lesions contrasted against the high intensity of CSF (myelogram effect) provided by T2 spin echo or T2/T2★ gradient echo techniques (Figs. 9-46 and 9-47). Occasionally CT without intrathecal iodinated contrast may assist in clarifying or confirming ossific septation, as well as providing further information regarding bony landmarks and other bony anomalies of the spinal column [2,6] (Fig. 9-51). In septate diastematomyelia, surgical repair consists of excision of the septum, dural reconstruction into a single tube, excision of associated developmental masses, and division of the tethering filum. Postoperative MRI should demonstrate a nonseptated split cord within the reconstructed single dural tube.

CAUDAL DYSPLASIA SYNDROMES

Caudal dysplasia refers to a spectrum of caudal cell mass disorders that result in a range of varying caudal spinal, anorectal, urogenital, and lower limb abnormalities.* At one extreme there is the caudal regression syndrome with lumbosacral agenesis, fused lower extremities, anal atresia, and abnormal genitalia. This may be seen in infants of diabetic mothers or associated with Potter's syndrome. At the other end of the spectrum there may be foot deformity, lower limb motor and sensory impairment, other hindgut and genitourinary anomalies, and neurogenic bladder. The spinal anomalies range from partial or unilateral sacral

*References 4, 6, 11, 13, 15, 17, 25, 52, 63.

agenesis to sacral or lumbosacral agenesis. Often there is bony, fibrous, or dural sac stenosis with fused vertebral segments just cephalad to the agenesis. (Figs. 9-45, 9-52, and 9-53).[13,63] There may be dysplasia, hypoplasia, or aplasia of the caudal spinal cord (Figs. 9-45 and 9-53). As a result there is a relatively high level of termination of the blunt or wedge-shaped caudal cord.[4,63] The myelodysplasia in this syndrome probably results from abnormal caudal neural tube development (defective secondary neurulation). Faulty retrogressive differentiation likely results in absence of the distal conus medullaris and filum terminale. Caudal to the incomplete and malformed spinal segments, disorganized nerve roots are dispersed within dense fibrous tissue. Other myelodysplasias in the caudal dysplasia spectrum include anterior or presacral meningoceles, cord tethering with filar thickening or developmental tumor, myelocystocele, and lipomyelomeningocele[13,63] (Figs. 9-31, 9-38, and 9-41).

DEVELOPMENTAL TUMORS

According to the revised WHO classification of tumors (see Chapter 7), malformative tumors of the CNS that occur within the spinal neuraxis include hamartomas, lipomas, epidermoid or dermoid cysts, enterogenous and respiratory

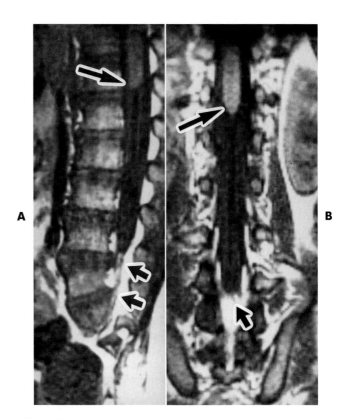

Fig. 9-53 Caudal dysplasia syndrome with sacral agenesis shown by sagittal **(A)** and coronal **(B)** T1 MRI with absent sacral segments, lumbosacral dural sac atresia-stenosis *(short arrows)*, more proximal dural ectasia, and high dysplastic caudal cord termination *(long arrows)* at T11-12.

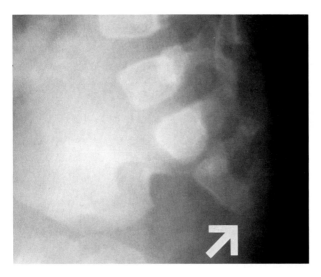

Fig. 9-52 Caudal dysplasia syndrome with sacral dysplasia and imperforate anus complex. Lateral plain film shows hypoplastic sacrum with absent lower segments *(arrow)* and fused middle segments.

(neurenteric) cysts, as well as arachnoid, ependymal, and neuroglial cysts.[4,6,14] Other congenital tumors include germ cell neoplasms such as teratomas. Some classifications would also include vascular malformations. The modified classification of congenital cerebral, cerebellar, and spinal malformations by van der Knaap and Valk (see Chapter 3) categorizes most of the congenital tumors and congenital vascular malformations of the nervous system as disorders of neuronal proliferation, differentiation, and histogenesis.[65] In that same scheme, arachnoid cysts are listed in the unclassified category.

Lipomas

Lipomas are by far the most common developmental intraspinal tumor of childhood. These have often been considered mesenchymal hamartomas composed of mature fat cells and frequently containing fibrous strands. These may also contain muscle, cartilage, calcification, or ossification. Other evidence suggests that these are developmental malformations that arise from persistence and maldifferentiation of the primitive meninges.[4] Lipomas in childhood primarily occur in the dysraphic states (95%), particularly in the form of lipomyelomeningoceles and filar lipomas (Figs. 9-29 to 9-33, 9-36, and 9-37). The rarer intradural lipoma is really a paramedullary or juxtamedullary tumor and usually not associated with spinal dysraphism, except that there may be occasional canal or foraminal widening or a minimally bifid neural arch. This type of lipoma usually occurs in the cervical or thoracic region after childhood and presents with gradually advancing myelopathy. The lipoma actually arises in an intramedullary location and has a subpial extramedullary component dorsally, laterally, or anterolaterally. Similar to the lipomyelomeningocele, the lipoma often occupies a dorsal cleft in the incompletely neurulated cord, and there may be associated hydrosyringomyelia.

Dermoids and epidermoids

Dermoids are usually cystic tumors of ectodermal origin composed of epidermal and dermal elements, including a squamous epithelial lining, skin appendages, hair follicles, and sweat and sebaceous glands. The cyst often contains glandular secretions and squamous epithelial breakdown products such as keratin and cholesterol. Epidermoids also are usually cystic lesions, but they consist of epidermal elements only. These are squamous epithelial-lined cysts containing keratin, cholesterol, or both. Intraspinally, dermoids are more common than epidermoids.[4,14,29,31] Dermoids or epidermoids may be associated with dermal sinuses, as discussed earlier, or may occur as congenital rests or iatrogenic implants. There may be associated dysraphic cord tethering or compression, suppuration with abscess formation, or chemical meningitis from leakage of content. The majority occur in the lumbar or lumbosacral region; they occur less often in the thoracic region. A dermoid may not be readily distinguished from an epidermoid by neuroimaging, even when exhibiting findings suggesting fat or calcification (Fig. 9-34). The epidermoid or dermoid may be especially difficult to separate from CSF or the cord, since the tumor often exhibits similar intensities throughout the MRI sequences. Iodine or gadolinium enhancement is not expected unless there is an inflammatory reaction or suppuration (such as an abscess).

Teratomas

Teratomas are germ cell tumors that may be histologically classified as mature, immature, or anaplastic (see Chapter 7). These may arise from multipotential cell rests, displaced germ cells, or along the path of germ cell migration. Teratomas most commonly occur in the sacrococcygeal region, usually as an external perineal or gluteal mass with or without pelvic involvement and less often as a pelvoabdominal or entirely presacral tumor[4,14,29,38] (Figs. 9-54 and 9-55). Two thirds are of the mature variety; the other third are of the immature or anaplastic type. These are usually encapsulated and lobulated and may be solid, cystic, or both. Fat or calcification may be present along with sacral bony erosion, although spinal canal invasion is unusual. A familial form has been reported that is of autosomal dominant inheritance and consists of sacrococcygeal defects, anorectal stenosis, vesicoureteral reflux, and cutaneous stigmata.[4] Spinal teratomas arising outside the sacrococcygeal region are exceedingly rare in childhood. These are more often benign than malignant and may occur at the thoracic or lumbar level as intramedullary or extramedullary masses, and occasionally with associated syrinx (Fig. 9-56). The tumors may be solid or cystic, contain fat, bone, cartilage, or dental elements, and often produce spinal canal widening.

Hamartomas

Hamartomas other than lipomas are rarely reported.[4] These are usually of mixed neuroectodermal or mesodermal composition including neuroglial tissue, meningeal tissue, bone, cartilage, fat, and muscle. Hamartomas may occur as dorsal solid or cystic subcutaneous masses at the thoracic, thoracolumbar, lumbar, or sacrococcygeal levels and are associated with cutaneous angiomas (Figs. 9-57 and 9-58). Spina bifida and spinal canal widening are common. A hamartoma containing choroid plexus and producing hydrosyringomyelia has been described.[4]

Arachnoid cysts

Arachnoid cysts are actually a very rare cause of spinal neurological dysfunction in childhood.[4,18,26,62] Although occasionally accompanying other dysraphic myelodysplasias, arachnoid cysts are usually primary and isolated, or secondary and postinflammatory. Primary arachnoid cysts of developmental etiology may be intradural or extradural in location. Secondary arachnoid cysts of acquired etiology are usually intradural in location and associated with arachnoiditis. Primary intradural arachnoid cysts probably arise as a result from a developmental deficiency in the formation of the arachnoid, which is of combined mesodermal and

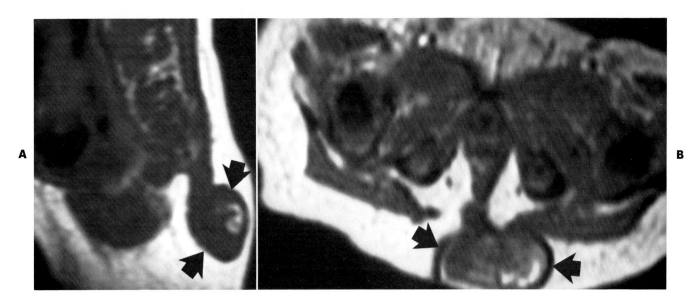

Fig. 9-54   Caudal or gluteal teratoma in an infant shown by sagittal **(A)** and axial **(B)** T1 MRI as an isointense to hypointense mass *(arrows)* containing fatty high intensities.

Fig. 9-55   Pelvoabdominal teratoma in an infant shown by sagittal T1 **(A)** and axial T2 **(B)** MRI as a huge mixed intensity mass *(arrows)* filling the pelvis and displacing the bladder *(asterisks)*. The internal high and low intensities represent a combination of fatty content, calcification, and hemorrhage.

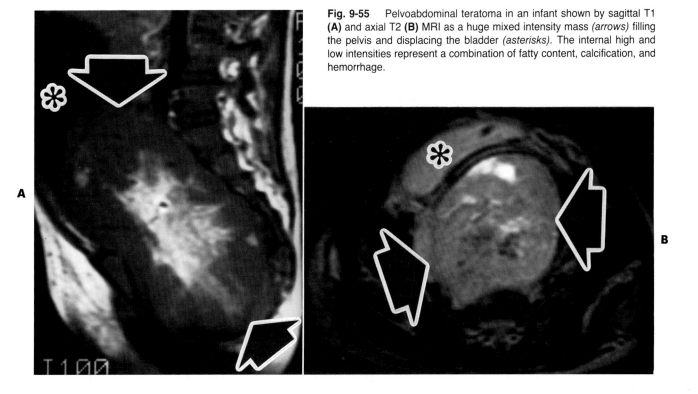

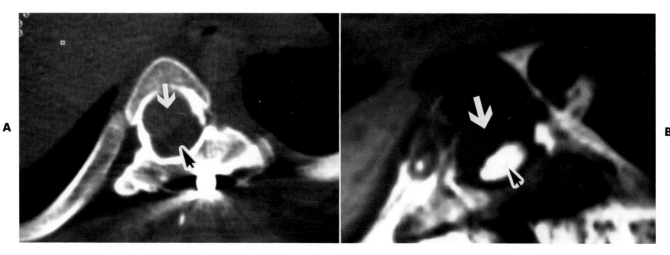

Fig. 9-56   Recurrent thoracic intraspinal teratoma shown by axial myelographic CT **(A)** with isodense *(white arrow)* and hypodense *(black arrow)* components. **B,** Axial T1 MRI demonstrates the isointense cord expansion *(white arrow)* along with the associated hyperintense fatty component *(black arrow)*.

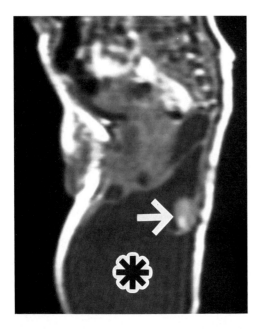

Fig. 9-57   Caudal sacrococcygeal neuroepithelial hamartoma shown by sagittal T1 MRI with CSF hypointense cystic *(asterisk)* and isointense to hyperintense solid *(arrow)* components.

neural crest origin. Extradural arachnoid cysts probably result from developmental dural defects with herniation of arachnoid and CSF extradurally (Fig. 9-59). Arachnoid cysts have also been described as either communicating or noncommunicating in relation to the subarachnoid spaces. The communicating cysts are actually arachnoid diverticulae, whereas the noncommunicating cysts are true cysts.

Arachnoid cysts may occur anteriorly or posteriorly within the spinal canal. These are usually found in the dorsal thoracic region, but may be seen in the lumbar or sacral region, at multiple levels, or, rarely, in the cervical region. Clinical presentations include radiculopathy or myelopathy with pain, paresis, or scoliosis. Plain films may be negative or demonstrate nonspecific scoliosis, spinal canal enlargement, or pedicle thinning. It may be very difficult to "directly" demonstrate arachnoid cysts by MRI, since the intensity characteristics are often similar to that of CSF throughout the spin echo sequences. Because of the lack of "CSF flow" within the cyst as compared with CSF in the subarachnoid space, occasionally the cyst may appear of higher intensity relative to CSF, especially on the T2-weighted spin echo images, depending on the influence of flow compensation techniques. Confusing CSF intensity variations may normally be seen dorsolaterally to the cord where arachnoid trabeculae exist between the septum posticum and dentate ligaments. Otherwise, the cyst may be directly identified or suspected only by mass effect upon the cord or nerve roots (Figs. 9-59 and 9-60). Dorsal extradural cysts may be identified not only by mass effect but also by the interface between the CSF-intensity cyst and the epidural fat (Fig. 9-59). For intradural or extradural arachnoid cysts, other diagnostic considerations include dural ectasia, neurenteric cyst, and intraspinal meningocele (Figs. 9-40, 9-42, and 9-60). Differentiating a communicating arachnoid cyst from a meningocele may not be possible by neuroimaging and may in fact be a matter of semantics, especially for intradural lesions. However, extradural arachnoid cysts, in contrast to meningoceles, do not ordinarily project beyond the bony confines of the spinal canal. Water-soluble myelography or myelographic CT may assist in diagnosis, although confusing patterns may appear after injection and require delayed imaging for possible clarification.

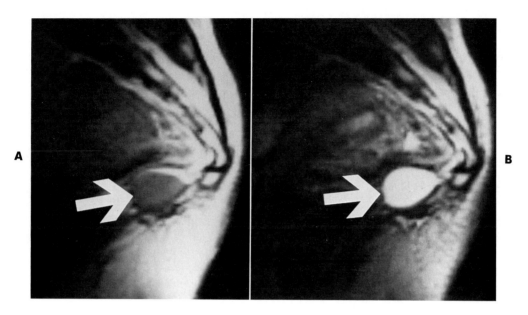

Fig. 9-58   Coccygeal cyst *(arrows)* shown by sagittal p **(A)** and T2 **(B)** MRI as a CSF intensity cyst.

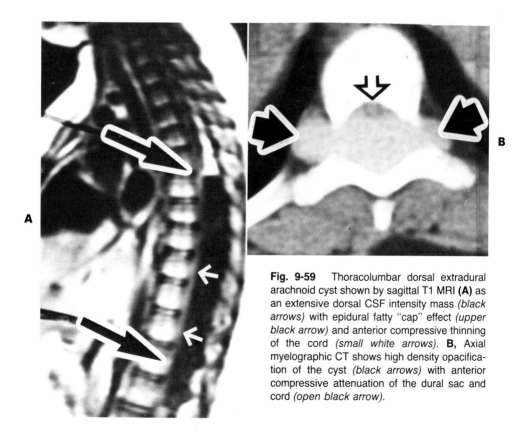

Fig. 9-59   Thoracolumbar dorsal extradural arachnoid cyst shown by sagittal T1 MRI **(A)** as an extensive dorsal CSF intensity mass *(black arrows)* with epidural fatty "cap" effect *(upper black arrow)* and anterior compressive thinning of the cord *(small white arrows)*. **B,** Axial myelographic CT shows high density opacification of the cyst *(black arrows)* with anterior compressive attenuation of the dural sac and cord *(open black arrow)*.

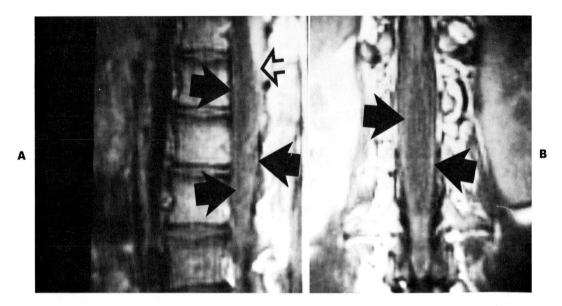

Fig. 9-60   Lumbar enterogenous (neurenteric) cyst shown by sagittal **(A)** and coronal **(B)** T1 MRI as an isointense to hypointense mass displacing the conus medullaris *(open arrow)* and cauda equina nerve roots *(arrows)*. The cyst was markedly hyperintense on T2 MRI.

REFERENCES
Dysraphic myelodysplasias

1. Altman NR, Altman DH: MR imaging of spinal dysraphism, *AJNR* 8:533, 1987.
2. Arredondo F, Haughton VM, Hemmy DC, et al: The computed tomographic appearance of the spinal cord in diastematomyelia, *Radiology* 136:685, 1980.
3. Banna M: Syringomyelia in association with posterior fossa cysts, *AJNR* 9:867, 1988.
4. Barkovich A: *Pediatric neuroimaging*, New York, 1980, Raven.
5. Barkovich AJ, Sherman JL, Citrin CM, et al: MR of postoperative syringomyelia, *AJNR* 8:319, 1987.
6. Barnes P: Imaging in spinal dysraphism, *Contemp Diagn Radiol* 13:1, 1990.
7. Barnes P, Lester P, Yamanashi W, et al: MR imaging in spinal dysraphism, *AJNR* 7:465, 1986.
8. Barnes PD, Lester PD, Yamanashi WS, et al: MRI in infants and children with spinal dysraphism, *AJR* 147:339, 1986.
9. Barnes PD, Reynolds AF, Galloway DC, et al: Digital myelography of spinal dysraphism in infancy: preliminary results, *AJNR* 5:208, 1984.
10. Batnitzky S, Price HI, Gaughan MJ, et al: The radiology of syringohydromyelia, *Radiographics* 3:585, 1983.
11. Brooks BS, El Gammal T, Hartlage P, et al: Myelography of sacral agenesis, *AJNR* 2:319, 1981.
12. Brunberg JA, Latchaw RE, Kanal E, et al: Magnetic resonance imaging of spinal dysraphism, *Radiol Clin North Am* 26:181, 1988.
13. Carson JA, Barnes PD, Tunell WP, et al: Imperforate anus: the neurologic implications of sacral abnormalities, *J Pediatr Surg* 19:838, 1984.
14. Cohen M, Edwards M: *MR imaging of children*, Philadelphia, 1990, BC Decker.
15. Currarino G, Coln D, Votteler T: Triad of anorectal, sacral, and presacral anomalies, *AJR* 137:395, 1981.
16. Davis PC, Hoffman JC, Ball TI, et al: Spinal abnormalities in pediatric patients: MR imaging findings compared with clinical, myelographic, and surgical findings, *Radiology* 166:679, 1988.
17. deVries PA, Friedland GW: The staged sequential development of the anus and rectum in human embryos and fetuses, *J Pediatr Surg* 9:755, 1974.
18. Duncan A, Hoare R: Spinal arachnoid cysts in children, *Radiology* 126:423, 1978.
19. Enzmann DR, O'Donohue J, Rubin JB, et al: CSF pulsations within nonneoplastic spinal cord cysts, *AJNR* 8:517, 1987.
20. Filly R, Cordoza J, Goldstein R, et al: Detection of fetal CNS anomalies: a practical level of effort for a routine sonogram, *Radiology* 172:403, 1989.
21. Fitz CR, Harwood-Nash DC: The tethered conus, *AJR* 125:515, 1975.
22. Fredericks B, Boldt D, Tress B, et al: Diseases of the spinal canal in children with noncontrast CT, *AJNR* 10:1233, 1989.
23. Gabriel R, McComb J: Malformations of the CNS. In Menkes J, editor: *Textbook of child neurology*, ed 3, Philadelphia, 1985, Lea & Febiger.
24. Geremia GK, Russell EJ, Clasen RA: MR imaging characteristics of a neurenteric cyst, *AJNR* 9:978, 1988.
25. Hafeez M, Tihansky DP: Intraspinal tumor with lumbosacral agenesis, *AJNR* 5:481, 1984.
26. Harwood-Nash D, Fitz C: *Neuroradiology in infants and children*, St Louis, 1976, Mosby – Year Book.
27. Heinz ER, Rosenbaum AW, Scarff TB, et al: Tethered spinal cord following meningomyelocele repair, *Radiology* 131:153, 1979.
28. Hilal SK, Marton D, Pollack E: Diastematomyelia in children, *Radiology* 112:609, 1974.
29. Hoffman H, Epstein F, editors: *Disorders of the developing nervous system: diagnosis and treatment*, Boston, 1986, Blackwell.
30. Holmes GL, Trader S, Ignatiadis P: Intraspinal enterogenous cysts, *Am J Dis Child* 132:906, 1978.
31. Holzman R, editor: *The tethered spinal cord*, New York, 1985, Thieme-Stratton.
32. Hood RW, Riseborough EJ, Nehme A-M, et al: Diastematomyelia and structural spinal deformities, *J Bone Joint Surg* 62:520, 1980.
33. James C, Lassman L: *Spinal dysraphism*, London, 1972, Butterworths.
34. Kangarloo H, Gold RH, Diament MJ, et al: High-resolution spinal sonography in infants, *AJR* 142:1243, 1984.
35. Kaplan JO, Quencer RM: The occult tethered conus syndrome in the adult, *Radiology* 137:387, 1980.
36. Lee BCP, Zimmerman RD, Manning JJ, et al: MR imaging of syringomyelia and hydromyelia, *AJR* 144:1149, 1985.
37. McConnell JR, Mawk JR, Kendall JD: Percutaneous balloon myelotomy for treatment of hydromyelia: technical note, *AJNR* 9:875, 1988.

38. McLaurin R, Schut L, Venes J, et al, editors: *Pediatric neurosurgery,* ed 2, Philadelphia, 1989, WB Saunders.

39. Naidich TP, Harwood-Nash DC: Diastematomyelia: hemicord and meningeal sheaths; single and double arachnoid and dural tubes, *AJNR* 4:633, 1983.

40. Naidich TP, Fernbach SK, McLone DG, et al: Sonography of the caudal spine and back: congenital anomalies in children, *AJNR* 5:221, 1984.

41. Naidich TP, McLone DG, Mutluer S: A new understanding of dorsal dysraphism with lipoma (lipomyeloschisis): radiologic evaluation and surgical correction, *AJR* 140:1065, 1983.

42. Naidich T, Quencer R, editors: *Clinical neurosonography,* New York, 1987, Springer-Verlag.

43. Nelson MD, Bracchi M, Naidich TP, et al: The natural history of repaired myelomeningocele, *Radiographics* 8:695, 1988.

44. Neuhauser EBD, Harris GBC, Berrett A: Roentgenographic features of neurenteric cysts, *AJR* 79:235, 1958.

45. Nokes SR, Murtagh FR, Jones JD, et al: Childhood scoliosis: MR imaging, *Radiology* 164:791, 1987.

46. Packer RJ, Zimmerman RA, Sutton LN, et al: Magnetic resonance imaging of spinal cord disease in childhood, *Pediatrics* 78:251, 1986.

47. Petterson H, Harwood-Nash D: *CT and myelography of the pediatric spine and cord,* New York, 1982, Springer-Verlag.

48. Pojunas K, Williams AL, Daniels DL, et al: Syringomyelia and hydromyelia: magnetic resonance evaluation, *Radiology* 153:679, 1984.

49. Quencer RM, Montalvo BM, Naidich TP, et al: Intraoperative sonography in spinal dysraphism and syringohydromyelia, *AJNR* 8:329, 1987.

50. Raghaven N, Barkovich AJ, Edwards M, et al: MR imaging in the tethered spinal cord syndrome, *AJNR* 10:27, 1989.

51. Resjo IM, Harwood-Nash DC, Fitz CR, et al: Computed tomographic metrizamide myelography in syringohydromyelia, *Radiology* 131:405, 1979.

52. Roller GJ, Pribram HFW: Lumbosacral intradural lipoma and sacral agenesis, *Radiology* 84:507, 1965.

53. Rubin J, DiPietro M, Chandler W, et al: Spinal ultrasonography: intraoperative and pediatric applications, *Radiol Clin North Am* 26:1, 1988.

54. Samuelsson L, Bergstrom K, Thuomas K-A, et al: MR imaging of syringohydromyelia and Chiari malformations in myelomeningocele patients with scoliosis, *AJNR* 8:539, 1987.

55. Sarwar M, Crelin ES, Kier EL, et al: Experimental cord stretchability and the tethered cord syndrome, *AJNR* 4:641, 1983.

56. Sarwar M, Virapongse C, Bhimani S: Primary tethered cord syndrome: a new hypothesis of its origin, *AJNR* 5:235, 1984.

57. Scatliff JR, Kendall B, Kingsley DPE, et al: Closed spinal dysraphism: analysis of clinical, radiological, and surgical findings in 104 consecutive patients, *AJR* 152:1049, 1989.

58. Scatliff JH, Till K, Hoare RD: Incomplete, false, and true diastematomyelia, *Radiology* 116:349, 1975.

59. Schlesinger AE, Naidich TP, Quencer RM: Concurrent hydromyelia and diastematomyelia, *AJNR* 7:473, 1986.

60. Scotti G, Musgrave MA, Harwood-Nash DC, et al: Diastematomyelia in children: metrizamide and CT metrizamide myelography, *AJR* 135:1225, 1980.

61. Sherman JL, Barkovich AJ, Citrin CM: The MR appearance of syringomyelia: new observations, *AJR* 148:381, 1987.

62. Sundaram M, Awwad E: MRI of arachnoid cysts of the sacrum, *AJR* 146:359, 1986.

63. Tunell WP, Austin JC, Barnes PD, et al: Neuroradiologic evaluation of sacral abnormalities in imperforate anus complex, *J Pediatr Surg* 22:58, 1987.

64. Vade A, Kennard D: Lipomeningomyelocystocele, *AJNR* 8:375, 1987.

65. van der Knaap MS, Valk J: Classification of congenital abnormalities of the CNS, *AJNR* 9:315, 1988.

66. Weinstein MA, Rothner AD, Duchesneau P, et al: Computed tomography in diastematomyelia, *Radiology* 118:609, 1975.

67. Wolpert SM, Anderson M, Scott RM, et al: Chiari II malformation: MR imaging evaluation, *AJNR* 8:783, 1987.

68. Zieger M, Dorr V, Schulz R: Pediatric spinal sonography. Part II. Malformations and mass lesions, *Pediatr Radiol* 18:105, 1988.

Spinal vascular anomalies

DEVELOPMENTAL AND ANATOMICAL ASPECTS

Embryologically, primitive vessels arise from angioblasts of mesodermal origin. The vessels extend from the yolk sac or primitive gut to reach the neural plate as it closes to form the neural tube.[1,9] The arteries, veins, and capillaries are formed from the primitive extraneural vascular plexus and subsequently undergo vascular wall development and intercommunicate. Three basic layers of vessels develop, that is, for the integument, the dura, and the pial-covered CNS. An adult pattern of vascular branching with vessel wall maturation ensues. More specifically for the spine, there is segmental aortic origin of paired vessels at 2 to 3 weeks of gestation that extend toward the neural tube along nerve roots and form branches to the skin, spinal column, meninges, and spinal cord. A subpial capillary network is formed on the cord surface with multiple anastomoses. Between 3 and 6 weeks separation occurs into anterior and posterior capillary systems along with formation of longitudinal perimedullary venous channels. There is capillary penetration of the cord anteriorly and posteriorly with formation of the central artery in the anterior median sulcus. From 6 weeks to 4 months there is craniocaudal formation of the adult vascular pattern with final maturation resulting in a single anterior spinal artery and double posterior spinal arteries (Figs. 9-61 and 9-62).

The anterior spinal artery has double origin from the terminal paired vertebral arteries. It lies within the anterior median sulcus extending the entire length of the cord and provides arterial supply to the anterior 80% of the cord.[1,9] Other contributions to the anterior spinal artery arise from the ascending cervical and deep cervical branches of the subclavian arteries, the intercostal and lumbar branches of the aorta, and the large artery of Adamkiewicz arising from the aorta in the thoracolumbar region usually from the left side. Large branch contributions may also be encountered at C5-6, or at T5 from the bronchial arteries. The posterior spinal arteries originate from the posterior inferior cerebellar arteries bilaterally and also as 8 to 12 pairs arising dorsolaterally from the intercostal and lumbar arteries. The paired arteries extend along the entire cord length supplying the posterior 20% of the cord. The conus loop at the cord termination is formed by anastomoses between the distal segments of the anterior and posterior spinal arteries.

In the lower cervical, thoracic, and lumbar spine the intercostal and lumbar arteries, respectively, originate from the dorsal aorta and randomly give rise to radiculomedullary branches, which segmentally anastomose with the anterior and posterior spinal arteries (Fig. 9-63). The midthoracic portion of the spinal cord is the largest and most critical arterial border zone because of the smaller calibre of the anterior and posterior spinal arteries and because of fewer radiculomedullary branches at this level. The spinal column is supplied by nutrient branches arising from these same intercostal and lumbar branches. As a result of ontogenic

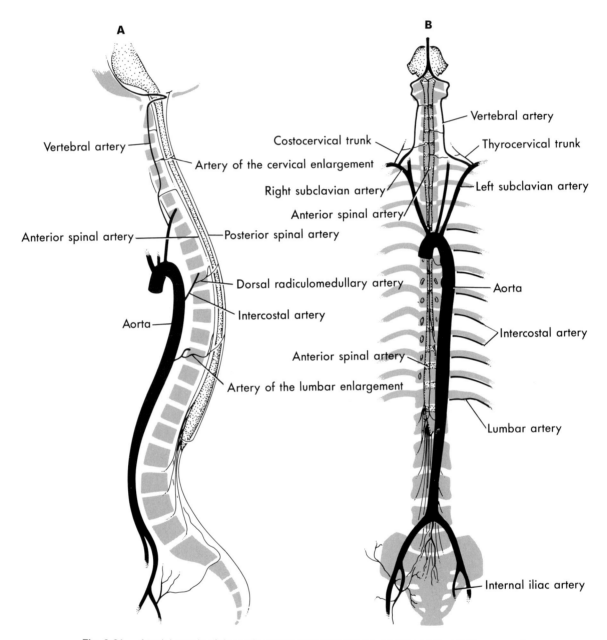

Fig. 9-61   Arterial supply of the entire spinal cord from the lateral **(A)** and frontal **(B)** perspectives. (Modified from Doppman J, et al: *Selective arteriography of the spinal cord,* St Louis, 1969, Warren H. Green.

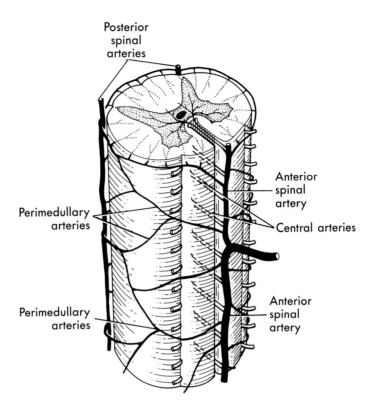

Fig. 9-62   The spinal cord arterial network. (Modified from Pia H, Djindjin R: *Spinal angiomas,* New York, 1978, Springer-Verlag.)

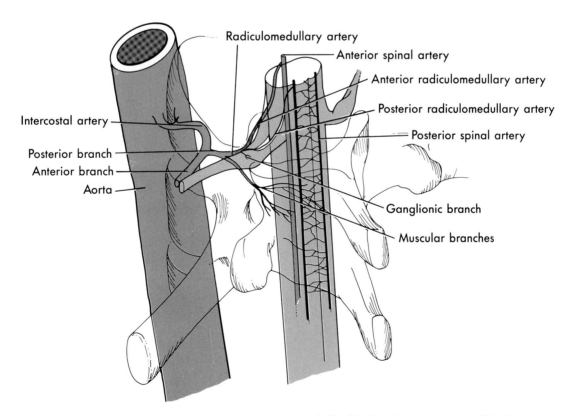

Fig. 9-63   Segmental arterial supply of the spinal cord. (Modified from Doppman J, et al: *Selective arteriography of the spinal cord,* St Louis, 1969, Warren H. Green.)

ascension of the lower cord, there is progressively steeper ascent of the arterial feeders at the lower spinal levels, with more acute hairpin configurations.

Venous drainage of the spinal cord is directed into the anterior and posterior spinal veins.[1,9] The posterior spinal vein is the major venous channel of the cord; it is a single large midline vessel within the posterior median sulcus that extends the entire cord length, draining the posterior 70% of the cord. Smaller veins follow the posterior spinal arteries and drain into the posterior main trunk. The smaller single or double anterior spinal vein follows the anterior spinal artery. All of these are drained by a series of numerous anastomosing radiculomedullary veins that drain into segmental intervertebral veins and then into the ascending lumbar or azygos systems. The epidural and external vertebral venous plexuses also drain via the intervertebral veins but without direct transdural anastomoses between the intradural and epidural systems.

BIOLOGICAL BASIS OF VASCULAR ANOMALIES

Vascular anomalies are infrequent but important causes of spinal neurological deficits in childhood. Most if not all of the vascular anomalies are of maldevelopmental origin. It is theorized that the primary developmental disorder probably occurs in the second stage of vascular formation at around 6 weeks of gestation.[9] As a result, there is persistence of thin-walled, tortuous vessels with defective media and elastica, primitive capillary and precapillary channels, and abnormal arteriovenous shunts. Also, there are often persistent supernumerary segmental arterial feeders or occasional segmental neurocutaneous vascular anomalies of the skin, dura, and CNS. Vascular anomalies of childhood in general may be classified according to the Mulliken and Glowacki classification based on biological criteria including histological and clinical characteristics as follows: vascular malformations, vascular tumors, and angiodysplastic syndromes[3,7,8] (see box above).

Vascular malformations

Vascular malformations are true structural anomalies representing inborn errors of vascular morphology and characterized by normal rates of endothelial turnover. These are congenital (that is, present at birth), although some may go undetected until later in life. These may begin as subtle vascular wall abnormalities and subsequently undergo progressive ectasia and increase in size commensurate with growth of the child. Sudden increases in size may be caused by changes in flow or pressure, collateral vascularization, hormonal changes, trauma, infection, or hemorrhage. Histologically, there is progressive ectasia of structurally abnormal vessels or channels lined with flat endothelium. Transient cellular hyperplasia is occasionally seen only as reactive after trauma, surgery, or other insult.

Vascular malformations may be subdivided into capillary, venous, arterial (with or without fistulae), and lymphatic subtypes.[8] Malformations may be of a single

---

VASCULAR ANOMALIES
VASCULAR MALFORMATIONS
Arterial ± fistulae
Capillary
Telangiectasias
Venous
Lymphatic
Combined
Cavernous angioma
VASCULAR TUMORS
Hemangiomas
ANGIODYSPLASTIC SYNDROMES
Sturge-Weber
Osler-Weber-Rendu
Klippel-Trenaunay-Weber

---

morphology, although combined morphologies are common. The anomalies may be further subclassified according to dynamics as low flow malformations (capillary, venous, lymphatic, or combined) or high flow malformations (for example, combined arteriovenous). These are diffuse lesions that increase in size by progressive ectasia, not by cellular proliferation, and as a rule do not undergo involution and do not respond to steroid therapy. Angiographically, low flow malformations demonstrate ectatic channels and phleboliths (for example, venous malformation), whereas high flow anomalies reveal enlarged tortuous arteries with arteriovenous shunting (that is, arteriovenous malformations [AVMs]). Low flow malformations may be associated with bony hypertrophy, distortion, elongation, or hypoplasia, whereas high flow malformations may produce osteopenic destruction, distortion, or occasional hypertrophy.

Vascular tumors

Hemangiomas are common benign vascular neoplasms of infancy.[8] These are rarely present at birth but characteristically undergo rapid postnatal enlargement or growth with endothelial proliferation, followed by a prolonged period of involution. Commonly there is proliferation forming a large hypercellular tumor with secondary formation of tortuous, dilated, feeding arterial and draining venous channels within and around the mass. These occasionally may be seen in older children or adolescents. These are usually expanding circumscribed tumors exerting mass effect on adjacent structures, often with bony changes. Platelet trapping and profound thrombocytopenia (Kasabach-Merritt syndrome) may occur along with occasional secondary consumptive coagulopathy. A true disseminated intravascular coagulation syndrome, however, is more often associated with vascular malformations, particularly the venous type. During the initial rapid proliferative phase, hemangi-

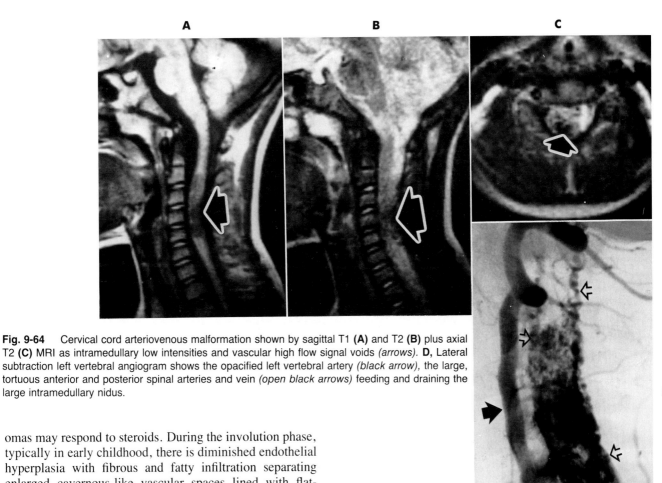

Fig. 9-64   Cervical cord arteriovenous malformation shown by sagittal T1 **(A)** and T2 **(B)** plus axial T2 **(C)** MRI as intramedullary low intensities and vascular high flow signal voids *(arrows)*. **D**, Lateral subtraction left vertebral angiogram shows the opacified left vertebral artery *(black arrow)*, the large, tortuous anterior and posterior spinal arteries and vein *(open black arrows)* feeding and draining the large intramedullary nidus.

omas may respond to steroids. During the involution phase, typically in early childhood, there is diminished endothelial hyperplasia with fibrous and fatty infiltration separating enlarged cavernous-like vascular spaces lined with flattened-appearing endothelium. Angiographically, hemangiomas are circumscribed masses with prominent staining and large peripheral vessels. Angiodysplastic syndromes are primarily discussed in Chapter 8.

SPINAL VASCULAR ANOMALIES

Vascular anomalies are infrequent but important causes of spinal neurological symptoms and signs in childhood.[1,3,9] Spinal vascular anomalies may be further classified according to spine level, anatomical involvement, and morphologic type. Vascular anomalies may occur at the cervical, thoracic, lumbar, or at multiple levels. These may be isolated and arise in extradural, intradural, or intramedullary locations. Multiple or contiguous multilayer anomalies may occur along the same segmental distribution (metameric malformations). The most common morphologic types include combined arteriovenous malformations, hemangiomas, cavernous angiomas, and, less often, arterial, capillary (telangiectatic), venous (variceal), or lymphatic malformations.[3,9] More than one morphologic type may occur in the same patient, especially in the angiodysplastic syndromes.

Arteriovenous malformations

Arteriovenous malformations (AVMs) are by far the most common type of vascular anomalies involving the spinal

neuraxis.[1-3,5,6,9] Three main groups have been described: spinal cord (intramedullary), spinal dural (radiculomedullary), and metameric (segmental multilayer).[3] Clinical presentations include pain, myelopathy, or radiculopathy due to intramedullary hemorrhage (hematomyelia), subarachnoid hemorrhage, posthemorrhage arachnoiditis, thrombotic vascular occlusion, cord or nerve root compression, steal ischemia, or venous congestive ischemia. Characteristic clinical syndromes associated with spinal AVMs include angiodysplasias, Cobb syndrome (metameric angiomatosis), and Foix-Alajouanine syndrome (subacute necrotizing myelitis).

SPINAL CORD AVMS. Spinal cord AVMs are the most common type of AVMs occurring in childhood and adolescence.[9] This juvenile form is a subpial perimedullary or intramedullary malformation of the high flow type, usually supplied by multiple arterial pedicles arising more often from the anterior than the posterior spinal arteries (Figs. 9-64 to 9-66). There are multiple AV shunts with

A B C

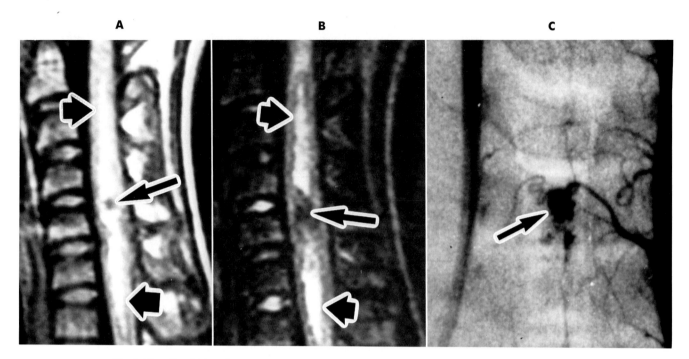

Fig. 9-65 Cervical cord arteriovenous malformation with intramedullary hemorrhage (hematomyelia) shown by sagittal T1 **(A)** and T2 **(B)** MRI as a large intramedullary high intensity hemorrhage *(short arrows)* with more central vascular flow signal voids *(long arrows)*. **C,** Anterior subtraction left vertebral angiogram demonstrates the AVM nidus *(arrow)*.

A B C

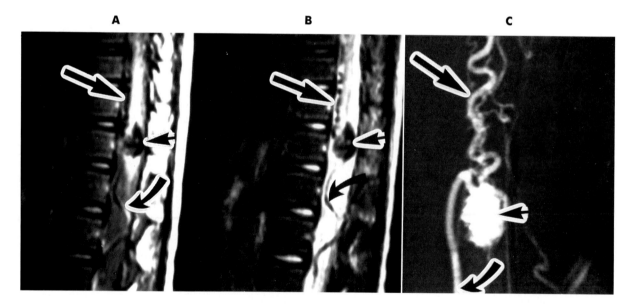

Fig. 9-66 Glomus-type intramedullary arteriovenous malformation of the conus medullaris with hematomyelia. Sagittal p **(A)** and T2 **(B)** MRI show the intramedullary ferrous hypointensities and vascular flow signal voids *(arrowheads)* with a large tortuous anterior spinal artery *(straight arrows)* and a large sinuous draining vein *(curved arrow)*. **C,** Digital subtraction angiography confirms the feeding arterial *(straight arrow)*, nidus *(arrowhead)*, and draining venous *(curved arrow)* components. (Courtesy Dachling Pang, M.D., Children's Hospital of Pittsburg.)

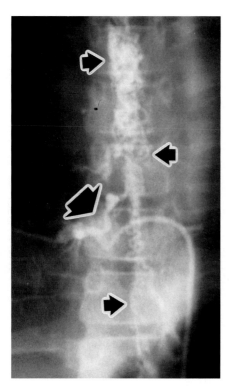

Fig. 9-67 A rare radiculomedullary (dural) arteriovenous malformation in a juvenile male demonstrated by frontal angiography including the nidus or fistula *(large arrow)* and the arterialized longitudinal perimedullary venous plexus *(smaller arrows).*

aneurysmally dilated venous channels. These usually occur at the cervical, cervicothoracic, or thoracolumbar level, are occasionally voluminous and fill the entire canal, or involve long segments. The clinical presentations are usually related to subarachnoid hemorrhage, intramedullary hemorrhage, or steal ischemia.

SPINAL DURAL AVMS. Spinal dural AVMs primarily occur after childhood and may actually be acquired, especially in the later decades.[5,9] These are slow flow malformations usually with single, or occasionally multiple, arterial feeders and slow circulation time via the minute AV fistulae or as an angiomatous network (glomus) with perimedullary venous drainage (Fig. 9-67). The arterial feeder usually originates from a normal-sized intercostal or lumbar segmental artery and supplies the caudal end, cranial end, or, rarely, the center of the AVM. Often there is a direct microscopic fistula between the dural branch of the radiculomedullary artery and the arterialized dorsal extramedullary posterolateral and longitudinal coronal venous plexus. The AVM nidus or fistula is usually found along the nerve root sleeve within the intervertebral foramen. Occasionally the nidus is a localized glomus (angiomatous or telangiectatic network) involving a short segment of the cord. Spinal dural AVMs are also referred to as *radiculomeningeal AVMs* and may present with Foix-Alajouanine syndrome, an advanced radiculomyelopathy

resulting from subacute necrotizing myelitis due to draining venous congestion and thrombosis with edema or infarction of the cord at that level.

METAMERIC AVMS. Metameric AVMs (Cobb's syndrome) are vascular malformations involving any or all layers along a spinal segment, including the cord, meninges, vertebral column, paraspinal muscles, subcutaneous tissues, and skin.[3,6,9] There may be subarachnoid hemorrhage or root compression due to enlarged veins, or obvious cutaneous malformations along the corresponding dermatome.

Arterial malformations

Pure arterial malformations in this region are rare. This category may include the hypertrophied spinal artery syndrome.[9] This syndrome refers to collateral high flow dilatation and tortuosity of the anterior spinal artery, which produces compressive myelopathy. This is usually associated with chronic aortic occlusive disease (for example, coarctation), but should not to be confused with the ischemic myelopathy that occasionally follows surgery for coarctation. The syndrome has also been described for other arterial occlusive processes, as well as for highly vascular tumors and vascular malformations producing low pressure run-off from anterior spinal artery collaterals.

Telangiectasias and cavernous angiomas

Other less common or rare vascular anomalies of the spinal column or neuraxis that may present with hemorrhage include the so-called occult vascular malformations, that is, telangiectasias and cavernous angiomas.[4,9] As opposed to arteriovenous and venous malformations that can be demonstrated angiographically, telangiectasias and cavernous angiomas characteristically are not revealed by angiography. Telangiectasias are capillary malformations that may be isolated, segmental or diffuse, and subpial or intramedullary. These often present with subarachnoid hemorrhage, hematomyelia, or myelomalacia. Telangiectasias often are associated with radiculomedullary AVMs and cavernous angiomas. Cavernous angiomas have been classified as both a subtype of hemangioma and a subtype of venous malformation. These are usually solitary and circumscribed malformations composed of blood-filled, thin-walled channels. Occasionally there are multiple lesions, particularly in familial cases. These may occur extradurally as vertebral angiomas in the thoracic, cervical, or, less often, lumbar regions and may present with pathological fracture or extradural extension with root or cord compression. The rare intramedullary cavernous angiomas may present with acute or recurrent subarachnoid hemorrhage or intramedullary hemorrhage with dissection and myelopathy (Fig. 9-68).

Venous malformations

Venous malformations are rare cirsoid or racemose varices consisting of one large vein and one or more draining pedicles or as a compact group of veins.[8,9] Occasionally these are cavernous in appearance and have

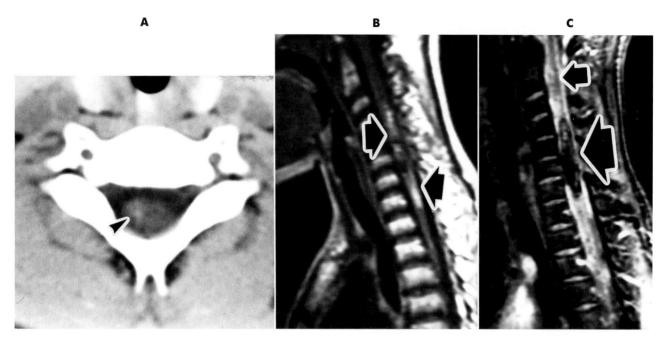

Fig. 9-68 Cervicothoracic intramedullary cavernous angioma with old and recent hemorrhage. **A,** Axial CT shows focal high density within the cord *(arrowhead)*. **B,** Sagittal T1 MRI shows intramedullary high intensities *(arrows)* consistent with methemoglobin. **C,** Sagittal T2 MRI shows low intensity consistent with the combination of deoxyhemoglobin, intracellular methomoglobin, and hemosiderin *(arrows)*. There is extension into the central canal *(smaller arrow)*. Focal gadolinium enhancement was also demonstrated.

been associated with the disseminated intravascular coagulation syndrome. These are slow flow but angiographically demonstrable malformations that are compressible and expand with increased venous pressure (for example, Valsalva maneuver). Often there is a hyalinized or collagenous and adipose stroma, occasionally with secondary inflammation or thrombosis and phlebolith formation (see Chapter 7). These malformations may occur within the vertebral bodies, extradural soft tissues, or, rarely, the intradural or intramedullary compartments. When arising in the latter sites these are probably more often the venous side of a low shunt AVM (for example, radiculomedullary AVM).

Lymphatic malformations

Lymphatic malformations of the spinal column or neuraxis are also unusual in childhood.[8,9] These malformations are composed of anomalous channels and cysts of varying size, shape, and extent (Fig. 9-69). The term *lymphangiectasia* is probably more appropriate than the terms *lymphangioma* or *cystic hygroma*, the latter implying cellular proliferation. Occasionally, extradural or parameningeal lymphatic malformations of the neck or mediastinum may secondarily involve the spinal column or neuraxis. Combined malformations other than the common arteriovenous type include capillary-lymphatic and venous-lymphatic. For instance, Klippel-Trenaunay-Weber syndrome refers to a combined capillary-venous-lymphatic malformation with skeletal overgrowth.

Hemangiomas

Hemangiomas are also rarely encountered along the spinal neuraxis or spinal column in childhood, although they are a common vertebral tumor of adulthood[8,9] (Fig. 9-70). Only rarely do paraspinal hemangiomas extend to involve the intraspinal structures. Hemangioma usually is not included in the differential diagnosis of other blood-vessel origin or vascular tumors (hemangioblastoma, hemangiopericytoma, angiosarcoma, or aneurysmal bone cyst).

Spinal vascular anomalies may be associated with other neural or extraneural vascular lesions, or other dysplastic lesions, in up to 25% of cases.[9] These include metameric and nonmetameric cutaneous, vertebral, visceral, extremity, and other CNS vascular anomalies. Spinal vascular anomalies may also be part of angiodysplastic syndromes, as listed in the box on p. 380, and are more fully presented in Chapter 8. Other CNS abnormalities reportedly occurring with spinal vascular anomalies include CNS neoplasms such as hemangioblastoma, ependymoma, neuroma, and lipoma, as well as CNS dysplastic lesions such as syringohydromyelia, spinal dysraphism, and kyphoscoliosis.

NEUROIMAGING

Plain film abnormalities associated with vascular anomalies range from nonspecific findings of scoliosis, vertebral deformity, paraspinal mass, canal or foraminal widening, pedicle erosion, and rare calcification to the more specific striated appearance characteristic of vertebral involvement in hemangioma.[9]

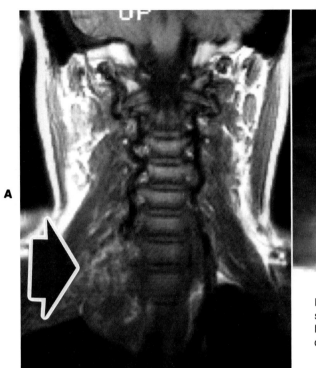

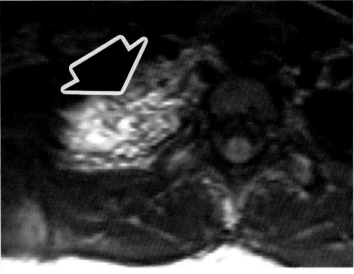

Fig. 9-69 Cervicothoracic paraspinal lymphatic malformation *(arrow)* shown by coronal T1 MR **(A)** as a large mixed isointense to hyperintense lesion. On axial p/T2 MRI **(B)** there is mixed isointensity and hyperintensity consistent with lymph-filled channels and a fibrofatty stroma.

AVMs

High flow AVMs, whether intradural or extradural in location, are demonstrated by MRI (Figs. 9-64 to 9-66) as serpiginous and nodular signal voids on all spin echo sequences using presaturation. High intensity flow enhancement is characteristically present on vascular flow-sensitive gradient echo sequences using gradient moment nulling. AVMs typically have no recognizable soft tissue parenchymal component. The signal voids represent the feeding arteries, nidus, and draining veins, which often cannot be distinguished from one another. In cord AVMs intramedullary and perimedullary vascular signal voids are demonstrated ventrally or ventrally and dorsally[2,6] (Figs. 9-64 to 9-66). There may be associated cord enlargement, hemorrhage, edema, infarction, syrinx, atrophy, or scoliosis (Figs. 9-65 and 9-66). Gradient echo sequences may assist in distinguishing spin echo vascular flow voids (gradient echo high intensity) from acute hemorrhage (deoxyhemoglobin) or mineralization that is also of low intensity on spin echo MRI (gradient echo low intensity.) Methemoglobin in subacute-chronic hemorrhage is readily recognized as high intensity on T1 spin echo images (Fig. 9-65). In dural AVMs the vascular signal voids are demonstrated primarily dorsally as long, serpiginous, posterolateral perimedullary or dorsal intramedullary circumferential flow voids representing the dilated arterialized coronal venous plexus. There may be vascular grooving or scalloping of the cord.[5,6]

Axial T1 or T2 images may be needed to distinguish the intramedullary from the extramedullary type of AVM (Fig.

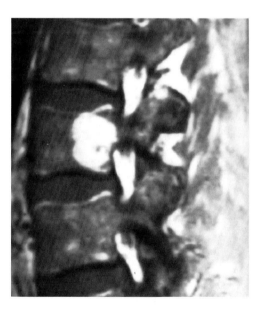

Fig. 9-70 Lumbar vertebral hemangioma shown by sagittal T1 MRI with characteristic fatty hyperintensity. The anomaly remained high intensity on sagittal p image but was low intensity on sagittal T2 MRI. (Courtesy J. Kramer, Beth Israel Hospital, Boston).

9-64). Low intensity CSF pulsation artifacts may cause confusion, particularly on T2-weighted images. These artifacts may be minimized or eliminated using vascular flow compensation techniques (such as gating, presaturation, or gradient moment nulling). Cord edema, infarction, or myelomalacia appear as low intensity lesions on T1-

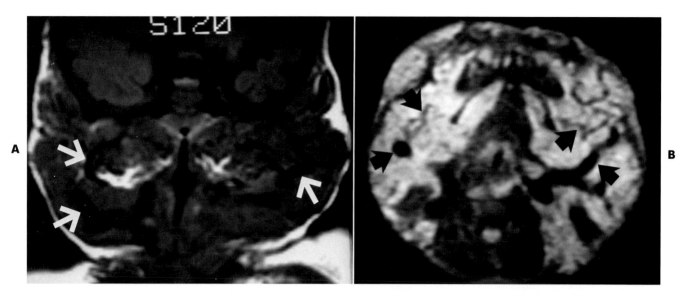

Fig. 9-71 Diffuse proliferating paraspinal hemangioma of the head and neck. **A,** Coronal T1 MRI shows the isointense to hypointense tumor parenchyma with multiple high flow vascular signal voids *(arrows)* and extending to the temporal skull base. **B,** Axial T2 MRI demonstrates diffuse high intensity tumor parenchyma, again with multiple vascular flow signal voids *(arrows)* and cervical paraspinal involvement.

weighted images and as high intensity on proton density and T2-weighted images. Cord enlargement may be present with edema, and cord thinning may be present with chronic infarction or myelomolacia. Syrinx or hydrosyringomyelia may appear as low intensity on T1 and proton density images, with high or low intensity on T2-weighted images depending upon the presence or absence of pulsatile CSF signal voids. The cord may or may not be expanded by the hydrosyrinx. Metameric AVMs are demonstrated as vascular flow signal voids involving more than one compartment or layer.

Telangiectasias and cavernous angiomas

Telangiectatic malformations may be difficult to directly identify as minute signal voids on spin echo images or as small areas of signal high intensity on flow-sensitive gradient echo images. This is particularly true when telangiectasias are associated with other malformations or hemorrhage. Spinal cavernous angiomas have imaging characteristics similar to those arising in the brain (see Chapter 6).[4] These may be identified by CT as high density and iodine-enhancing lesions with or without cord expansion or atrophy (Fig. 9-68). By MRI a rather characteristic pattern often is present including central high intensity with peripheral circumferential low intensity on all sequences plus gadolinium enhancement (Fig. 9-68). The imaging findings correlate with stagnant blood elements and breakdown products of hemoglobin from repeated hemorrhage. There are central methemoglobin high intensities and peripheral hemosiderin low intensities, the latter particularly exaggerated on longer TR sequences. There may be

intramedullary dissection or extension into the central canal. Other diagnostic considerations may include thrombosed AVM, hemorrhagic tumor, trauma, or the rare hemorrhage related to infection.

Venous and lymphatic malformations

Venous malformations of the variceal type may occasionally be demonstrated as branching signal voids on spin echo images and branching high intensities on gradient echo images. The more cavernous-appearing extradural venous malformations and lymphatic malformations are slow flow anomalies and are readily distinguished from AVMs and hemangiomas because of absence of vascular flow voids. However, the cavernous type of venous malformation may be difficult to distinguish from lymphatic malformations, since both contain cystlike areas of watery low intensity on T1 and proton density images that are of high intensity on T2 spin echo and T2/T2* gradient echo images (Fig. 9-69). The more homogeneous-appearing cavernous type of venous malformation may exhibit relatively higher intensity on gradient echo images than on T2 spin echo images. Venous and lymphatic malformations may also exhibit a heterogeneous pattern due to a fibrofatty stroma, calcification, or hemorrhage (Fig. 9-69). Phleboliths and gadolinium enhancement may distinguish venous from lymphatic malformations (see Chapter 7).

Hemangiomas

Extradural paraspinal hemangiomas are circumscribed masses demonstrating a heterogeneous intensity pattern with isointensity to low intensity on T1 images plus isointensity to high intensity on proton density and T2 spin echo sequences (Fig. 9-71). The vertebral hemangiomas are often of high intensity on T1-weighted images due to associated fat (Fig. 9-70). Particularly in the paraspinal hemangiomas there is evidence of rapid blood flow as spin echo signal voids and gradient echo flow enhancement corresponding to enlarged arterial and venous channels. Parenchymal gadolinium enhancement is expected.

Vascular anomalies may be treated by surgical excision, endovascular embolization, or by combined interventional and surgical techniques.[1,3,8-11] The goal is obliteration of the anomaly with preservation of blood flow to normal structures.

REFERENCES
Spinal vascular anomalies

1. Doppman J, DiChiro G, Ommaya A: *Selective arteriography of the spinal cord,* St Louis, 1969, Warren H. Green.
2. Dormant D, Gelbert F, Assouline E, et al: MR imaging of spinal cord AVMs, *AJNR* 9:833, 1988.
3. Eskridge J: Interventional neuroradiology, *Radiology* 172:991, 1989.
4. Fontaine S, Melanson D, Cosgrove R: Cavernous hemangiomas of the spinal cord: MR imaging, *Radiology* 166:839, 1988.
5. Masaryk T, Ross J, Modic M, et al: Radiculomeningeal vascular malformations of the spine: MR imaging, *Radiology* 164:845, 1987.
6. Minami S, Sasoh T, Nishimura K, et al: Spinal arteriovenous malformations: MR imaging, *Radiology* 169:109, 1988.
7. Mulliken J, Glowacki J: Hemangiomas and vascular malformations in infants and children: A classification based on endothelial characteristics, *Plast Reconstr Surg* 69:412, 1982.
8. Mulliken J, Young E: *Vascular birthmarks: hemangiomas and malformations,* Philadelphia, 1988, WB Saunders.
9. Pia H, Djindjian R, editors: *Spinal angiomas,* New York, 1978, Springer-Verlag.
10. Theron J, Cosgrove R, Melanson D: Spinal AVMs: advances in therapeutic embolization, *Radiology* 158:163, 1986.
11. Vinuela F, Dion J, Lylyk P, et al: Update on interventional neuroradiology, *AJR* 153:23, 1989.

Craniocervical anomalies

Abnormalities of the craniocervical junction and cervical spine are relatively frequent causes of neurological symptoms and signs in childhood and adolescence.* A working knowledge of the development, anatomy, and physiology of this region is important in the clinical and radiological management of patients with these anomalies. The basic developmental and anatomical aspects have been presented in the initial section of this chapter. The more important abnormalities of this region are listed in the box above. The most common anomalies are those resulting from faulty assimilation, atlantooccipital and cervical fusion, occipital dysplasia, and ligamentous laxity.† More often than not, multiple anomalies occur in the same patient. Also, it is important to remember that ligamentous deficiency commonly accompanies bony anomalies in this region. In this section, each anomaly is discussed in the order of frequency of occurrence.

---

*References 4, 16, 18, 28, 29, 37, 39, 41.
†References 5, 16, 18, 27, 30, 37, 41

CRANIOCERVICAL ANOMALIES

FAULTY ASSIMILATION (OCCIPITAL VERTEBRAE)
Odontoid anomalies, including os odontoideum
Basioccipital fissures
Third occipital condyle
Basilar processes
Bipartite atlantal facets

ATLANTOOCCIPITAL AND CERVICAL FUSION
Klippel-Feil anomaly
Occipitalization of the atlas
Paracondylar process
Epitransverse process

OCCIPITAL DYSPLASIAS
Constricted foramen magnum
Basilar impression
Condylar hypoplasia

LIGAMENTOUS LAXITY
Atlantoaxial instability
Atlantooccipital instability

CLINICAL MANIFESTATIONS

Clinical presentations in childhood and adolescence include torticollis, craniofacial and craniocervical dysmorphism, abnormal range of motion, headache, neck pain, neck mass, or clicking.[6,9,16,18] Craniocervical anomalies are commonly associated with genetic or chromosomal syndromes including Down's syndrome, achondroplasia, and others. Often there is associated kyphosis or scoliosis. Neural, vascular, or CSF compromise often occurs at the craniocervical junction and leads to motor or sensory radiculopathy or myelopathy, cerebellar or vestibular symptoms or signs, brain stem level deficits, or vertebral basilar insufficiency. Occasionally the anomalies are discovered incidentally on plain films after head and neck trauma or when there are neurological deficits out of proportion to the history of trauma. Occasionally there is the initial clinical suspicion of neurodegenerative disorder, neoplastic process, or trauma.

IMAGING CONSIDERATIONS

Radiological evaluation includes frontal and lateral plain films of the cervical spine and skull base. The open-mouth frontal view of the atlantooccipital and atlantoaxial articulations is particularly important. Occasionally, oblique views are helpful to assess the facets and foramina. The nature and extent of the anomalies may not be obvious in infancy because of incomplete ossification.[16,41] Voluntary flexion and extension lateral films or fluoroscopy is important to evaluate mobility or instability. Frontal and lateral tomography or CT with coronal, sagittal, or oblique reformatting is usually necessary for diagnosis and complete delineation of the anomaly or complex of anomalies. Axial CT may be preferable to Towne's or submentovertex plain films to evaluate the foramen magnum. Direct coronal CT may in fact be contraindicated, particularly in cases of

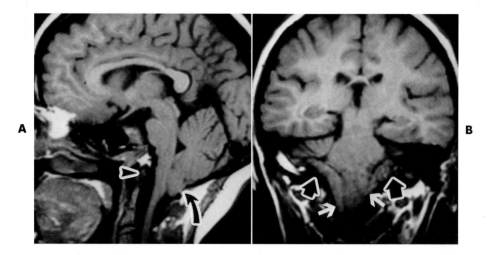

Fig. 9-72   Symptomatic basilar impression of unknown origin demonstrated by sagittal **(A)** and coronal **(B)** T1 MRI including upward angulation of the margins of the foramen magnum *(black arrows,* **B** *)* and high position of the dens *(arrowhead,* **A** *)* with relatively low position and compressive deformity of the medulla, pons, inferior cerebellar vermis, and tonsils *(curved arrow,* **A**; *white arrows,* **B***).*

instability. MRI is now preferred to myelography or myelographic CT to evaluate neuroanatomy for neural, vascular, and CSF compartment involvement or for underlying neural dysplasias.[25,26,38] There may be brain stem, cerebellar, outlet fourth ventricular, cervical cord, vertebrobasilar arterial or anterior spinal artery compromise, and infarction, atrophy, hydrocephalus, or hydrosyringomyelia. Dural ectasia, Chiari I malformation, or diastematomyelia may be present. The latter neural dysplasias may be suggested on plain films by spinal canal enlargement. It is critically important to fully delineate the primary and associated anomalies in each case. Multiple imaging modalities are usually required, especially for surgical planning.

BASILAR IMPRESSION

Basilar impression (BI), or basilar invagination, refers to occipital dysplasia with upward displacement of the margins of the foramen magnum into the posterior fossa.[2,16,18,37,41] The medial rims are curved upward, whereas the more lateral or paracondylar occipital bones are angled downward. There is reduced posterior fossa volume, an irregularly shaped foramen magnum, short vertical clivus, and high odontoid position relative to McGregor's line and McRae's line (Fig. 9-72). BI is not to be confused with platybasia, which refers to a flattened or increased base angle, that is, the intersection of the plane of the anterior cranial fossa with that of the clivus. This is usually of anthropomorphic interest only.

Primary BI may be of idiopathic, familial, or developmental in origin and is commonly associated with other craniocervical anomalies and syndromes, including occipitalization of the atlas, atlas hypoplasia (for example, absent C1 facet), bifid posterior C1 arch, odontoid anomalies, vertebral artery anomalies, Klippel-Feil syndrome, Down's syndrome, achondroplasia, mucopolysaccharidoses, cleidocranial dysplasia, and osteogenesis imperfecta. Secondary or acquired BI due to osseous softening has been reported with osteomalacia, rickets, renal osteodystrophy, rheumatoid arthritis, neurofibromatosis, ankylosing spondylitis, Paget's disease, fibrous dysplasia, hypothyroidism, hyperparathyroidism, and, rarely, neoplasia, infection, or trauma (for example, birth trauma).

BI occurs only in the upright child. Clinical manifestations usually are related to craniocervical dysmorphism and neural, CSF, or vascular compromise by bone (for example, the dens) or dural bands. Only occasionally will a localized indentation of the neural or vascular structures be apparent by MRI. Associated hydrocephalus, hydrosyringomyelia, and Chiari I malformation may be seen. Treatment may consist of occipital craniectomy with excision of the posterior rim of the foramen magnum, bilateral cervical laminectomy, lysis of dural-arachnoid bands or adhesions, dural grafting, and, if unstable, posterior cervical fusion.

KLIPPEL-FEIL ANOMALY

Klippel-Feil anomaly or syndrome refers to any congenital bony fusion of the cervical spine, whether localized, multisegmental, or diffuse.[*] The anomaly probably results from failure of normal segmentation of the cervical somites between the third and eighth weeks of gestation. The simplest form may be a single-level block vertebra (Fig. 9-73). Often, however, there is multilevel vertebral involvement with absent or hypoplastic disk spaces, as well as tall and narrow or flat and wide vertebral bodies (Fig. 9-74). The abnormal fusion may not be obvious in infancy because of incomplete ossification. There may be isolated or additional fusions of the posterior elements, especially of

---

*References 15, 16, 18, 19, 28, 33, 41.

A   B   C

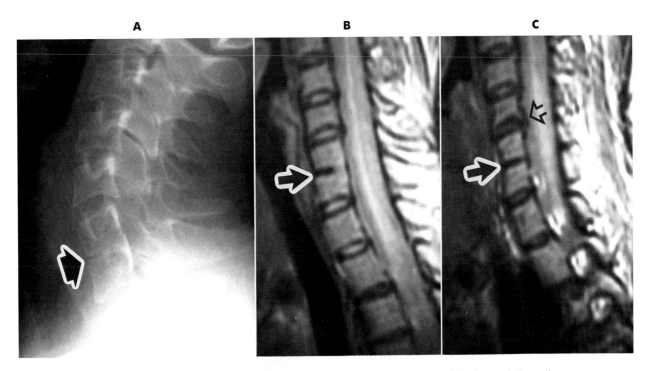

Fig. 9-73 Klippel-Feil anomaly with single block vertebral involvement at C6-7 *(arrows)* shown by lateral plain film **(A)** and sagittal p MRI **(B and C)**. Symptomatic disk protrusion *(open arrow, C)* is demonstrated at the hypermobile next higher level (C5-6).

the laminae. Occasionally the posterior arches are bifid or absent. Occipitalization of the atlas also may be a component of the syndrome, along with basilar impression or anomalies of the dens. The fusion anomalies may extend into the thoracic spine and produce congenital scoliosis.

The classical triad of Klippel-Feil syndrome—low posterior hairline, short webbed neck, and limited range of neck motion—is present in less than half of the cases, including the associated Sprengel's deformity of the scapula with a bridging omovertebral bone. Other reported associations are scoliosis, kyphosis, renal anomalies, congenital heart disease, hearing loss, petrous-temporal anomalies, and limb and digit anomalies.[18,19] Accompanying neurological syndromes include ptosis, Duane's contracture, lateral rectus palsy, facial nerve palsy, and synkinesis. Clinical manifestations more directly related to Klippel-Feil anomaly are those related to the craniocervical dysmorphia (for example, torticollis), hypermobility or instability at unfused segments, and early degenerative disease of the cervical spinal column (Figs. 9-73 and 9-74). There may be spinal canal or intervertebral foraminal narrowing due to any of the following alone or in combination: stenosis, osteophytic spurring, vertebral subluxation, facet arthropathy, disk protrusion, or ligamentous hypertrophy (Figs. 9-73 and 9-74).

As a result there may be nerve root, cord, or cervicomedullary compressive symptoms and signs, which are often exaggerated by minor trauma. Younger patients with upper segment instability are often at greater risk than patients with short segment or lower cervical spinal fusions. Patterns

of involvement that are high risk for early instability or degenerative disease include (1) C2-3 fusion with occipitalization of the atlas and odontoid hypermobility producing cervicomedullary compression, (2) long, multisegment fusion and abnormal craniocervical junction with dens-atlas ring anomaly, and (3) single open interspace between two fused segments.[18,19,33] Associated neural dysplasias (Fig. 9-75) that may further complicate management include Chiari I malformation, hydrosyringomyelia, and diastematomyelia (usually of the nonseptate type). Treatment may require surgical laminectomy for decompression, fusion for stabilization, or both. The clinical and radiological findings occasionally may be mimicked by the fusion deformities of childhood arthritis (juvenile rheumatoid arthritis, ankylosing spondylitis) or the fusion deformities following osteomyelitis (for example, tuberculosis).

OCCIPITALIZATION OF THE ATLAS

Occipitalization of the atlas refers to congenital fusion of the atlas to the occiput. The condition is also known as occipitocervical synostosis, assimilation of the atlas, and occipitocervical fusion.[9,16,18,37] The anomaly probably results from failure of segmentation of the last occipital and first cervical sclerotomes and the hypochordal bow. The fusion may be partial or complete and ranges from total occipital incorporation of the atlas to a bony or fibrous atlantooccipital band. The most common type is assimilation of the anterior arch into the anterior rim of the foramen magnum with a nonfunctioning atlantooccipital articulation and flexion occurring at the atlantoaxial joints (Fig. 9-76).

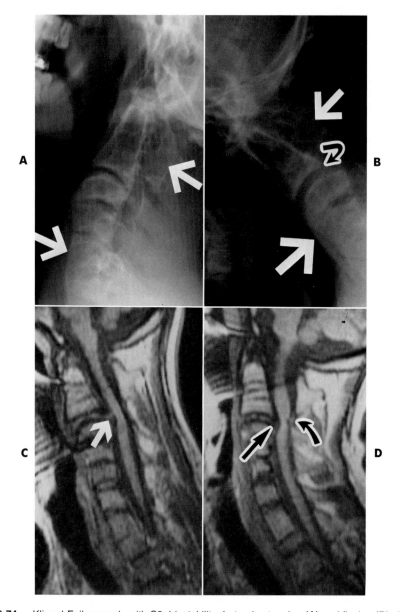

Fig. 9-74   Klippel-Feil anomaly with C3-4 instability. Lateral extension **(A)** and flexion **(B)** plain films show segmental fusions *(large white arrows)* above and below C3-4 with hypermobility in flexion at C3-4 *(curved black arrow,* **B** *)*. Flexion sagittal T1 MRI **(C)** shows C3-4 disk protrusion *(arrow)* and anterior cord impression, whereas extension sagittal T1 MRI **(D)** shows anterior disk protrusion *(straight arrow)* and additional ligamentum flavum buckling *(curved arrow)* with anterior and posterior cord impression, respectively, at the same level. (From Hall J, et al: *J Bone Joint Surg* 72:460, 1990.)

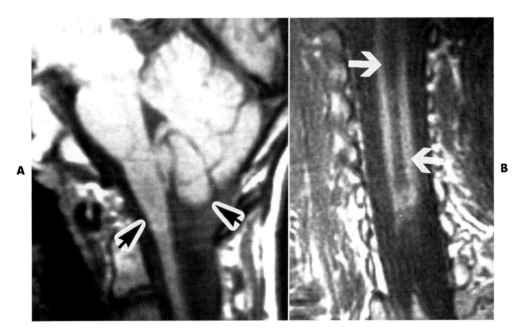

Fig. 9-75   Klippel-Feil anomaly shown by sagittal **(A)** and coronal **(B)** T1 MRI demonstrating Chiari I malformation *(black arrows)* and incomplete sagittal clefting of the cervical cord *(white arrows)*.

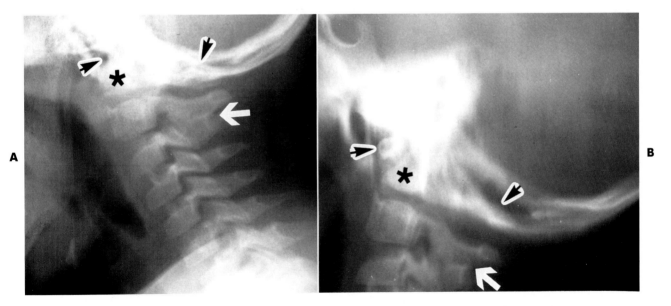

Fig. 9-76   Occipitalization of the atlas demonstrated by lateral plain film **(A)** and lateral tomography **(B)** with fusion of the C2-3 neural arches *(white arrows)*, assimilation of the anterior and the posterior atlas arch into the occiput *(black arrows)*, and high-placed dens *(asterisk)*.

Usually there is associated hypoplasia or absence of the posterior atlas arch. A high-positioned, hypoplastic dens at the anterior border of the foramen magnum may reduce the anteroposterior diameter of the foramen. Rarely is there isolated or associated assimilation of the posterior C1 arch. The occipitalization or fusion may be asymmetrical or unilateral, for example, involving the lateral mass or transverse process of C1. The fusion may be difficult to identify in infancy because of incomplete ossification. Often there is additional basilar invagination, Klippel-Feil anomaly including C2-3 fusion (in more than two thirds of cases), occipital vertebra, or condylar hypoplasia (Fig. 9-76).

Often there is transverse ligamentous laxity with atlanto-axial instability. A thickened posterior constricting dural band, representing a remnant of the posterior arch of C1 or C2, may encroach on and groove the cervical cord or medulla. Chiari I malformation, hydrosyringomyelia, or diastematomyelia (usually without a septum) occasionally may occur. The clinical manifestations are related to the craniocervical dysmorphia (such as torticollis), as well as neural, CSF, or vascular compression or constriction. This may occur anteriorly as related to the odontoid, or posteriorly as related to the posterior foramen magnum or to posterior dural bands. Treatment usually involves surgical decompression of the foramen magnum either by suboccipital craniectomy, posterior C1 laminectomy, lysis of dural bands, or odontoidectomy. Bony fusion may be necessary for associated atlantoaxial instability.

ODONTOID ANOMALIES

Important odontoid anomalies occurring in childhood and adolescence include aplasia, hypoplasia, and os odontoideum.* Aplasia is very rare and is recognized on frontal open-mouth views or frontal tomography as absence of the dens body to below the level of the lateral articular masses. Hypoplasia is more common and is recognized as a short dens projecting from the axis body to just above the lateral articular masses. The os odontoideum is probably a proatlas remnant and one variation of the persistent, nonassimilated occipital vertebra. Another theory of os odontoideum is that the ossicle represents a hypertrophied ossiculum terminale. Associated hypoplasia of the dens is almost always present and often there is a wide gap between the dens and the ossicle (Figs. 9-77 to 9-79). The ossicle is usually oval and of variable size in direct proportion to the degree of dens hypoplasia (larger os with severe dens hypoplasia). The ossicle may be located near the expected location of the dens tip (orthotopic os) or near the basion (dystopic os). The ossicle may be difficult to visualize on plain films, and tomography or CT may be required for confirmation. The dystopic ossicle may be fused to or articulate via pseudoarthrosis with the clivus at the basion (Fig. 9-77). In other cases the ossicle may appear fixed to the anterior arch of the atlas in flexion and extension. Occasionally there is

*References 12, 16, 18, 20, 37, 41.

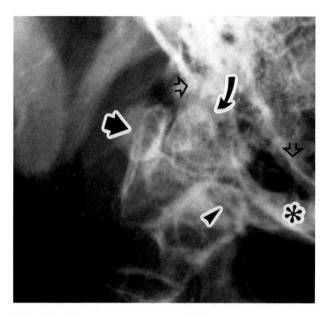

Fig. 9-77   Odontoid hypoplasia with os odontoideum and atlantoaxial dislocation in Down's syndrome. Lateral plain film shows the short dens *(arrowhead)* and the large dystopic os *(curved arrow)* fixed at the basion *(anterior open arrow)*, plus hypertrophy of the anterior atlas arch *(black arrow)*. Notice the separation of the hypoplastic dens from the anterior C1 arch with increased predental distance. There is decreased postdental distance from the hypoplastic dens *(arrow)* relative to the posterior margin of the foramen magnum *(posterior open arrow)* and the posterior arch of C1 *(asterisk)*.

associated hypertrophy of the anterior arch of C1 and hypoplasia with clefting or absence of the posterior arch.

Dens anomalies commonly produce craniocervical instability, which may be anterior, posterior, or multidirectional and result in neural or vascular compression. Normally the dens is stabilized primarily by the alar, apical, and transverse (cruciate) ligaments.[7,18] Consistent alignment of the dens tip with the clival tip in flexion and extension indicates intact alar and apical ligaments, whereas consistent alignment of the dens with the anterior arch of the atlas ensures transverse ligament integrity. Dens hypoplasia is often associated with ligamentous deficiency and atlantoaxial or occipitoaxial instability (that is, subluxation or dislocation) (Figs. 9-77 to 9-79). Dens anomalies and atlantoaxial subluxation occasionally are discovered incidentally on plain films obtained for evaluating head and neck trauma. Other clinical manifestations are related to craniocervical dysmorphia, pain, or neural and vascular compression or restriction. The anomaly may be idiopathic or part of the Down's syndrome, Morquio's syndrome, spondyloepiphyseal dysplasia, other skeletal dysplasia, or the Klippel-Feil spectrum.*

Often there is controversy or confusion over the developmental versus acquired origin or cause of these anoma-

*References 1, 3, 8, 10, 21, 23, 24, 40.

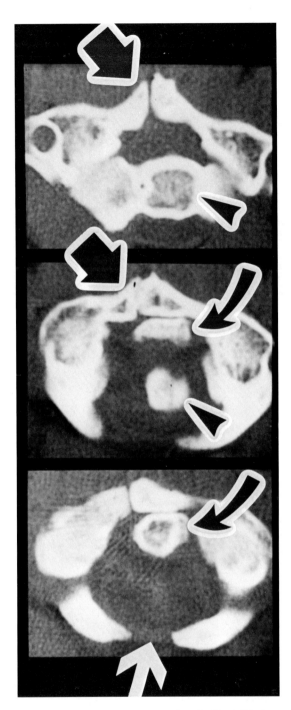

Fig. 9-78 Axial CTs in the same patient in Fig. 9-77 shows the hypertrophied and cleft anterior C1 arch *(large black arrow)*, the hypoplastic dens *(arrowhead)* separated from the anterior C1 arch, and the dystopic os *(curved arrow)* interposed, plus the unossified but cartilaginous posterior C1 arch *(white arrow)*.

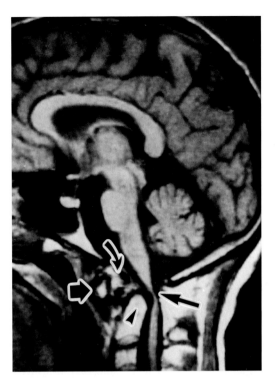

Fig. 9-79 Sagittal T1 MRI in the same patient in Fig. 9-78 showing the anterior C1 arch *(large arrow)*, the hypoplastic dens *(arrowhead)*, and the os odontoideum *(curved arrow)*. There is atlantoaxial dislocation with compressive cord thinning *(long arrow)* between the dens anteriorly and the C1 arch posteriorly.

of a fractured dens, but the gap between the axis and the dens fragment is often narrow and the detached or separate odontoid usually retains its normal dens shape. Establishing the origin of the anomaly is usually less important than determining the nature and degree of instability. Treatment of these anomalies often requires immobilization and traction for reduction followed by surgical stabilization (wiring and fusion) and postoperative traction and bracing.

CRANIOCERVICAL INSTABILITY

Craniocervical instability due to ligamentous laxity with an otherwise intact dens is a relatively common and particularly dangerous condition of childhood. The instability may take place at the atlantooccipital or atlantoaxial level.[16,18,41] Probably the most common predisposing condition is Down's syndrome, although instability has been reported with head and neck infections (for example, retropharyngeal abscess) and childhood arthritis (for example, juvenile rheumatoid arthritis)* The latter often produces dens erosion. Other rare causes include connective tissue disorders and steroid therapy.

lies, especially in odontoid hypoplasia with os odontoideum. It has been proposed that overgrowth of the ossiculum terminale may occur after dissolution of the dens from trauma (aseptic or ischemic necrosis) or infection (septic necrosis). Confusion also may occur with nonunion

*References 3, 8, 17, 24, 32, 34-36.

Atlantoaxial instability

Atlantoaxial subluxation or dislocation due to transverse ligamentous laxity is the most common cause of craniocervical instability and may occur in anteroposterior or rotary directions. With attenuation or disruption of the transverse ligament but intact apical and alar ligaments, the predental dimension, that is, the distance between the dens and the anterior arch of the atlas, may exceed 5 mm, but the subluxation may be initially asymptomatic. When the predental distance is 7 to 10 mm, symptoms or signs are usually present.[16,18,41]

Even though the natural history of atlantoaxial instability has not been clearly documented, it is the consensus that children with Down's syndrome undergo routine screening with flexion-extension lateral filming to distinguish minor hypermobility from instability.[8,18,34] If there is a predental distance of greater than 4.5 mm, an abnormal dens, or evidence of atlantooccipital instability, the children are excluded from activities that involve head and neck flexion. If neck symptoms or neurological symptoms or signs are present, stabilization becomes necessary. Peridontal reactive tissue of fibrous or synovial origin may be present in patients with chronic atlantoaxial dislocation, whether or not there is a coexisting odontoid anomaly. This may result in a relatively fixed dislocation that makes reduction more difficult if not impossible, or itself may be a cause of neural or vascular compression (see Chapter 10). In some cases, such as in rheumatoid arthritis with synovial hypertrophy, the reactive tissue mass may resolve partially or completely after immobilization or stabilization.

Atlantooccipital instability

Atlantooccipital instability may also be encountered, especially in Down's syndrome, whether anterior or posterior, and may be exaggerated after fusion for C1-2 instability.[11,14,22,36] The atlantooccipital instability results from laxity of the apical and alar ligaments. This is revealed by extension-flexion lateral plain films as malalignment of the dens tip with the basion (Fig. 9-80). Other predisposing conditions include infection, childhood arthritis, and other congenital craniocervical anomalies.

Rotary atlantoaxial displacement

Rotary atlantoaxial displacement is one of the commonest causes of torticollis in childhood.[16,18] The condition may be spontaneous, related to trivial trauma, associated with more severe trauma (see Chapter 10), or associated with head and neck inflammation (Fig. 9-81). When persistent, the condition is referred to as fixed displacement or rotary fixation. Fixation is probably caused by capsular or synovial interposition with muscle spasm and may progress to muscle contractures. Rotary displacement occurs within the normal range of motion, whereas rotary subluxation or dislocation occurs with anterior or posterior shift of the C1 lateral masses on the C2 lateral masses of greater than 3 to 4 mm or when there is an associated fracture (see Chapter

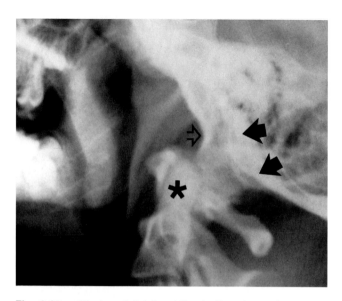

Fig. 9-80   Atlantooccipital instability in Down's syndrome with posterior subluxation in extension shown by lateral plain film including malalignment of the occipital condyles (black arrows) relative to the atlas, and malalignment of the basion (open arrow) relative to the tip of the dens (asterisk).

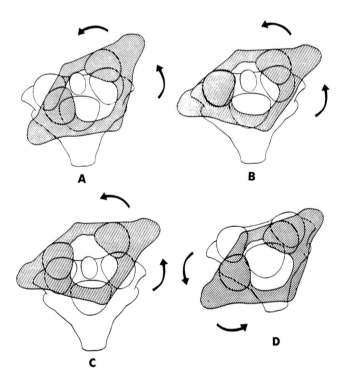

Fig. 9-81   The spectrum of rotary atlantoaxial displacement. (Atlas shaded): **A,** Type I; **B,** Type II; **C,** Type III; **D,** Type IV, see text. (From Gehweiler J, et al: *Radiology of vertebral trauma,* Philadelphia, 1980, WB Saunders.)

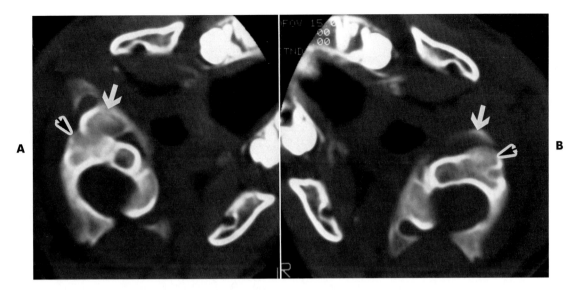

Fig. 9-82   Rotary displacement with combined mild instability and fixation demonstrated by axial CT with leftward **(A)** and rightward **(B)** head turning. There is mildly exaggerated anterior motion of the right lateral C1 mass *(white arrow,* **A***)* relative to the right lateral C2 mass *(black arrow,* **A***)*, but limited anterior motion of the left C1 lateral mass *(white arrow,* **B***)* relative to the left C2 lateral mass *(black arrow,* **B***)*.

10). Cord or vertebral artery compromise is rare unless there is extreme rotary dislocation with transverse ligament disruption and atlantoaxial instability.

The most common rotary deformity (Fig. 9-81) is that of simple rotary displacement without abnormal atlas shift (Type I rotary displacement ± fixation).[18] Recovery is often spontaneous or occurs after minimal treatment including simple bed rest and immobilization or traction and muscle relaxant therapy. Type II is rotary subluxation with less than or equal to 5 mm anterior atlas shift, and Type III is rotary dislocation with greater than 5 mm anterior atlas shift. In Type IV rotary dislocation there is additional posterior atlas offset. When rotary dislocation is accompanied by transverse ligamentous disruption, the dens becomes eccentrically separated from the anterior atlas arch. Surgical fusion may be considered for resubluxation, nonreducible subluxation, atlantoaxial instability, or persistent neurological symptoms and signs.

Frontal and lateral cervical spine films are usually difficult to obtain in anatomical projections and even more difficult to interpret. It may be desirable to obtain the views anatomically with respect to the skull. Lateral and open-mouth views show rotated, tilted, or asymmetrical C1 lateral masses relative to the dens, usually with normal relationship of the atlas and occiput. Axial CT is the preferred method for demonstrating and classifying the deformity and evaluating the range of motion by obtaining images with the head to one side and then to the other (Fig. 9-82). MRI is occasionally needed to evaluate neural or vascular compressive deformity.

OTHER ANOMALIES

Other less common or rare anomalies of the craniovertebral junction may occur as isolated defects or in association with other anomalies as outlined previously. Some of these are clinically unimportant variants; others may be very significant. Again, most of these may be further subclassified, with some overlap, as defects of incomplete assimilation; anomalies of atlantooccipital fusion, synostosis, or ossification; or occipital dysplasias.[16,37,41]

Occipital vertebra anomalies result from incomplete assimilation or persistence of sclerotomal segmentation. These are attempts at formation of an occipital vertebra (proatlas remnants) but without a foramen or groove for the vertebral artery or suboccipital nerve. *Basioccipital fissures* or clefts are transversely oriented defects that may be unilateral or bilateral, partial or complete, isolated and asymptomatic, or incidentally associated with other anomalies. The *third occipital condyle* is a single midline anterior ossicle that may remain separate or be attached to the basion and facetted for articulation with the dens or anterior arch of C1. This often accompanies occipitalization of the atlas and hypoplasia of the lateral condyles, and is associated with high position of the atlas and dens, short clivus, and restricted range of motion. *Basilar processes* are paramedian tubercles at the anterior foramen magnum that also may be separate or attached and articulate with the anterior C1 arch. Similar ossicles may be seen anteriorly in the midline between C1 and C2. *Bipartite atlantal facets* or cleft articular surfaces also may occur.

Anomalies of atlantooccipital fusion, synostosis, or

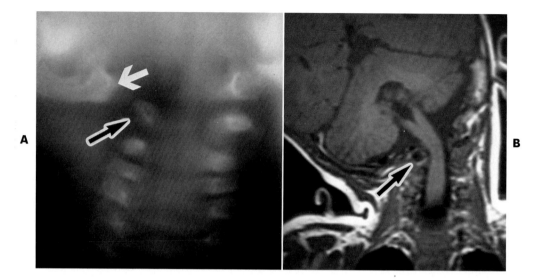

Fig. 9-83   Right occipital condylar hypoplasia *(white arrow)* shown by frontal tomography **(A)** with dysplastic C1 lateral mass *(black arrow)* and lateral atlantooccipital offset. Coronal T1 MRI **(B)** shows the offset C1 lateral mass *(black arrow)* and lateral cervicomedullary impression with right lateral flexion.

ossification result when there is failure of segmentation or lack of separation of the occiput and atlas. Occipitalization of the atlas is discussed earlier in this section. The *paracondylar process* is an accessory ossicle that extends from the lateral aspect of the occipital condyle toward the transverse process of the atlas. Its mirror image is known as the *epitransverse process,* which projects from the transverse process of the atlas toward the occipital condyle. These may be unilateral or bilateral and isolated or associated with complex abnormalities.

Anomalies resulting from occipital dysplasia, dysostosis, or dystrophy are basilar impression, condylar hypoplasia, and constricted foramen magnum. Basilar impression is discussed at the beginning of this section. *Condylar hypoplasia* results in unilateral or bilateral, symmetrical or asymmetrical flattening of the condyles with elevation of the atlas and dens, decreased angulation of the occipitoatlantal articulations, and possible anteroposterior instability or lateral offset (Fig. 9-83). Again, this may occur in isolation or in association with other anomalies. *Constriction of the foramen magnum* may result from premature synostosis of one or more occipital synchondroses and often accompanies occipitalization of the atlas or cervical spinal stenosis.[31] Foramen magnum stenosis also may occur as part of a skeletal dysplasia with skull base hypoplasia (such as achondroplasia). The result is condylar deformity with asymmetrical or symmetrical distortion and constriction of the foramen magnum. This deformity is unyielding to the growing and developing neural and vascular structures and is often further complicated by craniocervical instability (Fig. 9-84). Other dysplasias include those associated with Morquio's syndrome, spondyloepiphyseal dysplasia, and Conradi's syndrome.[16,18,41]

Other skeletal dysplasias often involving the skull base

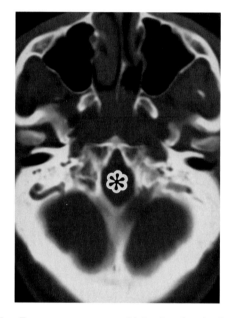

Fig. 9-84   Foramen magnum constriction in achondroplasia shown by axial CT with a small and deformed foramen magnum *(asterisk).*

foramina and resulting in neurovascular encroachment include osteopetrosis, pyknodysostosis, cleidocranial dysplasia, Englemann-Camurati disease, Van Buchem's disease, and craniometaphyseal dysplasia (Pyle's disease).[16,18,41] Other rare or unusual anomalies include atlantoaxial fusions (usually of the lateral masses), unilateral absence of the C1 arch or facet (hemiatlas), the ponticulus posticus variant (arcuate foramen of the atlas for the vertebral artery), and anterior or posterior atlas or axis dysraphic defects.

REFERENCES
Craniocervical anomalies

1. Banna M, Hollenberg R: Compressive meningeal hypertrophy in mucopolysaccharidosis, *AJNR* 8:385, 1987.
2. Bewermeyer H, Dreesbach HA, Hunermann G, et al: MRI of familial basilar impression, *J Comput Assist Tomogr* 8:953, 1984.
3. Burke S, French H, Roberts J, et al: Chronic atlantoaxial instability in Down syndrome, *J Bone Joint Surg* 67A:1356, 1985.
4. Burrows E: Clinical relevance of radiologic abnormalities of the craniovertebral junction, *Br J Radiol* 54:195, 1981.
5. Calvy TM, Segall HD, et al: CT anatomy of the craniovertebral junction in infants and children, *AJNR* 8:489, 1987.
6. Canale S, Griffin D, Hubbard C: Congenital muscular torticollis, *J Bone Joint Surg* 64A:810, 1982.
7. Daniels DL, Williams AL, Haughton VM: Computed tomography of the articulations and ligaments at the occipitoatlantoaxial region, *Radiology* 146:709, 1983.
8. Davidson R: Atlantoaxial instability in Down syndrome, *Pediatrics* 81:857, 1988.
9. Dubonsett J: Torticollis in children caused by congenital anomalies of the atlas, *J Bone Joint Surg* 68A:178, 1986.
10. Edwards MK, Harwood-Nash DC, Fitz CR, et al: CT metrizamide myelography of the cervical spine in Morquio syndrome, *AJNR* 3:666, 1982.
11. El-Khoury GY, Clark CR, Dietz FR, et al: Posterior atlantooccipital subluxation in Down syndrome, *Radiology* 159:507, 1986.
12. Fielding J, Hensinger R, Hawkins R: Os odontoideum, *J Bone Joint Surg* 62A:376, 1980.
13. Gehweiler JA Jr, Daffner RH, Roberts L Jr: Malformations of the atlas vertebra simulating the Jefferson fracture, *AJNR* 4:187, 1983.
14. Georgopoulos G, Pizzutillow P, Lee M: Occipito-atlantal instability in children, *J Bone Joint Surg* 69A:429, 1987.
15. Hall JE, Simmons ED, Danylchuk K, et al: Instability of the cervical spine and neurological involvement in Klippel-Feil syndrome, *J Bone Joint Surg* 72A:460, 1990.
16. Harwood-Nash D: Anomalies of the craniovertebral junction. In Hoffman H, Epstein F, editors: *Disorders of the developing nervous system*, Boston, 1986, Blackwell.
17. Hensinger R, Devito P, Ragsdale C: Changes in the cervical spine in juvenile rheumatoid arthritis, *J Bone Joint Surg* 68A:189, 1986.
18. Hensinger R, Fielding J: The cervical spine. In Morrissy R, editor: *Lovell and Winter's pediatric orthopaedics*, ed 3, Philadelphia, 1990, JB Lippincott.
19. Hensinger R, Lang J, MacEwen G: The Klippel-Feil syndrome, *J Bone Joint Surg* 56A:1246, 1974.
20. Holt RG, Helms CA, Munk PL, et al: Hypertrophy of C-1 anterior arch: useful sign to distinguish os odontoideum from acute dens fracture, *Radiology* 173:207, 1989.
21. Kao SCS, Waziri MH, Smith WL, et al: MR imaging of the craniovertebral junction, cranium, and brain in children with achondroplasia, *AJR* 153:565, 1989.
22. Kaufman RA, Carroll CD, Buncher CR: Atlantooccipital junction: standards for measurement in normal children, *AJNR* 8:995, 1987.
23. Kulkarni M, Williams J, Yeakley J, et al: MR imaging in craniocervical manifestations of the mucopolysaccharidosis, *Magn Reson Imaging* 5:317, 1987.
24. Larsson E-M, Holtas S, Zygmunt S: Preoperative and postoperative MR imaging of the craniocervical junction in rheumatoid arthritis, *AJR* 152:561, 1989.
25. Lee BCP, Deck MDF, Kneeland JB, et al: MR imaging of the craniovervical junction, *AJNR* 6:209, 1985.
26. McAfee P, Bohlman H, Han J, et al: Comparison of NMR imaging and CT in upper cervical cord compression, *Spine* 11:295, 1986.
27. McAlister A: Notes on development and variations of the atlas, *J Anat Physiol* 27:519, 1982.
28. McRae D: Craniovertebral junction. In Newton T, Potts D, editors: *Radiology of the skull and brain*, St Louis, 1971, Mosby–Year Book.
29. Menezes A, VanGilder J, Graf J, et al: Craniocervical abnormalities: a comprehensive surgical approach, *J Neurosurg* 53:444, 1980.
30. O'Rahilly R, Benson D: Development of the vertebral column. In Bradford D, Hensinger R, editors: *The pediatric spine*, New York, 1985, Thieme.
31. Pavlov H, Torg JS, Robie B, et al: Cervical spinal stenosis:

determination with vertebral body ratio method, *Radiology* 164:771, 1987.
32. Perovic MN, Kopits SE, Thompson RC: Radiological evaluation of the spinal cord in congenital atlantoaxial dislocation, *Radiology* 109:713, 1973.
33. Pizzutillo P, Woods M, Nicholson L: Risk factors in the Klippel-Feil syndrome, *Orthop Trans* 11:473, 1987.
34. Pueschel S, Suola F: Atlantoaxial instability in Down's syndrome, *Pediatrics* 80:555, 1987.
35. Roach J, Duncan D, Wenger D, et al: Atlantoaxial instability and spinal cord compression in children: diagnosis by CT, *J Bone Joint Surg* 66A:708, 1984.
36. Rosenbaum DM, Blumhagen JD, King HA: Atlantooccipital instability in Down syndrome, *AJR* 146:1269, 1986.
37. Shapiro R, Robinson F: Anomalies of the craniovertebral border, *Am J Roentgenol* 127:281, 1976.
38. Smoker WRK, Keyes WD, Dunn VD, et al: MRI versus conventional radiologic examinations in the evaluation of the craniovertebral and cervicomedullary junction, *Radiographics* 6:953, 1986.
39. Suss RA, Zimmerman RD, Leeds NE: Pseudospread of the atlas: false sign of Jefferson fracture in young children, *AJR* 140:1079, 1983.
40. Wang H, Rosenbaum AE, Reid CS, et al: Pediatric patients with achondroplasia: CT evaluation of the craniocervical junction, *Radiology* 164:515, 1987.
41. Wald S, McLaurin R: Anomalies of the craniocervical junction. In McLauren R, Schut L, Venes J, et al, editors: *Pediatric neurosurgery*, ed 2, Philadelphia, 1989, WB Saunders.

Spondylodysplasias

The term *spondylodysplasia* in this context refers to any developmental abnormality *(-dysplasia)* of the vertebral column *(spondylo-)*. This is used in contrast to the term *myelodysplasia*, which in general refers to any developmental abnormality of the spinal cord *(myelo-)*. The two may coexist, as discussed in earlier sections. Included in this section are a wide variety of spinal column malformations commonly encountered in childhood (see boxes on p. 398). The range of spondylodysplasias includes the common scoliosis or kyphosis syndromes and the less common skeletal dysplasias. The latter group is composed of a variety of conditions including chromosomal syndromes (such as Down's), osteochondrodysplasias (such as achondroplasia), metabolic disorders (such as mucopolysaccharidoses), connective tissue disorders (such as Marfan's), phacomatoses (such as neurofibromatosis), as well as other miscellaneous syndromes, sequences, defects, and associations.* The more common conditions are covered here in some detail; others are tabulated in the Appendix.

CLINICAL AND IMAGING CONSIDERATIONS

Common clinical and radiological manifestations include dwarfism, craniofacial dysmorphia, torticollis, scoliosis, kyphosis, kyphoscoliosis, and hyperlordosis.[4,7,14,15] Other manifestations are craniocervical anomaly, spinal instability, spinal canal or foraminal stenosis, and spinal canal ectasia. Other anomalies or deformities include platyspondyly (that is, vertebral body flattening), vertebral body beaking, wedging, or gibbus deformity, vertebral clefts, end plate irregularities, biconcave vertebral bodies, punctate mineralization, osteopenia, osteosclerosis, or patholog-

---

*References 4, 7, 14-18, 30, 31, 17

ical fracture. Other or additional findings may include spondylolysis, spondylolisthesis,[11] formation-segmentation anomalies, skull base sclerosis, and basilar impression.

Other than cosmetic spinal deformity, additional complications are those related to bony mechanical compression, constriction, or compromise of the cord, nerves, vascular structures, or CSF spaces.[14,17,24] Underlying myelodysplasias are rare unless there are formation-segmentation or dysraphic spinolaminal anomalies. There may be coexistent hydrocephalus or hydrosyringomyelia. Radiological evaluation includes frontal and lateral plain films, often flexion and extension or lateral bending films, and tomography or CT. MRI is important in assessing the mechanical effects on neural elements (cord and nerve compression or constriction), vascular structures (carotid, vertebrobasilar, or spinal arterial compromise), and CSF spaces (hydrocephalus and hydrosyringomyelia). Myelography is often difficult and hazardous, particularly in patients with impending or evolving cord compression. Neurological impairment due to spinal canal stenosis (such as in achondroplasia) may require occipital decompression, laminectomy, and foraminotomy.[4,5,14,15,17] Progressive curvature deformities or spinal instability may necessitate orthopedic instrumentation and fusion with or without vertebral resection. Symptomatic dural ectasia (for example, neurofibromatosis), hydrocephalus, or hydrosyringomyelia may require shunting.

In terms of spinal curvature evaluation and follow-up, the Cobb technique is the standard for curve angle measurement as applied to frontal and lateral upright films[7,13,22,32] (see Fig. 9-86). The end vertebral bodies of the scoliosis, kyphosis, or lordosis are the bodies at the top and bottom of the curve that are most tilted from the horizontal plane. Tangents are drawn along the upper end plate of the upper end body and along the lower end plate of the lower end body. Perpendicular lines from these are drawn, and the angle of intersection represents the angle of curvature. Standards for normal and abnormal vary from reference to reference. Scoliosis is usually defined as a standing lateral curvature greater than 10 degrees. Thoracic hyperkyphosis may be diagnosed when the sagittal curve exceeds 45 degrees as measured from T1 to T12. Kyphosis of any degree at any other level is considered abnormal. Thoracic hypokyphosis (straight back deformity) or lordosis refers to a curve of less than 20 degrees. Lumbar lordosis is normally quite variable. As measured from L1 to L5-S1, a lordotic curve beyond 50 degrees may be considered excessive.

IDIOPATHIC SCOLIOSIS

A classification of scoliosis is presented in the box on p. 399. Only some of the more important features are presented in this section. Idiopathic scoliosis refers to a lateral curvature of the spine of unknown origin and is by far the most common curvature abnormality of childhood.[1,6,7,22] There is a strong family occurrence (80%) with a female-to-male ratio ranging from 7:1 to 10:1, especially in adolescence and for larger and progressive curves. The most frequent patterns of idiopathic scoliosis in order are a right thoracic curve, a right thoracic and left lumbar curve, a right thoracolumbar curve, and a right lumbar curve. Left thoracic, left cervical, and left cervicothoracic curves are rare. Associated kyphosis is unusual, whereas lordosis is characteristic of severe or progressive curves. The uncommon infantile form (seen in children less than 3 years of age) tends to resolve spontaneously (90%), but progression may occur for curves persisting after the first year and for curves greater than 35 degrees. With such progression there is compensatory curve formation, increasing rib-vertebral angle differences, and characteristically a left kyphoscoliosis. The juvenile form (3 to 10 years of age) is less common than the adolescent form (greater than 10 years), usually with thoracic scoliosis only, and tends to progress.

The main complications or sequelae of idiopathic scoliosis include curve progression, painful curves, respiratory compromise, and cosmetic deformity. In general, curve progression tends to occur during growth spurts, that is, between birth and 2 years, and in the prepubertal period. Progressive curvature deformity tends to occur more often in skeletally immature females, especially when the curve is larger than 11 degrees at diagnosis, and for curves greater than 30 degrees after skeletal maturity (epiphyseal closure) is reached. Other indicators for progression include clinical deformity that is greater than radiological deformity, late prepubertal presentation, thoracic lordosis, and family history. Pain may occur as a result of curvature progression

---

CLASSIFICATION OF SCOLIOSIS

IDIOPATHIC

Infantile
Juvenile
Adolescent
Adult

NEUROMUSCULAR

Neuropathic

Upper motor neuron lesion (cerebral palsy, spinocerebellar degeneration, hydrosyringomyelia, cord trauma, cord tumor, other)
Lower motor neuron lesion (polio, trauma, spinal muscular atrophy, myelocele, other)
Dysautonomia
Other

Myopathic

Arthrogryposis
Muscular dystrophy
Other

CONGENITAL

Formation defects
Segmentation defects
Mixed
Associated myelodysplasia

NEUROFIBROMATOSIS

Dystrophic
Idiopathic
Scheuermann's disease

MESENCHYMAL

Marfan's syndrome
Homocystinuria
Ehlers-Danlos syndrome
Other

TRAUMATIC

Fracture-dislocation
Postradiation
Other

CONTRACTURES

Postburn

OSTEOCHONDRODYSTROPHIES

Achondroplasia
Spondyloepiphyseal dysplasia
Other

TUMOR

Benign
Malignant

RHEUMATOID

METABOLIC

Rickets
Juvenile osteoporosis
Osteogenesis imperfecta
Other

LUMBOSACRAL

Spondylolysis
Spondylolisthesis

THORACIC SURGERY

HYSTERICAL

FUNCTIONAL

Postural
Short leg
Muscular spasm

---

or associated degenerative disk or facet disease but is not unusual in childhood. Pain may also occur after spinal fusion. Degenerative changes usually are not encountered until after skeletal maturity and include disk degeneration and protrusion, facet sclerosis and hypertrophy, or transitory vertebral shift. The degenerative changes often result in a rigid curve with nerve entrapment. Vertebral shifts are lateral translocations (lystheses) associated with facet syndromes and often occur at the junction between curves with large rotational elements. Often there is root entrapment with pain, along with increased ligamentous laxity and increased risk of curvature progression. Respiratory compromise usually becomes a concern for curves greater than 60 degrees.

Treatment is nonoperative in the majority of cases. For patients with curvature progression, surgical instrumentation and fusion is usually employed.[1,6] Rarely, the procedure is complicated by paraplegia after Harrington rod distraction due to vascular compromise. The radiographic hallmark of idiopathic scoliosis is that of a rotatory curvature producing pedicle asymmetry. Other bony deformity is unusual unless the curve is severe or progressive. This results in additional lordosis.[7] Imaging beyond spine films is rarely indicated except for unusual or atypical signs or symptoms (such as pain, parasthesias, or paresis) that may otherwise indicate unsuspected neuropathology (such as neoplasm or hydrosyringomyelia), or a complication of curve progression (such as disk protrusion, nerve impingement, or cord thinning). In these situations MRI is the next procedure of choice, and CT or myelography is infrequently required (Fig. 9-85). Spinal cord imaging may be needed for the rare postoperative paraparesis or paraplegia (usually ischemic in origin) to rule out epidural hematoma. Atypical manifestations of idiopathic scoliosis that may be suggestive of other abnormalities (Fig. 9-86) include progressive or painful curves in younger children, curve abnormalities in males, a leftward curve, abnormal neurological signs, and atypical plain film findings such as spinal canal expansion, vertebral body or neural arch anomaly, bone destruction (pedicle erosion), or kyphosis component.[7,22] Other important conditions in the differential diagnosis of scoliosis occurring in childhood are listed in the box above.

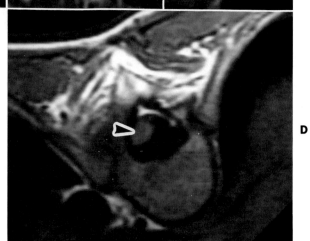

Fig. 9-85 Adolescent female with progressive idiopathic thoracic scoliosis and pain. **A-C,** Serial coronal T1 MRI showing characteristic rotatory thoracic lordoscoliosis with rightward convexity, bowstringing of the cord along the left concavity *(arrowhead)* and normal conus medullaris termination *(white arrow, C)*. **D,** The rotatory component and cord bowstringing are particularly evident on axial T1 MRI with eccentric cord position *(arrowhead)* and asymmetrical dural sac and epidural fatty landmarks.

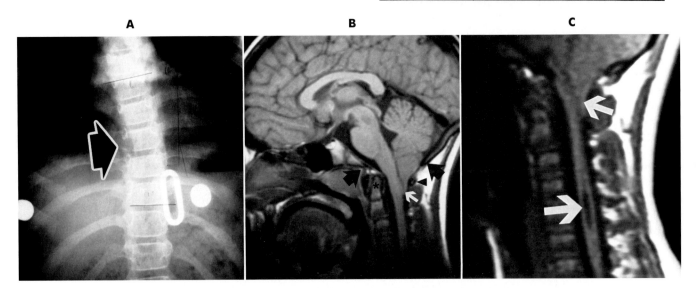

Fig. 9-86 Adolescent female with atypical idiopathic scoliosis. **A,** Frontal plain film shows mild leftward thoracic curvature abnormality as measured by the Cobb method. **B** and **C,** Sagittal T1 craniospinal MRI demonstrating Chiari I malformation with low-placed cerebellar tonsils *(smaller white arrows, B, C)* and cervicomedullary junction relative to the foramen magnum *(black arrows),* dens *(star),* and posterior C1 arch *(arrowhead).* Intramedullary longitudinal hypointensities *(larger white arrow, C)* are consistent with hydrosyringomyelia.

CONGENITAL SCOLIOSIS

Congenital scoliosis and kyphosis are coronal and sagittal plane curvature deformities, respectively, that result from formation or segmentation anomalies of the vertebral column.[7,14,20-23,33] Common anomalies of vertebral formation (Figs. 9-17, 9-87, and 9-88) that produce congenital scoliosis include wedge vertebra (partial unilateral failure of

formation) and hemivertebra (complete unilateral failure). Common segmentation anomalies are pedicle fusion bars (unilateral failure of segmentation) and block vertebra (bilateral failure). Mixed formation-segmentation anomalies (such as block hemivertebra) are also common. As emphasized earlier in this chapter, congenital scoliosis is commonly associated with spinal dysraphism (in 20% of

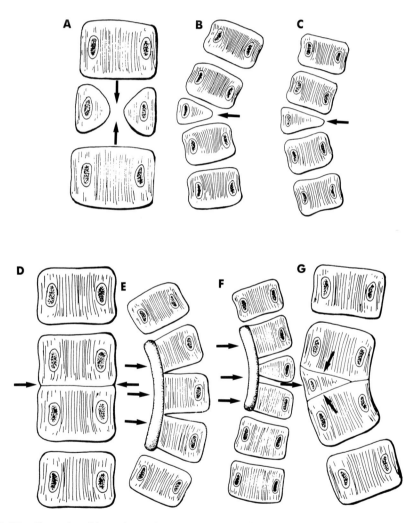

Fig. 9-87   Examples of formation and segmentation spinal anomalies. **A,** Partial or complete anterior central formational defect that may cause severe angular kyphosis or kyphoscoliosis, or the more benign butterfly vertebra anomaly. **B,** Hemivertebra formational defect with angular curve. **C,** Wedge vertebra formational defect with angular curve. **D,** Bilateral segmentation failure with block vertebra. **E,** Unilateral segmentation failure with pedicle bars and curve. **F,** Combined formational and segmentation defects with unilateral unsegmented bar and hemivertebra resulting in progressive curvature. **G,** Combined defects with block vertebra incorporating a hemivertebra and associated curvature deformity. (Modified from Hall J: Congenital scolisis. In Bradford D, Hensinger R, editors: *The pediatric spine,* New York, 1985, Thieme.)

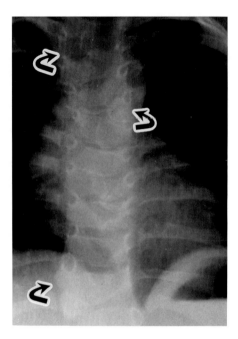

Fig. 9-88   Congenital thoracolumbar scoliosis in VATER syndrome with multiple vertebral formation anomalies (*arrows*).

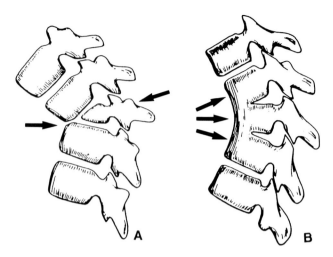

Fig. 9-89   Types of congenital kyphosis. **A**, Failure of formation. **B**, Failure of anterior segmentation. (From Winter R: Spinal problems in pediatric orthopedics, In Morrissy R, editor: *Lovell and Winter's pediatric orthopaedics*, ed 3, Philadelphia, 1990, JB Lippincott.)

cases), genitourinary anomalies (20%), and congenital heart disease (20%). Klippel-Feil anomaly may be considered a special subcategory of congenital scoliosis. Rib anomalies (absence, fusion, and the like) are common, as are pulmonary abnormalities. Approximately one half of the patients with congenital scoliosis demonstrate curve progression, especially those with unilateral fusion bars.

Spinal cord imaging, preferably by MRI, is indicated before orthopedic intervention or earlier if there are neuropathic manifestations such as bladder or bowel dysfunction and leg or foot deformity. As outlined in the dysraphism section, neurenteric spectrum anomalies are associated with vertebral formation-segmentation anomalies, especially diastematomyelia. Neurosurgical correction of the myelodysplasia is almost always required before orthopedic correction of the scoliosis. Spinal instrumentation and fusion in situ with spinal cord monitoring is often the procedure of choice. Reported complications of surgery include respiratory insufficiency, paraplegia, pseudoarthrosis, recurring curvature progression, short stature, and lordosis.

CONGENITAL KYPHOSIS

Congenital kyphosis refers to sagittal plane curvature deformity resulting from formation-segmentation anomalies of one or more vertebral segments.[7,14,22,35] This type of kyphosis may be associated with myelodysplasias or skeletal dysplasias, and the deformity is always progressive (Fig. 9-89). Congenital kyphosis is the most common noninfectious cause of spinal deformity causing paraplegia in childhood. Type I kyphosis results from failure of

vertebral formation with total or partial absence of one or more vertebral bodies (Fig. 9-90). The angular kyphosis produced, as well as the risk of cord injury, depends on the shape of the vertebral malformation, the spinal canal alignment, and also the status of the posterior arch (Fig. 9-91). Partial vertebral absence with an aligned spinal canal produces a rare, pure angular kyphosis, or occasional kyphoscoliosis, usually at the thoracic or thoracolumbar level, and is associated with gradually progressive bowstringing of the cord (Figs. 9-22, 9-45, and 9-90). Partial vertebral absence with a dislocated spinal canal has previously been labelled *congenitally dislocated spine*. The kyphosis usually occurs at the thoracolumbar junction and is associated with a step-off in canal alignment and a deficiency of the posterior arch. With this type there is a significant risk of cord compression with sudden paralysis. Total failure of vertebral formation produces an unstable, mobile kyphosis with or without absence of the neural arch. This anomaly occurs in the lumbar region and presents as congenital paraplegia with a thin or flattened cord segment (Fig. 9-92). Occasionally there is an associated lipoma.

Type II kyphosis results from a segmentation failure, usually at the lumbar or thoracolumbar level. The kyphosis or kyphoscoliosis is usually smooth, nonangular, and slowly progressive with minimal cord risk (Figs. 9-36 and 9-89). Spontaneous anterior fusion may occur beginning at 8 to 10 years of age. Type II congenital kyphosis is to be distinguished from Scheuermann's disease. Rotary vertebral dislocation is another type of mechanical deformity that may be associated with congenital curvature abnormalities. The rotary dislocation occurs at the kyphotic zone

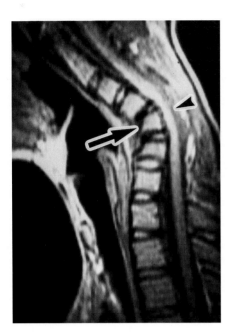

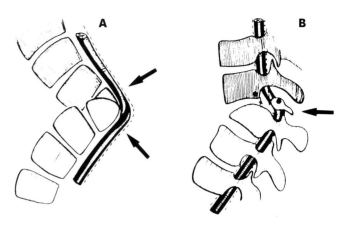

Fig. 9-91   Spinal alignment in congenital kyphosis. **A**, Aligned canal, **B**, Dislocated canal. (From Dubousset J: Congenital kyphosis, In Bradford D, Hensinger R, editors: *The pediatric spine*, New York, 1985, Thieme.)

Fig. 9-90   Progressive cervical kyphosis of unknown origin shown by sagittal MRI with dysplastic-hypoplastic C5 vertebral body (*arrow*), smooth kyphosis with aligned canal, and bowstringing of the cord (*arrowhead*).

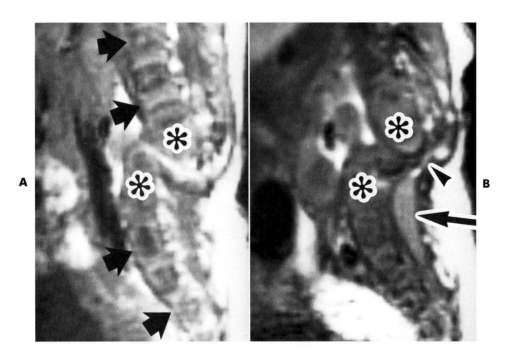

Fig. 9-92   Congenitally dislocated thoracolumbar spine (type I kyphosis) in a newborn demonstrated by sagittal T1 MRI. There is malalignment of the thoracic segments (*upper arrows*) in relation to the lumbar segments (*lower arrows*) with kyphotic dislocation at the thoracolumbar junction (*asterisks*) and marked cord attenuation (*arrowhead*) plus low-placed conus medullarais (*long arrow*).

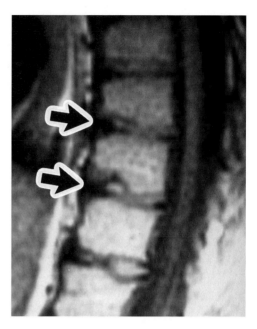

Fig. 9-93   Progressive thoracic Scheuermann's disease shown by sagittal proton density MRI with contiguous multilevel involvement including vertebral body wedging, irregular end plates, anterior disk space narrowing, and anterior Schmorl's nodes (*arrows*).

between two regions of congenital scoliosis, each often in lordosis and rotated opposite one another. An abrupt, angular kyphosis that is variably progressive results, and there is scissoring with vertebral collapse at the apex. This usually occurs at the upper thoracic level or at the thoracolumbar junction. Neurological complications are frequent with cord and nerve root twisting around the apex of the acute curve.

Complications or sequelae of congenital kyphosis include gradually progressive cord damage over time (aligned kyphosis), or acute cord injury (unstable or dislocated kyphosis), thoracic deformity with cardiopulmonary compromise, and cosmetic deformity. Prognosis depends on the clinical and radiological evaluation of stability, including neurological findings. Other important prognostic factors are instability on flexion and extension demonstrated by lateral plain films, plain film findings of an anterior vertebral "empty space" (fibrosis or nonossified elements), posterior vertebral malalignment, defective or absent posterior arch elements, and progression of vertebral deformities over time in the context of somatic growth. Surgical repair may require a combination of anterior and posterior instrumentation, fusion, and vertebral resection. The differential diagnosis of kyphosis (and lordosis) is provided in the box above.

SCHEUERMANN'S DISEASE

Scheuermann's disease is the commonest cause of thoracic kyphosis in the juvenile or adolescent patient.[7,22,29] It is the second commonest spinal deformity encountered in the pediatric orthopedic clinic (after idiopathic scoliosis) and the most common cause of thoracic spine pain, although pain is infrequent in this disease. A less common but more acute lumbar form also occurs.

Scheuermann's disease has been classified as one of the osteochondroses rather than a form of osteochondrodysplasia. In the osteochondroses there is a disturbance of enchondral ossification with degeneration or necrosis, followed by regeneration and reactive change including recalcification or reossification as manifested by vertebral end plate irregularities. The thoracic kyphosis presents as a curvature deformity and rarely progresses to produce neurological deficits.

The radiological diagnosis may be made according to Sorenson's criteria, that is, involvement of three or more adjacent vertebral bodies with wedging of greater than 5%, or Cobb's method, that is, greater than 35 degrees of thoracic kyphosis. Additional findings include end plate irregularities, disk space narrowing, and Schmorl's nodes (Fig. 9-93). The end plate and disk space changes relate to extensions or herniations of the disk (Schmorl's nodes) into the cancellous bone of the body via end plate fractures and the centrally thin margins of the ring apophyses. There is vertebral wedging and accentuation of kyphosis over time, including increased lumbar lordosis. The development of thoracic kyphosis is usually spontaneous and may be hereditary. The classical juvenile kyphosis occurs with the apex between T7 and T9, less commonly at T11-T12, and is slightly more common in females. A rigid kyphosis beyond 40 degrees may develop, and there may be associated thoracic scoliosis in about one fourth of cases. MRI is rarely indicated except for atypical pain or progression of kyphosis (Fig. 9-93). Other causes of childhood thoracic kyphosis include postlaminectomy, postspondylitis, posttrauma, spondyloepiphyseal dyspla-

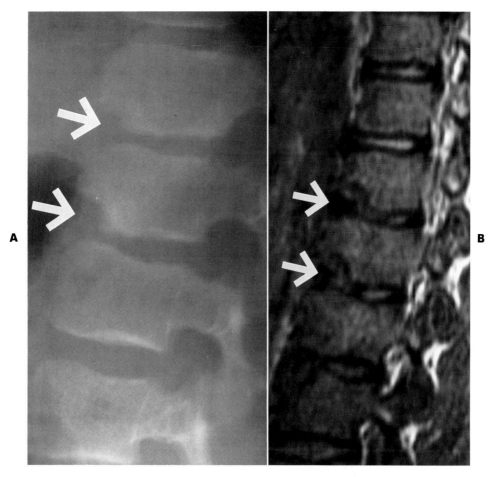

Fig. 9-94   Lumbar Scheuermann's disease with recurring pain. Lateral plain film **(A)** and sagittal proton density MRI **(B)** show anterior disk space narrowing and anterior Schmorl's nodes with limbus vertebra-like deformities (*arrows*). The MRI demonstrated no evidence of complicating posterior disk protrusions.

sias, muccopolysaccharidoses, and congenital kyphosis.

The lumbar form of Scheuermann's disease is usually painful and of traumatic origin.[7,22] It commonly occurs at the thoracolumbar junction or lower, and occasionally at more than one level. Often there is a history of acute strenuous activity or injury and pain with activity, especially on flexion and extension. This type occurs more often in males and young athletes. The radiological findings are similar to those of the thoracic type listed previously, including end plate irregularities and Schmorl's nodes but usually without vertebral wedging (Fig. 9-94). Occasionally the disk material extends peripherally and anteriorly beneath the apophyseal ring and separates the ring from the body. There is gradual healing but persistence of the Schmorl's node with anterior disk space narrowing, separate apophyseal fragment, and adjacent vertebral body corner defect (previously referred to as limbus vertebra). Symptomatic posterior lumbar disk protrusion may require further imaging (such as MRI or CT).

NEUROFIBROMATOSIS

The spinal curvature deformities associated with neurofibromatosis (see Chapter 8) have been subclassified as either dystrophic or nondystrophic.[7-10,19,22,34,38] The dystrophic type of curvature deformity includes the characteristic short-segment kyphoscoliosis of NF 1 resulting from and associated with the other manifestations of mesodermal dysplasia and neoplasia. These include vertebral scalloping and wedging, apical vertebral rotation, canal and foraminal enlargement and meningocele formation associated with dural ectasia, twisted ribbon or pencilled ribs, vertebral subluxation, and nerve sheath tumors (see Chapter 8). The dystrophic type of kyphoscoliosis is usually progressive and often produces cord impingement or compression, is usually unresponsive to nonoperative management, and tends to rapidly worsen especially after laminectomy for neoplasm.[10,34] Anterior and posterior instrumentation with fusion is often required. Such a procedure is routinely anticipated after laminectomy for tumor resection.

Another characteristic dystrophic spinal abnormality of NF 1 is cervical kyphosis with wedge or ''golf-tee'' vertebral body deformity[38] (see Chapter 8). This is one of the causes of cervical kyphosis, which is otherwise rare in childhood. Other causes of cervical kyphosis include congenital kyphosis, skeletal dysplasia, posttrauma, post-laminectomy, or neoplasm. The nondystrophic spinal curvature abnormalities of neurofibromatosis have a radiological appearance and clinical course very similar to that of idiopathic scoliosis and are not associated with other anomalies of mesodermal dysplasia or with tumor. Occasionally a secondary spinal curve abnormality occurs with limb deformity (such as pseudarthrosis) and leg length discrepancy. Other spondylodysplasias reportedly associated with neurofibromatosis include Scheuermann's kyphosis, postlaminectomy kyphosis, spondylolisthesis, and pedicle aplasia or hypoplasia. The latter is more commonly seen as an isolated developmental defect of vertebral formation, often associated with hypertrophy of the contralateral pedicle, and must be distinguished from neoplastic destruction.[36]

ACHONDROPLASIA

Achondroplasia is probably the most frequent form of dwarfism with axial skeletal involvement.[4,22,26] The dwarfism is primarily of the short-limbed type, but spinal complications produce truncal shortening also. Achondroplasia is of autosomal dominant inheritance, although sporadic cases are common because of the high genetic mutation rate. It is included in the spectrum of osteochondrodysplasias in which the basic abnormality is defective enchondral bone formation in the context of normal membranous ossification. In the axial skeleton there is characteristic involvement of the skull base and spinal column with normal cranial vault development. As a result craniofacial dysmorphia occurs with relative or absolute macrocephaly, frontal bossing, nasal bridge flattening, and constricted skull base. The skull base stenosis or synostosis probably is related to early fusion of the basal synchondroses and involves primarily the occipital bone. As a result there is a small, deformed, and sclerotic foramen magnum with short vertical clivus and stenotic jugular foramina (Fig. 9-95). Macrocephaly with hydrocephalus may occur secondary to impaired venous outflow with resulting subarachnoid and ventricular dilatation (external hydrocephalus). The hydrocephalus tends to stabilize with suture closure and collateral venous circulation, and rarely requires shunting. Subdural hematomas or hygromas also may occur, and hydrosyringomyelia has been reported.

Other neurological complications of axial skeletal involvement include neural compression or constriction from spinal canal stenosis or kyphoscoliosis. Foramen magnum or upper cervical canal stenosis occurs in about one third of cases (Figs. 9-95 and 9-96). The resulting cervicomedullary or upper cervical cord involvement tends to arise primarily in infancy and early childhood (under 5 years of age) and may require surgical decompression. Other frequently or

occasionally associated craniocervical abnormalities include occipitalization of the atlas with high position of the dens, odontoid hypoplasia, atlantoaxial instability, fibrous fusion of the C1 posterior arch to the occiput, and basilar impression. Symtoms due to spinal canal or foraminal stenosis at lower levels, or due to kyphoscoliosis, tend to arise during adolescence or adulthood. Symptomatic spinal stenosis occurs in the thoracolumbar or lumbar region in the majority of patients, whereas diffuse stenosis occurs in about 10%. The stenosis probably relates to premature fusion or ossification of the neurocentral synchondroses, which results in smaller than normal transverse and sagittal diameters of the spinal canal and small intervertebral foramina. There are short, flat vertebral bodies and short, thick pedicles with vertebral scalloping and narrowed interpediculate distances. The sagittal canal narrowing (short pedicles) usually occurs at all levels, whereas the transverse narrowing (short interpediculate dimension) occurs primarily at the lumbar levels. The lumbar stenosis tends to be progressive from L1 to L5. Achondroplasia and other spondylodysplastic causes of spinal stenosis are often readily distinguished from idiopathic spinal stenosis by the lack of vertebral deformities in the latter (Fig. 9-97).

Scoliosis, kyphosis, or kyphoscoliosis occurs in about one third of the patients. Vertebral wedging or gibbus deformity with kyphoscoliosis characteristically affects the thoracolumbar junction and may be progressive. Congenital disk hypertrophy with protrusion frequently accompanies the concave posterior vertebral bodies and bulging end plates. The canal stenosis frequently is worsened by disk protrusion or osteophytic spurring from associated degenerative spondylosis and arthrosis. Most commonly there is conus or cauda compression with progressive radiculopathy or myelopathy and neurogenic claudication with increasing age. Acute neurological symptoms and signs may occur with minor trauma.

Pseudoachondroplasia is another relatively common type of osteochondrodysplasia that may mimic achondroplasia.[22] This form of short-limbed dwarfism may be of either autosomal or recessive inheritance and manifests as thoracolumbar kyphosis with excessive lumbar lordosis. There are additional anterior midvertebral bony projections, platyspondyly, vertebral end plate grooving, biconcave body deformities, atlantoaxial instability, as well as hand and foot deformities. The condition is distinguished from achondroplasia by the normal craniofacial structures and the normal interpediculate dimensions.

MUCOPOLYSACCHARIDOSES

Craniocervical junction and spinal column involvement is common in mucopolysaccharidoses (MPS) especially in the Hurler (MPS I-H), Morquio (MPS IV), and Maroteaux-Lamy (MPS VI) syndromes* (see Chapter 4). Similar involvement may occur less commonly or to a milder

---

*References 2, 7, 12, 16, 17, 22, 31.

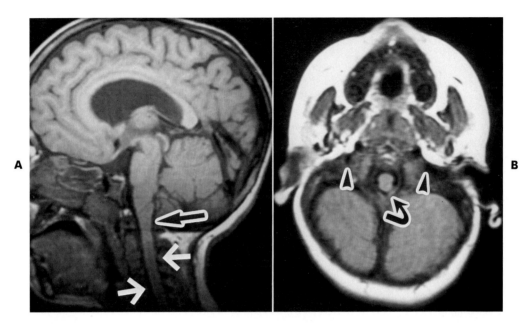

Fig. 9-95   Achondroplasia in a juvenile girl with foramen magnum and cervical spinal canal stenosis. Sagittal **(A)** and axial **(B)** T1 MRI demonstrate macrocephaly with ventricular dilatation, a small and deformed foramen magnum (*straight and curved black arrows*), stenotic jugular foraminal vascular flow voids (*arrowheads*), short vertical clivus, and narrow cervical spinal canal (*white arrows*).

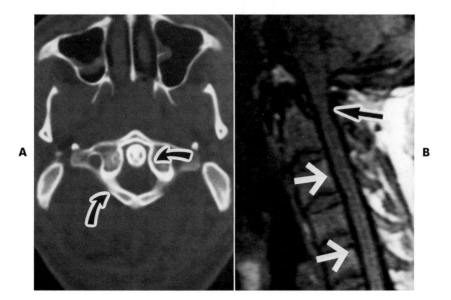

Fig. 9-96   Achondroplasia in an adolescent male with foramen magnum and cervical spinal canal stenosis. **A,** Axial CT shows the reduced sagittal and transverse dimensions of the canal at C1 (*arrows*). **B,** Sagittal T1 MRI demonstrates the diffuse sagittal canal narrowing (*white arrows*) in relationship to the spinal cord. The narrowing is most pronounced at the C1-2 level (*black arrow*) with anterior and posterior cord impressions.

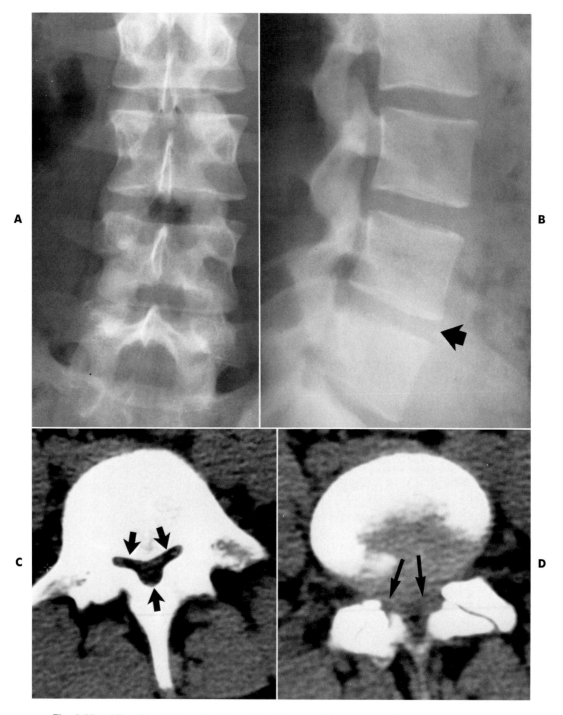

Fig. 9-97   Idiopathic lumbar spinal stenosis with acute disk protrusion. Frontal **(A)** and lateral **(B)** plain films show progressive narrowing of the transverse and sagittal spinal canal dimensions from L2 to L5 and disk space narrowing at L4-5 (*arrow*,**B**) without vertebral deformities. **C** and **D**, Axial CT scans demonstrate the characteristic triangular stenosis (*short arrows*) of the lumbar spinal canal with a paucity of epidural fat. Diffuse disk protrusion is shown at the L4-5 level (*long arrows*).

degree in the Hurler-Scheie (MPS I-H/S), Hunter (MPS II), San Filippo (MPS III), and Sly (MPS VIII) syndromes. Craniocervical abnormalities (see Chapter 4) include skull base thickening and occipital hypoplasia, odontoid hypoplasia, ligamentous laxity with atlantoaxial instability, occasional C3-C4 subluxation, and dural sac stenosis. Often there is a gradual and subtle progressive myelopathy that may be falsely attributed to the lower extremity deformities. Complications include foraminal and canal neurovascular compression, as well as altered CSF dynamics producing hydrocephalus or hydrosyringomyelia. The dural sac stenosis results from epidural and dural mucopolysaccharide deposition with elastic and collagenous proliferation.

Other important spinal abnormalities in MPS are platyspondyly (especially Morquio's syndrome), anterior vertebral beaking, vertebral wedging, gibbus deformity, and kyphosis or kyphoscoliosis. Cord compression may occur as a result of progressive kyphosis or scoliosis, posterior vertebral slip (such as in Morquio's syndrome) or large disk protrusion (such as Maroteaux-Lamy syndrome). Other deformities include osteoporosis, biconvex vertebral bodies, narrow bodies, long pedicles, ovoid bullet-shaped or rectangular bodies, and irregular vertebral margins. Findings similar to those of the Hurler and Hunter syndromes may be seen in mucolipidosis III (pseudoHurler polydystrophy) including vertebral breaking, upper lumbar gibbus, and dens hypoplasia.

DOWN'S SYNDROME

Down's syndrome, or trisomy 21, the most common of the chromosomal disorders, frequently is complicated by craniocervical instability due to ligamentous and bony abnormalities.[7,27,28] These include atlantoaxial subluxation with intact dens, atlantooccipital subluxation, odontoid hypoplasia, and os odontoideum. These are presented in detail in the previous section. Other spinal abnormalities in Down's syndrome include subluxations at other cervical levels, vertebral fusions, flat cervical vertebra, degenerative cervical spine disease, tall vertebral bodies, and scoliosis.

SPONDYLOEPIPHYSEAL DYSPLASIAS

The spondyloepiphyseal dysplasias (SED) may occur in the congenita form (autosomal dominant more common than autosomal recessive inheritance) or the tarda form (sex-linked recessive, autosomal dominant, or recessive inheritance).[4,7,16,31,37] The congenita form is characterized by short-trunk dwarfism, flexion contractures of the hip, marked lumbar lordosis, and thoracolumbar kyphosis that may be progressive. The vertebral bodies appear ovoid or pear-shaped with late platyspondyly and end plate irregularities. The major problem, however, in SED congenita is odontoid hypoplasia with atlantoaxial instability (seen in one third of patients), which may produce cord compression early in life and require spinal fusion (Fig. 9-98). The tarda form of SED is characterized by platyspondyly with

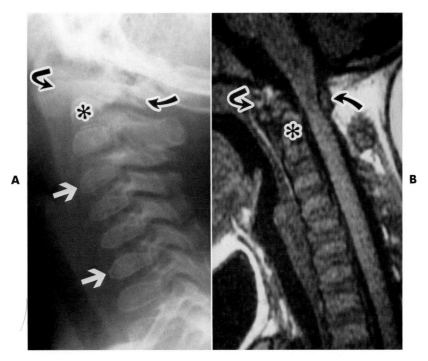

Fig. 9-98   Spondyloepiphyseal dysplasia congenita with odontoid hypoplasia, anterior atlantoaxial subluxation, and cord impingement demonstrated by lateral plain film **(A)** and sagittal T1 MRI **(B)** including the abnormal relationships of the short dens (*asterisk*) to the anterior C1 arch (*anterior curved black arrow*) and the posterior C1 arch (*posterior curved black arrow*). Also shown is multilevel platyspondyly (*white arrows*, **A**).

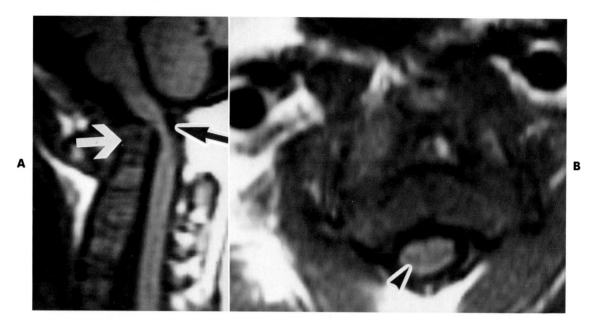

Fig. 9-99   Larsen's syndrome with progressive quadriplegia due to occipitalization of the atlas and anterior atlantoaxial dislocation. Sagittal **(A)** and axial **(B)** T1 MRI showing compressive attenuation of the cord between the hypoplastic dens (*white arrow*) anteriorly and the posterior C1 arch posteriorly (*black arrow*). An intramedullary low intensity (*arrowhead*, **B**) is consistent with cord infarction.

short-trunk dwarfism, lumbar vertebral end plate humps, and early degenerative spine (and hip) disease. This includes spondyloarthrosis with disk narrowing, calcification, and vacuum phenomenon. Thoracic kyphosis, lumbar lordosis, scoliosis, and odontoid hypoplasia occur less often than in SED congenita. Canal stenosis is infrequent in either form.

OTHER SPONDYLODYSPLASIAS

Diastrophic dysplasia is an autosomal recessively inherited form of short-limbed dwarfism with common spinal involvement.[4,7,16,31,37] Cervical vertebral hypoplasia with kyphosis may be progressive. There may be other associated formation-segmentation anomalies (for example, hemivertebra, unsegmented bar) with limited range of motion or cervical spina bifida. Craniocervical anomaly (for example, odontoid hypoplasia) with instability may occur rarely. Thoracic spinal deformities include platyspondyly, sharp-angled kyphosis, kyphoscoliosis, or lordoscoliosis. Although many curvatures do not require treatment, others progress to severe rigid deformities. Abnormal anterior vertebral body ossifications may occur at L1 or L2, or there may be L5 vertebral wedging with exaggerated lumbar lordosis. Lumbar or sacral interpediculate narrowing is common, especially at L5 and S1, although symptomatic spinal stenosis is rare.

Metatropic dysplasia is an autosomal recessive form of short-limbed dwarfism with abnormal vertebral ossification progressing to ankylosis and producing the most severe progressive kyphoscoliosis of all the dwarf syndromes.[4,7,16,31,37] The latter complication converts this to a short-trunk type of dwarfism with age. Radiological findings include dense, waferlike vertebral bodies, anterior vertebral wedging, coccygeal tail, dens hypoplasia, atlantoaxial subluxation, and hydrocephalus or hydrosyringomyelia. This condition may be confused with achondroplasia at birth or Morquio's syndrome later.

The Kozlowski type is the most common form of *spondylometaphyseal dysplasia*.[4,7,16] Spinal involvement includes severe platyspondyly, especially cervical and thoracic, with disk widening, kyphosis or kyphoscoliosis, canal narrowing, and early osteoarthrosis. Other abnormalities are thoracic spina bifida and sphenoid and basioccipital hypoplasia.

Kneist's dysplasia may be confused with metatrophic dwarfism or spondyloepiphyseal dysplasia, although the platyspondyly with anterior vertebral beaking and thoracolumbar kyphosis tends to be less severe.[4,7,16] Other abnormalities include lordosis, irregular end plates, coronal vertebral clefts, narrowing of the lumbar canal, dens hypoplasia, tall dens, anterior atlantoaxial fusion, and macrocephaly.

Larsen's syndrome is characterized by flat facies, multiple major joint dislocations (arthrogryposis), and club feet. Spinal abnormalities include segmental vertebral anomalies, flattened bodies, cervical vertebral hypoplasia, cervical kyphosis, cervicothoracic scoliosis or lordosis, and upper cervical and atlantoaxial dislocation (Fig. 9-99).[4,7,16]

Conradi-Hünermann syndrome is the most common form of *chondrodysplasia punctata* (chondrodysplasia calcificans congenita). Spinal involvement includes the characteristic stippled or dense punctate calcific vertebral deposits, vertebral clefting or wedging, congenital scoliosis (such as hemivertebra, unsegmented pedicle bar), odontoid hypoplasia, os odontoideum, and atlantoaxial instability.[4,7,16] Other syndromes associated with congenital scoliosis include *Robinow* and *Goldenhar syndromes*.

Craniometaphyseal dysplasia (Pyle's disease) is a genetically heterogeneous group of skeletal dysplasias characterized by bony overgrowth of the face, cranium, and peripheral skeleton due to failure of normal bony resorption and remodeling. There is hyperostosis of the vault and skull base and cervical spine deformities producing foraminal, foramen magnum, and canal encroachment.[4,17] The bony deformities result in cranial nerve constriction, cervicomedullary compression, vascular compromise, hydrocephalus, or hydrosyringomyelia.

Osteogenesis imperfecta is a heterogeneous group (types I to IV) of connective tissue diseases resulting from disorders of collagen metabolism with osteoporosis as a major feature.[17,31] There are congenita and tarda forms of autosomal dominant, recessive, and sporadic occurrences. Axial skeletal abnormalities include skull base involvement with basilar impression and foramen magnum distortion producing neural and vascular compromise, as well as hydrocephalus or hydrosyringomyelia. Other axial skeletal involvement includes biconcave vertebral bodies, vertebral collapse with severe kyphoscoliosis and cord compression, spondylolisthesis, or spondyloptosis.

Osteopetrosis, or Albers-Schönberg disease, is a generalized hereditary bone disorder in which there is failure of normal bone resorption (osteoclastic malfunction) with resultant diffuse sclerosis. The extent or severity of skull base and spinal column involvement varies from mild to moderate in the ''benign'' autosomal dominant form, and severe in the ''malignant'' autosomal recessive form.[3,17,31] With marrow encroachment there is pancytopenia or infection, as well as fractures and osteomyelitis. Skull base hypoplasia results in neural and vascular foraminal stenosis including foramen magnum constriction. This often results in multiple cranial nerve palsies, including optic atrophy, compromised venous return, and impaired CSF absorption resulting in hydrocephalus or hydrosyringomyelia. Cervicomedullary compression is infrequent. *Marfan's syndrome* is a connective tissue disorder with relatively common spinal involvement.[16,25,31] This includes kyphoscoliosis, wide canal with dural ectasia, meningocele, lumbar interfacet laxity, and atlantoaxial instability.

REFERENCES
Spondylodysplasias

1. Akbarnia B: Selection of methodology in surgical treatment of adolescent idiopathic scoliosis, *Orthop Clin North Am* 19:319, 1988.
2. Banna M, Hollenberg R: Compressive meningeal hypertrophy in mucoplysaccharidosis, *AJNR* 8:385, 1987.
3. Bartynski WS, Barnes PD, Wallman JK: Cranial CT of autosomal recessive osteoporosis, *AJNR* 10:543, 1989.
4. Bassett G, Scott C: The osteochondrodysplasias. In Morrissy R, editor: *Lovell and Winter's pediatric orthopedics*, ed 3, Philadelphia, 1990, JB Lippincott.
5. Ben-David B: Spinal cord monitoring, *Orthop Clin North Am* 19:427, 1988.
6. Benson DR: Idiopathic scoliosis: The last 10 years and state of the art, *Orthopedics* 10:1691, 1987.
7. Bradford D, Hensinger R: *The pediatric spine*, New York, 1985, Thieme.
8. Braffman B, Bilaniuk L, Zimmerman R: The CNS manifestations of the phakomatosis on MR, *Radiol Clin North Am* 26:773, 1988.
9. Casselman ES, Mandell GA: Vertebral scalloping in neurofibromatosis, *Radiology* 131:89, 1979.
10. Crawford A: Neurofibromatosis. In Morrissy R, editor: *Lovell and Winter's pediatric orthopedics*, ed 3, Philadelphia, 1990, JB Lippincott.
11. Edelson J, Nathan H: Nerve root compression in spondylolysis and spondylolisthesis, *J Bone Joint Surg* 68B:596, 1986.
12. Edwards MK, Harwood-Nash DC, Fitz CR, et al: CT metrizamide myelography of the cervical spine in Morquio syndrome, *AJNR* 3:666, 1982.
13. Fearon T, Vucich J, Butler P, et al: Scoliosis examinations: organ dose and image quality with rare-earth screen-film systems, *AJR* 150:359, 1988.
14. Gillespie R *Disorders of the developing nervous system*, Boston, 1986, Blackwell.
15. Hoffman H, Epstein F, editors: *Disorders of the developing nervous system*, Boston, 1986, Blackwell.
16. Jones KL: *Smith's recognizable patterns of human malformation*, ed 4, Philadelphia, 1988, WB Saunders.
17. Kooh S: Metabolic abnormalities of the skull and axial skeleton. In Hoffman H, Epstein F, editors: *Disorders of the developing nervous system*, Boston, 1986 Blackwell.
18. Kumar R, Guinto FC, Madewell JE, et al: The vertebral body: Radiographic configurations in various congenital and acquired disorders, *Radiographics* 8:455, 1988.
19. Leeds NE, Jacobson HG: Spinal neurofibromatosis, *AJR* 126:617, 1976.
20. McMaster M: Occult intraspinal anomalies and congenital scoliosis, *J Bone Joint Surg* 66A:588, 1984.
21. McMaster M, Ohtsuka K: The natural history of congenital scoliosis, *J Bone Joint Surg* 64A:1128, 1982.
22. Morrissy R, editor: *Lovell and Winter's pediatric orthopaedics*, ed 3, New York, 1990, JB Lippincott.
23. Pavlov H, Torg JS, Robie B, et al: Cervical spine stenosis: determination with vertebral body ratio method, *Radiology* 164:771, 1987.
24. Perovic MN, Kopits SE, Thompson RC: Radiological evaluation of the spinal cord in congenital atlantoaxial dislocation, *Radiology* 109:713, 1973.
25. Petterson H, Harwood-Nash D: *CT and myelography of the spine and cord*, New York, 1982, Springer-Verlag.
26. Pierre-Kahn A, Sainte-Rose C, Hirsch J: Neurological manifestations in achondroplasia. In Hoffman H, Epstein F, editors: *Disorders of the developing nervous system*, Boston, 1986, Blackwell.
27. Pueschel S, Scola F: Atlantoaxial instability with Down syndrome, *Pediatrics* 80:555, 1987.
28. Rosenbaum DM, Blumhagen JD, King HA: Atlantooccipital instability in Down syndrome, *AJR* 146:1269, 1986.
29. Sachs B, Bradford D, Winter R, et al: Scheuermann's kyphosis, *J Bone Joint Surg* 69A:50, 1987.
30. Tachdjian MO: *Pediatric orthopedics*, ed 2, Philadelphia, 1990, WB Saunders.
31. Taybi H, Lachman RS: *Radiology of syndromes, metabolic disorders, and skeletal dysplasias*, ed 3, Chicago, 1990, Mosby–Year Book.
32. Wilkinson RH, Willi UV, Gilsanz V, et al: Radiographic evaluation of the spine after surgical correction of scoliosis, *AJR* 133:703, 1979.
33. Winter R: Congenital scoliosis, *Orthop Clin North Am* 19:395, 1988.
34. Winter R, Lonstein J: Neurofibromatosis hyperkyphosis, *J Spinal Disord* 1:39, 1988.
35. Winter R, Moe J, Lonstein J: The surgical treatment of congenital kyphosis, *Spine* 10:224, 1985.
36. Wortzman G, Steinhardt MI: Congenitally absent lumbar pedicle: a reappraisal, *Radiology* 152:713, 1984.
37. Wynne-Davies R, Hall CM, Apley AG: *Atlas of skeletal dysplasias*, Edinburgh, 1985, Churchill Livingstone.
38. Yaghmai I: Spine changes in neurofibromatosis, *Radiographics* 6:261, 1986.

10 · Acquired Abnormalities of the Spine and Spinal Neuraxis

Patrick D. Barnes

Spine trauma

CLINICAL AND IMAGING CONSIDERATIONS

Traumatic spinal column and cord injuries occur less frequently in childhood than in adulthood. Less than 10% of all spine trauma occurs during childhood, with one peak occurrence in children under 5 years of age and the other peak in those over 10 years of age.[*] About one half of the incidents are related to vehicular accidents including motor vehicle–pedestrian, bicycle, and motorcycle mishaps. About one third are sustained during sports-related activities, especially diving. Less common but important causes include falls, gunshot wounds, and child abuse.[1,3,44] Multiorgan system injury may occur in up to one fourth of

spine trauma cases. A large percentage of spinal column injuries are not associated with neurological deficit. On the other hand, a significant number of cord injuries occur without demonstrating abnormal radiographic findings, especially in the neonate and infant.[1,44,60]

Because anatomical and biomechanical changes take place from birth to adolescence, the types and patterns of injury differ for the infant and young child compared with that for the adolescent and adult. The immature spine is in transition as a cartilaginous and incompletely ossified column including the relatively weak cartilaginous synchondroses that connect ossifying centers. Ligamentous, muscular, articular, and other soft tissue laxities also exist. By 8 to 10 years of age, after closure of the major synchondroses (for example, neurocentral, spinolaminal,

---

[*]References 1, 3, 28, 44, 49, 60.

and subdental), the spine has attained adult form, especially in the cervical region.[1,2,18,60]

In childhood spine injury occurs at the cervical level more commonly than at the thoracic or lumbar level.[1,2,20,28,60] In the infant and young child upper cervical injury occurs much more frequently than lower cervical injury, the latter usually associated with very severe trauma. Because of the larger relative head size in younger children, the structural spinal immaturity, and the higher fulcrum for flexion-extension above C2-3, the range of injuries for this group tends to include synchondrosis fractures of the atlas, axis, and dens, as well as occipitoatlantal and atlantoaxial dislocations.[1,18,44] Neurocentral and posterior synchondrosis fractures also may occur at other levels. In the older juvenile and adolescent there is relatively equal distribution between upper and lower cervical injuries similar to that in the adult. Burst fractures, facet fractures, facet dislocations, and ligamentous disruptions are more characteristic of adolescence and adulthood.[7,53] Other important traumatic lesions of childhood include spondylolysis and spondylolisthesis, rare disk herniations including acute Scheuermann's disease, slipped vertebral apophysis, and disk space calcification.

Plain films are the procedure of choice for initial imaging of spine trauma, followed by computed tomography (CT) or conventional tomography.[10,11,39,45,60] The first film obtained after protective immobilization for head and neck trauma is usually a cross-table lateral film of the cervical spine that includes the craniocervical and cervicothoracic junctions. This film serves as a guide for further, safe filming that includes frontal cervical and open-mouth views of the atlantooccipital and atlantoaxial structures. Oblique views are occasionally indicated to evaluate the neural arches, especially the facet articulations and intervertebral foramina. Clinically guided or voluntary flexion and extension radiography or fluoroscopy may be necessary, however, to evaluate stability. This is additionally important for patients with persistent symptoms and otherwise negative static films to evaluate ligamentous disruption. Initial supine cross-table lateral and frontal films usually suffice for thoracic and lumbar spine trauma. Occasionally, lateral plain films may be obtained after carefully logrolling the patient into the decubitus position. Adequate lateral views of the cervicothoracic junction and upper thoracic spine may require careful repositioning with oblique views, overexposed views, or tomography. After plain filming CT or tomography may be indicated to further characterize and better define the fractures and malalignment, including intraspinal fragments and spinal canal or foraminal encroachment. Isotope bone scanning is important in the assessment of occult spine injury, such as spondylolysis.[8]

Radiological abnormality or clinical signs of spinal cord or nerve dysfunction are indicators for immediate spinal immobilization. Spinal cord imaging, that is, myelography or MRI, is not usually indicated initially when total cord dysfunction is present. The most widely accepted indication for spinal cord imaging in acute trauma is partial or

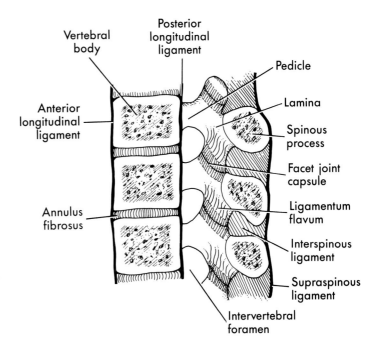

Fig. 10-1   Ligamentous structures of the spine. (Modified from Gehweiler J, et al: *The radiology of vertebral trauma*, Philadelphia, 1980, WB Saunders.)

progressive myelopathy or radiculopathy.[1-3,44] In patients with total cord dysfunction or normal neurological status, spinal imaging may be indicated when there is column instability (ligamentous injury) and surgical stabilization is anticipated. Neurological symptoms or signs and imaging findings out of proportion to the "history" of trauma should suggest the possibility of a preexisting anomaly (for example, craniocervical anomaly, dysraphism), tumor (for example, pathological fracture, neural tumor), or child abuse. MRI often obviates the need for myelography in acute trauma to assess disk protrusion, bony encroachment, pathological fracture, ligamentous injury, intraspinal hematoma, cord hemorrhage or edema, contusion or transection, and nerve root avulsion or plexus injury.* This is particularly true now that magnet-compatible vital monitoring and support devices are available. MRI is the procedure of choice for imaging the sequelae of spinal cord injury, including syrinx, cyst, and myelomalacia. MRI provides preoperative guidance, whereas ultrasonography is the choice for intraoperative guidance.[50-52,58,65]

BASIC MECHANISMS OF SPINE TRAUMA

As a fundamental approach to understanding spinal trauma, the three-column concept of Denis, as applied by Rogers and others, is presented.[16,17,29,53] The bony and ligamentous spinal column is subdivided into three longitudinal columns (Fig. 10-1). The posterior column comprises the bony neural arch, ligamentum flavum, inter-

---

*References 6, 13, 14, 19, 27, 37, 38, 46.

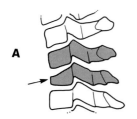
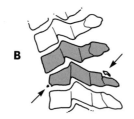
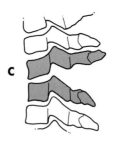
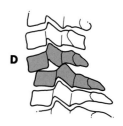

Fig. 10-2   The spectrum of flexion spine injuries. **A,** Anterior body wedge fracture *(arrow).* **B,** Anterior apophyseal dislocation with corner body fracture *(small arrow),* spinous avulsion fracture *(large arrow),* anterior disk space narrowing, and interspinous widening. **C,** Posterior ligamentous disruption with widening of the posterior disk space and widening of the interfacet, interlaminar, and interspinous distances. **D,** Bilateral or unilateral (rotational) facet dislocation. (Modified from Swischuk C: *Emergency radiology of the acutely ill or injured child,* ed 2, Baltimore, 1986, Williams & Wilkins.)

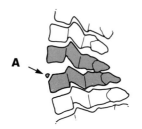
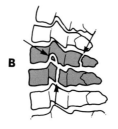
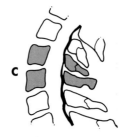

Fig. 10-3   The spectrum of extension spine injuries. **A,** Anterior longitudinal ligament disruption with avulsion corner body fracture *(arrow),* wide disk space, wide interfacet distance, and posterior dislocation with potential cord injury. **B,** Various neural arch fractures *(arrows),* for example, facet, pedicle, laminar, or spinous, with anterior subluxation on flexion. **C,** Ligamentum flavum buckling *(jagged line)* with potential cord injury. (Modified from Swischuk C: *Emergency radiology of the acutely ill or injured child,* ed 2, Baltimore, 1986, Williams & Wilkins.)

spinous and supraspinous ligaments, and the facet joint capsules. The anterior column consists of the anterior vertebral body, anterior longitudinal ligament, anterior disk, and anterior annulus fibrosis. The middle column, which comprises the posterior vertebral body, posterior longitudinal ligament, posterior disk, and posterior annulus fibrosis, functions as a pivot, or fulcrum, between the anterior and posterior columns. The term *posterior ligamentous complex* refers to the critically important ligamentous structures of the middle and posterior columns, which are responsible for spinal stability, especially important in the cervical spine. Hyperflexion tends to produce anterior column compression and posterior column tension or distraction (Fig. 10-2), whereas hyperextension tends to result in anterior column tension and posterior column compression (Fig. 10-3). Other basic forces of injury include axial or vertical compression (that is, burst injuries), axial or vertical distraction, shearing injury (anteroposterior direction), horizontal rotational trauma, and translation (that is, anterior, posterior, rotary, or lateral dislocation).[66] Spinal column stability may be defined according to the status of the middle column and integrity of the anterior and posterior ligamentous structures.[17,29,53] An

injury is considered unstable if there is evidence of abnormal translation, that is, anteroposterior malalignment on flexion and extension filming, lateral offset with lateral flexion, or rotary misalignment with right and left head turning.

With hyperflexion trauma (Fig. 10-2) the spectrum of injuries, depending on severity, may include anterior body wedge fracture, anterior disk narrowing, posterior disk widening, neural arch avulsion fractures, posterior ligamentous complex disruption, facet joint disruption, and anterior subluxation or dislocation with widening of the interlaminar and interspinous distances. With hyperextension trauma (Fig. 10-3) the range includes anterior body avulsion fracture, anterior ligamentous disruption, anterior disk widening, posterior disk narrowing, neural arch compression fractures, and interlaminar and interspinous narrowing. Posterior or lateral vertebral translation is very rare except in severe trauma. With a predominant burst injury, or flexion trauma with additional burst component, there may be an atlas or axis ring fracture, teardrop anterior body fracture with retropulsed posterior body fragment, vertebral body and laminar fractures, and wide interpediculate distance. With a predominant distraction injury, or flexion-extension trauma with additional distraction, there may be horizontal posterior body and neural arch fractures or posterior ligamentous complex disruption. With shearing or rotation injury there is vertebral malalignment in the axial plane (anteroposterior, lateral, or rotary), which may include unilateral or bilateral facet subluxation or dislocation. Shearing trauma may also produce an anterior body avulsion fracture or an avulsion facet fracture.

Static imaging findings that indicate potential or real spinal instability include vertebral body malalignment, vertebral corner avulsion or teardrop fragments, a retropulsed body fragment, burst fracture (wide interpediculate distance), lateral or rotary C1 lateral mass offset, a dens fracture, wide predental space, interlaminar or interspinous widening (except C1-2), widening or narrowing of the disk space, interfacet widening, interfacet narrowing, rotary interfacet offset, and widening of the Luschka joints.[60]

CERVICAL SPINE TRAUMA

When applying the fundamental concepts of imaging cervical spine trauma in childhood, it is important to be familiar with the normal variations to avoid confusion. The variations relate to incomplete ossification of the developing spine in early childhood, as well as the normal soft tissue laxities.[1,2,29,44,60] Lack of the expected lordotic cervical contour with uneven vertebral angulation is often normal in infants and young children as is pseudosubluxation (angulation without displacement) at C2-3 or C3-4 when there is maintained spinolaminal alignment. Spinolaminal malalignment at C1-2 and C2-3 may indicate bilateral C2 neural arch fracture or posterior ligamentous complex disruption.[60] Slight pseudosubluxation of the bodies and rotation of the facets and spinous processes uniformly over several segments are normal occurrences. Abrupt segmental angulation, displacement, or rotation is abnormal, especially at the lower cervical levels.[60] Normally prominent prevertebral thickening is common in infancy, and prevertebral fat stripe changes are a less reliable sign of abnormality in infants than in older patients. Marked prevertebral swelling, however, is an important indicator of anterior column injury. The interspinous distance at C1-2 is normally wide in flexion, and the anterior arch of C1 may normally override the dens in extension. The predental space may normally approach a maximum of 5 mm with an excursion of up to 2 mm between flexion and extension. An abnormally increased predental space is not expected in pediatric cervical spine trauma, since compromise of the stronger transverse ligament is much rarer than dens injury.[60] In dens fracture the intact transverse ligament carries the dens fragment with the anterior arch of the atlas. Occasionally an increased predental space may occur with a Jefferson fracture, whereas an apparent increase may be evident with rotary atlantoaxial injury. A wide predental space otherwise may indicate a nontraumatic condition such as a developmental anomaly or inflammation. In the frontal plane the relationship of the dens and C2 lateral masses to the C1 lateral masses varies with head tilt and rotation.

Lateral offset of one or both C1 lateral masses relative to the C2 lateral masses may be seen as a normal variant in infancy (atlas pseudospread or pseudoJefferson effect).[22,59,64] CT or tomography, however, may be needed to distinguish this variant from a true Jefferson fracture.

Other important variants and anomalies that may simulate fracture or other injury include an unfused anterior arch of C1, medial tubercles of the lateral masses of C1, arcuate foramina of the C1 posterior arch, unilateral C1 posterior arch hypoplasia, and partial or complete absence of the C1 posterior arch with hypertrophy of the C2 spinous process. Others may include facet notching, anomalous horizontal facet joints, ununited secondary ossification centers of the transverse processes, ring apophyses, asymmetrical transverse processes, spina bifida occulta, and congenital body or arch fusions with obliterated disks or obliterated interlaminar spaces.[29,60] Potential imaging pitfalls include difficulties in distinguishing preossified bony structures or synchondroses from fractures (for example, undisplaced dens fracture versus subdental synchondrosis), and in detecting posterior ligamentous complex disruption in the absence of abnormal plain film findings in the neutral to extended neck position.[60] Flexion-extension filming may be required in these instances.

Neonate and young infant

Regarding detailed delineation of the types of cervical spine injury encountered in childhood (see box on p. 416), a developmental approach according to age-related injury patterns is presented.[1,2,18,44,60] The three groups considered are the infantile, young juvenile (up to 8 to 10 years of age), and the older juvenile and adolescent. Cervical spine injury in the infant may occur as a result of obstetrical trauma, accidents, or child abuse. The immature spine is primarily cartilaginous and ligamentous and more flexible or elastic than the dura and spinal cord. As a result, meningeal, cord, or nerve injury often occurs without obvious fracture or dislocation. The range of injury includes atlantooccipital or atlantoaxial dislocation, dens fracture, neurocentral synchondroses fractures, epidural or subdural hematoma, subarachnoid hemorrhage, and cord or nerve root injury.

Upper cervical and cervicothoracic junction injuries may occur in birth trauma, especially with breech position, transverse lie, or difficult cephalic deliveries.[1,5,40,44] Often there is neck hyperextension and head or shoulder torsion resulting in stretching, elongation, and angulation of the spinal column without fracture. As a result, there may be meningeal injury with epidural hematoma. A second type of injury is that of excessive longitudinal traction on the spinal cord that results in distortion, compression, laceration, or vascular injury. As a result there may be edema, contusion, hemorrhage, and necrosis or cord transection. The third type of injury is nerve root laceration and avulsion with dural tear and extraarachnoid leakage of CSF.[47] With difficult breech presentations the injury usually occurs at the lower cervical or upper thoracic level. Lower thoracic or

TYPES OF SPINAL COLUMN INJURY ACCORDING TO REGION AND MECHANISM[29,53,60]

CRANIOCERVICAL JUNCTION

Flexion	Dens fracture, lateral mass C1 or C2 fracture (lateral flexion)
Extension	C1 posterior arch fracture, C1 anterior arch avulsion, hangman's fracture, dens fracture, C2 teardrop fracture
Burst	Jefferson C1 fracture, C2 teardrop fracture
Distraction	Atlantoaxial, atlantooccipital disassociation
Translation	Atlantoaxial, atlantooccipital subluxation-dislocation

CERVICAL

Flexion	Compression fracture, clay shoveler's fracture, uncinate or transverse process avulsion (lateral flexion), hyperflexion sprain
Extension	Hyperextension sprain, spondylitic fracture, spinous fracture, anterior vertebral corner avulsion, pillar fracture
Burst	Teardrop fracture, classic burst fracture, sagittal body fracture
Distraction	Hyperflexion sprain
Translation	Unilateral/bilateral facet subluxation-dislocation, anterior vertebral corner avulsion

THORACOLUMBAR

Flexion	Compression fracture
Extension	Pedicle or laminar fracture
Burst	Classic burst fracture
Distraction	Classic seat belt (Chance) fracture, fulcrum fracture, hyperflexion sprain
Translation	Fracture-dislocation, dislocation without fracture

lumbar injury is infrequent. With traumatic cephalic deliveries the injury usually occurs at the cervical level above the origin of the brachial plexus roots. Injuries above C3-4 are usually fatal.

Cord, nerve, or brachial plexus damage may result in partial or complete dysfunction. There may be shock with respiratory distress, truncal and extremity hypotonia, and absent reflexes. The clinical diagnosis may be difficult, since hypoxic-ischemic CNS insult, neuromuscular disease, or sepsis may produce similar signs. Plain film findings are usually negative, although marked prevertebral swelling or, rarely, fracture-dislocation may be evident. Chronically there is cord atrophy with or without fibrosis. The diagnosis is confirmed with ultrasonography or MRI[5,40] (Fig. 10-4). Other types of cervical spine trauma in infancy are similar in mechanisms and manifestations to those in the young juvenile.

Older infant and juvenile

In the infant and young juvenile (up to 8 to 10 years) there remains a strong predilection for upper cervical spine injury (Fig. 10-5) because of the developmental factors emphasized earlier.[1,2,18,44,60] In addition to the supportive tissue laxities the upper three segments have horizontal articular interfaces (atlantooccipital and atlantoaxial) that allow increased translation. Also, incomplete uncinate development allows increased flexion and rotation. Trauma to the immature, incompletely ossified cervical spine tends to result in avulsions, apophyseal separations, epiphyseal growth plate fractures, and synchondrosis fractures, involv-

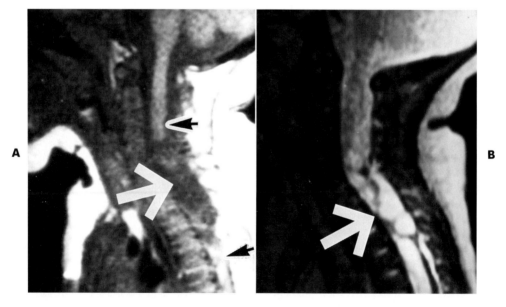

Fig. 10-4   Traumatic cord transection shown by sagittal T1 **(A)** and T2 **(B)** MR. Chronic, mixed intensity cystic and fibrotic changes are evident *(white arrows)* at the level of the cord disruption with more intact cord intensities above and below *(black arrows).*

ing the dens, atlas ring, and axis ring. Occipitoatlantal and atlantoaxial dislocations are also common.

ATLAS INJURIES. Atlas injuries include Jefferson fracture, posterior arch fractures, and anterior arch fractures.[*] *Jefferson fracture* is an axial compressive or burst injury that results in bilateral or unilateral anterior and posterior arch fractures. There may be associated vertical or oblique fractures of the axis body, dens, or lower cervical bodies. There is unilateral or bilateral outward displacement of the C1 lateral masses relative to the C2 lateral masses on frontal and axial images (Figs. 10-5 and 10-6). This traumatic spread or offset is to be distinguished from the normal atlas pseudospread variant (3 months to 4 years of age).[22,59,64] The normally faster neural growth pattern of the atlas is similar to that of the skull base during the first year of life as contrasted with the normally slower somatic growth pattern of the axis, which is similar to that of the lower cervical segments. In the normal pseudospread variant, CT demonstrates an intact atlas ring (absence of fracture). Catch-up growth of the axis occurs from 3 to 6 years. Occasionally, congenital atlas clefts and arch aplasias cause confusion and may be associated with lateral mass offsets of

1 to 2 mm. Jefferson fractures usually produce offsets of greater than 3 mm. Displacements of greater than 7 mm indicate transverse ligament rupture with atlantoaxial instability.

Posterior atlas arch fractures are hyperextension injuries resulting from compression of the posterior arch between the occiput above and axis spinous process below. The fractures appear as unilateral or bilateral narrow defects that occur in isolation or in association with other C1-C2 injury (Fig. 10-5). These are to be distinguished from developmental arch anomalies, which are usually wide defects with odd-shaped and tapered ossification centers. The rare *avulsion injury of the anterior arch* appears as a horizontal fracture with associated prevertebral swelling (Figs. 10-5 and 10-7).

AXIS INJURIES. *Odontoid fractures* tend to occur at the subdental synchondrosis below the level of the articular surfaces of the lateral masses of the axis (low dens fracture, subtype III).[*] The fracture usually occurs as a hyperflexion injury with anterior angulation and displacement of the dens (Figs. 10-5 and 10-8), which moves with the anterior arch of the atlas (anterior atlantoaxial dislocation). Cord com-

---

[*]References 1, 18, 23, 25, 29, 60, 64.

[*]References 1, 18, 23, 25, 29, 60.

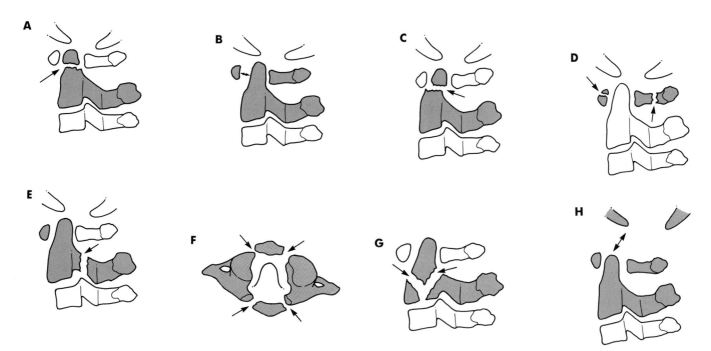

Fig. 10-5   The spectrum of craniocervical junction injuries. **A,** Flexion dens fracture *(arrow).* **B,** Flexion or rotational transverse ligament rupture with anterior or rotatory atlantoaxial dislocation *(arrow).* **C,** Extension dens fracture *(arrow).* **D,** Extension horizontal fracture of the C1 anterior arch *(anterior arrow)* or compressive posterior C1 arch fracture *(posterior arrow).* **E,** Extension C2 neural arch fracture, that is, Hangman's fracture *(arrow).* **F,** Burst fracture of anterior and posterior C1 arches, that is, Jefferson fracture *(arrows).* **G,** Burst fracture of the C2 body *(arrows).* **H,** Atlantooccipital disassociation with dens-basion malalignment *(arrows).* (Modified from Swischuk C: *Emergency radiology of the acutely ill or injured child,* ed 2, Baltimore, 1986, Williams & Wilkins.)

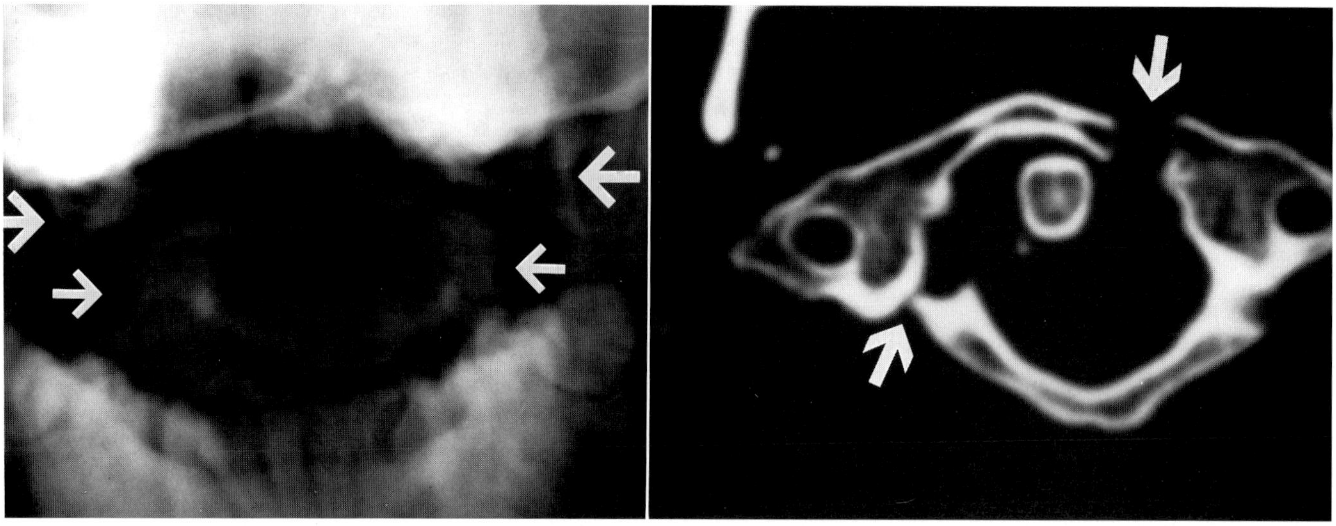

Fig. 10-6   Jefferson fracture in an adolescent male with open mouth frontal plain film **(A)** demonstrating lateral offset of the C1 lateral masses *(large arrows)* relative to the C2 lateral masses *(smaller arrows).* **B,** CT demonstrates the displaced anterior and posterior C1 arch fractures *(arrows)* and the slightly eccentric dens relative to the anterior C1 arch.

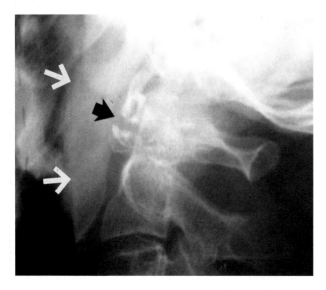

Fig. 10-7   Avulsion fracture of the anterior C1 arch *(black arrow)* shown by lateral plain film along with associated prevertebral swelling *(white arrows).*

pression occurs between the axis base anteriorly and the posterior arch of C1 or the posterior margin of the foramen magnum posteriorly. Hyperextension dens fracture with posterior atlantoaxial dislocation or posterior atlas arch fracture is rare. An undisplaced dens fracture may be difficult to distinguish from the normal subdental synchondrosis early in life without flexion-extension images.[60] Indicators of fracture include widening of the subdental

line, the presence of a subdental line after the age of expected ossification, angulation or tilting of the dens, and reactive change or resorption of the dens. Ischemic necrosis of the dens body with overgrowth of the os terminale (acquired os odontoideum) has been observed.[30] Other types of dens fracture have been described in this age group, as well as in older groups. Type I dens fracture is an avulsion of the dens tip, which is very rare but occurs with occipitoatlantal disassociation. Type II is a superior transverse fracture occurring above the axis lateral masses (high dens fracture). Type III, as discussed earlier, is an axis body fracture extending across the dens base (low dens fracture) and is often associated with fracture of one or both articular pillars and disruption of the axis ring.

Hangman's fracture is another type of axis injury that occurs in the infant or young child as a result of traumatic hyperextension. There is unilateral or bilateral traumatic spondylolysis with or without anterior axis body and dens displacement or dislocation (spondylolisthesis).[*] The fractures may involve the pars, pedicle, laminae, superior facets, or synchondroses (Figs. 10-5 and 10-9). Another more unusual or rare axis fracture is the hyperextension axis teardrop fracture. This is an avulsion triangular corner fracture of the anterior-inferior axis body. Lateral mass axis or atlas fractures are very rare but may be associated with the rare laterally displaced dens fracture.

TRAUMATIC ATLANTOAXIAL AND ATLANTOOCCIPITAL INSTABILITY. Traumatic craniocervical instability without fracture is very rare in childhood but may occur at the atlantoaxial or occipitoatlantal articulations (Fig. 10-5).

*References 1, 18, 23, 25, 29, 60

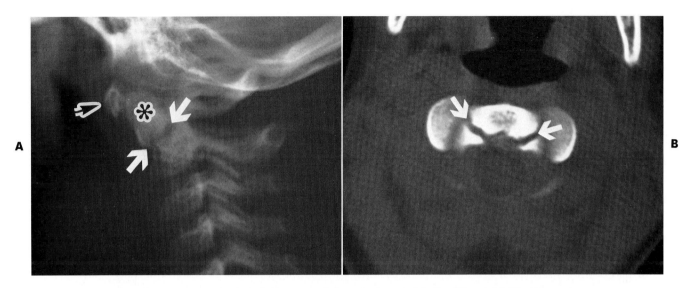

Fig. 10-8   Odontoid fracture *(white arrows)* shown by lateral plain film **(A)** and CT **(B)** with anterior dens angulation *(asterisk)* and displacement with the anterior C1 arch *(black arrow)*.

Disruptions of the synovial joints, transverse ligament, apical and alar ligaments result in increasing degrees of *atlantoaxial subluxation* or *dislocation*. As mentioned earlier, however, traumatic instability is more commonly caused by dens fracture (or Jefferson fracture) than by ligamentous disruption alone. Causes of anteroposterior atlantoaxial instability other than trauma should be considered including inflammatory processes (infection, arthritis) and congenital anomalies (dens hypoplasia, os odontoideum, Down's syndrome), as presented in Chapter 9.[60] Nevertheless, even with the relatively large canal at the C1 level, the normal or abnormal ligamentous laxity of early childhood predisposes to instability with increased risk of spinal cord injury when the displacement is greater than one dens width. In anterior atlantoaxial dislocation cord encroachment occurs between the dens anteriorly and the posterior arch of the atlas or posterior margin of the foramen magnum posteriorly.

Rotary atlantoaxial displacement, fixation, subluxation, and dislocation are discussed in Chapter 9.[1,23,36] In traumatic cases there is often an angled, tilted, or dislocated appearance of C1 relative to C2 as seen on the lateral film. A normal or slightly widened predental space is seen but is usually less than 5 mm with rotary displacement or fixation. On the frontal view the C2 spinous process is displaced to the same side as the tip of the mandible, since the head and lateral masses of the atlas are rotated together (usually less than 40 degrees) on the C2 lateral masses. Rotary subluxation or dislocation (greater than 40 degrees) is suspected if an abnormally widened predental space is apparent on the lateral view, and inward offset of the rotated lateral mass of C1 relative to C2 is seen on the frontal view. In this

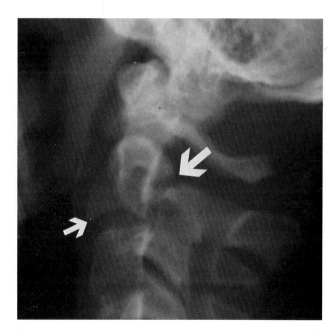

Fig. 10-9   Hangman's fracture shown by lateral plain film with fracture defects through the C2 pedicles *(large arrow)*, anterior subluxation of C2 on C3 *(small arrow)*, and C1-C2-C3 neural arch malalignment.

situation there is expected transverse ligament rupture with anterior or posterior rotary articular offset and the risk of cord compression (Fig. 10-10). CT may demonstrate the full range of abnormalities, as detailed in Chapter 9. More importantly, in acute trauma CT definitively establishes the presence of associated fractures (Fig. 10-11). In the

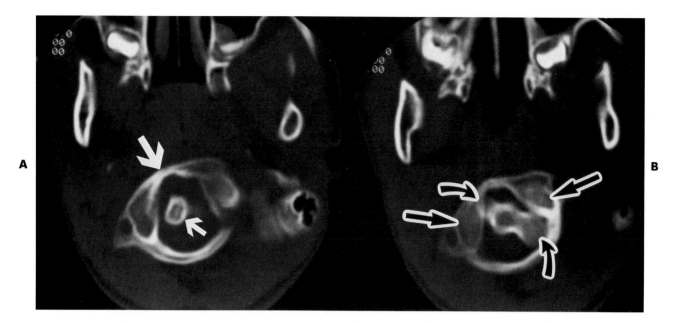

Fig. 10-10   Traumatic rotary atlantoaxial dislocation shown by axial CTs **(A** and **B)** with counter-clockwise rotatory offset of the C1 lateral masses *(straight black arrows)* relative to the C2 lateral masses *(curved black arrows)* plus separation of the rotated dens *(small white arrow)* from the anterior arch of C1 *(large white arrow)* with increased predental and decreased postdental distances and canal-cord encroachment.

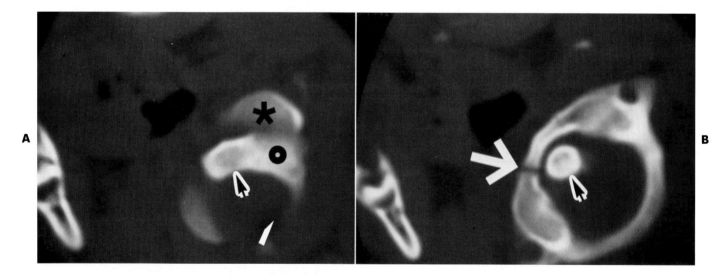

Fig. 10-11   Traumatic rotary atlantoaxial displacement with fixed subluxation shown by axial CT including counterclockwise offset of the left C1 lateral mass *(star)* relative to the left C2 lateral mass *(bull's-eye),* although the rotated dens *(black arrows)* approximates the anterior C1 arch. Fracture diastasis of the right anterior neurocentral synchondrosis is also shown *(large white arrow).*

postacute stages, particularly after resolution of associated spasm and with careful clinical guidance, CT with right and left head rotation confirms rotary fixation, subluxation, or dislocation, whereas flexion-extension lateral filming or MRI confirms anteroposterior atlantoaxial instability.

Atlantooccipital or *occipitoatlantal dislocation* or *disassociation* is a hyperflexion or hyperextension injury with

concomitant craniocervical distraction.* There is a high mortality with disassociation trauma because of cervicomedullary injury (for example, transection), but partial or complete neurological injury including cranial nerve avulsion may sometimes occur. Small children are particularly

---

*References 1, 29, 33, 41, 44, 60.

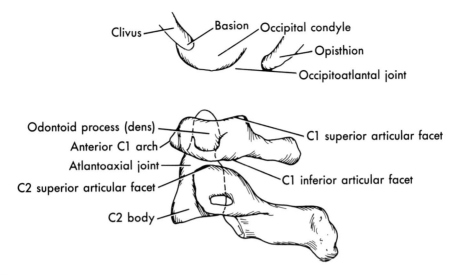

Fig. 10-12   Occipitoatlantal disassociation. There is superior and anterior dislocation with separation of the occipital condyles from the superior articular surfaces of the C1 lateral masses and separation of the dens tip from the basion. (Compare with Fig. 10-13.) (Modified from Gerlock A, et al: *The cervical spine in trauma,* Philadelphia, 1978, WB Saunders.)

susceptible to anteroposterior occipitoatlantal injuries, especially those resulting from autopedestrian collisions, because of the horizontal plane of articulation and the small occipital condyles. Patients with Down's syndrome are also prone to this injury because of ligamentous laxity. With anterior or posterior occipitoatlantal dislocation the dens tip is malaligned relative to the basion as the occipital condyles sublux anteriorly or posteriorly relative to the condylar fossae or superior articular surfaces of the C1 lateral masses (Figs. 10-12 and 10-13). With occipitoatlantal disassociation there is disruption of the tectorial membrane and apical and alar ligaments. Large prevertebral and retropharyngeal hematomas are characteristic. The occiput is vertically separated from the atlas and there is anterior or posterior displacement of the dens from the basion. There may be associated fractures of the occipital condyles or dens tip, and atlantoaxial or C2-3 dislocation or disassociation. The occipital condyles and atlas fossae appear bare with longitudinal separation of the occipital condyles from the atlas condylar facets of greater than 5 mm (normal: 1.5 to 3.5 mm).

Older juvenile and adolescent

In the older juvenile and adolescent (after 8 to 10 years of age), traumatic cervical spine injuries follow a pattern or spectrum similar to that of the skeletally mature adult.[*] Any of the upper cervical or craniocervical injuries just described occur in this older age group, although lower cervical injuries (below C2-3) occur more commonly than in the younger age group. In the 8- to 16-year-old range,

---

[*]References 1, 7, 21, 23, 25, 29, 53.

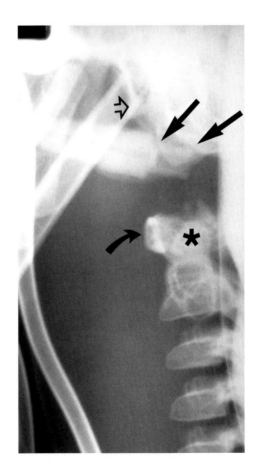

Fig. 10-13   Traumatic occipitoatlantal disassociation with dramatic separation of the atlas *(curved arrow)* and dens *(asterisk)* relative to the occipital condyles *(straight arrows)* and basion *(open arrow)*. Massive prevertebral hemorrhage and edema are present.

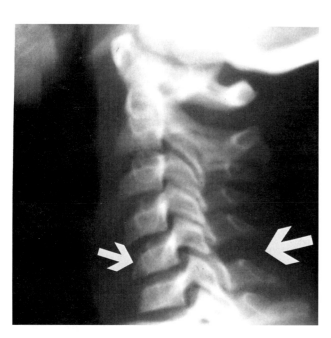

Fig. 10-14   Cervical vertebral wedge fracture *(small arrow)* shown by lateral plain film with associated posterior ligamentous disruption and interspinous widening *(large arrow)*.

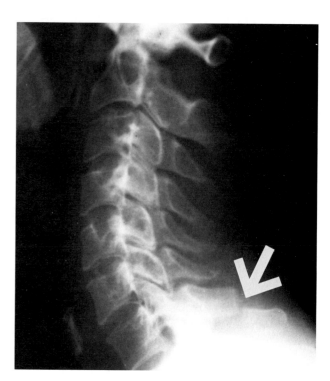

Fig. 10-15   Clay shoveler's fracture of C7 *(arrow)* shown by lateral plain film.

cervical injuries make up 60% to 80% of all spine trauma. Hyperflexion injuries include the simple wedge compression fracture, clay shoveler's fracture, hyperflexion sprain, flexion teardrop fracture, and bilateral interfacet dislocation. Simultaneous hyperflexion and rotation leads to unilateral interfacet dislocation. Vertical compression produces the burst fracture, whereas lateral flexion injuries are often associated with brachial plexus damage.

HYPERFLEXION AND COMPRESSION INJURIES. With hyperflexion and anterior compression, *simple wedge fracture* of the anterior vertebral body occurs (Figs. 10-2 and 10-14) with superior end plate impaction and angulation.[23,29,53,60] Subluxation or dislocation does not occur unless there is posterior ligamentous complex disruption. *Clay shoveler's fracture* is an avulsive, oblique spinous process fracture (Figs. 10-2 and 10-15) usually occurring at C6, C7, or T1.[23,29,53,60] *Hyperflexion sprain* is a combined distraction and flexion injury that results in kyphotic vertebral angulation and anterior subluxation as a result of posterior ligamentous disruption.[23,29,53,60] There may be temporary or partial dislocation of the facet joints with or without associated body, spinous, or subjacent body fractures. Horizontal body and neural arch (Chancelike) fractures have also been observed. Without demonstrable fracture the hyperflexion sprain may be misdiagnosed on supine cross-table lateral or upright extension lateral films. On upright flexion lateral films there is interfacet, interlam-

inar, and interspinous widening along with anterior vertebral angulation and subluxation (Figs. 10-2 and 10-16). Occasionally there is persistent vertebral flexion, angulation, and subluxation with the neck in the extended position. This injury is associated with a 30% to 50% incidence of delayed or chronic instability, which may include vertebral body wedge or beak deformity and posterior ligamentous calcification.

The *flexion teardrop fracture* is a flexion and axial compression injury that produces a shearing teardrop fracture of the anteroinferior body with displacement of the postero-inferior body fragment into the spinal canal[29,34] (Figs. 10-2 and 10-17). The injury usually occurs at the C4, C5, or C6 level and results in a kyphotic deformity. The anterior fragment is aligned with the lower spine, and the displaced posterior fragment is aligned with the upper spine. The appearance may change with traction. The lower disk is disrupted and narrowed, and there is posterior ligamentous complex disruption with facet joint, interlaminar, and interspinous widening. There is anterior longitudinal ligament disruption with marked prevertebral swelling. There may also be posterior displacement of the inferior facet along with sagittal body or laminar fractures. The patient may be neurologically intact or there may be partial or complete deficits (quadriparesis) associated with this highly unstable injury. Classically the flexion teardrop fracture produces anterior cord syndrome, that is, quadri-

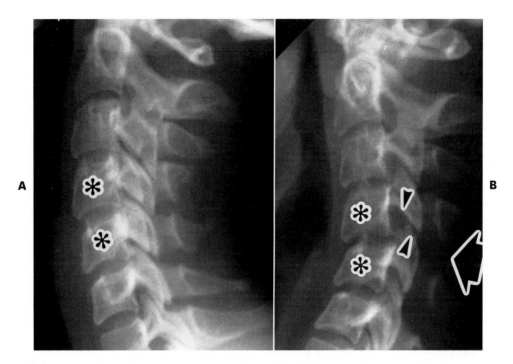

Fig. 10-16   Cervical hyperflexion sprain with C4-5 instability *(asterisks)* demonstrated by lateral extension-flexion plain films. **A,** The extension film reveals normal alignment with developmentally short C4 and C5 spinous processes. **B,** The flexion film shows abnormal angulation and subluxation of C4 body relative to C5 along with facet subluxation *(arrowheads)* and interlaminar plus interspinous widening *(large arrow).*

paresis with loss of pain, temperature, and touch, but intact posterior column function (position, motion, vibratory sense). This type of bony injury is to be distinguished from the burst fracture and the extension avulsion body fracture, discussed later, and from distraction-flexion injury with axial loading. The latter injury consists of sagittal body and laminar fractures with a disrupted posterior ligamentous complex and kyphosis. In that injury the upper spine is displaced anteriorly and often there is unilateral or bilateral facet lock.

Severe hyperflexion trauma may result in *bilateral interfacet dislocation* with posterior ligamentous complex disruption and occasionally with associated avulsion body, facet, or arch fractures.[23,25,29,60] The inferior facets above lie anterior to the superior facets below and project into the foramina in this unstable injury (Fig. 10-2). In bilateral facet dislocation the anterior body displacement is equal to or greater than one half the anteroposterior (A-P) diameter of the body below. With *unilateral interfacet dislocation*[23,25,29,60] there is disruption of the posterior ligaments and joint capsule with attenuation of the anterior and posterior longitudinal ligaments and disk. The anterior body displacement is less than one half the A-P diameter of the body below. On lateral views there is an abrupt rotational offset or malalignment of the facet joints with a bow tie appearance and vertebral body rotation (Fig. 10-18). In the frontal projection there is an abrupt offset or malalignment

of the spinous processes to the same side at and above the facet dislocation (Fig. 10-18). Occasionally there is lateral body displacement and dislocation of the joint of Luschka. Oblique views show perched or overriding facets.

When the predominant mechanism is vertical compression, then a *burst fracture* results.[4,12,23,25,29] There is comminution of the vertebral body with smaller anterior fragments and larger retropulsed posterior fragments. Vertical body and laminar fractures are present with widening of the interpediculate distance. Usually there is normal posterior element alignment (intact posterior ligaments) with a straight cervical spine (see Fig. 10-23). The injury commonly occurs at C6-7, is frequently unstable, and is often associated with severe neurological dysfunction. *Lateral flexion trauma* may produce lateral body compression with avulsion fractures of the contralateral transverse or uncinate processes and widening of the opposite joint of Luschka.[29,60] This lateral column injury often accompanies contralateral brachial plexus avulsion injury and limb paralysis resulting from excessive lateral flexion-rotation of the spine or posterior stretching of the arm. Extraarachnoid extravasation of water-soluble contrast media may be present on myelography or CT.[47] Lateral flexion injury may also accompany other types of injury.

HYPEREXTENSION INJURIES. Hyperextension injuries of the cervical spine include hyperextension sprain and hyperextension fracture-dislocation with pillar or neural

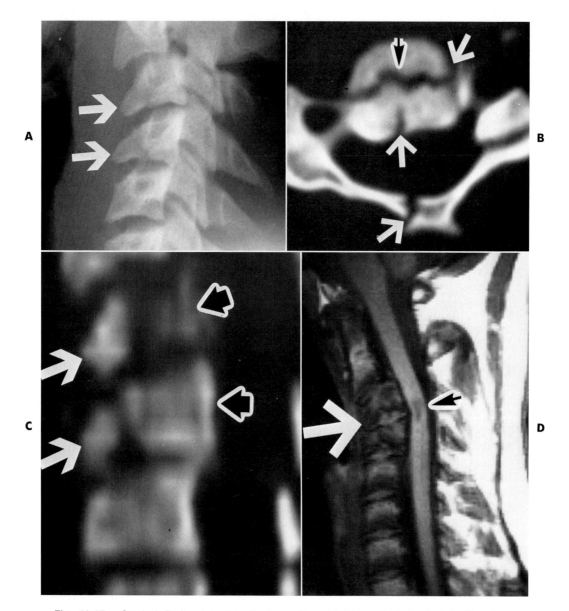

Fig. 10-17 Cervical flexion tear-drop fracture with cord injury. **A,** Lateral plain film shows anteroinferior vertebral body fractures at C3 and C4 *(arrows)* with angular kyphotic malalignment at C2-C3 and C3-C4. There is marked prevertebral soft tissue swelling. **B,** Axial CT shows the associated sagittal *(white arrows)* and coronal *(black arrow)* body and neural arch fractures. **C,** Sagittal CT reformatting demonstrates the tear-drop body fractures *(white arrows)* and retropulsed fragments *(black arrows)*. **D,** Follow-up sagittal T1 MRI shows residual upper cervical kyphosis and retropulsed fragments *(white arrow)* with anterior cord impression and intramedullary hypointensity *(black arrow)* consistent with segmental myelomalacia.

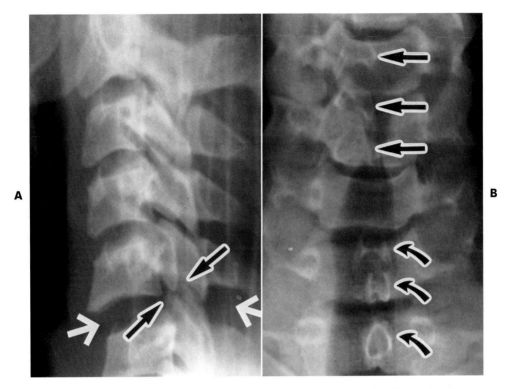

Fig. 10-18   Unilateral cervical interfacet dislocation shown by lateral plain film **(A)** involving the right C5 and C6 facets *(black arrows)*. There is anterior rotatory malalignment of C5 body relative to C6 with disk space and interspinous widening *(white arrows)*. **B,** Frontal plain film demonstrates abrupt rightward offset of the spinous processes at and above C5 *(straight arrows)* relative to those at and below C6 *(curved arrows)* with marked C5-C6 interspinous widening.

arch fractures. *Hyperextension sprain* or dislocation involves disruption of the anterior longitudinal ligament and disk with avulsion of the anteroinferior vertebral body endplate (see Fig. 10-3 and 10-22). Separation of the posterior longitudinal ligament from the lower body also occurs.[23,29,60] Occasionally, there is a horizontal body fracture or posterior element fractures. The spinal cord may be pinched between the posteriorly displaced body anteriorly and the subjacent lamina or buckled ligamentum flavum posteriorly in this unstable injury (see Fig. 10-3 and 10-22). An anterior, central, or complete cord syndrome may result. Marked prevertebral swelling (edema or hemorrhage) is present with anterior disk widening, and an avulsed corner fracture is identified in more than one half of the cases. Occasionally the film findings are deceptively negative because the injury is primarily ligamentous and the dislocation transient.

Hyperextension fracture-dislocation injury with pillar fracture results from combined hyperextension, compression, and rotation.[23,29,60] There is unilateral vertical fracture of the inferior articular pillar with retropulsed fragment resulting from impaction by the superior articular pillar (Fig. 10-3). Occasionally this injury occurs at more than one level. There is anterior vertebral body displacement,

disk narrowing, slight vertebral rotation, and distorted foramina. A lateral column fracture line or displaced pillar is seen on frontal views and is distinguished from unilateral facet dislocation by the lack of spinous process displacement. In *hyperextension fracture-dislocation with arch comminution* there are fractures of the articular pillar, pedicle, and lamina with pillar rotation similar to that just described.[23,29,60] In other cases there is severe posterior arch comminution bilaterally. There may be bilateral articular pillar fractures or a pillar fracture with contralateral facet dislocation, anterior body displacement, disorganized posterior elements, and disrupted lateral columns.

THORACOLUMBAR SPINE TRAUMA
Younger children

Thoracolumbar spine injury occurs less often than cervical trauma in childhood (see box on p. 416). As with cervical trauma there are age-related developmental patterns for injury that occur at the thoracic and lumbar levels.[*] Normal anatomical variants that may be confused for trauma include ring apophyses and bipartite or accessory transverse processes. As mentioned before, spinal cord

---

[*]References 3, 17, 23, 28, 44, 54, 60, 61.

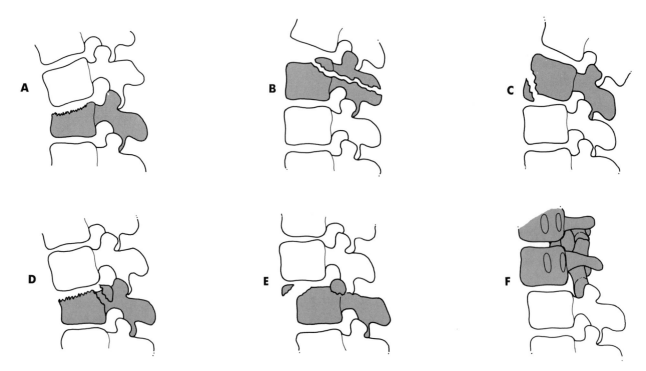

Fig. 10-19   The spectrum of thoracolumbar spine injury. **A,** Flexion injury. **B,** Chance mechanism. **C,** Extension injury. **D,** Burst injury. **E,** Shearing mechanism. **F,** Rotational injury. (Modified from Rogers L: The pathomechanics of spine imaging. Categorical course syllabus on spine imaging, American Society of Neuroradiology meeting, Chicago, May 12, 1988.)

injury in the infant and young child may occur without obvious radiographical abnormality. In children under 10 years of age, cord injury without evidence of radiological abnormality may be seen after autopedestrian collisions, in children thrown from motor vehicles, after falls, and following sports injuries. With either a hyperflexion or hyperextension mechanism there is longitudinal cord traction that may result in transection, infarction, or contusion from ligamentum flavum buckling.[1,3,44] Disk protrusion and epidural hematoma are infrequent. This type of injury may occur at the cervical, upper thoracic, lower thoracic, or, rarely, the lumbar level. There is usually little or no evidence of spinal column abnormality or instability. There may be partial or complete cord dysfunction, and the onset of neurological deficits may be delayed for hours or even a few days. Chronically there is segmental cord atrophy. The proper use of infant car seats can prevent this type of injury.

Older children and adolescents

In the older group (5 to 14 years of age) the use of lap belts is more often associated with lumbar injury.[3,17,60,61] The belt is usually secured about the abdomen of the child instead of over the pelvis and iliac crest as in the adults. With a higher center of gravity in the child, upper body flexion on the lap belt often results in lumbar spinal injury in addition to abdominal injuries. In older adolescents and adults the fulcrum is over the pelvis and the injury more often occurs at the thoracolumbar junction.

HYPERFLEXION AND HYPEREXTENSION INJURIES. The spectrum of hyperflexion injuries (Figs. 10-19 and 10-20) includes anterior vertebral compression fractures, occasional teardrop vertebral fractures, posterior element distraction with facet dislocation, avulsion arch fractures, or

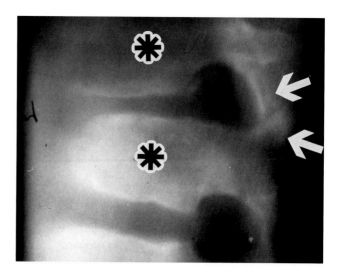

Fig. 10-20   Hyperflexion thoracolumbar spine injury shown by lateral tomogram with T12 anterior wedge vertebral compression *(lower asterisk),* anterior angular subluxation of T11 body *(upper asterisk)* relative to T12, and bilateral facet dislocation *(arrows).*

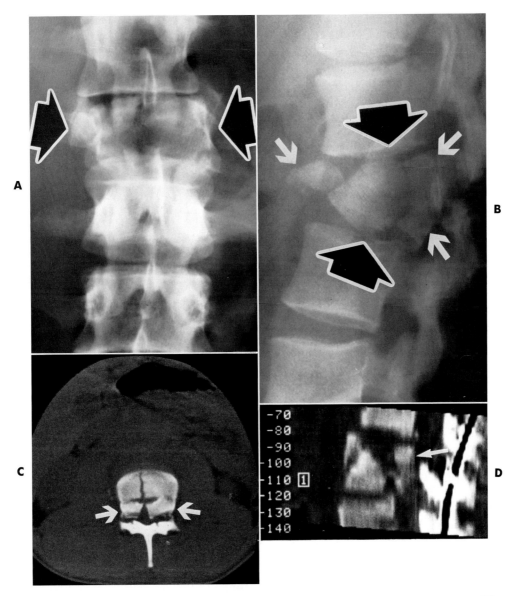

Fig. 10-21   Thoracolumbar burst fracture *(black arrows)* in an adolescent male shown by frontal **(A)** and lateral **(B)** plain films plus axial **(C)** and sagittally reformatted **(D)** CT images including retropulsed fragments *(posterior white arrows).*

posterior ligamentous disruption with interlaminar and interspinous widening. Hyperflexion lap belt trauma with distraction may also produce the classic Chance fracture, that is, horizontal fracture of the body and neural arch with posterior element separation (Fig. 10-19). Hyperextension thoracolumbar injuries are uncommon at any age and are usually associated with severe or fatal trauma.[3,44,60] The spectrum of injury (Fig. 10-19) may include posterior arch or spinous fractures, anterior vertebral body avulsion fractures (that is, lumbar limbus or corner fracture) with ligamentous injury and instability, anterior disk widening, posterior body displacement, or the rare traumatic spondylolysis with spondylolisthesis and anterior body displacement.

BURST FRACTURES. Axial compression combined with hyperflexion, rotation, or both produces the common burst fracture.[3,44,60] There is centripetally directed disruption of the body with vertical fractures, marked anterior body wedging, and a retropulsed posteroinferior or posterosuperior corner body fragment with canal impingement (Figs. 10-19 and 10-21). Instability (that is, ligamentous disruption) is often indicated by severe body compression, posterior element fractures, increased interpediculate distance, and A-P or lateral translation. Neurological deficit occurs at the level of the burst injury in the majority of cases. In more than half of the cases, body or arch fractures occur at other levels. Spinal canal impingement due to body displacement and posterior ligamentous complex disruption are the major determinants of neurological injury and prognosis. Sequelae include pain, angular vertebral deformity with kyphosis, instability, and residual neurological impairment.

Other uncommon types of spinal injury in childhood include rotation injuries, lateral flexion injuries, sacral and coccygeal fractures, and gunshot injuries. Rotation injury combined with angular bending and shearing commonly occurs at the thoracolumbar junction and produces a fracture-dislocation with ligamentous disruption, instability, and injury of the conus medullaris or cauda equina.[3,44,60] Lateral flexion trauma produces compression lateral body fractures with contralateral transverse process avulsion. Sacral fractures usually occur with pelvic trauma, whereas, coccygeal fractures may occur with falls upon the buttocks. Gunshot injury of the spine is rare in childhood and usually results in incomplete neurological injury.[24,62]

Unstable spinal injuries may include fracture-dislocation with ligamentous rupture and facet interlock, rotation-hyperflexion fracture-dislocation with posterior ligamentous disruption and lateral body displacement, and burst injury with neural arch fractures. Another unstable injury is the sagittal vertebral body fracture that extends into the subjacent body. There may be associated lateral displacement of the lower body fragment, or anterior and posterior ligamentous rupture with disk disruption and spinal dislocation. Most thoracolumbar junction fractures associated with conus-caudae injury are considered unstable, especially in cases of severe body compression (Fig. 10-21). Rotary fracture-dislocations occurring at this level are also highly unstable. Common thoracic or lumbar spinal injury patterns associated with cord injury (Figs. 10-19 and 10-21) include anterior vertebral fracture-dislocations with subjacent vertebral body compression and anterior triangular fragment, vertebral fracture-dislocations with additional comminution and upper body dislocation, and vertebral fracture-dislocations with additional compression fractures of one or more bodies below.[54] Apophyseal disruption with facet subluxation or dislocation is commonly present. Cervical spine injury may be associated with thoracolumbar injury in these cases. Upper thoracic spine injury with fracture-dislocation may be stabilized by the rib cage, although neurological deficit is common because of the small canal at this level.

SPINE TRAUMA IN CHILD ABUSE

The spectrum of injury in spine trauma due to child abuse overlaps that due to accidental trauma. However, often there are patterns of injury that may indicate abuse.[35,57,60] In fact, spinal fracture or fracture-dislocation in a child without a history of major trauma should be viewed with suspicion. Vertebral compression deformities of varying severity may be seen often with intact end plates and disk spaces. The majority of the deformities are seen at the lower thoracic or upper lumbar levels, although multilevel involvement is common. Thoracolumbar kyphosis may result. With severe hyperflexion trauma there may be anterior disk herniation into the vertebral end plate superiorly or

inferiorly resulting in anterior disk space narrowing and vertebral corner notching with sclerosis. Sequelae include spinal growth disturbance, ununited ring apophyses, kyphoscoliosis, scoliosis, or hyperlordosis.

Spinous process fractures may be seen with or without vertebral fractures and associated with shaking at the waist. There are avulsions of cartilage and bone occurring at ligamentous attachments, and are usually located mid to lower thoracic or, occasionally, upper lumbar. Progressive calcification or ossification may be seen on follow-up films. The wandering vertebral body injury occurs when the posterior arch separates from the vertebral body at the neurocentral synchondroses, resulting in anterior body displacement. Other types of injury reported with child abuse include hangman's fracture of C2, clay shoveler's fracture of the lower cervical spine, paraspinal hemorrhage with calcification, and cord injury without obvious spinal column abnormality.

SPINAL CORD INJURY
Clinical aspects

Spinal cord injury may be clinically manifested as complete or incomplete loss of sensory and motor function.[1,3,19,28,44] Early transient symptoms and signs may precede the more permanent deficits of delayed cord injury for up to 4 days. Often there is a poor correlation between spinal column injury and neural injury. Traumatic myelopathy or radiculopathy may be classified as *complete* with total loss of motor, sensory, and autonomic function distally, or *partial* as with posterior cord syndrome (crude touch present only), anterior cord syndrome (touch and proprioception intact only), central cord syndrome (arms more affected than legs), Brown-Sequard syndrome (ipsilateral motor loss with contralateral pain and temperature loss), or root syndrome (pain with or without sensory, motor, or reflex loss). The Frankel classification categorizes spinal cord injury as (1) complete motor and sensory loss, (2) preserved sensation only, (3) preserved nonfunctional motor activity, (4) preserved functional motor activity, and (5) complete neurological recovery.[19]

Complete cord injury is more common than incomplete or partial injury, and occurs more frequently at the cervical level (quadriparesis) than at the thoracolumbar level (paraparesis).[1,3,44] More than three fourths of cervical and thoracic cord injuries are initially complete and remain so. Up to one fourth of severe partial lesions show recovery. Thirty percent of patients with thoracolumbar junction injuries and the initial complete loss of function regain motor function. Other important sequelae include chronic spinal instability at the trauma site with progressive deformity, paralytic scoliosis, kyphosis or lordosis, especially before skeletal maturity, and exacerbation of preexisting idiopathic scoliosis. Most spinal cord injuries involving permanent loss of neurological function are caused by compression and contusion with hemorrhage, edema, and ischemic cord destruction. The greatest neurological loss usually occurs at impact, although the process evolves. In fact, the outcome of spinal cord injury is often determined

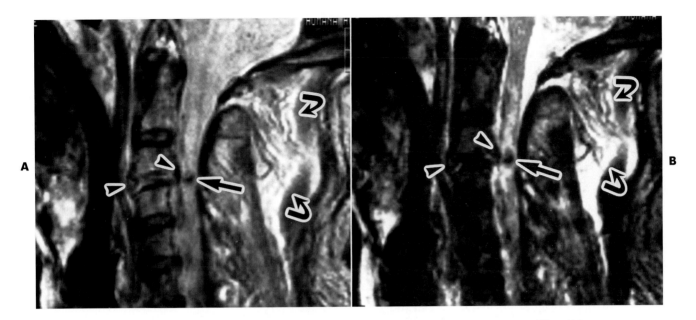

Fig. 10-22   Acute complex cervical spine trauma with cord injury. Sagittal proton density **(A)** and T2 **(B)** MRI demonstrate C3-4 vertebral body fractures with anterior corner fragment *(anterior arrowhead)*, posterior retropulsed fragment *(posterior arrowhead)*, and disrupted C3-4 disk space. Acute cord hemorrhage *(long arrow)* is demonstrated as an intramedullary hypointensity (deoxyhemoglobin) with surrounding hyperintensity (edema). Posterior ligamentous injury is also shown as diffuse hyperintensities *(curved arrows)*. (From Beers GJ, et al: *J Comput Assist Tomogr* 12:755, 1988.)

in the immediate posttrauma period by a combination of primary or direct injury effects and secondary or reactive effects.[1,3,19,28,44] The direct effects of acute injury include vascular tears with petechial hemorrhage and pial disruption with infusion of CSF into the cord. Also, there is axonal disruption with shift of intracellular fluid into the extracellular spaces. Reactive changes are those related to postcapillary vascular stasis with the early occurrence of edema and decreased perfusion of the gray matter. White matter changes occur later, and the process extends rostrally and caudally. There is variable gross hemorrhage within the gray matter that spreads peripherally to the white matter. The edema occurs by about 4 hours and continues to the end of the second day. Necrosis may occur as early as 2 hours with extension beyond the original injury site by about 4 hours. This hemorrhagic infarction is followed by intramedullary cavitation with gliosis and adhesive arachnoiditis. As mentioned earlier, spinal cord injury often occurs in the younger child without evidence of radiographical abnormality. In these instances the injury may result from transient subluxation without bone injury, reversible disk prolapse, longitudinal cord distraction, ligamentum flavum buckling, anterior spinal artery spasm or occlusion, or radiculomedullary arterial injury.

The management of spinal cord injury includes immediate immobilization and medical stabilization while maintaining spinal alignment.[1,3,44] With complete neurological dysfunction, treatment is primarily supportive. With incomplete or partial dysfunction, spinal cord imaging is indicated and spinal canal decompression anticipated. Traction is often employed for nonreducible or neurologically unstable lesions, although there is often the risk of overdistraction, especially in injuries with ligamentous compromise. Posttraction filming is therefore critical. Other important aspects are management of instability and residual deformity, including spinal column realignment and stabilization, often through instrumentation and fusion. Surgical fusion is indicated for posturally unstable injuries, injuries with compromised ligamentous continuity, or when motion threatens neurological function.

Neuroimaging considerations

Neuroimaging of acute spinal cord injury involves the combination of plain films, CT, tomography (occasionally), and MRI. The x-ray based techniques are best for demonstrating fractures and fragment displacement. Although MRI often shows these, particularly the latter, its major contribution is the detection of ligamentous injury, disk protrusion, and intraspinal injury including contusion, hemorrhage, and edema.[*] MRI evaluation of acute spinal cord injury should include sagittal spin echo (SE) T1-weighted images followed by sagittal SE proton density and T2 (p/T2) images or sagittal gradient echo (GE) T2*-weighted images. Axial images are also important to obtain especially for localizing compressive lesions. Ligamentous disruption is demonstrated by MRI as high intensity lesions on p and T2 images in the anatomical distribution of specific ligamentous structures (Figs. 10-22 to 10-24) such as the

---

[*]References 6, 13, 19, 27, 37, 38, 42, 46.

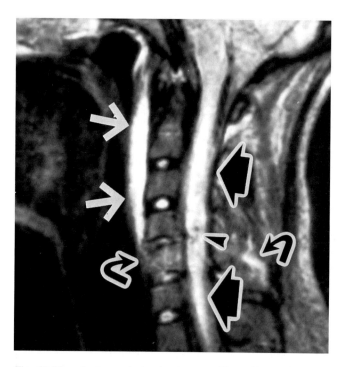

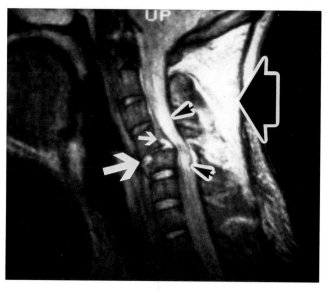

Fig. 10-23   Acute cervical spine trauma with cord injury. Sagittal T2 MRI shows diffuse prevertebral high intensity hemorrhage *(white arrows),* C5 vertebral body burst fracture *(anterior curved arrow)* with disruption of the disk spaces above and below, canal encroachment, and diffuse intramedullary high intensity edema *(large black arrows)* and minute hypointensities *(arrowhead),* which may indicate contusion (deoxyhomoglobin). More localized high intensity posterior ligamentous injury is also shown *(posterior curved arrow).* (From Beers GJ, et al: *J Comput Assist Tomogr* 12:755, 1988.)

Fig. 10-24   Acute cervical trauma with epidural hemorrhage and cord injury. Sagittal T2 MRI shows C4-C5 fracture-dislocation *(large white arrow)* with anterior cord impression, anterior epidural high intensity hemorrhage *(small white arrow),* intramedullary high intensity edema *(black arrows),* and high intensity posterior ligamentous injury *(large black arrow).* (Courtesy GJ Beers, The New York Neurologic Institute, New York.)

posterior ligamentous complex (posterior longitudinal ligament, facet joint capsules, ligamentum flavum, and the interspinous and supraspinous ligaments). Although MRI readily shows dural sac deformities, it is often nonspecific regarding bone fragments, disk protrusion, or hematoma. In the acute or subacute phase (less than 1 week) spinal epidural hematoma may appear isointense to hypointense as contrasted against epidural fat. In the more subacute-chronic phase the high intensity hemorrhage may be difficult to distinguish from fat except on T2 images (Fig. 10-24). Bone hemorrhage associated with vertebral fractures may also be apparent.

Acute spinal cord injury

Acute spinal cord injury (less than 24 hours) is readily identified by MRI and may conform to one of three patterns.[6,13,19,27,37,38] Acute intramedullary hemorrhage (hematomyelia) is often of inhomogeneous or mixed intensity on T1 images and appears as a central hypointensity at the gray-white junction with a surrounding hyperintense thin rim on T2 SE images (Fig. 10-22) or T2* GE images (deoxyhemoglobin). Acute edema appears isoin-

tense to hypointense on T1 images and hyperintense on T2 images and often extends above and below the injury site (Fig. 10-23 and 10-24). Contusion, or mixed injury, may appear isointense relative to the cord on T1 images. Central isointensity to hypointensity with a thick peripheral high intensity halo is seen on T2 SE (Fig. 10-23) or T2* GE images (hemorrhage plus edema). Acute cord hemorrhage may be difficult to distinguish from acute contusion, and both tend to evolve in a manner similar to that for intracerebral hemorrhage and contusion. Acute edema tends to show resolution on follow-up MRI. Although MRI usually distinguishes hemorrhage (or contusion) from edema, necrosis may not be differentiated from edema except on follow-up imaging as a lack of resolution of the hyperintensity, as a cavitation, or as focal atrophy (see Fig. 10-17). The acute cord hemorrhage pattern has been correlated with complete or incomplete injury and poor recovery. The acute edema pattern has been associated with normal function or partial dysfunction and good recovery. The acute contusion pattern has been correlated with a variable but often more favorable outcome as compared with acute cord hemorrhage.

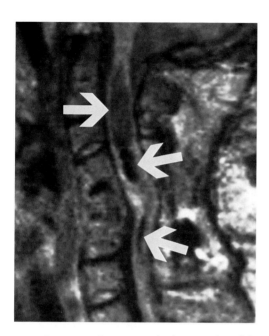

Fig. 10-25   Posttraumatic macrocystic degeneration of the spinal cord shown by sagittal proton density MRI as a hypointense intramedullary expansion *(upper arrow)* with flow signal voids *(lower arrows).*

Chronic spinal cord injury

The sequelae of spinal cord injury include myelomalacia, posttraumatic cord cysts or syringomyelia, arachnoiditis, arachnoid cyst, and neuroarthropathy.[15,50-52,58,65] In chronic spinal cord injury with quadriplegia or paraplegia, there may be new or worsening symptoms or signs including pain. Imaging is indicated to distinguish myelomalacia from posttraumatic cord cyst or syringomyelia and to rule out cord or nerve root compression related to column instability, disk protrusion, osteophytic impingement, or complications of instrumentation and fusion. With the exclusion of cord or root encroachment, the major task is then to distinguish myelomalacia from cystic degeneration.[52] The clinical significance is that cephalad extension of the cyst beyond the level of initial injury into the normal cord may be responsible for neurological deterioration but amenable to shunting. Myelomalacia is primarily a combination of microcystic degeneration and gliosis (see Fig. 10-17) and appears hypointense on T1 MRI, isointense with the cord on p images, and as hypointense as the cord relative to CSF on T2 images. Also, there may be cord thinning. Macrocystic degeneration of the cord (Fig. 10-25)

also appears hypointense on T1 images but appears hypointense relative to the cord on p images and as hyperintense as CSF relative to the cord on T2 images. Often, vascular pulsatile flow signal voids are present, especially on T2 images when flow compensation software is not used. Cord expansion may be present also. Ultrasonography is an important intraoperative guide for shunting of these cysts. (Arachnoiditis is discussed later in this chapter, and arachnoid cysts are presented in Chapter 10.) Postparaplegic neuroarthropathy is characterized by juxtaarticular bone destruction, dense new bone formation, large osteophytes, and soft tissue debris.

SPONDYLOLYSIS AND SPONDYLOLISTHESIS
Clinical aspects

Spondylolysis refers to a defect or defects of the neural arch at the level of the pars interarticularis.[*] The defect may be unilateral (20%) or bilateral and associated with anterior translation (or *spondylolisthesis*) of the involved vertebral segment on the lower segment, most commonly at L5-S1 and less often at L4-5. Spondylolysis is often implicated as the most common cause of low back pain in childhood and is usually encountered after 7 or 8 years of age. Often there is a history of minor trauma during the adolescent growth spurt with resultant stress fracture of the pars interarticularis. The abnormality may be exacerbated or exaggerated by lumbar lordosis, hyperextension, or tumbling. The low back pain is often related to mechanical instability and extends to the buttocks and thighs. The pain is especially prominent with strenuous athletic activity involving repetitive flexion and extension of the back.

The isthmic type with pars defect or elongation is the most common variation of spondylolysis. The dysplastic type of spondylolysis is much rarer and refers to congenitally inadequate facet joints and disk, with or without elongation or attenuation of the pars, and posterior facet subluxation.[9,48] The risk of spondylolisthesis or slippage is higher for females during the adolescent growth spurt (10 to 15 years of age) and especially with the rare dysplastic type. Spondylolisthesis may be associated with idiopathic scoliosis, or the scoliosis may be caused by progressive slippage. Dysplastic spondylolisthesis may be associated with spinal dysraphism, whereas acute traumatic spondylolisthesis often demonstrates neural arch fragmentation. The degree of slippage of the upper vertebral body on the lower body is graded according to Meyerding's classification as the percentage of body length slipped on lateral viewing: grade I (less than 25%), grade II (25% to 50%), grade III (50% to 75%), and grade IV (greater than 75%).

Imaging aspects

The diagnosis may be made by obtaining plain films (frontal, lateral, or oblique), isotope scanning, tomography,

---

*References 3, 8, 9, 26, 31, 32, 48, 55, 56, 63.

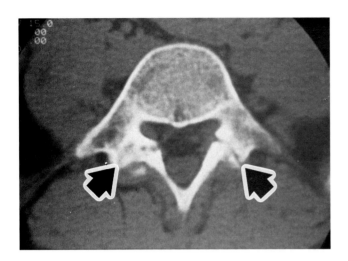

Fig. 10-26   Bilateral L5 spondylolysis and L5-S1 spondylolisthesis shown by axial CT as bilateral irregular pars defects *(arrows)* and associated sclerotic changes.

or CT.[8,9,48,63] Spondylolisthesis is easily determined by MRI, although the spondylolytic defects may not be readily delineated. Acutely there may be a narrow pars defect with irregular edges, whereas the chronic lesion may have smooth and rounded margins. There may be reactive sclerosis with pedicle and laminar hypertrophy (Fig. 10-26) ipsilateral, contralateral, or bilateral to the pars defect(s). Differentiation from the sclerotic nidus of an osteoid osteoma is occasionally required. With healing there may be an intact but sclerotic pars. The pars may be elongated and thinned, with or without a defect, and associated with a malformed lamina, with dysraphic defects, or with deficient facets. There may be neural arch asymmetry and unilateral body wedging. With severe spondylolisthesis angular slippage of L5 on S1 occurs with a trapezoid configuration of the L5 body and superior doming of S1 (Fig. 10-27). This may result in a lumbosacral kyphosis.

CT, MRI, or, rarely, myelography may be indicated for atypical pain (for example, radicular) or for rare neurological deficits.[9,26,32] With slippage greater than 25% to 30%, pars defects or elongation must be present to avoid caudae compression. With severe slippage, nerve root compression may occur at L5 between the pars remnant above and the body or disk below (Fig. 10-27). Nerve root involvement may occur with foraminal stenosis, fibrocartilaginous callus, bony hypertrophy, ligamentum flavum hypertrophy, or rare disk herniation. MRI may be indicated, also, to rule out other sources of pain such as a tumor. The treatment of spondylolisthesis may include surgical fusion. Depending on the surgical technique used, further slippage or pseudarthrosis may occur postfusion. Reduction of severe spondylolisthesis may involve traction or casting plus arthrodesis with or without L5 vertebrectomy to reduce severe pain or prevent deformity.[48,56]

OTHER TRAUMATIC SPINE LESIONS

Other unusual or rare traumatic causes of spine pain in childhood include disk herniation, slipped vertebral apophysis, and disk space calcification.[3,9,43]

Disk herniation

Disk herniation is much less commonly encountered in childhood than in adulthood, but may occur in adolescence in association with the acute or chronic exertion required for participating in some athletic activities. The most common levels of involvement are L4-5 and L5-S1. There may be low back pain with activity, muscle spasm, scoliosis, and gait abnormality, but neurological deficits are rare. Plain film findings are often normal. The diagnosis may be made by obtaining CT or MRI images, but myelography is rarely necessary (Fig. 10-28). The imaging findings are similar to those for adult disk disease.

Slipped vertebral apophysis

Occasionally, disk herniation is associated with slipped vertebral apophysis. This often occurs in teenage males, especially with heavy lifting, weight-lifting, or gymnastics, and with symptoms and signs similar to those of acute disk herniation. Imaging demonstrates avulsion of the posteroinferior apophysis with displacement of the bone fragment and adjacent disk into the spinal canal (Fig. 10-29). The injury more often occurs at L4 than at L5 or L3. Surgical removal of the disk and bone fragment is usually indicated.

Disk space calcification

Disk space calcification[43] occasionally occurs in childhood, usually at the cervical level but occasionally at the thoracic, lumbar, or at multiple levels. The calcification is often of uncertain origin although trauma and inflammation

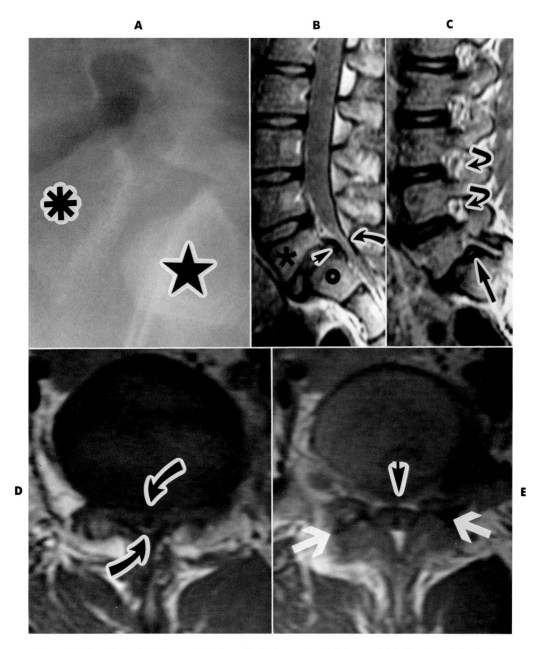

Fig. 10-27   Bilateral L5 spondylolysis with high grade L5-S1 spondylolisthesis and kyphosis.
A, Lateral plain film shows severe anterior angular displacement of the L5 body *(asterisk)* relative to the deformed S1 body *(star)*. Sagittal proton density **(B** and **C)** and axial T1 **(D** and **E)** MRI also show the L5 *(asterisk)* upon S1 (bull's-eye) kyphotic displacement with disk pseudoprotrusion *(arrowhead)*, dural sac narrowing *(curved arrows)*, narrowing of the L5-S1 intervertebral foramina *(straight black arrow)* compared with the normal foramina above *(curved arrows)*, and the bilateral hypointense pars defects *(white arrows)*.

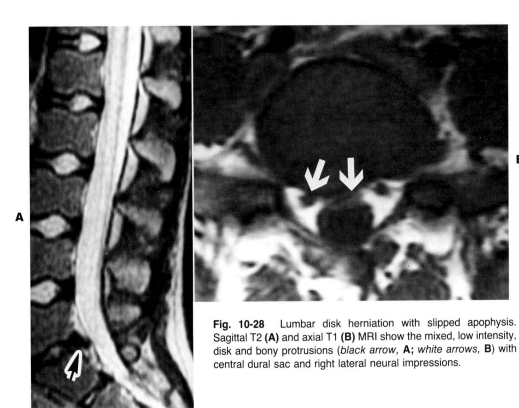

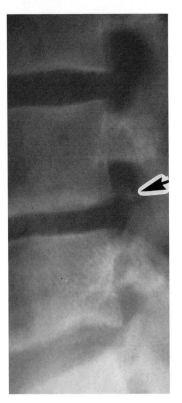

Fig. 10-28 Lumbar disk herniation with slipped apophysis. Sagittal T2 **(A)** and axial T1 **(B)** MRI show the mixed, low intensity, disk and bony protrusions (*black arrow,* **A;** *white arrows,* **B**) with central dural sac and right lateral neural impressions.

Fig. 10-29 Lumbar disk herniation with slipped vertebral apophysis. Lateral plain film shows L4-5 disk space narrowing and the apophyseal fragment *(arrowhead)* displaced into the canal.

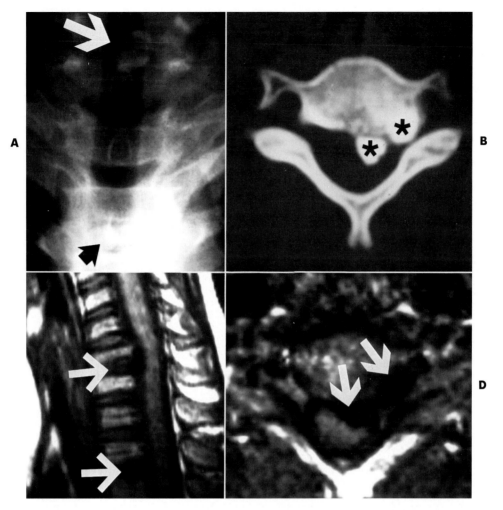

Fig. 10-30   Cervicothoracic disk space calcifications with disk protrusion. **A,** Frontal plain film shows the C6-7 *(white arrow)* and T2-3 *(black arrow)* calcific densities. **B,** Axial CT at C6-7 shows the calcific nodular hyperdensities *(asterisks)* with left foraminal and central canal encroachment. **C** and **D,** Sagittal and axial T1 MRI show the calcific disk space nodular hypointensities *(arrows)* with left foraminal and central canal encroachment at C6-C7.

have been implicated. It occurs more commonly in males and often around the age of 7 years. There may be pain, stiffness, or occasional herniation with neurological signs. The diagnosis is usually made by obtaining plain films (Fig. 10-30). CT or MRI is indicated to evaluate the herniation (Fig. 10-30).

REFERENCES
Spine trauma

1. Allen B, Ferguson R: Cervical spine trauma in children. In Bradford D, Hensinger R, editors: *The pediatric spine,* New York, 1985, Thieme.
2. Apple J, Kirks D: Cervical spine fractures and dislocations in children, *Pediatr Radiol* 17:45, 1987.
3. Asher M, Jacobs R: Pediatric thoracolumbar spine trauma. In Bradford D, Hensinger R, editors: *The pediatric spine,* New York, 1985, Thieme.
4. Atlas SW, Regenbogen V, Rogers LF, et al: The radiographic characterization of burst fractures of the spine, *AJR* 147:575, 1986.
5. Babyn P, Chuang S, Daneman A, et al: Sonographic evaluation of spinal cord birth trauma with pathologic correlation, *AJNR* 9:765, 1988.
6. Beers G, Raque G, Wagner G, et al: MR in acute cervical spine trauma, *J Comput Assist Tomogr* 12:755, 1988.
7. Berquist TH: Imaging of adult cervical spine trauma, *Radiographics* 8:667, 1988.
8. Bodner RJ, Heyman S, Drummond DS, et al: The use of single photon emission computed tomography (SPECT) in the diagnosis of low-back pain in young patients, *Spine* 13:1155, 1988.
9. Bradford D, Hensinger R, editors: *The pediatric spine,* New York, 1985, Thieme.
10. Brant-Zawadzki M, Miller EM, Federle MP: CT in the evaluation of spine trauma, *AJR* 136:369, 1981.
11. Brown BM, Brant-Zawadzki M, Cann CE: Dynamic CT scanning of spinal column trauma, *AJR* 139:1177, 1982.
12. Chakera TMH, Bedbrook G, Bradley CM: Spontaneous resolution of spinal canal deformity after burst-dispersion fracture, *AJNR* 9:779, 1988.

13. Chakeres DW, Flickinger F, Bresnahan JC, et al: MR imaging of acute spinal cord trauma, *AJNR* 8:5, 1987.
14. Cotler H, Kulkarni M, Bondurant F: MR imaging of acute spinal cord trauma, *J Orthop Trauma* 2:1, 1988.
15. Crim JR, Bassett LW, Gold RH, et al: Spinal neuroarthropathy after traumatic paraplegia, *AJNR* 9:359, 1988.
16. Denis F: The three column spine and its significance in the classification of acute thoracolumbar spine injuries, *Spine* 8:817, 1983.
17. Denis F: Spinal instability as defined by the three-column spine concept in acute spine trauma, *Clin Orthop* 189:65, 1984.
18. Ehara S, El-Khoury G, Sato Y: Cervical spine injury in children: radiologic manifestations—pictorial essay, *AJR* 151:1175, 1988.
19. Flanders AE, Schaefer DM, Doan HT, et al: Acute cervical spine trauma: correlation of MR imaging findings with degree of neurologic deficit, *Radiology* 177:25, 1990.
20. Fuchs S, Barthel MJ, Flannery AM, et al: Cervical spine fractures sustained by young children in forward-facing car seats, *Pediatrics* 84:348, 1989.
21. Gehweiler JA, Clark WM, Schaaf RE, et al: Cervical spine trauma: the common combined conditions, *Radiology* 130:77, 1979.
22. Gehweiler JA, Daffner RH, Roberts L: Malformations of the atlas vertebra simulating the Jefferson fracture, *AJNR* 4:187, 1983.
23. Gehweiler JA, Osborne R, Becker R: *The radiology of vertebral trauma*, Philadelphia, 1980, WB Saunders.
24. Gellad FE, Paul KS, Geisler FH: Early sequelae of gunshot wounds to the spine: radiologic diagnosis, *Radiology* 167:523, 1988.
25. Gerlock A, Kirchner S, Heller R, et al: *The cervical spine in trauma*, Philadelphia, 1978, WB Saunders.
26. Grenier N, Kressel HY, Schiebler ML, et al: Isthmic spondylolysis of the lumbar spine: MR imaging at 1.5 T, *Radiology* 170:489, 1989.
27. Hackney DB, Asato R, Joseph PM, et al: Hemorrhage and edema in acute spinal cord compression: demonstration by MR imaging, *Radiology* 161:387, 1986.
28. Hadley M, Zabramski J, Browner C, et al: Pediatric spinal trauma, *J Neurosurg* 68:18, 1988.
29. Harris J, Edeiken-Monroe B: *The radiology of acute cervical spine trauma*, ed 2, Baltimore, 1987, Williams & Wilkins.
30. Holt RG, Helms CA, Munk PL, et al: Hypertrophy of C-1 anterior arch: useful sign to distinguish os odontoideum from acute dens fracture, *Radiology* 173:207, 1989.
31. Johansen JG, McCarty DJ, Haughton VM: Retrosomatic clefts: computed tomographic appearance, *Radiology* 148:447, 1983.
32. Johnson DW, Farnum GN, Latchaw RE: MR imaging of the pars interarticularis, *AJR* 152:327, 1989.
33. Kaufman RA, Dunbar JS, Botsford JA, et al: Traumatic longitudinal atlantooccipital distraction injuries in children, *AJNR* 3:415, 1982.
34. Kim KS, Chen HH, Russell EJ, et al: Flexion teardrop fracture of the cervical spine: radiographic characteristics, *AJR* 152:319, 1989.
35. Kleinman P: *Diagnostic imaging of child abuse*, Baltimore, 1987, Williams & Wilkins.
36. Kowalski HM, Cohen WA, Cooper P, et al: Pitfalls in the CT diagnosis of atlantoaxial rotary subluxation, *AJNR* 8:697, 1987.
37. Kulkarni MV, Bondurant FJ, Rose SL, et al: 1.5 tesla magnetic resonance imaging of acute spinal trauma, *Radiographics* 8:1059, 1988.
38. Kulkarni MV, McArdle CB, Kopanicky D, et al: Acute spinal cord injury: MR imaging at 1.5 T, *Radiology* 164:837, 1987.
39. Lally KP, Senac M, Hardin WD, et al: Utility of the cervical spine radiograph in pediatric trauma, *Am J Surg* 158:540, 1989.
40. Lanska MJ, Roessmann U, Wiznitzer M: Magnetic resonance imaging in cervical cord birth injury, *Pediatrics* 85:760, 1990.
41. Lee C, Woodring JH, Goldstein SJ, et al: Evaluation of traumatic atlantooccipital dislocations, *AJNR* 8:19, 1987.
42. McArdle CB, Crofford MJ, Mirfakhraee M, et al: Surface coil MR of spinal trauma: preliminary experience, *AJNR* 7:885, 1986.
43. McGregor J, Butler P: Disc calcification in childhood: CT and MR, *Br J Radiol* 59:180, 1986.
44. Menezes A, Godersky J, Smoker W: Spinal cord injury. In McLaurin R, Schut L, Venes J, et al, editors: *Pediatric neurosurgery*, ed 2, Philadelphia, 1989, WB Saunders.
45. Mirvis SE, Diaconis JN, Chirico PA, et al: Protocol-driven radiologic evaluation of suspected cervical spine injury: efficacy study, *Radiology* 170:831, 1989.
46. Mirvis SE, Geisler FH, Jelinek JJ, et al: Acute cervical spine trauma: evaluation with 1.5 T MR imaging, *Radiology* 166:807, 1988.
47. Morris RE, Hasso AN, Thompson JR, et al: Traumatic dural tears: CT diagnosis using metrizamide, *Radiology* 152:443, 1984.
48. Pederson A, Hagen R: Spondylolysis and spondylolisthesis, *J Bone Joint Surg* 70A:15, 1988.
49. Posman H, Gilmore H: Acute brain and spinal cord injury. In Swaiman K: *Pediatric neurology*, St Louis, 1989, Mosby–Year Book.
50. Quencer RM, Ayyar DR, Angus E, et al: Somatosensory-evoked potential measurements in percutaneous fluid aspiration from intraspinal cystic lesions, *AJNR* 9:551, 1988.
51. Quencer RM, Green BA, Eismont FJ: Posttraumatic spinal cord cysts: clinical features and characterization with metrizamide computed tomography, *Radiology* 146:415, 1983.
52. Quencer RM, Sheldon JJ, Donovan Post MJ, et al: Magnetic resonance imaging of the chronically injured cervical spinal cord, *AJNR* 7:457, 1986.
53. Rogers L: The spine. In Rogers L, editor: *Radiology of skeletal trauma*, New York, 1982, Churchill Livingstone.
54. Rogers LF, Thayer C, Weinberg PE, et al: Acute injuries of the upper thoracic spine associated with paraplegia, *AJR* 134:67, 1980.
55. Rothman SLG, Glenn WV: CT multiplanar reconstruction in 253 cases of lumbar spondylolysis, *AJNR* 5:81, 1984.
56. Saraste H: Long-term clinical and radiological evaluation of spondylolysis and spondylolisthesis, *J Pediatr Orthop* 7:631, 1987.
57. Sato Y, Yuh WTC, Smith WL, et al: Head injury in child abuse: evaluation with MR imaging, *Radiology* 173:653, 1989.
58. Seibert CE, Dreisbach JN, Swanson WB, et al: Progressive posttraumatic cystic myelopathy: neuroradiologic evaluation, *AJR* 136:1161, 1981.
59. Suss RA, Zimmerman RD, Leeds NE: Pseudospread of the atlas: false sign of Jefferson fracture in young children, *AJNR* 4:183, 1983.
60. Swischuk C: *Emergency radiology of the acutely ill or injured child*, ed 2, Baltimore, 1986, Williams & Wilkins.
61. Taylor GA, Eggli KD: Lap-belt injuries of the lumbar spine in children: a pitfall in CT diagnosis, *AJR* 150:1355, 1988.
62. Teitelbaum G, Yee C, VanHorn D, et al: Metallic ballistic fragments: MR imaging, *Radiology* 175:855, 1990.
63. Teplick JG, Laffey PA, Berman A, et al: Diagnosis and evaluation of spondylolisthesis and/or spondylolysis on axial CT, *AJNR* 7:479, 1986.
64. Wirth RL, Zatz LM, Parker BR: CT detection of a Jefferson fracture in a child, *AJR* 149:1001, 1987.
65. Yamashita Y, Takahashi M, Matsuno Y, et al: Chronic injuries of the spinal cord: MR imaging, *Radiology* 175:849, 1990.
66. Young JWR, Resnik CS, DeCandido P, et al: The laminar space in the diagnosis of rotational flexion injuries of the cervical spine, *AJR* 152:103, 1989.

Neoplastic processes of the spine and spinal neuraxis

CLINICAL ASPECTS

In childhood spinal tumors occur much less commonly than intracranial tumors. Tumors of the spine and spinal neuraxis may be classified according to the revised WHO classification[108] (see box on p. 437). and according to the anatomical compartment of origin or involvement, that is, extradural, intradural, or intramedullary (see box on p. 437). Clinical presentations include local pain, tenderness, palpable mass, or acute painful scoliosis, especially for extradural and intradural tumors. Chronic nonpainful but

---

CLASSIFICATION OF SPINAL NEOPLASIA ACCORDING TO HISTOPATHOLOGY[108,115]

I. **NEUROEPITHELIAL TUMORS**
   A. Glial tumors
      1. Astrocytic
      2. Ependymal
      3. Mixed glial
   B. Neuronal tumors
      1. Ganglioglioma
   C. Primitive neuroepithelial tumors

II. **TUMORS OF MENINGEAL AND RELATED TISSUES**
   A. Meningiomas (see Chapter 8)
   B. Meningeal sarcomas
   C. Melanocytic tumors

III. **NERVE SHEATH CELL TUMORS** (see Chapter 8)
   A. Schwannoma
   B. Neurofibroma

IV. **LYMPHOMAS**

V. **TUMORS OF BLOOD VESSEL ORIGIN**
   A. Hemangioblastoma (see Chapter 8)

VI. **GERM CELL TUMORS**
   A. Teratomas (see Chapter 9)

VII. **MALFORMATIVE TUMORS** (see Chapter 9)
   A. Lipomas
   B. Epidermoid-dermoid
   C. Neurenteric cyst
   D. Arachnoid cyst
   E. Hamartoma

IX. **LOCAL EXTENSIONS FROM REGIONAL TUMORS**
   A. Extradural or parameningeal tumors

X. **METASTATIC TUMORS**

CLASSIFICATION OF SPINAL TUMORS BY ANATOMICAL COMPARTMENT

EXTRADURAL TUMORS AND TUMORLIKE CONDITIONS

Benign tumors

Osteoid osteoma
Osteochondroma
Osteoblastoma
Aneurysmal bone cyst
Vascular anomalies
Giant cell tumor

Sarcomas

Ewing's sarcoma
Osteosarcoma
Chondrosarcoma
Rhabdomyosarcoma
Other rare sarcomas

Chordoma

Pseudoneoplastic tumors

Histiocytosis
Fibromatosis

Leukemias and lymphomas

Neural crest origin neoplasms

Neuroblastoma
Ganglioneuroblastoma
Ganglioneuroma

Primitive neuroectodermal tumors

Metastases

INTRADURAL TUMORS

Nerve sheath cell tumors

Schwannoma
Neurofibroma

Meningeal tumors

Meningioma
Meningeal sarcoma
Melanocytic tumors

Seeding

Medulloblastoma
Primitive neuroectodermal tumors
Germ cell tumors
Anaplastic ependymoma
Malignant glial tumors (for example, glioblastoma)
Lymphoma

Developmental tumors

Lipomas
Epidermoid-dermoid
Neurenteric cyst
Arachnoid cyst
Hamartoma

INTRAMEDULLARY TUMORS

Astrocytoma
Ependymoma
Mixed glial tumors
Hemangioblastoma
Ganglioglioma

---

progressive scoliosis may be the presentation, particularly with intramedullary tumors. Radiculopathy may occur with paresthesia, pain, or motor paresis. Progressive myelopathy may produce motor deficits including paraparesis or quadriparesis, bladder or bowel dysfunction, sensory levels, or Brown-Séquard syndrome (unilateral motor paresis with contralateral pain and temperature loss).*

The symptoms may be vague and long-standing including back stiffness, back pain, gait abnormality, or spinal deformity. There may be a history of trauma, usually trivial, as well as motor regression with refusal to walk or crawl. The gait abnormality may be related to lower extremity weakness. Occasionally there is severe local pain due to neural tube distention or epidural venous congestion, or radicular pain with scoliosis from nerve root irritation. The nonpainful progressive curvature deformity may be related to denervation and paraspinal muscle imbalance as a neuropathic, neuromuscular, or paralytic scoliosis. Cervical level tumors may cause neck pain, head tilt or torticollis, upper extremity monoparesis, intrinsic hand muscle atro-

---

*References 19, 35, 48, 62, 67, 117.

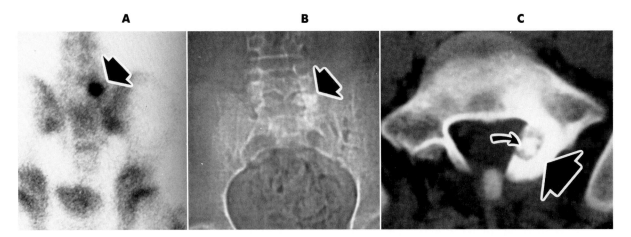

Fig. 10-31   Lumbar osteoid osteoma shown as a focus of intense uptake *(arrow)* on isotope bone scan **(A)**. **B,** Frontal CT scout projection image shows a focal sclerotic high density *(arrow)*. **C,** Axial CT demonstrates the high density calcified nidus *(curved arrow)* with low density collar and surrounded by intense high density sclerosis *(large arrow)*.

phy, and lower extremity hyperreflexia. With thoracic level tumors scoliosis is common and there may be pain, spasm, ataxia, lower extremity weakness, dysesthesias, and late bladder (or bowel) dysfunction. A very rare sign is increased intracranial pressure from obstructive hydrocephalus due to hemorrhage, altered CSF protein, or tumor seeding. There may be signs of meningeal irritation suggesting meningitis or subarachnoid hemorrhage, or systemic signs such as fever, fatigue, or weight loss (for example, with neuroblastoma). Atypical idiopathic scoliosis, such as a leftward curve, or idiopathic scoliosis inappropriate for age, gender, or progression should be a red-flag for cord tumor or syringohydromyelia[16] (see Fig. 10-51).

IMAGING CONSIDERATIONS

Plain film findings of the spine are abnormal in 50% to 70% of pediatric patients with spinal column or neuraxis tumors.[35,62,94,117] This is the first examination recommended because the findings often give an indication of the category of tumor and serve as guides for further imaging and for surgery and radiotherapy. Extradural tumors may produce vertebral bony destruction, paraspinal soft tissue masses, calcifications, and foraminal or spinal canal enlargement (see Figs. 10-35, 10-36, and 10-40). A bony lytic expansion of the neural arch, or body and arch, often indicates a solitary benign tumor such as an aneurysmal bone cyst, osteoblastoma, or giant cell tumor[66] (see Fig. 10-35). A destructive bone lesion with volume loss or collapse may indicate a more aggressive or malignant neoplastic process (see Fig. 10-36). This often occurs with tumors of reticuloendothelial origin such as neuroblastoma, histiocytosis, sarcoma (for example, Ewing's), leukemia, lymphoma, or metastases (for example, rhabdomyosarcoma). A paraspinal mass with or without foraminal or spinal canal enlargement may indicate a neurogenic tumor (see Fig. 10-40), such as a neuroblastoma, ganglioneuro-

blastoma, or ganglioneuroma, a nerve sheath cell tumor, such as a Schwannoma or neurofibroma, or a vascular anomaly, such as a hemangioma or a vascular malformation. Spinal column infection (diskitis, osteomyelitis) must be excluded, especially when there is disk space involvement. Pedicle or laminar sclerosis with or without scoliosis may be seen with osteoid osteoma and must be distinguished from pedicle hypertrophy related to spondylolysis (Fig. 10-31). Intradural extramedullary tumors such as nerve sheath cell tumors (for example, neurofibroma) may produce pedicle erosion, foraminal enlargement, or canal widening with or without scoliosis. Intramedullary tumors such as astrocytoma or ependymoma often produce scoliosis, canal widening, and pedicle thinning (see Fig. 10-51). Hydrosyringomyelia without tumor may produce similar plain film findings.

Isotope bone scanning is important for evaluating extradural tumors (Fig. 10-31), especially to delineate single versus multifocal disease (for example, metastases). CT scanning may be indicated for single level benign lesions (for example, osteoid osteoma) as a real-time guide for needle biopsy or as a preoperative guide for surgical excision.[8] MRI is often the more sensitive and precise imaging modality for demonstrating soft tissue and bone marrow involvement, anatomical delineation, (especially neural and vascular), and tissue characterization (for example, hemorrhage).[*] MRI is certainly the procedure of choice for displaying intraspinal extent and cord involvement. For extradural bone and soft tissue involvement, sagittal spin echo T2-weighted images are superior to T1-weighted images, especially to determine marrow involvement (see Fig. 10-43). The fat signal (short T2) is decreased on long TR/long TE images relative to the higher intensity water signal (long T2) of many neoplastic and inflammatory processes. Gradient echo sequences with fat

---
*References 32, 33, 55, 80, 88, 127, 140.

suppression (short T2*) relative to water (long T2*) may also be used. The most sensitive technique, however, may be the short TI inversion recovery sequence (STIR) in which fat suppression is combined with the additive T1 and T2 high intensity character of water (see Chapter 1). Other sensitive fat-suppression techniques may include chemical shift imaging or RF saturation of the fat-peak combined with gadolinium enhancement. Axial sections are important for planning surgical approaches.

For intradural and intramedullary processes MRI is the definitive procedure. Sagittal and coronal T1 sections are preferred in patients with myelopathy for longitudinal screening of intramedullary expansion or intradural masses. Gadolinium-DTPA is a requirement for demonstrating subarachnoid tumor seeding, such as medulloblastoma, as well as for intramedullary tumor, especially when attempting to differentiate neoplastic (for example, astrocytoma or ependymoma) from benign causes of hydrosyringomyelia[*] (see Figs. 10-49 and 10-53). MRI is also the procedure of choice for follow-up after therapy even when there is severe kyphoscoliotic deformity following surgery or radiotherapy. Newer surgical techniques using laminotomy with bone replacement have been introduced to minimize the curvature deformity. Also, orthopedic instrumentation with fusion may be required. In the latter case MRI is still worth attempting to evaluate residual or recurrent intraspinal tumor.[78] Using T1-weighted sequences with as short TE as possible and intravenous gadolinium administration, MRI sections may be obtained in sagittal or coronal planes that do not directly intersect the instrumentation.

EXTRADURAL OR PARAMENINGEAL TUMORS

Extradural or parameningeal compartment tumors are those of spinal column or paraspinal origin.[†] These include benign and malignant bone and soft tissue tumors or tumorlike conditions (see box on p. 437). These tumors may grow into the spinal canal directly, extend within the canal by epidural venous spread, or disseminate to the spine by hematogeneous or lymphatic routes. Benign tumors and tumorlike conditions include osteoid osteoma, osteochondroma, osteoblastoma, aneurysmal bone cyst, and vascular anomalies, such as hemangioma (see Chapter 9). The more malignant-acting conditions include giant cell tumor, sarcomas, chordomas, histiocytoses, fibromatosis, leukemia, lymphoma, neural crest tumors, primitive neuroectodermal tumors, and metastases. Other abnormalities of importance in the differential diagnosis include inflammatory processes, treatment effects, and bone marrow disorders.

Osteoid osteoma

Osteoid osteoma is a benign, usually solitary, osteoblastic tumor with a vascular fibrous connective tissue nidus surrounded by an osteoid matrix that is bone producing.[‡]

Often there is central calcification within the nidus and characteristic surrounding reactive bone sclerosis. Less than 10% of all osteoid osteomas occur in the spine. These usually involve the pedicle or lamina in the lumbar region and less often in the thoracic or cervical region. The majority occur between 5 and 25 years of age, and are usually manifested by local pain and tenderness that is worse at night but relieved with aspirin. There may be associated scoliosis with the lesion occurring along the concavity of the curve opposite the apex. Plain films, tomography, or CT may demonstrate a radiolucent or low density nidus, usually smaller than 1.0 to 1.5 cm, with surrounding radiodense or high density sclerosis and occasional central calcific density (Fig. 10-31). The nidus may be obscured by the sclerosis. The lesion may have an atypical appearance with central sclerotic density and surrounding lucency or low density when arising primarily within cancellous bone (for example, vertebral body). MRI is rarely needed unless there is confusion or uncertainty regarding the diagnosis or there are neurological signs and another lesion must be ruled out. The reported findings by MRI include intense and often extensive marrow edema seen as T1 low intensity and T2 high intensity.[43,82] The calcific center and surrounding sclerosis appear as low intensity on T1 and T2 images, whereas the nidus may appear isointense to hypointense on T1-weighted images and hypointense or hyperintense on T2-weighted images. Gadolinium enhancement of the nidus may be evident, especially on T1 images using fat suppression. Important differential diagnoses include subacute or chronic osteomyelitis (Brodie's abscess), which often demonstrates an irregular sequestrum, and spondylolysis with reactive sclerosis. The osteoid osteoma is treated by resection of the nidus.

Osteochondroma

Osteochondroma is a benign osteocartilaginous exostosis that is a hamartoma of subperiosteal cartilage cell origin.[*] The osteochondroma contains mature cancellous, cortical, and cartilaginous elements that are organized and continuous with the mature elements of the parent bone. It is the most common benign bone tumor encountered in patients under 20 years of age, although only 5% occur in the spinal column, usually at the cervical or thoracic level. These are usually solitary growths that arise from the posterior elements (spinous or transverse process). Multiple lesions may occur, especially in familial cases. Spinal exostoses in childhood or adolescence may occur years after radiation therapy for other diseases, such as Wilms' tumor or neuroblastoma. Malignant degeneration to chondrosarcoma or osteosarcoma with increased pain and growth is rarely reported, although it is a more common occurrence in familial cases.

The plain film and CT appearances of osteochondromas are often characteristic (Fig. 10-32). The growth has the

---

[*]References 92, 97, 127, 131-133, 138.
[†]References 1, 5, 6, 53, 63, 93, 117, 136, 143, 145, 147.
[‡]References 4, 40, 43, 74, 82, 136.

[*]References 21, 59, 60, 71, 73, 75, 82, 89, 136, 137.

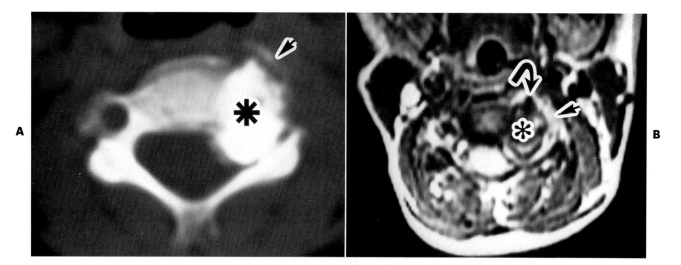

Fig. 10-32   Cervical osteochondroma occurring years after radiotherapy for neuroblastoma. **A,** Axial CT shows the high density ossific mass *(asterisk)* with calcified isodense cartilaginous rim *(arrow).* **B,** Axial proton density MRI shows the mixed intensity cortical and medullary elements *(asterisk)* and the high intensity cartilaginous cap *(arrow).* There is encroachment on the left intervertebral foramen and central spinal canal, and anterior compressive encasement of the vertebral artery flow signal void *(curved arrow).*

appearance of a sessile or pedunculated miniature metaphysis and epiphysis with marrow and cortical elements continuous with the bone of origin. MRI is indicated for surgical planning, especially if neurological signs are present or if malignant degeneration is suspected. By MRI the continuity of mature marrow and cortical elements is demonstrated along with the cartilaginous cap, which is isointense to hyperintense on T1 images and hyperintense on T2 images[71,82] (Fig. 10-32). The calcified-ossified components are of low intensity on both T1 and T2 images, whereas the marrow or cancellous components such as fat follow the normal intensity patterns of the parent bone throughout the sequences. Malignant degeneration is indicated by a disorganized appearance with cap disruption, soft tissue mass, and parent bone marrow involvement (T1 low intensity and T2 high intensity).[60,82] Surgical excision is carried out for lesions producing pain or mass effect with root or cord signs.

Osteoblastoma

Osteoblastoma is a benign bone tumor with a hyperemic fibrovascular matrix and osteoblastic mesenchyme with giant cells and rich capillary and sinusoidal vascularization.[*] Osteoblastomas contain a larger number of osteoblasts and giant cells than does osteoid osteoma, and the nidus is often larger than 1.5 to 2.0 cm. Most lesions occur in the first or second decade, and there is a predilection for the axial skeleton including the sacrum, lumbar spine, and, less often, the cervical or thoracic spine. These are usually

solitary lesions involving the neural arch or body and arch. Malignant degeneration is very rare. Plain films and CT usually show a lytic, expansile-appearing lesion containing bone matrix or calcified flecks with cortical erosion, a soft tissue mass, and a thin calcified shell (Fig. 10-33). MRI often shows the lesion as isointense to hypointense on T1 images with heterogeneous high intensity on T2 images.[65,82] Hemorrhage may be present (Fig. 10-33), and gadolinium enhancement has been described. Surgical excision is performed in most cases. Radiotherapy is rarely needed except for recurrences not controlled by surgery.

Aneurysmal bone cysts

Aneurysmal bone cysts are nonneoplastic, usually solitary lesions consisting of nonendothelial-lined, blood-filled cystic cavities.[*] These may arise as a result of a local sudden hemodynamic disturbance, probably a local venous outflow occlusion or arteriovenous shunt. These are circumscribed cavernous spaces or sinusoids filled with nonclotted blood. Reactive and reparative changes are common and similar to that with eosinophilic granuloma including giant cells, histiocytes, fibroblasts, osteoblasts, and osteoid. There may be a fibrous wall or a solid fibrotic mass. The majority occur in the first two decades, with up to 30% arising within the axial skeleton, lumbar more often than sacral or cervical. Usually there is involvement of the neural arch (spinous or transverse process) or the neural arch and posterior body. The early presentation is that of local pain and swelling that may be acute. With progression there may

*References 4, 65, 82, 86, 135, 136.

*References 7, 10, 22, 24, 82, 85, 136, 141.

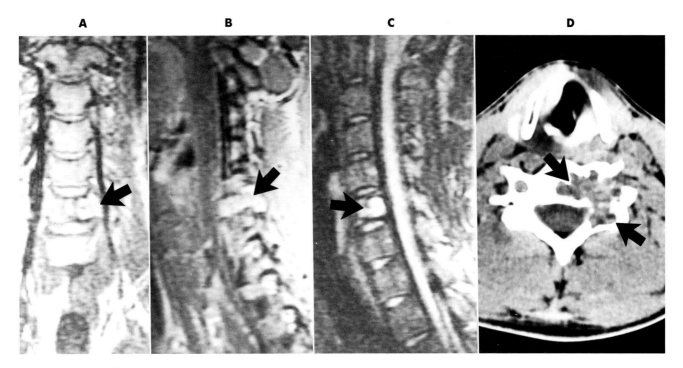

Fig. 10-33   Cervical osteoblastoma with giant cell and aneurysmal bone cyst elements. Coronal T1 **(A)**, sagittal T1 **(B)**, and sagittal T2 **(C)** MRI demonstrate C6 vertebral body and neural arch expansion with hyperintense areas *(arrows)* consistent with methemoglobin. **D**, Axial CT shows isodense destructive expansion of the left body and neural arch *(arrow)*.

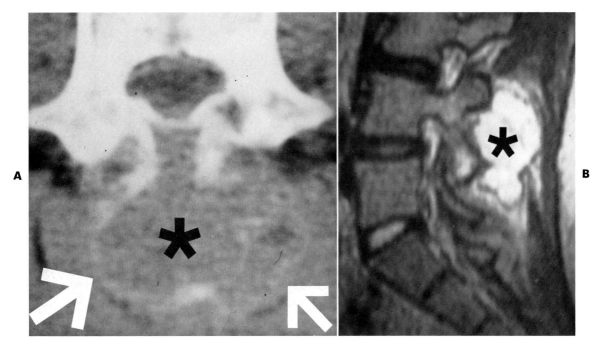

Fig. 10-34   Lumbar aneurysmal bone cyst with giant cell, osteoid, and fibrous elements. **A,** Axial CT shows an isodense spinous process mass *(asterisk)* with calcified margins *(arrows)*. **B,** Sagittal proton density MRI shows the tumor as markedly hyperintense *(asterisk)* with isointense to hypointense margins and surrounding hyperintensities.

A   B   C   D

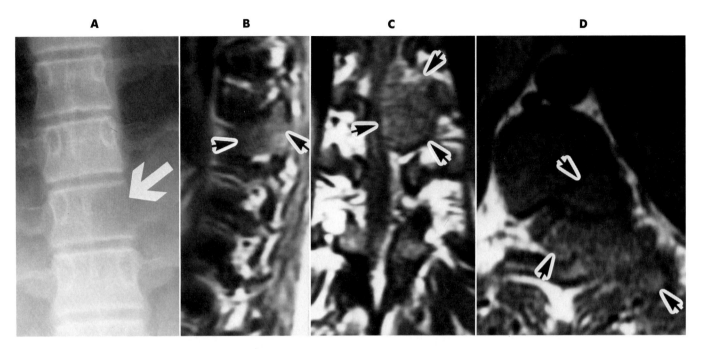

Fig. 10-35   Thoracic giant cell tumor with aneurysmal bone cyst elements. **A,** Frontal plain film shows a lytic expansile destruction *(arrow)* of the left body, pedicle, and transverse process of T10. Sagittal **(B),** coronal **(C),** and axial **(D)** T1 MRI show the isointense to hypointense tumor *(arrows)* involving the body and neural arch with intraspinal (dural sac and cord displacement), foraminal, and paraspinal extension.

be radicular symptoms and signs or myelopathy with rapid vertebral destruction, hemorrhage, scoliosis, and a palpable mass. Aneurysmal bone cysts may be isolated lesions or may occur in association with giant cell tumor, osteoblastoma, or hemangioma.

During the active growth phase the lesions have a lytic and rapidly destructive blow-out appearance on plain films and CT (Figs. 10-33 to 10-35). The process may involve contiguous levels across the disk space with body collapse or vertebral dislocation. During the mature phase there is a septated, trabecular soap-bubble appearance with a peripheral bony shell. In the healing phase there is increasing calcification and ossification to a mature dense mass. The mass tends to project from the parent bone into the soft tissues.

On T1 and p/T2 MRI the lesion may appear isointense, hyperintense, or hypointense, or as a heterogeneous intensity mass depending on the evolutionary stage and dominant pathological elements[7,22,82,85,136] (Figs. 10-33 to 10-35). Fibrous, ossific, calcific, and hemosiderin components appear as low intensity on T1 and T2 images. Methemoglobin content may appear as low intensity on T1 and T2 images. Methemoglobin content may appear as high intensity on T1 and T2 images. Gadolinium enhancement has also been reported. There is often a multilocular appearance with a low intensity fibrous or bony rim, internal fluid levels, and surrounding edema during the acute phase. The fluid levels display varying intensities as related to content (for example, serous, proteinaceous, or hemorrhagic). The

fluid-fluid levels often occur after hemorrhage with a serous supernatant and cellular precipitant including varying concentrations of hemoglobin breakdown products (deoxyhemoglobin, methemoglobin, hemosiderin). The appearance of an expanding, lytic, loculated mass with fluid-fluid levels and a low intensity rim has been described as characteristic for aneurysmal bone cyst. However, a similar appearance has been reported in other lesions. The differential diagnosis may include lymphatic or venous malformations and telangiectatic osteosarcoma. Treatment of aneurysmal bone cyst is primarily surgical, with preoperative transcatheter embolization preferred. Radiotherapy is an important consideration for treating recurring cysts. Malignant degeneration after radiotherapy is rare.

Giant cell tumors

Giant cell tumors are often considered benign, although occasionally there is malignant degeneration with late metastasis.[9,49,82,136] This osteoclastoma is composed of multinucleated giant cells with a fibroblastic mesenchymal stroma and tends to be vascular. These occur in the second decade, usually after epiphyseal closure, with rare involvement of the spine. The tumor most often occurs at the thoracic level and is locally aggressive. Plain films and CT show an osteolytic, expansile mass involving the neural arch, or arch and body, with cortical thinning and occasional soft tissue extension (Fig. 10-35). MRI demonstrates an isointense to hypointense mass on T1 images that is isointense to hypointense on T2 images[49,82,136] (Fig.

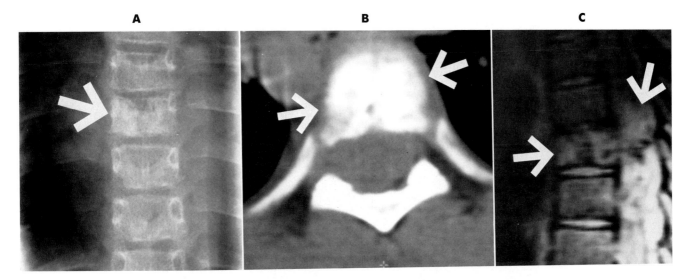

Fig. 10-36   Thoracic round cell tumor. **A,** Frontal plain film shows a mixed lytic and sclerotic permeative destruction of T6 vertebral body *(arrow)* with partial collapse and paraspinal soft tissue thickening. **B,** Axial CT shows the bony destruction *(arrows)* with obliteration of the intraspinal epidural fat. **C,** Sagittal T2 MRI shows isointense to hyperintense tumor involvement of the partially collapsed body *(anterior arrow)* with intraspinal extension *(posterior arrow).* The stagnant CSF below the intraspinal mass is markedly hyperintense. The pathological considerations *(round cell tumors)* include Ewing's sarcoma, PNET, neuroblastoma, rhabdomyosarcoma, leukemia (for example, chloroma), and lymphoma. The final diagnosis was PNET.

10-35). Patchy T2 high intensities may correlate with hemorrhage (T1 high intensity) or cystic components. Gadolinium enhancement has been reported. (Vascular anomalies including hemangiomas and vascular malformations [arterial, venous, capillary, lymphatic, combined][*] are presented in Chapter 9.)

Ewing's sarcoma

Ewing's sarcoma is the second most common primary malignant neoplasm of bone after osteosarcoma in childhood.[†] It is a tumor that probably arises from the primitive reticulum stem cell of bone marrow origin. It is characterized by a small round cell infiltration similar to other tumors of childhood (neuroblastoma, rhabdomyosarcoma, leukemia, lymphoma, primitive neuroectodermal tumor). Ewing's sarcoma tends to occur late in the first decade or early in the second decade with infrequent spine involvement that may be primary or metastatic. Systemic symptoms are common in addition to local pain, tenderness, and mass effect with neural involvement. There may be involvement at multiple sites as with other round cell tumors.

Plain films and CT in Ewing's sarcoma demonstrate a permeative, lytic destructive process of bone (Fig. 10-36). Sclerotic or calcified components are occasionally identified. Classically this is a lesion of medullary origin with cortical involvement, loss of bone volume, cortical erosion,

and soft tissue mass effect. Occasionally there is a soft tissue mass only (extraosseous Ewing's). With MRI the process appears similar to that of other round cell tumors [13,39,82,136] (Fig. 10-36). These are hypercellular tumors that are isointense to hypointense on T1 images and isointense to hypointense on T2 images. Associated tumor edema appears hyperintense on T2 images. The intensity patterns may be homogeneous or heterogenous depending on associated hemorrhage, necrosis, or cysts. Gadolinium enhancement has been observed. Treatment often involves a combination of surgical decompression, radiotherapy, and chemotherapy.

Osteosarcoma

Osteosarcoma is the most common primary bone malignancy of childhood. It is a neoplasm of undifferentiated mesenchyme with bone-forming neoplastic osteoid composed of primitive malignant osteoblasts.[*] Histological subtypes include osteoblastic, chondroblastic, fibroblastic, and telangiectatic varieties. The majority of cases present in the 10- to 25-year age group with pain, swelling, systemic symptoms, and early metastasis. Spine involvement occurs infrequently and may be metastatic. Osteosarcoma may occur years after radiotherapy for another neoplasm or it may arise from a preexisting osteochondroma.

Osteosarcoma is a destructive, lytic lesion of bone, as demonstrated by plain film and CT, with or without

[*]References 58, 69, 70, 84, 112, 120.
[†]References 13, 36, 38, 39, 82, 136.

[*]References 13, 36, 41, 82, 128, 136, 146.

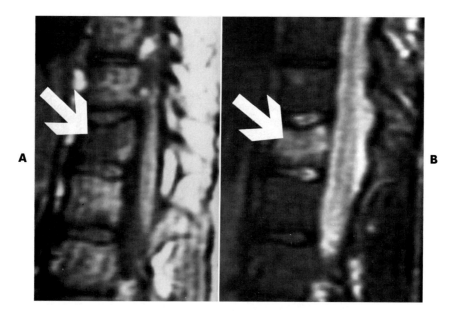

Fig. 10-37 Thoracic rhabdomyosarcoma, probably metastatic, shown by sagittal T1 **(A)** and T2 **(B)** MRI as T1 isointense to hypointense and T2 hyperintense involvement *(arrows)* of the T12 vertebral body with partial collapse but no intraspinal extension.

sclerotic or blastic components. Cortical penetration with a soft tissue mass and tumor bone formation is frequent as is marrow infiltration and pathological fracture. There may be associated necrosis, hemorrhage, calcification, or fibrosis. Areas of soft tissue tumor on MRI appear isointense to hypointense on T1 images and hyperintense on T2 images (see Chapter 7). Sclerotic, calcified, or fibrotic areas often appear isointense or hypointense on T1 and T2 images.[13,41,82,128,146] The telangiectatic subtype may have a similar appearance to aneurysmal bone cyst. Chondroid elements may appear as high intensity on T1-weighted images. Gadolinium enhancement often correlates with the vascular noncalcified and nonnecrotic tumor areas.

Chondrosarcoma

Chondrosarcoma is a malignant bone neoplasm of cartilage origin that may arise de novo, from a preexisting cartilage-matrix lesion (for example, osteochondroma in multiple familial exostoses), or following radiation therapy.[*] The spine is only occasionally involved. Plain films and CT usually demonstrate a lobular lytic bone lesion (see Chapter 7) with variable chondroid calcifications (floccules, rings, pinpoints). MRI may show a mass that is isointense to hypointense or hyperintense on T1 images with T2 hyperintensity[17,34,82,136] (see Chapter 7). The higher grade tumors often show even greater signal heterogeneity on T1 and T2 images. Gadolinium enhancement has been observed. MRI findings that indicate malignant degeneration

of a preexisting cartilaginous tumor include disorganized morphology with medullary and cortical disruption, soft tissue mass, and reportedly a cartilaginous cap thicker than 1 cm.

Rhabdomyosarcoma

Rhabdomyosarcoma is a malignant neoplasm of embryonic mesenchyme with rhabdomyomatous differentiation.[5,42,51,82,136] The tumor is made up of small round rhabdomyoblasts of variable size and maturation. The most common subtypes are embryonal and alveolar. This is one of the commonest solid tumors of childhood, with peak occurrence in the first decade. This aggressive neoplasm usually occurs in the head and neck region or pelvis but may also arise in the thorax, abdomen, or retroperitoneum. Recurrence and metastasis are common. There may be a paraspinal mass with direct extension and spinal or intraspinal involvement, or more commonly, lymphatic or hematogenous metastasis to the spinal marrow with or without soft tissue masses[5,82,83] (Figs. 10-37 and 10-38). On plain films and CT these are usually solid, lobular tumor masses that secondarily erode or destroy adjacent bone. By MRI these are similar to other round cell tumors and are usually isointense to hypointense on T1 images and isointense to hypointense with high intensity areas on T2 images. Gadolinium enhancement has also been observed. Treatment usually involves a combination of surgery, radiotherapy, and chemotherapy. Other very rare sarcomas that may involve the spine include liposarcoma, fibrosarcoma, and angiosarcoma.

---

[*]References 2, 17, 60, 82, 136, 137.

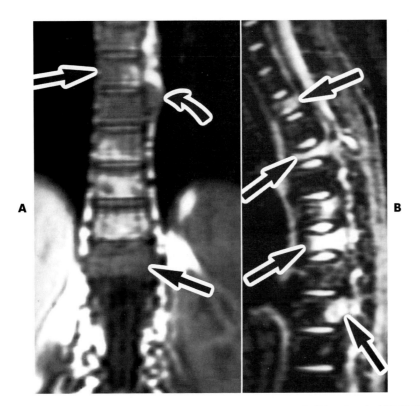

Fig. 10-38   Metastatic spinal rhabdomyosarcoma shown by coronal T1 **(A)** and sagittal T2 (STIR) **(B)** MRI as multiple T1 isointense to hypointense and T2 hyperintense lesions *(straight arrows)* of the spinal vertebral marrow including multilevel body collapse and paraspinal masses *(curved arrow).* Any of the round cell tumors may produce a similar appearance including leukemia or lymphoma (see text).

Chordoma

Chordoma is a malignant neoplasm of primitive notochordal origin, presumably arising from intraosseous notochordal remnants that may occur at any point from the clivus to the sacrum.* These are often subclassified as typical and chondroid types. Chordoma of sacral and clival origin is much more common than those arising from the vertebrae, with the cervical level involved more often than the lumbar or thoracic level. This is an extremely rare tumor that occurs before the second or third decade. Chordoma tends to be slow growing and locally invasive with infrequent metastasis or seeding (see Chapter 7). Vertebral chordomas tend to be more malignant than clival or sacral lesions. Plain films and CT show bone destruction and a soft tissue mass often with calcification. Disk space involvement may occur. MRI demonstrates these tumors as isointense to low intensity on T1 images, gadolinium enhancing, and hyperintense on T2 images.[5,11,27,134,136] There may be isointense or low intensity septations and encapsulation. Hemorrhage and cystic changes may also be apparent. Treatment of chordoma includes surgical excision and radiotherapy.

*References 5, 27, 79, 111, 134, 136.

Leukemia

Leukemia is the most common malignancy of childhood with the majority of cases occurring as either the acute lymphoblastic form (ALL, 80%) or the acute monoblastic form (AML, 10%).[77,83,91,136] The peak incidence is in the first decade with systemic symptomatology and complications related to bone marrow infiltration including infection, anemia, hemorrhage, and organomegaly. CNS involvement, that is, leukemic meningitis, is also common. The diffuse bone marrow involvement may be apparent on plain films or CT as osteopenia with decreased trabeculation, lucent bands, and permeative lytic vertebral destruction with or without areas of sclerosis or pathological fracture. Leukemic masses (chloromas) may rarely arise as epidural intraspinal or paraspinal masses and are usually associated with AML. These may produce local pain, mass effect, meningeal irritative symptoms, and nerve root or cord compressive symptoms or signs. The marrow process is similar in appearance to that of other round cell tumors and is demonstrated by MRI usually as diffuse and uniform involvement that is isointense to hypointense on T1 images and isointense to slightly hyperintense on T2 images.[77,83,91] Gadolinium enhancement has been observed. Chloromas are often isodense to hyperdense on CT with marked iodine enhancement (see Chapter 7). By MRI the masses are usually isointense to hypointense on T1 images and markedly enhance with gadolinium, whereas on T2 images the tumors may also be isointense to hypointense with or without areas of hyperintensity (see Chapter 7).

Lymphoma

Lymphoma in childhood may be of the Hodgkin's disease (HD) type or the nonHodgkin's lymphoma (NHL) type, the latter including the undifferentiated Burkitt type lymphomas.[77,83,91] The HD type is more often focal with involvement of contiguous structures, whereas the NHL type is more often diffuse and widespread. There may rarely be primary or secondary spinal involvement by direct extension or by hematogeneous or lymphatic dissemination.

Plain film and CT findings of lymphoma may show permeative and lytic or sclerotic bony vertebral involvement, including pathological fracture and soft tissue masses. By MRI the bone marrow involvement may be focal, multifocal, or diffuse,[83] as with other round cell tumors. The lesions are usually isointense to hypointense on T1 images relative to muscle and enhance with gadolinium. On T2 images the lesions are usually isointense to hypointense or hyperintense. The intensity pattern may be homogeneous or heterogeneous depending on the mix of pathological elements. Hypercellular areas and sclerotic areas are often isointense to hypointense on both T1 and T2 images. Associated edema is usually T2 hyperintense.

Langerhans cell histiocytosis

Langerhans cell histiocytosis is a pseudoneoplastic process characterized by a granulomatous proliferation of lipid-laden reticulum cells (reticuloendotheliosis) at single or multiple sites within the reticuloendothelial system.[*] The most benign form is eosinophilic granuloma. The disease is usually encountered in the 5- to 10-year age group. Spinal involvement is common and more often thoracic or lumbar than cervical. There may be local pain in addition to systemic symptoms, but radicular or myelopathic symptoms and signs are rare. There may be intracranial or intraspinal involvement with leptomeningeal spread (see Chapter 7).

On plain films and CT there may be lytic destruction usually without sclerosis. Often there is involvement of one or more vertebral bodies with pathological fracture and uniform body collapse (vertebra plana) with wide disk spaces and often without associated soft tissue mass or scoliosis. The lesions appear on MRI (Fig. 10-39) as isointense or hypointense on T1 images and enhance with gadolinium.[5,82,136] On T2 images the lesions are usually hyperintense. Mixed intensity patterns may be seen, however, especially with associated hemorrhage or necrosis. Treatment often requires radiotherapy or chemotherapy after biopsy, although spontaneous healing is well documented. The differential diagnosis often includes neuroblastoma and Ewing's sarcoma.

Juvenile fibromatosis

Juvenile fibromatosis is a locally infiltrating pseudoneoplastic process characterized by fibroelastic proliferation.[82,117] The congenital form is widespread with multiple infiltrating visceral and bone lesions, but usually no metastases. The less aggressive, juvenile form usually

---

[*]References 5, 31, 47, 82, 94, 117, 136.

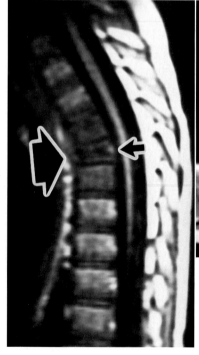
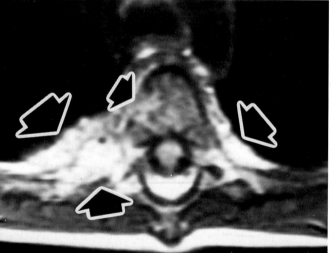

Fig. 10-39   Thoracic spinal histiocytosis demonstrated by sagittal T1 MRI **(A)** as isointense to hypointense involvement of three contiguous levels *(large arrow)* including vertebra planum-like collapse at one level *(small arrow)* with intact intervening disk spaces and localized kyphosis. **B,** Axial proton density MRI shows hyperintense vertebral and paraspinal soft tissue tumor *(large arrows).*

involves musculoskeletal structures without visceral involvement. Fibromatosis appears as infiltrating soft tissue masses that obliterate tissue plains and secondarily involve bone. The masses may be isointense to hypointense on both T1 and T2 images,[129] although T2 hyperintensity may also be seen (see Chapter 7).

Tumors of neural crest origin

Tumors of neural crest origin may include neuroblastoma, ganglioneuroblastoma, ganglioneuroma, nerve sheath cell tumors, and meningeal tumors. (Nerve sheath and meningeal tumors are presented in the next section and in Chapters 7 and 8).

NEUROBLASTOMA. Neuroblastoma is the most common solid tumor of childhood arising outside of the central nervous system.* The tumor is of neuroblast origin and usually arises from the adrenal medulla, paraspinal sympathetic chain, or, less frequently, from autonomic primordia within other organs (for example, carotid or aortic body, organ of Zuckerkandl). Histologically these tumors are characterized by small round cell infiltration with necrosis, hemorrhage, and calcification. The majority arise intraabdominally, although these also occur in the thoracic region (posterior mediastinum), pelvis, and cervical region. Neuroblastoma is a malignancy of infancy and early childhood (usually less than 5 years of age). Metastases are often present at initial diagnosis including bone marrow and meningeal involvement. Spinal involvement is very common, either by direct extension with epidural intraspinal spread caudad and cephalad, or by hematogenous or

---

*References 3, 5, 29, 37, 82, 83, 99, 121, 136.

lymphatic metastasis to the spinal marrow.

Plain films and CT may show paraspinal masses with calcification and lytic or sclerotic bone destruction and vertebral collapse (Fig. 10-40). Infrequently there may be bony expansion or disk involvement. Intraspinal extension often produces foraminal and spinal canal widening, obliteration of the epidural fat planes, and displacement or compression of the dural sac and spinal cord (Fig. 10-41). By MRI the tumor often appears isointense to hypointense on T1 images and enhances with gadolinium.[5,29,82,83,136]

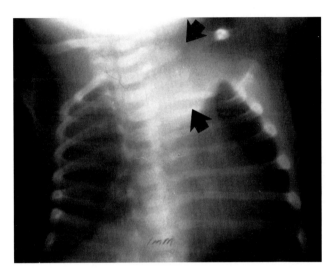

Fig. 10-40 Cervicothoracic neuroblastoma shown by frontal plain film as a paraspinal mass *(arrows)* with calcification and bony vertebral and rib destruction.

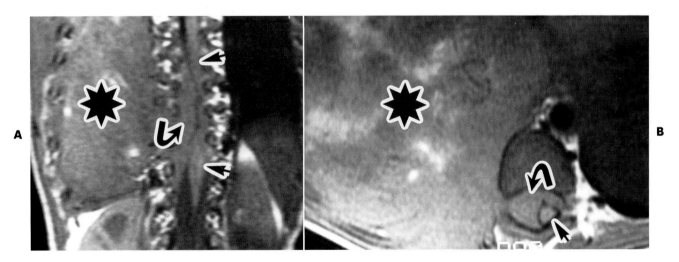

Fig. 10-41 Thoracic tumor in an infant evaluated for neuroblastoma and shown by coronal **(A)** and axial **(B)** T1 MRI as an isointense to hypointense mass *(asterisk)* filling the right thorax with intraspinal extension *(curved arrow)* and compressive displacement of the dural sac and spinal cord *(arrowheads)*. The high intensities within the huge tumor represent a combination of hemorrhage and mineralization.

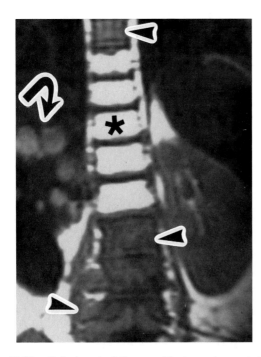

Fig. 10-42 Spinal metastatic neuroblastoma demonstrated by coronal T1 MRI as isointense to hypointense spinal column and paraspinal masses *(arrowheads)* and contrasted against the vertebral fatty hyperintensities *(asterisk)* related to prior radiotherapy. High intensity hepatic metastases *(curved arrow)* are also seen as contrasted against the intrahepatic ferrous hypointensities. It may be difficult to distinguish marrow metastases from marrow iron overload without additional T2 MRI.

On T2 and T1 images the tumor may have a heterogenous appearance depending on the presence and amount of hemorrhage, calcification, necrosis, edema, and hypercellular tumor elements. Spinal marrow involvement produces T1 isointensity to hypointensity and T2 hyperintensity relative to muscle (Figs. 10-42 and 10-43). Treatment involves surgical resection, including excision of intraspinal tumor, chemotherapy, and radiotherapy.

Maturation of neuroblastoma may occur with transformation to ganglioneuroblastoma or to ganglioneuroma, either spontaneously or following therapy.[3,5,82,83,136]

GANGLIONEUROBLASTOMA. Ganglioneuroblastoma contains both immature neuroblast cells and mature ganglion cells. Its behavior and imaging characteristics are similar to neuroblastoma including regional extension and metastasis. Posterior mediastinal and abdominal involvement are most common.

GANGLIONEUROMA. Ganglioneuroma is a benign tumor of neural crest origin composed of mature ganglion cells that occurs in later childhood and adolescence. This is a slow-growing tumor and arises more often in the thoracic paraspinal region than in the abdomen. The tumor may be of huge dimensions at discovery. Clinical presentations include respiratory compromise, local pain or tenderness, scoliosis, and radicular or myelopathic symptoms and signs. Plain films, CT, or MRI imaging demonstrate a paraspinal mass of variable size with or without calcification (Fig. 10-44). Often there is intraspinal extension with foraminal and spinal canal enlargement and compressive displacement of the dural sac contents (Fig. 10-45).

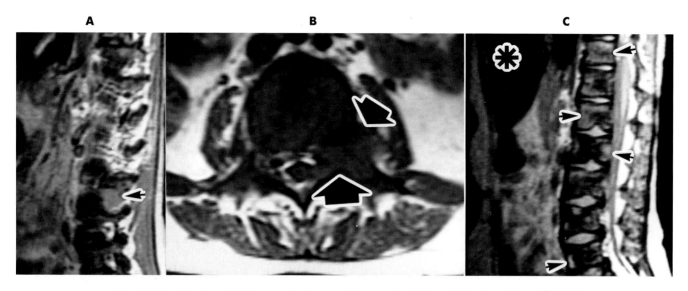

A   **B**   **C**

Fig. 10-43 Spinal metastatic neuroblastoma and iron overload after multiple transfusions. Sagittal **(A)** and axial **(B)** T1 MRI show isointense to hypointense vertebral involvement and a left paraspinal-intraspinal soft tissue mass at L2-3 *(arrows)* with tumor obliteration of the epidural fat within the intervertebral foramen *(arrowhead)*. **C,** Sagittal p/T2 MRI separates the presumed tumor (marrow hyperintensities, *arrowheads*) from the iron deposits (marked hypointensities). Ferrous hypointensities are also demonstrated within the liver *(asterisk)*.

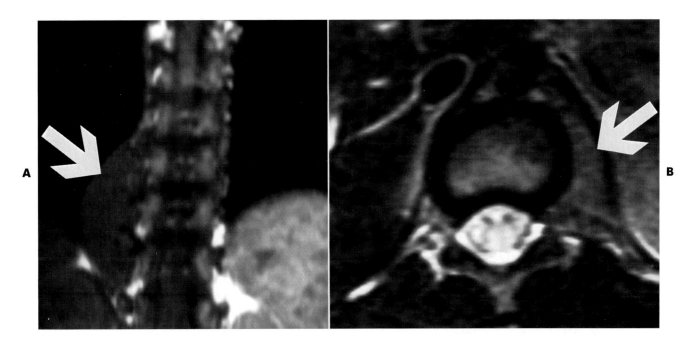

Fig. 10-44   Thoracic ganglioneuroma demonstrated by coronal T1 **(A)** and axial T2 **(B)** MRI as a three-level T1 isointense to hypointense and T2 isointense to hyperintense paraspinal mass *(arrows)* without intraspinal extension.

Calcification may help distinguish this tumor from nerve sheath cell tumors. By MRI the tumor is often isointense or hypointense on T1 images and enhances with gadolinium.[5,136] On T2 images the tumor appears isointense or hyperintense with or without low intensities related to calcification.

Primitive neuroectodermal tumors

Primitive neuroectodermal tumors (PNET) are rare malignancies of primitive neuroepithelial origin arising outside of the CNS.[*] These are characterized by small round cell infiltrations similar to that of neuroblastoma and other round cell tumors mentioned previously. Neurosecretory granules are identified by electron microscopy. The clinical and imaging characteristics are similar to the other tumors of this group (see Fig. 10-36) and include soft tissue mass with calcification and bone destruction and a high incidence of early metastasis.

Spinal metastases

Spinal metastases in childhood most commonly occur with neuroblastoma, rhabdomyosarcoma, leukemia, and histiocytosis.[5,15,83,124,136] Other sources of metastases in childhood include lymphoma, Ewing's sarcoma, osteosarcoma, Wilms' tumor, PNET, and, rarely, medulloblastoma or retinoblastoma. Spread is common via hematogenous or lymphatic routes to the vascularized red marrow of the vertebral column. Plain films or CT may show lytic or sclerotic bone destruction, pathological fracture with body

collapse, paraspinal masses, or epidural intraspinal masses. The MRI intensity patterns may vary according to the mix of infiltrative tumor hypercellularity, marrow edema, hemorrhage, and sclerotic or fibrous reactive changes[*] (Figs. 10-38, 10-42, and 10-46). Often there is T1 isointensity or

---

[*]References 5, 20, 23, 56, 77, 83, 91, 105, 136.

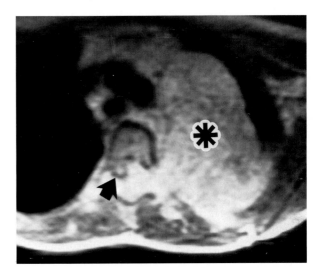

Fig. 10-45   Thoracic mixed ganglioneuroma and ganglioneuroblastoma demonstrated by axial proton density MRI as a huge high intensity tumor occupying the left hemithorax *(asterisk)* with intraspinal extension producing displacement and compression of the dural sac and cord *(arrow)*.

---

[*]References 5, 42, 108, 113, 115, 136.

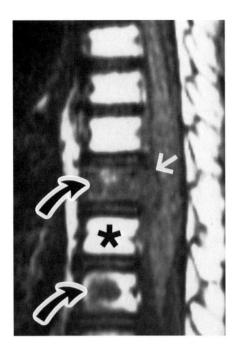

Fig. 10-46   Spinal metastatic Wilms' tumor shown by sagittal T1 MRI as isointense to hypointense vertebral involvement *(curved arrows)* contrasted against the postradiation fatty hyperintensities *(asterisk)*. Intraspinal extension with cord compression *(small arrow)* is demonstrated at T11.

hypointensity with T2 hyperintensity representative of tumor and edema, the latter a frequent component of metastases arising from primary tumors outside the bone marrow. Leukemia or lymphoma may appear isointense or slightly hyperintense on T2 images. Blastic metastasis may appear hypointense on both T1 and T2 images. Gadolinium enhancement is common.

Other disease processes of bone marrow

For the accurate interpretation of neoplastic spinal marrow involvement by MRI, the physician should also be aware of other disease processes that commonly involve the bone marrow and produce similar MRI findings.* These include myeloproliferative disorders, hemolytic anemias, marrow depletion disorders, hemosiderosis, ischemia, and treatment effects related to radiation therapy, chemotherapy, and transplantation.†

Myeloproliferative disorders, or preleukemias, are neoplasias of multipotential hematopoetic cells. These include chronic myelogenous leukemia and polycythemia vera. On MRI the spinal marrow may appear diffusely isointense or hypointense on T1 images and isointense or slightly hyperintense on T2 images.[52,83] Common *hemolytic anemias* include sickle cell anemia, thalassemias, and spherocytosis. In sickle cell anemia spinal abnormalities as demonstrated by MRI may result from marrow hyperplasia, ischemia, or infection.[76,83,102,119] Marrow hyperplasia ap-

pears as focal or diffuse isointensity or hypointensity on T1 images and isointense to hyperintense on T2 images. Ischemic edema, infarction, and infection (that is, osteomyelitis) usually appear as focal or diffuse hypointensity on T1 images and hyperintensity on T2 images. Thalassemias often produce the most prominent changes of marrow hyperplasia including extramedullary hematopoiesis often with multiple bilateral paraspinal masses that are T1 isointense and T2 isointense to slightly hyperintense.[83]

Disorders of marrow depletion include aplastic anemia and myelofibrosis. In aplastic anemia the marrow is hypocellular or acellular with fatty replacement and areas of fibrosis. There is marked T1 hyperintensity with T2 isointensity or hypointensity.[57,83] Often there is a patchy or heterogeneous intensity pattern especially in treated cases caused by areas of cellular recovery and other areas of fibrosis. Myelofibrosis may occur in association with a myeloproliferative disorder, or more commonly in childhood, as a sequela of treatment for leukemia or metastases. On MRI there is usually patchy or diffuse low intensity on T1 and T2 images that may be difficult to distinguish from hemosiderosis.[68,83] *Excessive iron deposition* may occur with primary or secondary hemochromatosis, especially after iron therapy and blood transfusions for erythropoietic disorders such as thalassemia.[83] Hemosiderosis may occur as ferritin or hemosiderin deposition within the reticuloendothelial system and involve the liver, spleen, pancreas, heart, pituitary, and bone marrow. Progressive hypointensity is seen on MRI from T1 images to T2 images (Figs. 10-42 and 10-43). *Ischemic marrow edema and infarction* commonly occur in sickle cell anemia and Gaucher's disease and may result in pathological fracture.[50,83,110,119] There may be homogeneous or heterogeneous T1 isointensity or hypointensity and T2 hypointensity or hyperintensity.

Therapeutic bone marrow changes include those related to radiotherapy, chemotherapy, and bone marrow transplantation.* Increased T2 intensity on MRI has been observed up to 3 to 4 weeks after 2000 to 4000 rad to the bone marrow and correlates with sinusoidal destruction, decreased hematopoiesis, and marrow edema. T2 hyperintensity persisting beyond this time may reflect radiation necrosis. After 3 to 4 weeks increased marrow fat and fibrosis appear as homogeneous or heterogeneous T1 hyperintensity and T2 isointensity or hypointensity (Fig. 10-42, 10-43, and 10-46)[101,106,126] Areas of fibrosis may appear as low intensity on T1 and T2 images. Partial or complete recovery of hematopoiesis has been documented in as high as 60% of patients at 6 to 9 months. Children often exhibit more rapid recovery with yellow to red marrow reconversion that results in T1 isointensities. Reactive changes reported with chemotherapy[83] include marrow cellular hypoplasia with increased fat content (T1 hyperintensity), marrow edema (T1 hypointensity and T2 hyperintensity), fibrosis (T1 and T2 hypointensity), and yellow to red marrow conversion (T1 isointensity). Short-

---

*References 26, 45, 81, 90, 95, 98, 107, 123, 130, 139, 142.
†References 52, 57, 68, 76, 83, 101, 102, 109, 119, 125.

---

*References 46, 83, 101, 106, 125, 126.

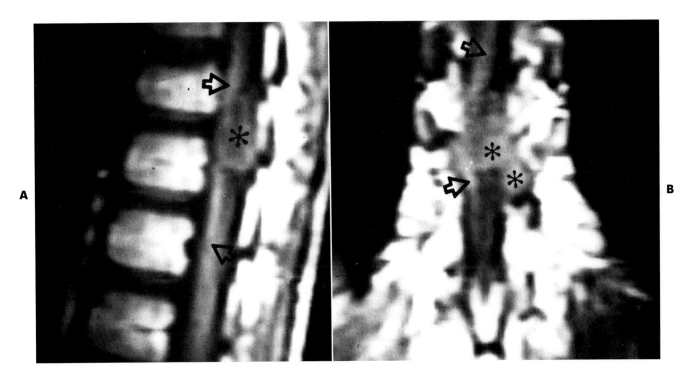

Fig. 10-47   Thoracic dumbbell Schwannoma shown by sagittal **(A)** and coronal **(B)** T1 MRI as an intradural extramedullary isointense mass *(asterisk)* displacing and compressing the cord *(open arrows)*. The extradural component is also shown on the coronal image *(lower asterisk)*. (From Barnes P: *Neurol Clin North Am* 8:741, 1990.)

term changes after bone marrow transplantation have also been described.[83,125] T1 hyperintensity is present up to 3 months after marrow ablation with chemotherapy or radiotherapy. Beyond that period a "band pattern" has been observed within the vertebral bodies as peripheral T1 isointensity (red marrow repopulation) and central T1 hyperintensities (yellow marrow).

INTRADURAL TUMORS
Nerve sheath, meningeal, and developmental tumors

Tumors involving the intradural extramedullary compartment include nerve sheath cell tumors, meningeal tumors, developmental tumors, and neoplastic seeding* (see box on p. 437). *Nerve sheath cell tumors* include schwannomas (neurinomas, neurilemmomas) and neurofibromas.[12,14,18,72,108] These are the most common benign tumors of this compartment, but they may also occur extradurally or transdurally (dumbbell type). These are infrequent in childhood except in neurofibromatosis and following radiotherapy for other tumors (for example, Wilms' tumor, neuroblastoma). Schwannomas may occur with or without neurofibromatosis, whereas neurofibromas, especially of the plexiform type, are characteristic of neurofibromatosis (Figs. 10-47 and 10-48). Plain films, CT, or MRI may show a paraspinal soft tissue mass, foraminal

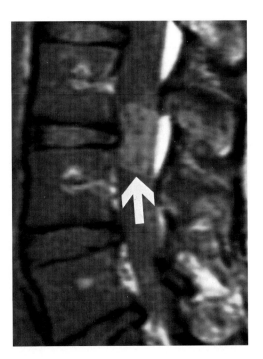

Fig. 10-48   Lumbar intradural neurofibroma *(arrow)* best shown by sagittal proton density MRI as an isointense to hyperintense mass at L2-3. The mass is poorly separated from CSF on sagittal T1 and T2 MRI without gadolinium enhancement (see Chapter 8).

*References 5, 47, 62, 94, 118, 136.

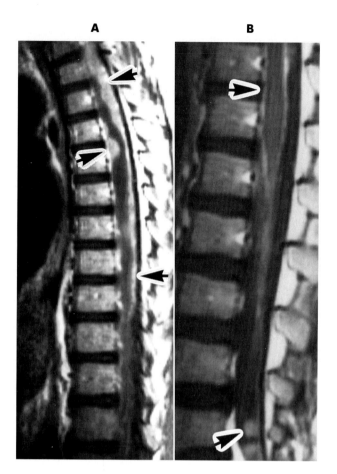

Fig. 10-49   Thoracolumbar spinal neuraxis seeding of cerebral glioblastoma shown by sagittal T1 MRI with nodular and laminar gadolinium-enhancing cord and nerve root deposits *(arrows)*.

enlargement, spinal canal widening, pedicle erosion, laminar thinning, vertebral body scalloping, rib erosion, or kyphoscoliosis. (The MRI findings are described in greater detail in Chapters 7 and 8.) *Meningeal tumors* include meningiomas, meningeal sarcomas, and melanocytic tumors.[108] Again, these are rare in childhood and adolescence but may occur with neurofibromatosis or after radiotherapy. The imaging findings are described in Chapter 7. Developmental or malformative tumors and germ cell tumors include lipomas, epidermoid and dermoid tumors, teratomas, hamartomas, neurenteric cysts, and arachnoid cysts.[108] These are presented in greater detail in Chapter 9.

Neoplastic seeding

Neoplastic seeding of the subarachnoid space is a common occurrence in childhood.[5,25,61,64,136] It occurs most commonly with medulloblastoma, other primitive neuroectodermal tumors (for example, pineoblastoma), germ cell tumors, recurrent anaplastic ependymoma, any highly malignant glial neoplasm (for example, glioblastoma), and lymphoma. Other less common sources for seeding are choroid plexus tumors (for example, carcinomas), oligodendrogliomatosis, neuroblastoma, retinoblastoma, rhabdomyosarcoma, and leukemia. Seeding may be present at the time of initial discovery of the primary tumor, especially in medulloblastoma, or may occur later after treatment with or without recurrence of the primary tumor. The seeding may be demonstrated at the lumbosacral, thoracic, or cervical levels and with or without evidence of intracranial spread. MRI before and after intravenous gadolinium administration is the procedure of choice and has replaced myelography.[5,97,136] The seeding is demonstrated as laminar or nodular enhancement along the cord surfaces and nerve roots, dorsally more often than ventrally (Fig. 10-49). Tumor seeding must be distinguished from operative intradural hemorrhage, which may appear as high

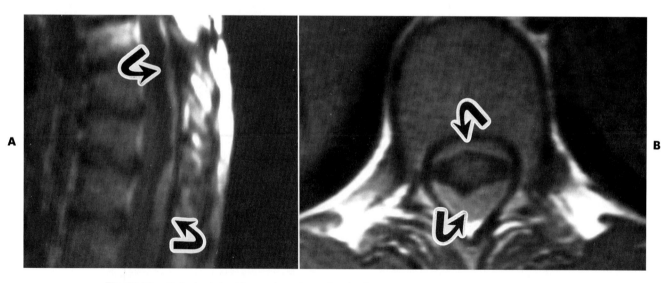

Fig. 10-50   Spinal subdural hemorrhage immediately after resection of intracranial germ cell tumor. Sagittal **(A)** and axial **(B)** T1 MRI show high intensity, irregular, laminar, dural-based collections *(curved arrows)* without cord deposits.

intensity on T1 images (methemoglobin). The distribution of hemorrhage is usually subarachnoid or subdural in location with a peripheral or dural-based layering, rather than the pial-based nodular or laminar effect of seeding, and clears within a few weeks (Fig. 10-50). Clinical presentations include pain, meningeal irritation, and nerve root or spinal cord symptoms and signs.

INTRAMEDULLARY TUMORS
Astrocytomas and ependymomas

Astrocytomas and ependymomas constitute the majority of cord tumors in childhood and adolescence[*] (see box on p. 437). Other less common tumors are mixed gliomas, neuronal tumors, and hemangioblastomas. Hematogenous metastases to the cord are very rare in childhood.[96] Subarachnoid tumor seeding with cord deposition is often associated with subpial invasion. The peak incidence for primary cord tumors is in the second decade. The tumors may be focal or extend to involve multiple segments. Holocord involvement is common, as are associated cysts or hydrosyringomyelia. Clinical presentations include progressive myelopathy with gait disturbance, lower extremity weakness, vague sensory symptoms, scoliosis, and subsequent paraparesis or quadriparesis with loss of bladder or bowel control. Plain films may show spinal canal widening,

[*]References 5, 35, 47, 94, 136, 148.

pedicle thinning, and scoliosis. Solid tumor components often correlate with the level of neurological signs, scoliosis, and pedicle thinning. *Astrocytomas* (50% to 60% of intramedullary tumors) are often well differentiated (grade I or II) but may be of a higher grade of malignancy.[5,35,104,136] Usually these are poorly demarcated and infiltrating tumors arising from and involving the cervical or cervicothoracic spinal cord. There is usually irregular or nonuniform cord expansion, occasionally with exophytic components. Holocord involvement occurs more commonly with astrocytoma than with ependymoma or mixed tumors (Figs. 10-51 and 10-52). In fact, in more than one half of the cases the entire cord is involved from the medulla or cervicomedullary junction to the conus medullaris. There is variable solid and cystic involvement. Often there is a solid column of intramedullary tumor posteriorly with rostral and caudal reactive cysts containing gliosis but no tumor. Occasionally there is a large cyst or syrinx containing small tumor nodules. Intratumoral cysts usually result from tumor necrosis.

Ependymomas (20% to 30% of intramedullary tumors) often involve the lower spinal cord, conus medullaris, filum terminale, or cauda equina.[5,35,136] Less often there is holocord involvement. Ependymomas arise from the central canal, terminal ventricle of the conus, or from ependymal cells of the filum terminale. The myxopapillary subtype typically arises from the filum and may be associated with

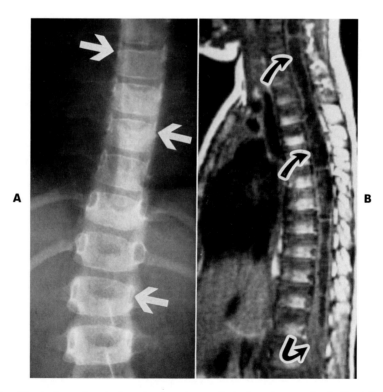

Fig. 10-51   Cervicothoracic spinal cord astrocytoma with hydrosyringomyelia. **A,** Frontal plain film shows thoracic scoliosis with canal widening and pedicle thinning *(arrows).* **B,** Sagittal T1 MRI shows isointense intramedullary solid tumor at the conus level *(lower arrow)* with expanding cervicothoracic cystic intramedullary hypointensities *(upper arrows)* consistent with secondary hydrosyringomyelia.

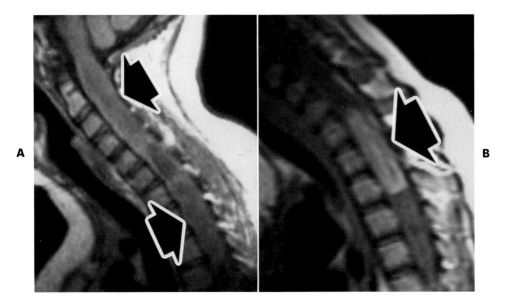

Fig. 10-52   Cervicothoracic junction cord astrocytoma with proximal and distal hydrosyringomyelia. **A,** Sagittal T1 MRI shows lower cervical and upper thoracic expanding intramedullary hypointensities *(lower arrow)* with upper cervical intramedullary isointensities *(upper arrow).* **B,** Sagittal T1 MRI after gadolinium administration shows high intensity enhancement only of the cervicothoracic junction component *(arrow).*

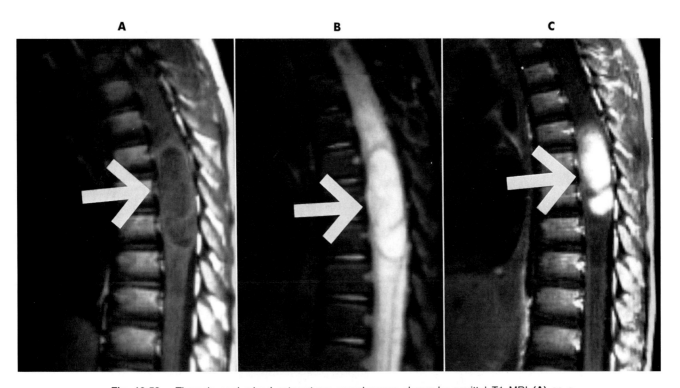

Fig. 10-53   Thoracic cord mixed astrocytoma-ependymoma shown by sagittal T1 MRI **(A)** as a circumscribed isointense to hypointense expansion *(arrow).* **B,** Sagittal T2 MRI demonstrates marked hyperintensity *(arrow).* **C,** Sagittal T1 MRI after gadolinium administration demonstrates marked high intensity tumor enhancement *(arrow)* with nonenhancing intramedullary hypointensity expansion above and below consistent with hydrosyringomyelia.

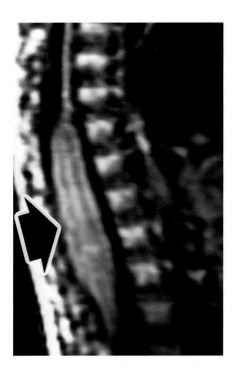

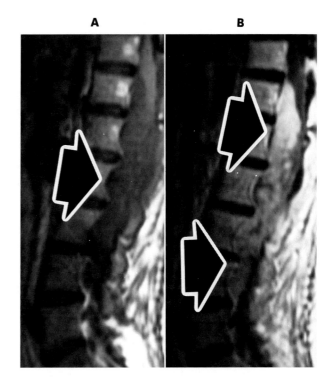

Fig. 10-54   Lower thoracic cord and conus medullaris mixed astrocytoma-ependymoma shown by sagittal T1 MRI as an isointense intramedullary expansion *(arrow)* with hypointense longitudinal striations (see text) and normal to small cord dimensions above.

Fig. 10-55   Ependymoma of the conus medullaris and cauda equina shown by sagittal T1 MRI **(A)** as a poorly defined, isointense intraspinal expansion *(arrow)* with vertebral scalloping. The mass was poorly shown by proton density and T2 MRI. **B,** After gadolinium administration sagittal T1 MRI shows marked and extensive high intensity enhancement of the tumor from T11 to L5 *(arrows).*

subarachnoid hemorrhage (see Fig. 10-55). Again, there is focal or long segment and irregular or nonuniform cord expansion often with cystic components or syringomyelia (Figs. 10-53 to 10-55). Commonly there is a pseudocapsule producing a cord-tumor plane. Subarachnoid seeding has been reported with this tumor.

The MRI findings in astrocytoma and ependymoma are similar and include irregular or nonuniform cord expansion that is isointense or hypointense on T1 images, often with gadolinium enhancement, and isointense to hyperintense on T2 images* (Figs. 10-51 to 10-55). The intensity patterns may be similar for soft tissue tumor components, cystic components, edema, or necrosis, although gadolinium enhancement usually identifies the solid tumor (Figs. 10-52 and 10-53). The cysts may contain CSF, proteinaceous fluid, or hemorrhage. Infrequently the tumor shows no enhancement at all, or not all of the tumor enhances. In addition to abnormal enhancement, nonuniform cord expansion assists in differentiating neoplastic cysts or syrinx from benign hydrosyringomyelia, the latter usually producing a more uniform and tapering cord expansion.

Treatment of cord astrocytomas and ependymomas usually involves excision of as much tumor as possible. The procedure is facilitated by intraoperative ultrasonography

and sensory-evoked potential monitoring.[35,87,100,114] Ependymomas are often demarcated, and excision may be carried out from top to bottom along the cyst-tumor-cord interfaces. Astrocytomas occasionally have an interface and are excised by dissection beginning at the midportion of the tumor and proceeding in an inside-out fashion to the tumor-glial interface. The reactive cystic components often resolve with resection of the solid tumor components. Repeat resection may be preferred to radiotherapy for recurrence.[46]

Hemangioblastomas

Hemangioblastomas are rarely encountered in childhood but may occur in association with von Hippel–Lindau syndrome, as presented in Chapter 8.[54,103,116] These may be single or multiple and may occur at the cervical, cervicothoracic, or thoracolumbar levels as intramedullary, intradural, or extradural tumors. These are vascular tumors, often with cysts and hemorrhage, and are composed of endothelial cells with a fatty and hemosiderin stroma. By MRI the intramedullary lesion may be identified as a cord expansion with varying intensity abnormalities including flow signal voids related to the feeding arterial, vascular nidus, and draining venous components, plus edema, cyst, and hemorrhagic elements. Gadolinium enhancement is usually a prominent feature (see Chapter 8).

*References 5, 28, 30, 44, 122, 136, 144.

REFERENCES
Neoplastic processes of the spine and spinal neuraxis

1. Aisen AM, Martel W, Braunstein EM, et al: MRI and CT evaluation of primary bone and soft tissue tumors, *AJR* 146:749, 1986.
2. Aprin H, Riseborough EJ, Hall JE: Chondrosarcoma in children and adolescents, *Clin Orthop* 166:226, 1982.
3. Armstrong EA, Harwood-Nash DCF, Fitz CR, et al: CT of neuroblastomas and ganglioneuromas in children, *AJR* 139:571, 1982.
4. Azouz EM, Kozlowski K, et al: Osteoid osteoma and osteoblastoma of the spine in children: report of 22 cases with brief literature review, *Pediatr Radiol* 16:25, 1986.
5. Barkovich A: Neoplasms of the spine. In Barkovitch A, editor: *Pediatric neuroimaging,* New York, 1990, Raven.
6. Beltran J, Noto AM, Chakeres DW, et al: Tumors of the osseous spine: staging with MR imaging versus CT, *Radiology* 162:565, 1987.
7. Beltran J, Simon DC, Levy M, et al: Aneurysmal bone cysts: MR imaging at 1.5 T, *Radiology* 158:689, 1986.
8. Berger PE, Kuhn JP: Computed tomography of tumors of the musculoskeletal system in children, *Radiology* 127:171, 1978.
9. Bidwell JK, Young JWR, et al: Giant cell tumor of the spine: computed tomography appearance and review of the literature, *CT* 11:307, 1987.
10. Biescker JL, Marcove RC, Huvos AG, et al: Aneurysmal bone cyst: a clinical pathologic study of 66 cases, *Cancer* 26:615, 1970.
11. Bloem JL, Taminiau AHM, Eulderink F, et al: Radiologic staging of primary bone sarcoma: MR imaging, scintigraphy, angiography, and CT correlated with pathologic examination, *Radiology* 169:805, 1988.
12. Bourgouin PM, Shepard JAO, Moore EH, et al: Plexiform neurofibromatosis of the mediastinum: CT appearance, *AJR* 151:461, 1988.
13. Boyko OB, Cory DA, Cohen MD, et al: MR imaging of osteogenic and Ewing's sarcoma, *AJR* 148:317, 1987.
14. Burk DL, Brunberg JA, Kanal E, et al: Spinal and paraspinal neurofibromatosis: surface coil MR imaging at 1.5 T, *Radiology* 162:797, 1987.
15. Carmody RF, Yang PJ, Seeley GW, et al: Spinal cord compression due to metastatic disease: diagnosis with MR imaging versus myelography, *Radiology* 173:225, 1989.
16. Castillo M, Quencer RM, Green BA, et al: Syringomyelia as a consequence of compressive extramedullary lesions: postoperative clinical and radiologic manifestations, *AJR* 150:391, 1988.
17. Cohen EK, Kressel HY, Frank TS, et al: Hyaline cartilage-origin bone and soft tissue neoplasms: MR appearance and histologic correlation, *Radiology* 167:477, 1988.
18. Cohen LM, Schwartz AM, Rockoff SD: Benign schwannomas: pathologic basis for CT inhomogeneities, *AJR* 147:141, 1986.
19. Cohen M, Dufner P: Tumors of the brain and spinal cord. In Swaiman K: *Pediatric neurology,* St Louis, 1989, Mosby–Year Book.
20. Cohen MD, Klatte EC, Bachner R, et al: Magnetic resonance of bone marrow disease in children, *Radiology* 151:715, 1984.
21. Cohn RS, Fielding JW: Osteochondroma of the cervical spine, *J Pediatr Surg* 21:997, 1986.
22. Cory DA, Fritsch SA, Cohen MD, et al: Aneurysmal bone cysts: imaging findings and embolotherapy, *AJR* 153:369, 1989.
23. Daffner RH, Lupetin AR, Dash N, et al: MR in the detection of malignant infiltration of bone marrow, *AJR* 146:353, 1986.
24. Dahlin DC, McLeon RA: Aneurysmal bone cyst and other nonneoplastic conditions, *Skeletal Radiol* 8:243, 1982.
25. Davis PC, Griedman NC, Fry SM, et al: Leptomeningeal metastasis: MR imaging, *Radiology* 163:449, 1987.
26. Dawson KL, Moore SC, Rowland J: Spectrum of appearance of red and yellow marrow in the pelvis with age: magnetic resonance and pathologic correlation, *Radiology* 173:465, 1989.
27. de Bruine FT, Kroon HM: Spinal chordoma: radiologic features in 14 cases, *AJR* 150:861, 1988.
28. Di Chiro G, Doppman JL, Dwyer AJ, et al: Tumors and arteriovenous malformations of the spinal cord: assessment using MR, *Radiology* 156:689, 1985.
29. Dietrich RB, Kangarloo H, Lenarsky C, et al: Neuroblastoma: the role of MR imaging, *AJR* 148:937, 1987.
30. Dillon WP, Norman D, Newton TH: Intradural spinal cord lesions: Gd-DTPA–enhanced MR imaging, *Radiology* 170:229, 1989.
31. Drolshagen LF, Kessler R, Partain CL: Cervical meningeal histiocytosis demonstrated by magnetic resonance imaging, *Pediatr Radiol* 17:63, 1987.
32. Dwyer AJ, Frank JA, Sank VJ, et al: Short T1 inversion-recovery pulse sequence: analysis and initial experience in cancer imaging, *Radiology* 168:827, 1988.
33. Ehman RL, Berquist TH, McLeod RA: MR imaging of the musculoskeletal system: a 5-year appraisal, *Radiology* 166:313, 1988.
34. Ellis JH, Siegel CL, Martel W, et al: Radiologic features of well-differentiated sarcoma, *AJR* 151:739, 1988.
35. Epstein F, Wisoff J: Intramedullary tumors of the spinal cord. In McLaurin R, Schut L, Venes J, et al, editors: *Pediatric neurosurgery,* Philadelphia, 1989, WB Saunders.
36. Erlemann R, Sciuk J, Bosse A, et al: Response of osteosarcoma and Ewing sarcoma to preoperative chemotherapy: assessment with dynamic and static MR imaging and skeletal scintigraphy, *Radiology* 175:791, 1990.
37. Farrelly C, Daneman A, Chan HSL, et al: Occult neuroblastoma presenting with opsomyoclonus: utility of computed tomography, *AJR* 142:807, 1984.
38. Fletcher BD, Lemmi MA, Slade WT, et al: MRI signal changes associated with therapy of Ewing sarcoma, *AJR* 153:202, 1989.
39. Frouge C, Vanel D, Coffre C, et al: The role of magnetic resonance imaging in the evaluation of Ewing sarcoma, *Skeletal Radiol* 17:387, 1988.
40. Gamba JL, Martinez S, Apple J, et al: CT of axial skeletal osteoid osteomas, *AJR* 142:769, 1984.
41. Gillespy T, Manfrini M, Ruggieri P, et al: Staging of intraosseous extent of osteosarcoma: correlation of preoperative CT and MR imaging with pathologic macroslides, *Radiology* 167:765, 1988.
42. Ginaldi S, deSantos LA: Computed tomography in the evaluation of small round cell tumors of bone, *Radiology* 134:441, 1980.
43. Glass RB, Poznanski AK, Fisher MR, et al: Case report: MR imaging of osteoid osteoma, *J Comput Assist Tomogr* 10:1065, 1986.
44. Goy AMC, Pinto RS, Raghavendra BN, et al: Intramedullary spinal cord tumors: MR imaging, with emphasis on associated cysts, *Radiology* 161:381, 1986.
45. Hajek PC, Baker LL, Coobar JE, et al: Focal fat deposition in axial bone marrow: MR characteristics, *Radiology* 162:245, 1987.
46. Halperin E, Kun L, Constine L, et al: *Pediatric radiation oncology,* New York, 1989, Raven.
47. Harwood-Nash DC, Fitz CR: *Neuroradiology in infants and children,* St Louis, 1976, Mosby–Year Book.
48. Heideman R, Packer R, Albright L, et al: Tumors of the central nervous system. In Pizzo P, Poplack D, editors: *Pediatric oncology,* Philadelphia, 1989, JB Lippincott.
49. Herman SD, Mesgarzadeh M, Bonakdarpour A, et al: The role of magnetic resonance imaging in giant cell tumor of bone, *Skeletal Radiol* 16:635, 1987.
50. Hermann G, Wagner LD, Gendal ES, et al: Spinal cord compression in type I Gaucher disease, *Radiology* 170:147, 1989.
51. Holscher NC, Bloem JL, Nooy MA, et al: The value of MR imaging to monitor the effect of chemotherapy in bone sarcomas, *AJR* 154:763, 1990.
52. Jensen KE, Grube T, Thomsen C, et al: Prolonged bone marrow T1 relaxation in patients with polycythemia vera, *Magn Reson Imaging* 6:291, 1988.
53. Jones BE, Wood BP, Schwartz C, et al: MR appearances of childhood bone tumors, *AJR* 153:202, 1989.
54. Kaffenberger DA, Sah CP, Mortagh FR, et al: MR imaging of spinal cord hemangioblastoma associated with syringomyelia, *J Comput Assist Tomogr* 12:495, 1988.
55. Kanal E, Burk DL, Brunberg JA, et al: Pediatric musculoskeletal magnetic resonance imaging, *Radiol Clin North Am* 26:211, 1988.
56. Kangarloo H, Dietrich RB, Taira RT, et al: MR imaging of bone marrow in children, *J Comput Assist Tomogr* 10:205, 1986.
57. Kaplan PA, Asleson RJ, Klassen LW, et al: Bone marrow patterns in aplastic anemia: observations with 1.5 T MR imaging, *Radiology* 164:441, 1987.

58. Kaplan PA, Williams SM: Mucocutaneous and peripheral soft tissue hemangiomas: MR imaging, *Radiology* 163:163, 1987.

59. Karian JM, DeFilipp G, Buchheit WA, et al: Vertebral osteochondroma causing spinal cord compression, *Neurosurgery* 14:483, 1984.

60. Kenney PJ, Gilula LA, Murphy WA: The use of computed tomography to distinguish osteochondroma and chondrosarcoma, *Radiology* 139:129, 1981.

61. Kilgore D, Strother C, Starshak R, et al: Pineal germinoma: MR imaging, *Radiology* 158:435, 1986.

62. Klein D: Extramedullary spinal tumors. In McLaurin R, Schut L, Venes J, et al, editors: *Pediatric neurosurgery,* Philadelphia, 1989, WB Saunders.

63. Kozlowski K, Beluffi G, Masel J, et al: Primary vertebral tumours in children: report of 20 cases with brief review of the literature, *Pediatr Radiol* 14:129, 1984.

64. Krol G, Sze G, Malkin M, et al: MR of cranial and spinal meningeal carcinomatosis comparison with CT and myelography, *AJR* 151:583, 1988.

65. Kroon HM, Schurmans J: Osteoblastoma: clinical and radiologic findings in 98 new cases, *Radiology* 175:783, 1990.

66. Kumar R, Guinto FC, Madewell JE, et al: Expansile bone lesions of the vertebra, *Radiographics* 8:749, 1988.

67. Kumar S, Marks H, et al: Intraspinal tumors in children with hip symptoms, *J Pediatr Orthop* 8:529, 1988.

68. Lanir A, Aghai E, Simon JS, et al: MR imaging in myelofibrosis, *J Comput Assist Tomogr* 10:634, 1986.

69. Laredo JD, Assouline E, Gelbert F, et al: Vertebral hemangiomas: fat content as a sign of aggressiveness, *Radiology* 177:467, 1990.

70. Laredo JD, Reizine D, Bard M, et al: Vertebral hemangiomas: radiologic evaluation, *Radiology* 161:183, 1986.

71. Lee HK, Yao L, Wirth CR: MR imaging of solitary osteochondromas: report of eight cases, *AJR* 149:557, 1987.

72. Levine E, Huntrakoon M, Wetzel LH: Malignant nerve-sheath neoplasms in neurofibromatosis: distinction from benign tumors by using imaging techniques, *AJR* 149:1059, 1987.

73. Libshitz HI, Cohen MA: Radiation-induced osteochondromas, *Radiology* 142:643, 1982.

74. Mahboubi S: CT appearance of nidus in osteoid osteoma, *J Comput Assist Tomogr* 10:457, 1986.

75. Malat J, Virapongse C, Levine A: Solitary osteochondroma of the spine, *Spine* 11:625, 1986.

76. Mankad VN, Williams JP, Harpen MD, et al: Magnetic resonance imaging of bone marrow in sickle cell disease: clinical, hematologic, and pathologic correlations, *Blood* 75:274, 1990.

77. McKinstry CS, Steiner RE, Young AT, et al: Bone marrow in leukemia and aplastic anemia: MR imaging before, during, and after treatment, *Radiology* 162:701, 1987.

78. Mechlin M, Thickman D, Kressel HY, et al: Magnetic resonance imaging of postoperative patients with metallic implants, *AJR* 143:1281, 1984.

79. Meyer JE, Lepke RA, Lindfors KK, et al: Chordomas: their CT appearance in the cervical, thoracic, and lumbar spine, *Radiology* 153:693, 1984.

80. Moore SG: MR imaging evaluation of bone lesions: comparison of inversion-recovery and spin-echo images, *Radiology* 169:191, 1988.

81. Moore SG, Berry G, Smith JT, et al: Extent of marrow and soft tissue involvement in pediatric bone tumors: magnetic resonance and pathologic correlation, *AJR* 153:202, 1989.

82. Moore SG, Dawson K: Tumors of the musculoskeletal system. In Cohen M, Edwards M, editors: *MR imaging of children,* Philadelphia, 1990, BC Decker.

83. Moore SG, Sebag G: Primary disorders of bone marrow. In Cohen M, Edwards M, editors: *MR imaging of children,* Philadelphia, 1990, BC Decker.

84. Mulliken JB, Glowacki J: Hemangiomas and vascular malformations in infants and children: a classification based on endothelial characteristics, *Plast Reconstr Surg* 69:412, 1982.

85. Munk PL, Helms CA, Holt RG, et al: MR imaging of aneurysmal bone cysts, *AJR* 153:99, 1989.

86. Myles ST, MacRae ME: Benign osteoblastoma of the spine in childhood, *J Neurosurg* 68:884, 1988.

87. Naidich T, Quencer R, editors: *Clinical neurosonography,* New York 1987, Springer-Verlag.

88. Nokes S, Murtagh F, Jones J, et al: Childhood scoliosis: MR imaging, *Radiology* 164:791, 1987.

89. Novick GS, Pavlov H, Bullough PG: Osteochondroma of the cervical spine: report of two cases in preadolescent males, *Skeletal Radiol* 8:13, 1982.

90. Okada Y, Aoki S, Barkovich AJ, et al: Cranial bone marrow in children: assessment of normal development with MR imaging, *Radiology* 171:161, 1989.

91. Olson DO, Shields AF, Sheunch CJ, et al: Magnetic resonance imaging of the bone marrow in patients with leukemia, aplastic anemia, and lymphoma, *Invest Radiol* 21:540, 1986.

92. Parziel PM, Baleriaux D, Rodesch G, et al: Gd-DTPA–enhanced MR imaging of spinal tumors, *AJNR* 10:249, 1989.

93. Petersson H, Gillespy T, Hamlin DJ, et al: Primary musculoskeletal tumors: examination with MR imaging compared with conventional modalities, *Radiology* 164:237, 1987.

94. Petterson H, Harwood-Nash D: *CT and myelography of the pediatric spine and cord,* New York, 1982, Springer-Verlag.

95. Porter BA, Shields AF, Olson DO: Magnetic resonance imaging of bone marrow disorders, *Radiol Clin North Am* 24:269, 1986.

96. Post MJD, Quencer RM, Green BA, et al: Intramedullary spinal cord metastases, mainly of nonneurogenic origin, *AJR* 148:1015, 1987.

97. Powers T, Partain C, Kessler R, et al: CNS lesions in pediatric patients: Gd-DTPA–enhanced MR imaging, *Radiology* 169:723, 1988.

98. Price HI, Batnitzky S, Levine E, et al: The computed tomographic findings in benign disease of the vertebral column, *Radiographics* 4:283, 1984.

99. Punt J, Pritchard J, Pincott JR, et al: Neuroblastoma: a review of 21 cases presenting with cord compression, *Cancer* 45:3095, 1980.

100. Raghavendra BN, Epstein FJ, McClearly L: Intramedullary spinal cord tumors in children: localization by intraoperative sonography, *AJNR* 5:395, 1984.

101. Ramsey RG, Zacharis CE: MR imaging of the spine after radiation therapy: easily recognizable effects, *AJR* 144:1131, 1985.

102. Rao VM, Fishman M, Mitchell DG, et al: Painful sickle cell crisis: bone marrow patterns observed with MR imaging, *Radiology* 161:211, 1986.

103. Rebner M, Gebarski SS: Magnetic resonance imaging of spinal cord hemangioblastoma, *AJNR* 6:287, 1985.

104. Reimer R, Onofrio CM: Astrocytomas of the spinal cord in children and adolescents, *J Neurosurg* 63:669, 1985.

105. Reither M, Kaiser W, Zeitler E: Bone marrow diseases in children: significance of MRI in comparison to other imaging modalities, *Ann Radiol* 30:511, 1987.

106. Remedios PA, Colletti PM, Raval JK, et al: Magnetic resonance imaging of bone after radiation, *Magn Reson Imaging* 6:301, 1988.

107. Ricci C, Cova M, Kang YS, et al: Normal age-related patterns of cellular and fatty bone marrow distribution in the axial skeleton: MR imaging study, *Radiology* 177:83, 1990.

108. Rorke L, Gilles F, Davis R, et al: Revision of the WHO classification of brain tumors for childhood, *Cancer* 56:1869, 1985.

109. Rosen BR, Fleming DM, Kushner DC, et al: Hematologic bone marrow disorders: quantitative chemical shift MR imaging, *Radiology* 169:799, 1988.

110. Rosenthal DI, Scott JA, Barranger J, et al: Evaluation of Gaucher's disease using magnetic resonance imaging, *J Bone Joint Surg* 68A:802, 1986.

111. Rosenthal DI, Scott JA, Mankin HJ, et al: Sacrococcygeal chordoma: Magnetic resonance imaging and computed tomography, *AJR* 145:143, 1985.

112. Ross JS, Masaryk TJ, Modic MT, et al: Vertebral hemangiomas: MR imaging, *Radiology* 165:165, 1987.

113. Rousselin B, Vanel D, Terrier-Lacombe MJ, et al: Clinical and radiologic analysis of 13 cases of primary neuroectodermal tumors of bone, *Skeletal Radiol* 18:115, 1989.

114. Rubin J, DiPietro M, Chandler W, et al: Spinal ultrasonography: intraoperative and pediatric applications, *Radiol Clin North Am* 26:1, 1988.

115. Russell D, Rubenstein L: *Pathology of tumors of the nervous system,* ed 4, Baltimore, 1977, Williams & Wilkins.

116. Sato Y, Wazirim L, Smith W, et al: Hippel-Lindau disease: MR imaging, *Radiology* 166:241, 1988.

117. Savini R, Giunti A, Boriani S: Benign and malignant spinal tumors. In Bradford D, Hensinger R: *The pediatric spine*, New York, 1985, Thieme.

118. Scotti G, Scialfa G, Colombo N, et al: MR imaging of intradural extramedullary tumors of the cervical spine, *J Comput Assist Tomogr* 9:1037, 1985.

119. Sebes JI: Diagnostic imaging of bone and joint abnormalities associated with sickle cell hemoglobinopathies, *AJR* 152:1153, 1989.

120. Siegel MJ, Glazer HS, St Amour TE, et al: Lymphangiomas in children: MR imaging, *Radiology* 170:467, 1989.

121. Siegel MJ, Jamroz GA, Glazer HS, et al: MR imaging of intraspinal extension of neuroblastoma, *J Comput Assist Tomogr* 10:593, 1986.

122. Slasky B, Bydder G, Niendorf H, et al: MR imaging with gadolinium-DTPA in the differentiation of tumor, syrinx, and cyst of the spinal cord, *J Comput Assist Tomogr* 11:845, 1987.

123. Smith SR, Williams CE, Davies JM, et al: Bone marrow disorders: characterization with quantitative MR imaging, *Radiology* 172:805, 1989.

124. Smoker WRK, Godersky JC, Knutzon RK: The role of MR imaging in evaluating metastatic spinal disease, *AJNR* 8:901, 1987.

125. Stevens SK, Moore SG, Amylon MD: Repopulation of marrow after transplantation: MR imaging with pathologic correlation, *Radiology* 175:213, 1990.

126. Stevens SK, Moore SG, Kaplan I: Early and late bone marrow changes after irradiation: MR evaluation, *AJR* 154:745, 1990.

127. Stimac GK, Porter BA, Olson DO, et al: Gadolinium-DTPA–enhanced MR imaging of spinal neoplasms: preliminary investigation and comparison with unenhanced spin-echo and STIR sequences, *AJNR* 9:839, 1988.

128. Sundaram M, McGuire MH, Herbold DR: Magnetic resonance imaging of osteosarcoma, *Skeletal Radiol* 16:23, 1987.

129. Sundaram M, McGuire MH, Schajowicz F: Soft tissue masses: histologic basis for decreased signal (short T2) on T2-weighted MR images, *AJR* 148:1247, 1987.

130. Surimura K, Yamasaki K, et al: Bone marrow diseases of the spine: differentiation with T1 and T2 relaxation times in MR imaging, *Radiology* 165:541, 1987.

131. Sze G, Abramson A, Krol G, et al: Gadolinium-DTPA in the evaluation of intradural extramedullary spinal disease, *AJNR* 9:153, 1988.

132. Sze G, Krol G, Zimmerman RD, et al: Intramedullary disease of the spine: Diagnosis using Gadolinium-DTPA–enhanced MR imaging, *AJNR* 9:847, 1988.

133. Sze G, Krol G, Zimmerman R, et al: Malignant extradural spinal tumors: MR imaging with Gd-DTPA, *Radiology* 167:217, 1988.

134. Sze G, Uichanco LS, Brant-Zawadzki M, et al: Chordomas: MR imaging, *Radiology* 166:187, 1988.

135. Tonai M, Campbell CJ, Ahn GH, et al: Osteoblastoma: clarification and report of 16 patients, *Clin Orthop* 167:222, 1982.

136. Twohig M, Sze G: Spinal tumors. In Cohen M, Edwards M, editors: *MR imaging of children*, Philadelphia, 1990, BC Decker.

137. Unger EC, Kesler HB, Kowalyshyn MJ, et al: MR imaging of Maffucci syndrome, *AJR* 150:351, 1988.

138. Valk J: Gd-DTPA in MR of spinal lesions, *AJR* 150:1163, 1988.

139. Vogler JB, Murphy WA: Bone marrow imaging, *Radiology* 168:679, 1988.

140. Walker HS, Dietrich RB, Flannigan BD, et al: Magnetic resonance imaging of the pediatric spine, *Radiographics* 7:1129, 1987.

141. Wang A, Lipson S, Hay Kal HA, et al: Computed tomography of aneurysmal bone cyst of the CT vertebral body, *J Comput Assist Tomogr* 8:1186, 1984.

142. Weinreb JC: MR imaging of bone marrow: a map could help, *Radiology* 177:23, 1990.

143. Wetzel LH, Levine E, Murphey MD: A comparison of MR imaging and CT in the evaluation of musculoskeletal masses, *Radiographics* 7:851, 1987.

144. Williams AL, Haughton VM, Pojunas KW, et al: Differentiation of intramedullary neoplasms and cysts by MR, *AJNR* 8:527, 1987.

145. Yuh WTC, Zachar CK, Barloon TJ, et al: Vertebral compression fractures: distinction between benign and malignant causes with MR imaging, *Radiology* 172:215, 1989.

146. Zimmer WD, Berguist TH, McLeod RA, et al: Magnetic resonance imaging of osteosarcomas: comparison with computed tomography, *Clin Orthop* 208:289, 1986.

147. Zimmer WD, Berguist TH, McLeod RA: Bone tumors: MR imaging versus CT, *Radiology* 155:709, 1985.

148. Zimmerman RA, Bilaniuk LT: Imaging of tumors of the spinal canal and cord, *Radiol Clin North Am* 26:65, 1988.

Inflammatory processes of the spine and spinal neuraxis

CLINICAL AND IMAGING ASPECTS

Inflammatory diseases of the spinal column and neuraxis are relatively infrequent but important causes of childhood spinal deformity and neurological disability* The processes include infectious spondylitis (diskitis, vertebral osteomyelitis), epidural abscess or empyema, meningitis, arachnoiditis, myelitis, spinal cord abscess, and spinal involvement in childhood arthritis (noninfectious spondylitis). Clinical presentations include local or referred pain and tenderness, irritability, fever, and other systemic symptoms. There may be back, hip, or abdominal pain. The child may limp or refuse to walk, sit, or stand. There may be meningeal symptoms or signs, postural rigidity, spasm, scoliosis, kyphosis, or acute pain with pathological fracture. The course may be acute, rapidly progressive, or chronic. Radiculopathy or myelopathy may result. Causes include bacterial, viral, tuberculous, fungal, and, rarely, parasitic or sarcoid. (Meningitis is discussed in Chapter 5.) It is important to recall that leukemia and neoplastic seeding may be manifested as meningitis and that dermal sinus and epidermoid or dermoid tumor may be the cause of septic or aseptic (chemical) meningitis that may be recurrent. Recurrent infectious meningitis may also be related to otherwise occult parameningeal foci, such as osteomyelitis, sinus or otomastoid infection, posttrauma CSF leak, as well as immunodeficiency states (for example, AIDS) or immunosuppression (for example, posttransplant, chemotherapy). Furthermore, infections of the spine or spinal neuraxis may mimic neoplasm.

Initial imaging includes plain films or radionuclide bone scanning, especially for diskitis or osteomyelitis. CT or MRI may assist needle aspiration for biopsy and cultures in selected cases.[19] MRI may be indicated if there are neurological symptoms or signs indicative of spinal column deformity or instability with neural compression, including epidural or intradural suppuration, arachnoiditis, or myelitis.[4,13,14] Proton density and T2-weighted images are preferred for the evaluation of diskitis, osteomyelitis, epidural abscess, and myelitis. T1-weighted images alone may often be all that is needed to evaluate spondylitis associated with childhood arthritis. Gadolinium enhancement may be important for evaluating suppurative collections, arachnoiditis, or meningitis. For likely inflammatory

---

*References 4, 6, 11, 14, 36, 38, 40.

cord lesions such as myelitis, sagittal and coronal T1-weighted sequences may be used to rule out cord expansion or compression, whereas T2 SE or T2/T2* GE sections may be required to delineate the nature and extent of the inflammatory cord involvement, especially when there is minimal or no cord expansion.

SPINAL COLUMN INFECTIONS
Infectious spondylitis

Spinal column infection (infectious spondylitis) includes diskitis and vertebral osteomyelitis. The spectrum of column infection ranges from a self-limiting nonsuppurative disk space inflammation (diskitis) without specific organism to that of a pyogenic disk and vertebral end plate infection (vertebral osteomyelitis).[35] Bacteriological diagnosis is available in less than one half the cases. Bacterial (for example, *Staphylococcus aureus*), viral, and traumatic causes have all been implicated. Tuberculosis must always be ruled out. Diskitis usually occurs in children under 5 years of age, most often at the lumbar level and less often at the thoracic or cervical level.* Infrequently, more than one level is involved. The infection is of hematogenous origin. In the infant and younger child with persistence of the disk arterial microcirculatory pattern, the infection tends

---

*References 7, 15, 18, 28, 31, 35, 37.

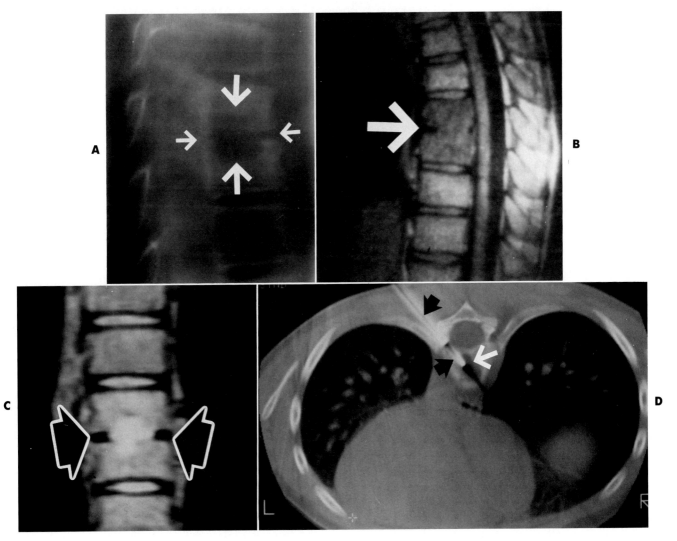

Fig. 10-56 Thoracic diskitis and vertebral osteomyelitis. **A,** Lateral tomogram shows disk space narrowing and end-plate destruction *(small arrows),* plus vertebral body lytic destruction *(large arrows).* **B,** Sagittal T1 MRI shows hypointensity obliteration *(arrow)* of the disk space and end-plates. **C,** Coronal T2 MRI demonstrates marked hyperintensity of the process *(arrows).* **D,** CT-guided needle biopsy *(black arrows)* of the lytic vertebral lesion *(white arrow)* was done for cultures *(Staphylococcus aureus).* (From Hoffer F, et al: *J Pediatr Orthopaedics* 8:442, 1988.)

A   B   C

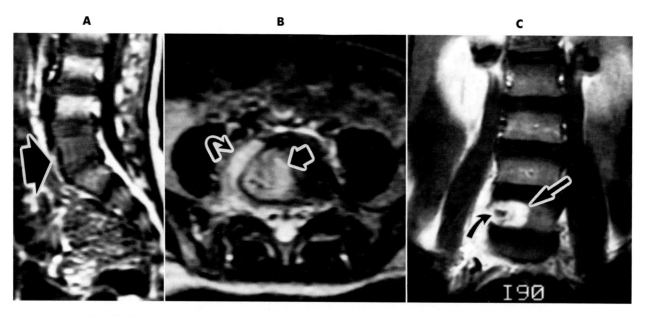

Fig. 10-57   Lumbar vertebral osteomyelitis with abscess. **A,** Sagittal T1 MRI shows L5 vertebral body hypointensity *(arrow).* **B,** Axial T2 MRI demonstrates high intensity involvement of the body *(straight arrow)* with a paravertebral subligamentous mass *(curved arrow).* **C,** Coronal T1 MRI shows marked high intensity gadolinium enhancement *(straight arrow)* with central hypointensity *(curved arrow)* consistent with abscess. A specific organism was not identified; however, the process responded to antibiotics, which was confirmed on follow-up MRI.

to involve the disk space initially and then the vertebral end plates. In older patients with a mature and relatively avascular disk, the end plate is initially involved. Plain film abnormalities may not appear for 2 to 4 weeks after the initial onset of symptoms, although isotope bone or gallium scanning may be positive.

The plain film, CT, and MRI findings include disk space narrowing, end plate irregularities, subsequent end plate erosions, Schmorl's nodes, and sclerosis[16,22,39] (Fig. 10-56). Other findings include paraspinal soft tissue masses (edema, cellulitis, abscess) or psoas abscess. MRI demonstrates inflammatory involvement of the disk, end plates, and marrow edema as T1 hypointensity and T2 hyperintensity[5,15,18,25,37] (Figs. 10-56 and 10-57). Usually there is loss of the intranuclear cleft. Associated soft tissue paraspinal masses are identified along with intraspinal involvement with dural sac compression. Gadolinium enhancement has also been reported (Fig. 10-57). Early diagnosis and treatment are important to prevent spinal deformity and neurological impairment. Conservative management in diskitis includes immobilization and rest with administration of antiinflammatory agents. Antibiotics are administered only if there are other signs of infection, such as sepsis, if there are positive blood cultures, or if conservative therapy fails. Aspiration biopsy and cultures are important especially if the process progresses to osteomyelitis with vertebral destruction and abscess or if tuberculosis is suspected[19] (Fig. 10-56). Sequelae include persistent disk narrowing or partial restoration, osseous disk bridging, secondary degenerative facet arthropathy, scoliosis, kyphosis, Schmorl's nodes, or vertebra magna (see Fig. 10-59).

Tuberculous spondylitis

Tuberculosis, or tuberculous spondylitis, is a disease primarily of children from underdeveloped or underserved areas but may occur at any age in any population and mimic other diseases, especially neoplasms.[9,12,20,32,34] Often the infection spreads to the spine from adjacent infected organs, such as the lung or kidney, although sometimes spinal disease is the first or only manifestation of the infection. The thoracolumbar spine is most commonly involved and the infection usually starts anteriorly in the vertebral body or anterior paradiskal region. The infection infrequently starts or involves the posterior elements only. Pott's paraplegia may result from active or healed disease. In the active phase there is vertebral bone destruction with caseous suppuration, granulation, and sequestra with or without secondary disk space involvement (Fig. 10-58). Subligamentous, subperiosteal, and epidural venous extension results in contiguous or skip involvement of other vertebral segments. Abscess formation occurs paraspinally and prevertebrally or within the psoas muscle. There may be extension of the abscess to remote areas such as the abdomen, pelvis, or thorax (empyema). Vertebral collapse results in kyphosis, kyphoscoliosis, vertebral dislocation, and epidural cord compression. Rarely, transdural extension results in pachymeningitis or meningomyelitis. With healing, there is fibrous, calcific, or bony ankylosis. In extreme cases there may be anterior bony bridging with increasing kyphosis and spinal cord transection or fibrous constriction of the dural sac, cord, or nerve roots. The resulting bony kyphosis may mimic congenital or dysplastic kyphosis (Fig. 10-59). Plain films, CT, and MRI show

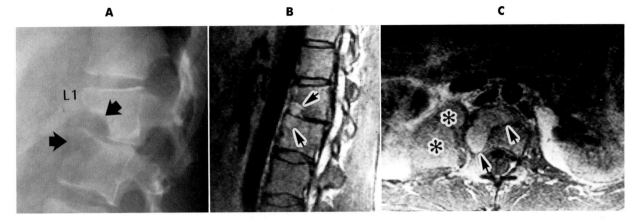

Fig. 10-58   Lumbar tuberculous spondylitis. **A,** Lateral plain film shows L1-L2 gibbus deformity with anteroinferior L1 body and anterosuperior L2 body erosion with disk space narrowing *(arrows).* Sagittal proton density **(B)** and axial T2 **(C)** MRI show L1 and L2 vertebral and disk space hyperintensities *(arrowheads)* and right paraspinal high intensity mass *(asterisks).* (From Smith A, et al: *AJR* 153:399, 1989.)

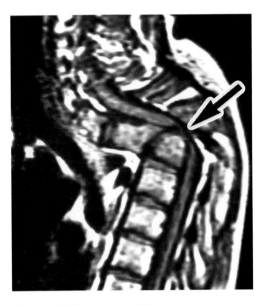

Fig. 10-59   Probable postspondylitis cervicothoracic kyphosis in an Ethiopian girl being evaluated for severe congenital kyphosis versus chronic tuberculous spondylitis. Sagittal T1 MRI shows gibbus vertebral deformity with severe kyphosis and marked cord thinning *(arrow).*

vertebral destruction, often without disk involvement, but with paraspinal calcified masses (cold abscesses), kyphotic deformity, and scalloped or eroded anterior bodies from subperiosteal spread (Fig. 10-58). The inflammatory process is isointense to hypointense on T1 MRI, and there is gadolinium enhancement.[12,34] The process usually appears T2 hyperintense. The fibrous, sclerotic, and calcific components are often isointense to hypointense on all sequences. Management includes antituberculous chemotherapy with surgical excision and decompression followed by bone grafting. Complications of treatment may include residual or recurrent infection, and bone graft slippage, resorption, fractures, or nonunion.

SPINAL NEURAXIS INFECTIONS
Epidural abscesses

Other less common or rare infections of the spine or neuraxis include epidural abscess, meningitis, arachnoiditis, myelitis, and spinal cord abscess. Epidural abscesses of pyogenic origin may occur with or without vertebral infection, by direct extension, or by the hematogenous route.[2,4,5,11,13] The thoracic or lumbar levels are most commonly involved, although cervical ventral epidural abscesses may occur secondary to nasopharyngeal infections. The infection may be in the form of a cellulitis or abscess, more often involves the dorsal canal, and may extend rostrally or caudally with dural sac compression. MRI shows displacement or replacement of the epidural fat and dural sac deformity with or without disk space or vertebral abnormalities (Figs. 10-57 and 10-60). The collection is usually isointense to hypointense relative to fat on T1 images, shows gadolinium enhancement, and is often heterogeneous high intensity on T2 images.[2,5,13] Treatment includes surgical drainage and antibiotics.

Meningitis and arachnoiditis

Meningitis is discussed in greater detail in Chapter 5. It is often a component of other inflammatory processes of the spine or neuraxis. MRI demonstrates meningeal thickening with gadolinium enhancement.[4,10,13] Arachnoiditis may occur after trauma, surgery, or infection.[4,11] There may be associated arachnoidal cysts (see Chapter 9) or hydrosyringomyelia. MRI may reveal aggregates of adherent nerve roots centrally within the sac or peripherally along the meninges, and CSF-replacing nodules or masses[30,33] (Fig. 10-60). The process often appears isointense to hypointense on T1 images, enhances with gadolinium, and appears isointense to hyperintense on T2 images. Often there is irregular narrowing of the subarachnoid space. Arachnoiditis is to be differentiated from neoplastic seeding (nodular enhancement usually with a normal or expanded dural sac) and hypertrophic neuropathy (smooth and regular nerve root enlargement with a normal dural sac).

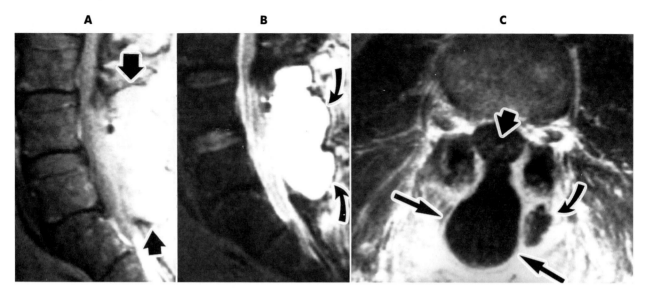

Fig. 10-60   Epidural abscess following surgery for lumbar spinal stenosis. Sagittal proton density **(A)** and T2 **(B)** MRI show a large dorsal lumbar collection with fluid level *(black arrows,* **A***)* and hypointense margins *(curved arrows,* **B***).* **C,** Axial T1 MRI after gadolinium administration shows the large hypointense pseudomeningocele collection *(long arrows)* with enhancement of the margins in addition to adjacent irregular low intensity collection with margin enhancement *(curved arrows).* The poor separation of the intradural nerve roots may suggest arachnoiditis *(arrowhead).* (Courtesy J. Kramer and R. Bajakian, Beth Israel Hospital, Boston.)

Myelitis and spinal cord abscess

Spinal cord infection, or *myelitis,* is an unusual cause of acute or progressive myelopathy in childhood (for example, transverse myelitis).* The causes are usually viral infection and postviral or postvaccinial immune-mediated inflammation (for example, acute disseminated encephalomyelitis, ADEM). Inflammatory myelopathy has also been reported in patients with AIDS (see Chapter 4).[17] There may be reversible or permanent white matter involvement. MRI may show T1 isointensity to hypointensity with or without cord expansion or gadolinium enhancement.[3,23,24] Hyperintensity may be demonstrated on T2 images. The clinical differential diagnosis includes Guillan-Barré syndrome and Devic syndrome. *Spinal cord abscess* is very rare but may occur with direct spread from a dermal sinus, from hematogenous or lymphatic sources, or may be associated with immunological compromise, such as AIDS.[4,11,14] The abscesses may be single or multiple, are often of staphylococcal or streptococcal origin, or occasionally fungal. Usually there is associated meningitis, back pain, and myelopathy. MRI demonstrates irregular cord expansion or intradural perimedullary masses (see Chapter 9). The process is often T1 isointense to hypointense, gadoliniumenhancing, and T2 isointense to hyperintense.[4,14]

SPINAL INVOLVEMENT IN CHILDHOOD ARTHRITIS

Spinal involvement in childhood arthritis is uncommon (less than 10% of cases). The *rheumatoid* designation is

_____
*References 3, 4, 11, 23, 24, 26.

often inappropriate in childhood and adolescence, since the rheumatoid factor is rarely positive.[14,21,29] The presence of HLA-B27 antigen often suggests but does not confirm ankylosing spondylitis. Often childhood arthritis is a diagnosis of exclusion, referring to a systemic inflammatory process with primary involvement of joints about the most actively growing bones including the knee, ankle, and wrist. Although spinal disease is infrequent, the cervical synovial joints are more often involved than the thoracic or lumbar joints. Cervical involvement occurs in about one fourth of the cases with systemic disease and in one third of the cases of polyarticular juvenile rheumatoid arthritis. Pain and restricted motion are common manifestations. Torticollis is uncommon but may result from spasm associated with the apophyseal disease, or less often from atlantoaxial subluxation. Trauma and infection should be excluded.

Plain films, CT, or MRI may show calcification about the anterior arch of C1, apophyseal joint fusion (ankyloses), especially in the upper cervical segments, arrested vertebral growth with shortened sagittal and vertical dimensions, and often narrowing or obliteration of the disk spaces.[1,8,21,27,29] Other findings include basilar impression, ligamentous calcification, osteophyte formation, and atlantoaxial subluxation or dislocation with or without dens erosion[1,8,27] (Fig. 10-61). The latter occurs much less frequently in children than in adults. The odontoid may appear flattened. Hypermobility may occur above or below fused segments. On MRI atlantoaxial instability may be associated with a sizeable peridontal mass that represents synovial inflammation (Fig. 10-62). The inflammatory mass may result in fixed subluxation but is often reduced after a period of

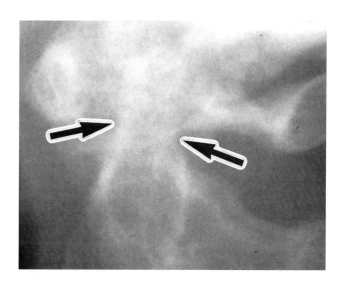

Fig. 10-61 Rheumatoid arthritis with cervical spinal involvement demonstrated by lateral plain film with erosions along the base of the dens *(arrows)* and atlantoaxial subluxation.

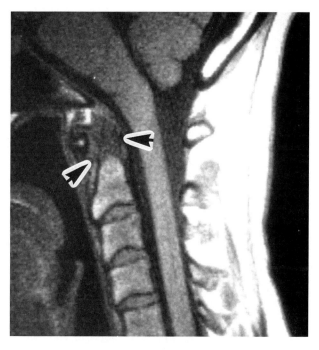

Fig. 10-62 Rheumatoid arthritis with cervical spine involvement shown by sagittal T1 MRI with peridental pannus *(arrows),* ligamentous thickening, loss of supradental fat, and dens erosions. (From Bundschuh C, et al: *AJNR* 9:565, 1988.)

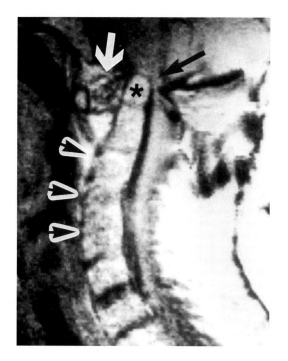

Fig. 10-63 Rheumatoid arthritis with cervical spine involvement shown by sagittal T1 MRI including multisegmental fusions *(arrowheads)* and marked pannus formation *(white arrow)* between the dens and anterior C1 arch preventing reduction of the anterior atlantoaxial dislocation. There is dens impression *(asterisk)* on the ventral cervicomedullary junction *(long black arrow).* (From Bundschuh C, et al: *AJNR* 9:565, 1988.)

immobilization[1,8,27] (Fig. 10-63).

Thoracic and lumbar involvement may be manifested as scoliosis, compression fractures, spondylitis with apophyseal erosion, osteoporosis due to disuse or steroids, ankylosis, and vertebral growth disturbance.[21] Sacroiliac involvement is often asymptomatic and without sclerosis, which often differentiates it from ankylosing spondylitis. Ankylosing spondylitis is characterized by symmetrical sacroiliac disease with sclerosis, and there may often be involvement of the lumbar, thoracic, and, less often, the cervical spine with synovial and ligamentous inflammation. There is a tendency for ankylosis with paraspinal ossification. The disease is symptomatic in about 10% of patients younger than 15 years of age. The diagnosis is made with plain films, bone scan, and a positive HLA-B27 antigen.

Treatment of spinal involvement in childhood arthritis may include observation, bracing, a cervical collar, or, rarely, surgery. Posterior cervical fusion may be necessary for atlantoaxial subluxation or for unstable mobile segments between fused levels. Occasionally the major radiological differential diagnosis in childhood arthritic involvement of the spine with extensive calcification or ossification is that of fibrodysplasia ossificans progressiva.[29]

REFERENCES
Inflammatory processes of the spine and spinal neuraxis

1. Aisen AM, Maetel W, Ellis JH, et al: Cervical spine involvement in rheumatoid arthritis: MR imaging, *Radiology* 165:159, 1987.
2. Angtuaco E, McConnell J, Chadduck W, et al: MR imaging of spinal epidural sepsis, *AJNR* 8:879, 1987.

3. Awerbuch G, Feinberg W, Ferry P, et al: Acute postviral myelitis with MR imaging, *Pediatr Neurol* 3:367, 1987.
4. Barkovich A: *Pediatric neuroimaging,* New York, 1990, Raven.
5. Bertino R, Porter B, Stimac G, et al: Imaging spinal osteomyelitis and epidural abscess with short T1 inversion recovery (STIR), *AJNR* 9:563, 1988.
6. Bradford D, Hensinger R, editors: *The pediatric spine,* New York, 1985, Thieme.
7. Brown T, Wilkinson RH: Chronic recurrent multifocal osteomyelitis, *Radiology* 166:493, 1988.
8. Bundschuh C, Modic MT, Kearney F, et al: Rheumatoid arthritis of the cervical spine: surface-coil MR imaging, *AJR* 151:181, 1988.
9. Chang K, Han M, Choi Y, et al: Tuberculous arachnoiditis of the spine: myelography, CT, and MR imaging, *AJNR* 10:1255, 1989.
10. Chang K, Han M, Roh J, et al: Gd-DTPA–enhanced MR imaging in patients with meningitis, *AJNR* 11:69, 1990.
11. Cheek W, Laurent J: Spinal infections. In McLaurin R, Schut L, Venes J, et al: editors: *Pediatric neurosurgery,* ed 2, 1989, WB Saunders.
12. de Roos A, van Persijn van Meerten EL, et al: MRI of tuberculous spondylitis, *AJR* 146:79, 1986.
13. Donovan Post M, Quencer R, Montalvo B, et al: Spinal infection: MR imaging and operative ultrasound, *Radiology* 169:765, 1988.
14. Edwards M, Harris T: Miscellaneous disorders of the spine. In Cohen M, Edwards M, editors: *MR imaging of children,* Philadelphia, 1990, BC Decker.
15. Forster A, Pothmann R, Winter K, et al: Magnetic resonance imaging in nonspecific discitis, *Pediatr Radiol* 17:162, 1987.
16. Golimbu C, Firooznia H, Rafii M: CT of osteomyelitis of the spine, *AJR* 142:159, 1984.
17. Haney P, Yale-Loehr A, Nussbaum A, et al: Imaging of infants and children with AIDS, *AJR* 152:1033, 1989.
18. Heller R, Szalay E, Green N, et al: Disc space infection in children: MR imaging, *Radiol Clin North Am* 26:207, 1988.
19. Hoffer FA, Strand RD, Gebhardt M: Percutaneous biopsy of pyogenic infection of the spine in children, *J Pediatr Orthopaedics* 8:442, 1988.
20. Hsu L, Yan A: Tuberculosis of the spine. In Bradford D, Hensinger R, editors: *The pediatric spine,* New York, 1985, Thieme.
21. Jones E: Childhood arthritis. In Bradford D, Hensinger R, editors: *The pediatric spine,* New York, 1985, Thieme.
22. Larde D, Mathieu D, Frija J, et al: Vertebral osteomyelitis: disk hypodensity on CT, *AJNR* 3:657, 1982.
23. Marks W, Bodensteiner J, Bobele G, et al: Parainflammatory leukoencephalomyelitis: clinical and MR imaging findings, *J Child Neurol* 3:205, 1988.
24. Merine D, Wang H, Kumar AJ, et al: CT myelography and MR imaging of acute transverse myelitis, *J Comput Assist Tomogr* 11:606, 1987.
25. Modic MT, Feiglin DH, Piraino DW, et al: Vertebral osteomyelitis: assessment using MR, *Radiology* 157:157, 1985.
26. Nesbit GM, Miller GM, Baker HL, et al: Spinal cord sarcoidosis: a new finding at MR imaging with Gd-DTPA enhancement, *Radiology* 173:839, 1989.
27. Pettersson H, Larsson EM, Holtas S, et al: MR imaging of the cervical spine in rheumatoid arthritis, *AJNR* 9:573, 1988.
28. Price AC, Allen JH, Eggers FM, et al: Intervertebral disk space infection: CT changes, *Radiology* 149:725, 1983.
29. Resnick D, Niwayama G: *Diagnosis of bone and joint disorders,* ed 2, Philadelphia, 1988, WB Saunders.
30. Ross JS, Masaryk TJ, Modic MT, et al: MR imaging of lumbar arachnoiditis, *AJNR* 8:885, 1987.
31. Sartoris DJ, Moskowitz PS, Kaufman RA, et al: Childhood diskitis: computed tomographic findings, *Radiology* 149:701, 1983.
32. Sharif HS, Clark DC, Aabed MY, et al: Granulomatous spinal infections: MR imaging, *Radiology* 177:101, 1990.
33. Sklar E, Quencer R, Green B, et al: Acquired spinal subarachnoid cysts, *AJNR* 10:1097, 1989.
34. Smith AS, Weinstein M, Mizushima A, et al: MR imaging characteristics of tuberculous spondylitis vs. vertebral osteomyelitis, *AJR* 153:399, 1989.
35. Smith T: Diskitis in children. In Bradford D, Hensinger R, editors: *The pediatric spine,* New York, 1985, Thieme.
36. Swaiman K: *Pediatric neurology,* St Louis, 1989, Mosby–Year Book.
37. Szalay EA, Green NE, Heller RM, et al: Magnetic resonance imaging in the diagnosis of childhood discitis, *J Pediatr Orthop* 7:164, 1987.
38. Sze G, Zimmerman R: MR imaging of infections and inflammatory diseases, *Radiol Clin North Am* 166:241, 1988.
39. Van Lom KJ, Kellerhouse LE, Pathria MN, et al: Infection versus tumor in the spine: criteria for distinction with CT, *Radiology* 166:851, 1988.
40. Weil M: Infections of the nervous system. In Menkes J: *Textbook of child neurology,* Philadelphia, 1985, Lea & Febiger.

Appendix

Neuroradiological Findings in Miscellaneous Syndromes, Disorders, and Dysplasias

Aarskog syndrome Cervical vertebral anomalies, scoliosis, atlantoaxial laxity, thoracic disk calcifications

Aase syndrome Scoliosis, craniofacial dysmorphia

Aase-Smith syndrome Hydrocephalus, Dandy-Walker syndrome, calvarial thickening

Abetalipoproteinemia Acanthocytosis; degenerative disease of the cerebellum, spinal cord, and peripheral nerves; bilateral caudate and putamen atrophy

Achard syndrome Calvarial thickening, brachycephaly, thoracic hypokyphosis

Achondrogenesis I, II Calvarial osteopenia, calvarial bony plaques, absent or poor vertebral ossification, nonossified sacrum, macrocephaly

Acrocraniofacial dysostosis Craniosynostosis, tall lumbar vertebra, spinal canal widening with scalloping

Acrocallosal syndrome Agenesis or hypoplasia of the corpus callosum, hydrocephalus, tentorial hypoplasia, cysts

Acrodermatitis enteropathica Brain atrophy, reversible

Acrodysostosis Optic atrophy, calvarial thickening, hydrocephalus, thoracolumbar vertebral end plate irregularities, thoracic kyphosis, canal narrowing, vertebral hypoplasia, vertebral collapse, scoliosis

Acrogeria Delayed suture closure, wormian bones, craniosynostosis after childhood

Acromegaly and gigantism Pituitary tumor, large sinuses and otomastoids, calvarial thickening, wide atlantoaxial joint, large, scalloped vertebral bodies, thoracic hyperkyphosis, spinal stenosis, cerebral arterial ectasia.

Acromesomelic dysplasia Scaphocephaly, hydrocephalus, low thoracic kyphosis, lumbar hyperlordosis, oval vertebral bodies, anterior vertebral beaking and wedging, lower spinal canal narrowing, platyspondyly, gibbus

Addison's disease Pituitary enlargement (primary) or destruction (secondary), or tumor (panhypopituitarism).

Adducted thumb syndrome Microcephaly, demyelination, atrophy, torticollis

Adenosine deaminase deficiency with severe combined immunodeficiency and chondroosseous dysplasia Recurrent infections, lymphoma, bone-in-bone vertebra, thoracic vertebral beaking, platyspondyly

Agammaglobulinemia, X-linked Recurrent infections, including sinus, otomastoid, and intracranial (for example, abscess)

Aicardi's syndrome Callosal agenesis, gray matter heterotopia, hydrocephalus, Chiari malformation, Dandy-Walker syndrome, porencephaly, holoprosencephaly, lissencephaly, polygyria, microgyria, choroid plexus papilloma, extracerebral fluid collections, microphthalmos, coloboma, optic atrophy, block vertebra, hemivertebra, butterfly vertebra, spina bifida, scoliosis.

Alagille syndrome Arteriohepatic syndrome; hemivertebra, butterfly vertebra, small vertebral bodies, narrow spinal canal, irregular end plates, anterior process of the atlas, fused vertebral bodies, spina bifida occulta

Alkaptonuria Loss of lumbar lordosis, kyphosis, scoliosis, osteopenia; disk narrowing, vacuum, calcification or ossification, protrusion, osteophytes, ligamentous calcification; vertebral fusion

Alport's syndrome Spina bifida, drusen

Aminopterin fetopathy Cranial dysplasia with poor ossification, Wormian bones, cranium bifidum, craniosynostosis

Aminopterin-like syndrome Parietal cranial defects, hydrocephalus, scoliosis, spina bifida

Amniotic band sequence Calvarial defects, hydrocephalus, anencephaly, encephalocele, microcephaly, craniosynostosis, myelomeningocele, facial cleft

Amyloidosis Cerebral amyloid angiopathy, hemorrhage, infarction

Anderson's syndrome Calvarial thinning, petrous hypoplasia, cervical vertebral spinous process pointing, thoracic scoliosis

Angelman's syndrome Happy puppet syndrome; microbrachycephaly, vertical skull base, occipital depression, brain atrophy

Aniridia–Wilms' tumor association Kyphoscoliosis

Anorexia nervosa Reversible ventricular and subarachnoid space dilatation, cerebral involvement more than cerebellar

Antley-Bixler syndrome Craniosynostosis, choanal atresia, tympanomastoid anomalies, sclerotic vertebral end plates

Apert's syndrome Acrocephalosyndactyly; craniosynostosis, hydrocephalus, brain atrophy, callosal agenesis, absent septum pellucidum, petrous temporal anomalies, hydromyelia

Aplasia cutis syndrome Adams-Oliver syndrome; skull defect beneath scalp lesion, wormian bones, anomalous scalp veins, hydrocephalus, atrophy, cerebral malformations, meningocele, dural defects, myelodysplasias

Arthrogryposis Brachycephaly, callosal agenesis, microcephaly, vermian agenesis, porencephaly, hydrocephalus, lissencephaly, micropolygyria, atrophy, gray matter heterotopia, moyamoya, congenital spinal epidural hematoma spinal cord hypoplasia-atrophy

Aspartylglucosaminuria   Microcephaly, calvarial thickening, hypoplastic frontal sinuses, small sella, thoracic kyphosis, scoliosis, vertebral osteochondritic changes, flat, beaked vertebral bodies, spondylolysis/spondylolisthesis, osteopenia, pathological fractures

Asphyxiating thoracic dysplasia   Craniosynostosis, hydrocephalus

Atelosteogenesis   Spondylohumerofemoral hypoplasia; encephalocele, coronal/sagittal vertebral clefts, thoracic vertebral hypoplasia, platyspondyly, scoliosis, cervical segmentation defects with double scoliosis

Azorean disease   Machado-Joseph-Azorean disease; pontine and cerebellar atrophy, basal ganglia and spinal cord atrophy

Baller-Gerold syndrome   Craniosynostosis, vertebral defects, scoliosis, spina bifida occulta

Bannayan-Riley-Ruvalcaba syndrome   Macrocephaly, meningioma

Bardet-Biedl syndrome   Skull defects, microphthalmia

Beals-Hecht syndrome   Congenital contractural arachnodactyly; short neck, vertebral anomalies, kyphoscoliosis

Bean's syndrome   Blue rubber bleb nevus syndrome; CNS hemangioma, calcifications, venous thrombosis, atrophy

Behçet's syndrome   Cerebral venous thrombosis and infarction, pseudotumor cerebri, meningoencephalitis, atlantoaxial subluxation

Bencze's syndrome   Scoliosis

Berk-Tabatznik syndrome   Optic atrophy, cervical kyphosis, hemivertebra, vertebral wedging

Biemond syndrome II   Hydrocephalus

Binder's syndrome   Cervical kyphosis and scoliosis, C1 arch anomalies, os odontoideum, spina bifida, block vertebra

Biotinidase deficiency   Diffuse brain atrophy

Bobble-head doll syndrome   Suprasellar arachnoid cyst, third ventricular cyst, aqueductal stenosis, cystic cavum velum interpositum, anterior third ventricular tumor

Boomerang dysplasia   Absent thoracolumbar vertebral ossification

Börjeson-Forssman-Lehmann syndrome   Microcephaly, brain atrophy, narrow cervical canal, scoliosis, kyphosis, Scheuermann's vertebral changes

Brachyolinia   Scoliosis, platyspondyly, disk narrowing, irregular vertebral end plates, canal narrowing

Branchiogenitoskeletal syndrome   C2-3 fusion

C syndrome   Opitz trigonocephaly, microcephaly

Calcium pyrophosphate dihydrate deposition disease   Cervical myelopathy, spinal and paraspinal crystal deposition with calcification (disk, ligamentous), spinal stenosis, atlantoaxial subluxation

Calvarial doughnut lesions – osteoporosis – dentinogenesis imperfecta   Osteoporosis, calvarial defects, vertebral defects and fractures

Calvarial hyperostosis, familial   Thickened calvaria

Campomelic dysplasia   Macrocephaly, scaphocephaly, CNS anomalies, kyphoscoliosis, cervical vertebral hypoplasia and poor ossification

Cantrell's syndrome   Anencephaly, hydrocephalus

Carbonic anhydrase II deficiency   Marble brain disease; osteopetrosis, basal ganglia and periventricular white matter calcifications

Carnitine deficiency   Encephalopathy with edema

Carpenter's syndrome   Acrocephalopolysyndactyly, craniosynostosis

Cataract – cerebellar atrophy – mental retardation – myopathy syndrome   Cerebellar atrophy

Cat's eye syndrome   Vertebral anomalies

Celiac disease   Cerebral atrophy, reversible

Cephaloskeletal dysplasia   Taybi-Linder syndrome; microcephaly, ventricular and subarachnoid space dilatation, platyspondyly

Cerebrocostomandibular syndrome   Microcephaly, brain defects, brain dysgenesis, vertebral anomalies, hydrocephalus

Cerebrooculofacioskeletal syndrome   Microcephaly, microphthalmia, basal ganglia and white matter calcifications, kyphosis, scoliosis

Ceroid lipofuscinosis (neuronal)   Neural destruction and gliosis with cerebral or cerebellar atrophy

Charcot-Marie-Tooth syndrome   Hereditary demyelinating motor and sensory neuropathy, nerve root enlargement, large intervertebral foramina, scoliosis, lumbar vertebral scalloping

CHARGE association   Coloboma, petrous temporal anomalies, choanal atresia, CNS anomalies

Cheiro-Oral syndrome   Thalamic and brain stem infarction or hematoma

Cherubism   Familial fibrous dysplasia of the mandible, multiloculated mandibular expansion

CHILD syndrome   Unilateral hypoplasia of brain and spinal cord, vertebral defects, scoliosis

Chondroectodermal dysplasia   Ellis – van Creveld syndrome; Dandy-Walker syndrome, heterotopia

Chromosome 1, long arm deletion   Microcephaly, partially fused cervical vertebra

Chromosome 1, partial deletion syndrome   Microcephaly

Chromosome 3, trisomy syndrome   Microcephaly

Chromosome 3, trisomy (3q+) syndrome   Microcephaly, trigonocephaly, hemivertebra

Chromosome 4p syndrome   Wolf syndrome; microcephaly, craniosynostosis, ventricular dilation, persistent cavum septum pellucidum, absent septum pellucidum, intraventricular cyst, microgyria, pachygyria, fused vertebra, bifid vertebra, kyphoscoliosis

Chromosome 4p trisomy (4p+) syndrome   Microcephaly, small sella, scoliosis, square vertebral bodies, kyphoscoliosis, vertebral anomalies

Chromosome 4q syndrome   Microcephaly

Chromosome 5p syndrome   Microcephaly, hemivertebra, scoliosis

Chromosome 7q+ syndrome   Kyphoscoliosis

Chromosome 8 trisomy syndrome   Macrocephaly, callosal agenesis, osteoporosis, vertebral anomalies, kyphoscoliosis, scoliosis, lumbar canal narrowing, spina bifida occulta, bifid vertebral bodies, extralumbar vertebra

Chromosome 9 trisomy syndrome   Microcephaly, cystic brain malformations, vertebral anomalies, kyphoscoliosis, meningocele

Chromosome 9 (p+) trisomy syndrome   Microcephaly, vertebral anomalies, osteoporosis, scoliosis, kyphosis

Chromosome 13 trisomy syndrome   Patau's syndrome; microcephaly, holoprosencephaly, myelomeningocele

Chromosome 18 p syndrome   Kyphoscoliosis

Chromosome 18 q syndrome   Microcephaly, atlantoaxial rotary displacement

Chromosome 18 trisomy syndrome   Thin calvaria, J-shaped sella, callosal agenesis, choroid plexus cyst, kyphoscoliosis, myelomeningocele

Chromosome 20 p trisomy syndrome   Microcephaly, partially fused vertebra, kyphoscoliosis

Chromosome 21 trisomy syndrome   Down's syndrome; Alzheimer's disease, moyamoya, microcephaly, calvarial thinning, delayed suture closure, basal ganglia calcification, cerebellar and brain stem hypoplasia, large sylvian fissures, prominent cavum septae, posterior fossa ependymal cyst, odontoid anomalies, atlantoaxial subluxation, atlantooccipital subluxation, other cervical subluxations, vertebral fusion, cervical vertebral hypoplasia, degenerative cervical spine disease, tall lumbar vertebra, scoliosis

Chromosome 22 trisomy syndrome   Microcephaly

Chromosome X, fragile   Cerebral gigantism, Down's syndrome, neurofibromatosis, ventricular dilation, macrocephaly, pontine and cerebellar vermian hypoplasia, torticollis, kyphoscoliosis

Chromosome X, monosomy syndrome   Parietal calvarial thinning, large pituitary fossa, petroclinoid calcifications, craniosynostosis, scoliosis, vertebral fusion, Scheuermann's changes, osteoporosis, spina bifida, kyphosis

Chromosome XXXXY syndrome   Calvarial thickening, craniosynostosis, square vertebral bodies, scoliosis, kyphosis

Chromosome XXY syndrome   Klinefelter's syndrome; myelodysplasia, aneurysm with subarachnoid hemorrhage, spina bifida occulta, scoliosis

Chronic granulomatous disease of childhood   Neutrophil dysfunction syndrome, chronic and recurrent suppurative infections, mediastinitis extension into vertebrae and spinal canal

Churg-Strauss syndrome   Cerebral hemorrhage, infarction

Cleidocranial dysplasia   Absent or partially absent clavicles, macrocephaly, brachycephaly, large fontanelle and sutures (delayed closure), wormian bones, sinus and tympanomastoid hypoplasia, notched posterior foramen magnum, sphenoid hypoplasia, curved clivus, persistent neurocentral synchondroses, scoliosis, kyphosis, hydrosyringomyelia, posterior thoracic vertebral wedging, lumbar spondylolysis

Clouston's syndrome   Skull thickening

Cloverleaf skull deformity   Kleeblattschädel syndrome; craniosynostosis, hydrocephalus, callosal agenesis, associated with other anomalies or syndromes

Cockayne's syndrome   Microcephaly, intracranial calcifications, hydrocephalus, demyelination, cerebellar and brain stem hypoplasia, small sella, ovoid vertebral bodies with anterior notching, biconcave or flat vertebral bodies, broad vertebral bodies, vertebral scalloping and wedging, thoracic kyphosis, disk calcifications

Coffin-Lowry syndrome   Frontal cranial thickening, anterior superior vertebral body defects, lumbar gibbus, narrow disks, thoracolumbar kyphoscoliosis

Coffin-Siris syndrome   Callosal agenesis, microcephaly, hindbrain dysgenesis, medulloblastoma, Dandy-Walker syndrome, disk narrowing, vertebral fusion, supernumerary vertebra and ribs, scoliosis

Cohen's syndrome   Microcephaly, petrous temporal anomalies, lumbar lordosis, thoracic scoliosis

Cowden's syndrome   Macrocephaly, neurofibroma, meningioma

Craniodiaphyseal dysplasia   Progressive craniofacial sclerosis, skull base foraminal obliteration, sinus obliteration, hydrocephalus, vertebral neural arch sclerosis, neural compression, vascular occlusion

Cranioectodermal dysplasia   Macrocephaly, osteoporosis, biconvex infantile vertebral bodies, narrow lumbar canal

Craniofrontonasal dysplasia   Craniosynostosis, scoliosis

Craniosynostosis–radial/fibular aplasia–cleft lip/palate syndrome   Craniosynostosis, vertebral anomalies

Craniotelencephalic dysplasia   Craniosynostosis, cerebral dysgenesis, agyria, microgyria, gray matter heterotopia, hydrocephalus, callosal agenesis, optic hypoplasia, lobar holoprosencephaly, microphthalmus

Cronkhite-Canada syndrome   Macrocephaly

Crouzon's syndrome   Craniofacial dysostosis, craniofacial dysmorphia, craniosynostosis, hydrocephalus, craniocervical junction anomalies, basilar impression

Currarino's triad   Sacral anomalies with hypoplasia, presacral meningocele, teratoma, neurenteric cyst, dysraphic myelodysplasias, anorectal malformations

Cushing's syndrome   Pituitary microadenoma or macroadenoma, neuroblastoma, craniopharyngioma, vertebral fractures and osteoporosis, epidural lipomatosis with dural sac stenosis, cerebral and cerebellar atrophy

Cutis laxa   Osteoporosis with vertebral fractures

Cutis verticis gyrata   Microcephaly, cerebellar hypoplasia, cerebral hypoplasia, ventricular dilation, hydranencephaly, optic atrophy

Cystic fibrosis   Pseudotumor cerebri, brain abscess, nasosinus polyps, neuroblastoma, retinoblastoma, kyphosis, scoliosis, spinal intradural hematoma

Cystinosis   Lysosomal cystine accumulation, hydrocephalus, brain atrophy

Degos' syndrome   Intracranial arterial narrowing and ectasia (beading), subarachnoid hemorrhage

Dejerine-Sottas syndrome Hypertrophic neuropathy; thickened nerve roots, vertebral anomalies, vertebral scalloping, canal widening, pedicle anomalies and erosion

de Lange's syndrome Microbrachycephaly, ventricular dilatation, optic atrophy, coloboma, choanal atresia

de Morsier syndrome Septooptic dysplasia; pituitary dwarfism, agenesis septum pellucidum, primitive optic ventricle, optic chiasm hypoplasia, optic nerve hypoplasia, agenesis corpus callosum, infundibular hyperplasia, brain atrophy, sphenoidal encephalocele

Deprivation dwarfism Brain atrophy before treatment and reversible, macrocephaly with wide sutures during treatment

De Sanctis-Cacchione syndrome Microcephaly, atrophy, secondary craniosynostosis

Diabetes insipidus Absence of posterior pituitary bright spot with or without hypothalamic tumor

Diabetes mellitus Cerebral edema associated with ketoacidosis, intracranial hemorrhage, cerebral infarction, atrophy

Diabetic mother, infant of Holoprosencephaly, neural tube defects, microcephaly, hydrocephalus, intracranial hemorrhage, absence of the pituitary, caudal regression syndrome, hemivertebra, spina bifida, meningocele

Diamond-Blackfan syndrome Klippel-Feil syndrome

Diaphyseal dysplasia Camurati-Engelmann disease; craniofacial and skull base sclerosis, posterior cervical vertebral sclerosis, neural and vascular foraminal constriction, hydrocephalus, hydrosyringomyelia

DiGeorge syndrome Brain abscess, glioma, vertebral anomalies

Distal osteosclerosis Calvarial hyperostosis, skull base sclerosis, vertebral pedicle sclerosis

Distal arthrogryposis syndrome Mild scoliosis

Distichiasis-lymphedema syndrome Epidermoid cyst, kyphoscoliosis, spina bifida

Dolichospondylic dysplasia Tall vertebral bodies

Door's syndrome Spinal anomalies

DR syndrome Duane/radial syndrome; Klippel-Feil anomaly, meningocele, syringomyelia

Dubowitz syndrome Microcephaly, neuroblastoma

Duchenne's muscular dystrophy Macrocephaly, scoliosis, kyphosis, muscle replacement by fat

Dyggve-Melchior-Clausen dysplasia Smith-McCort syndrome; microcephaly, dens hypoplasia, atlantoaxial subluxation, scoliosis, thoracic kyphosis, platyspondyly, anterior vertebral body beaking, double vertebral body hump with notched end plates, posterior vertebral scalloping, elongated lamina

Dyke-Davidoff-Masson syndrome Cerebral hemiatrophy, ipsilateral cranial thickening and sinus hyperpneumatization, unilateral ventricular dilatation, ipsilateral midline shift

Dyschondrosteosis Leri-Weill disease; lumbar spinal stenosis

Dyskeratosis congenita Intracranial calcifications

Dysosteosclerosis Cranial vault and skull base sclerosis, mastoid sclerosis, sinus hypoplasia, neural and vascular foraminal constriction, punctate vertebral body sclerosis, progressive platyspondyly

Dyssegmental dysplasia Encephalocele, hydrocephalus, Dandy-Walker syndrome, cerebellar hypoplasia, coronal vertebral clefts, oversized vertebral bodies, sagittal clefting, cervical spinal underossification, anisospondyly with severe segmental defects including absent, oversized, and clefted vertebral bodies

Eagle syndrome Ossified stylohyoid ligamentous compression of the carotid arteries with pain

Early amnion rupture sequence Scoliosis

Ectodactyly–ectodermal dysplasia–clefting syndrome Microcephaly, scoliosis, cervical vertebral anomaly

Ehlers-Danlos syndrome Intracranial aneurysm with or without hemorrhage, vascular malformation, dilated fourth and lateral ventricles, dilated supracerebellar cisterns, delayed calvarial ossification, scoliosis, kyphosis, thoracic lordosis, platyspondyly, disk herniation

Empty sella syndrome Subarachnoid space extension into enlarged sella with or without compression or atrophy of the pituitary gland; idiopathic, familial, postsurgery, postradiation, secondary to hydrocephalus, necrosis, or tumor; intrasellar chiasmatic herniation

Encephalocraniocutaneous lipomatosis Fishman's syndrome; neurocutaneous syndrome with scalp and neck lipomas, intracranial and intraspinal lipomas, leptomeningeal lipogranulomatosis, ipsilateral cerebral atrophy, porencephaly, calcifications, vascular malformations

Enchondromatosis I to VII *Ollier's disease:* multiple enchondromata, malignant transformation to chondrosarcoma (parasellar 30%), astrocytoma, rare scoliosis; *Maffucci's syndrome:* additional multiple cutaneous hemangiomata; metachondromatosis; spondyloenchondrodysplasia with generalized severe platyspondyly; irregular vertebral dysplasia; mild platyspondyly; vertebral anomalies (hemivertebra) with end plate irregularities

Endosteal hyperostosis *Van Buchem type:* cranial vault and skull base sclerosis with neural and vascular foraminal involvement, empty sella, hydrocephalus, vertebral sclerosis, aneurysmal bone cyst, cord compression; *Worth type:* cranial sclerosis with foraminal involvement, vertebral sclerosis, small posterior fossa and foramen magnum

Epidermal nevus syndrome Astrocytoma, glioma, leptomeningeal hemangioma, skull asymmetry, brain atrophy, porencephaly, hydrocephalus, aneurysm, white matter disease, calcifications, gray matter heterotopias, lateral ventricular coarctation, kyphoscoliosis, cord compression

Escobar's syndrome Bifid spinous processes, cervical vertebral fusions

Ethanalaminosis Hydrocephalus

Exostoses, multiple cartilaginous Osteochondromatosis;

malignant transformation, usually chondrosarcoma, spine or skull base involvement

Fabry's disease Angiokeratoma corporis diffusum universalis; glycolipid metabolic disorder, cerebrovascular disease, hemorrhage, infarction

Facioauriculoradial dysplasia Vertebral fusion

Fahr's disease Ferrocalcinosis; vascular and perivascular calcifications (basal ganglia, periventricular white matter, cerebellar dentate)

Fanconi's anemia Microcephaly, moyamoya, Klippel-Feil anomaly

Femoral-facial syndrome Vertebral anomalies including absent vertebra, hemivertebra, sacralization, scoliosis, sacral dysplasia

Fetal alcohol syndrome Microcephaly, microphthalmia, optic hypoplasia-atrophy, choanal stenosis, migrational anomalies, hydrocephalus, anencephaly, porencephaly, callosal agenesis, Dandy-Walker syndrome, medulloblastoma, neuroblastoma, ganglioneuroblastoma, sacrococcygeal teratoma, scoliosis, hemivertebra, Klippel-Feil anomaly, myelomeningocele, lumbosacral lipoma

Fetal cytomegalovirus infection Chorioretinitis, optic atrophy, calcifications, atrophy, migrational anomalies, germinal matrix cysts, ventricular dilation, periventricular inflammation

Fetal herpes simplex infection Microcephaly, microphthalmia, chorioretinitis, calcifications, atrophy

Fetal hydantoin syndrome Microcephaly, anencephaly, myelomeningocele, melanotic neuroectodermal tumor, neuroblastoma, ganglioneuroblastoma

Fetal isotretinoin syndrome Hydrocephalus, fourth ventricular cyst, holoprosencephaly, cerebral dysgenesis, cerebellar hypoplasia (vermian agenesis), agyria, heterotopia, calcifications, microphthalmia

Fetal rubella syndrome Microphthalmia, white matter disease, white matter and basal ganglia calcifications, germinal matrix cyst, craniosynostosis, aqueductal stenosis, myelomeningocele

Fetal toxoplasmosis infection Hydrocephalus, microcephaly, chorioretinopathy, cerebritis, encephalomalacia, porencephaly, aqueductal stenosis, hydranencephaly, calcifications (basal ganglia and periventricular white matter), atrophy, microphthalmia

Fetal trimethadione syndrome Microcephaly, brachycephaly, myelomeningocele, scoliosis

Fetal valproate syndrome Meningocele, myelomeningocele

Fetal varicella syndrome Optic atrophy, microcephaly, chorioretinitis, microphthalmia, hydrocephalus, atrophy, cerebral hypoplasia, basal ganglia and brain stem calcifications, scoliosis, lacunar skull

Fetal warfarin effects Stippled vertebral epiphyses, scoliosis

FG syndrome Opitz-Kaveggia syndrome; megalencephaly, heterotopias, pachygyria, cortical dysgenesis, agenesis of the corpus callosum, spinal anomalies, lumbar hyperlordosis

Fibrochondrogenesis Cranial osteopenia, platyspondyly, posterior vertebral hypoplasia, sagittal vertebral cleft

Fibrodysplasia ossificans progressiva Fibrous dysplasia with progressive ossification, small vertebral bodies, large pedicles, vertebral fusions (arches then bodies), spinal canal narrowing

Fibrous dysplasia Skull base hyperostosis, cranial calvarial osteolysis, orbitosphenoid sclerosis, bony sinus obliteration, osseous sarcoma, vascular malformations, scoliosis, lordosis, cord compression

Filippi syndrome Microcephaly

Fluorosis Ground-glass calvaria, thick, dense skull, wide vertebral bodies with dense end plates, thick disks, vertebral sclerosis, ligamentous calcifications, vertebral osteophytes, thoracic kyphosis, cord compression

Flynn-Aird syndrome Kyphoscoliosis

Foster Kennedy syndrome Optic neuritis-atrophy, contralateral papilledema, ipsilateral frontoorbital tumor

Fountain syndrome Cochlear dysplasia, brain atrophy

Fraser's syndrome Cryptophthalmos-syndactyly syndrome; tympanomastoid anomalies, coloboma, microcephaly, ocular anomalies, encephalocele

Freeman-Sheldon syndrome Craniocarpotarsal dysplasia; microcephaly, brachycephaly, dolichocephaly, tall, narrow vertebral bodies, flat vertebrae, kyphosis, kyphoscoliosis, spina bifida occulta

Friedreich's ataxia Progressive spinocerebellar degeneration, cerebellar and cord atrophy, kyphoscoliosis

Frontofacionasal dysplasia Cranium bifidum, encephalocele, frontal lipoma, microphthalmia, coloboma

Frontometaphyseal dysplasia Large foramen magnum and cervical canal, anterior dens, cervical vertebral fusion, scoliosis, wide lumbar canal

Fryns syndrome CNS anomalies

Fucosidosis Disorder of fucosyl metabolism; cranial thickening, craniosynostosis, sinus hypoplasia, odontoid hypoplasia, cervical platyspondyly, thoracolumbar anterior vertebral beaking, thoracolumbar kyphosis, L5 vertebral hypoplasia, vacuum disk, sacral hypoplasia with square vertebrae, coccygeal hypoplasia, lumbar hyperlordosis

Fukuyama-type muscular dystrophy Cerebral dysgenesis, cerebral and cerebellar micropolygyria, leptomeningeal fibroglial proliferation, hydrocephalus

G syndrome Opitz-Frias syndrome: agenesis of the corpus callosum, wide sutures

Galactosemia Brain edema in neonate, brain atrophy in childhood

Gangliosidosis GM_1: sphingolipidosis, Norman-Landing disease, brain atrophy, white matter degeneration, cranial sclerosis, gibbus, vertebral beaking, vertebral hypoplasia, thoracic kyphoscoliosis; GM_2: Tay-Sachs disease; Sandhoff disease; macrocephaly, cerebral cortical thickening

Gapo's syndrome Optic atrophy, intracranial venous occlusion with dilated scalp veins

Garcin's syndrome   Hemibasis syndrome; skull base tumor with multiple cranial nerve palsies

Gardner's syndrome   Scoliosis

Gaucher's disease   Cerebroside lipidosis; bone infarction with pathological fracture and vertebral collapse

Geroderma osteodysplastica hereditaria   Walt Disney dwarfism; platyspondyly, biconcave bodies, bone-in-bone appearance, scoliosis

Gilles de la Tourette's syndrome   Porencephaly, basal ganglia abnormality

Glenoid hypoplasia   Spina bifida, hemivertebra

Glycogen storage disease type I   von Gierke's disease; osteoporosis, pathological fracture; brain necrosis and atrophy (hypoglycemia)

Golden-Lakim syndrome   Defective laminar ossification, kyphoscoliosis

Goldenhar's syndrome   Facioauriculovertebral dysplasia; coloboma, tympanomastoid anomalies, occipital encephalocele, callosal/pericallosal lipoma, dermoid, falx calcification, encephalocele, hydrocephalus, aqueductal stenosis, callosal agenesis, vermian agenesis, porencephaly, cerebral hypoplasia, cranium bifidum, microcephaly, hemivertebra, block vertebra, supernumerary vertebra, spina bifida, occipitalization of the atlas

Goltz syndrome   Coloboma, microphthalmia, anophthalmia, microcephaly, scoliosis, vertebral segmentation anomalies

Goodman camptodactyly syndrome A and B   Scoliosis

Goodman syndrome   Acrocephalopolysyndactyly; craniosynostosis

Gordon's syndrome   Spinal stenosis, narrow disks

Gorlin's syndrome   Cervical or thoracic vertebral fusion, scoliosis

Gorlin-Chaudhry-Moss syndrome   Craniosynostosis

Gradenigo's syndrome   Petrositis, mastoiditis, bone destruction, dural collection, cerebritis, thrombophlebitis

Grant's syndrome   Wormian bones, brachycephaly

Greig's cephalopolysyndactyly syndrome   Macrocephaly

Grisel's syndrome   Torticollis and atlantoaxial subluxation with pharyngitis

Guillain-Barré syndrome   Acute inflammatory demyelinating polyradiculoneuropathy; edematous, exudative, or fibrous thickening of nerves and roots

Hajdu-Cheney syndrome   Arthrodentoosteodysplasia; tympanomastoid anomalies, optic atrophy, basilar impression, wormian bones, osteopenia, kyphosis, tall lumbar vertebra, disk narrowing, Schmorl's nodes, vertebral collapse, biconcave vertebra

Hallermann-Streiff syndrome   Oculomandibulofacial syndrome; microcephaly, falx calcification, osteopenia, vertebral anomalies, scoliosis, lordosis, platyspondyly, spina bifida

Hemihypertrophy   Cerebellar hemangioblastoma, cerebral aneurysm, hemangioma, arteriovenous malformation

Hemochromatosis   Primary or secondary, disk mineralization, osteoporosis, vertebral collapse, marrow iron deposition, pituitary iron deposition

Hemolytic-uremic syndrome   Disseminated intravascular coagulation and microangiopathy with hemolytic anemia and thrombocytopenia plus microthrombi; cerebral infarction, hemorrhage

Hemophilia   Intracranial hemorrhage, intraspinal hemorrhage, increased atlantoaxial ligamentous laxity, cystic changes, and end plate irregularities in vertebral bodies of cervical spine

Hemorrhagic shock–encephalopathy syndrome   Cerebral edema, infarctions

Henoch-Schönlein syndrome   Allergic necrotizing arteritis, intracranial infarction, hemorrhage

Hepatic fibrosis–renal cystic disease   Intracranial hemorrhage (aneurysm, hemangioma)

Hereditary hemihypotrophy-hemiparesis-hemiathetosis syndrome   Right cerebral atrophy or hypoplasia

Herrmann-Opitz syndrome   Acrocephalosyndactyly; craniosynostosis

Hirschsprung's disease   Microcephaly, macrocephaly, neuroblastoma, ganglioneuroblastoma

Holt-Oram syndrome   Cardiac-limb syndrome; vertebral anomalies, hemivertebra, vertebral fusion, scoliosis

Homocystinuria   Optic atrophy, microcephaly, dural calcification, calvarial thickening, cerebral infarction, osteopenia, vertebral collapse, platyspondyly, scoliosis, kyphosis

Hughes-Stovin syndrome   Jugular venous or dural sinus thrombosis

Humerospinal dysostosis   Lumbar hyperlordosis, coronal cleft vertebra

Hydrolethalus syndrome   Occipitoschisis, hydrocephalus, cerebral dysgenesis including midline defects, migration anomalies, brain stem malformation, hypothalamic hamartoma, pituitary aplasia, Dandy-Walker syndrome

Hydrops calcification—moth-eaten skeletal dysplasia   Cranial osteopenia, platyspondyly with multiple ossification centers

Hyperammonemic disorders   Propionic acidemia, methylmalonic acidemia, isovaleric acidemia, multiple carboxylase deficiency, glutaric acidemia II, betaketothiolase deficiency, chronic liver disease, drug-induced, Reye's syndrome, hepatoxicity, primary systemic carnitine deficiency; hyperammonemia-hyperornithinemia-homocitrullinemia syndrome: brain edema, atrophy, delayed myelination or hypomyelination

Hyperimmunoglobulinemia E syndrome   Chronic sinus and tympanomastoid infection, craniosynostosis, osteoporosis with fractures

Hyperinsulinism   Beckwith-Wiedemann syndrome; CNS injury, edema, atrophy

Hyperostosis generalisata with striations   Cranial base sclerosis

Hyperparathyroidism   *Primary:* calvarial osteopenia, basilar invagination, biconcave vertebral bodies, kyphosis, scoliosis, pathological fractures; *Secondary:* discovertebral joint bone resorption, vertebral Brown tumor, sellar/parasellar Brown tumor, spinal osteosclerosis, cerebral calcifications

Hyperphosphatasemia Cranial thickening, platyspondyly, kyphoscoliosis, biconcave vertebral bodies, large disks

Hypertelorism, microtia, facial clefting syndrome Microcephaly, vertebral anomaly

Hyperthermia-induced spectrum Myelomeningocele

Hyperthyroidism Craniosynostosis, osteoporosis, fractures, cervical osteophytes, cervical kyphosis, ophthalmopathy with extraocular muscle thickening, optic nerve swelling

Hypochondrogenesis Ossified ovoid or flat vertebral bodies

Hypochondroplasia Macrocephaly, foramen magnum narrowing, delayed fontanelle closure, scoliosis, lordosis, narrow lumbar canal, posterior vertebral scalloping, platyspondyly, posterior sacral tilt, exaggerated lumbar lordosis

Hypomelanosis of Ito Incontinentia pigmenti achromians; brain atrophy, gray matter heterotopias, gliosis, white matter degeneration, optic atrophy, macrocephaly, microcephaly, microphthalmia, coloboma, porencephaly, kyphosis, scoliosis

Hypoparathyroidism Idiopathic, infant of diabetic mother, DiGeorge syndrome; calvarial thickening, brain edema (pseudotumor cerebri), calcifications (basal ganglia, cerebellar, choroid plexus, vascular/perivascular, white matter), vertebral body hyperdense bands

Hypophosphatasia Poor cranial and vertebral ossification with multiple fractures and wide sutures followed by craniosynostosis, thoracolumbar vertebral wedging

Hypothyroidism, juvenile Wormian bones, wide sutures, brachycephaly, large fontanelles, short sclerotic skull base, large sella, delayed closure of basal synchondroses, sinus and tympanomastoid hypoplasia, craniosynostosis with replacement therapy; pituitary microadenoma, hyperplasia, or macroadenoma; cerebral atrophy, flat hypoplastic vertebral bodies, wide disks, gibbus, thoracolumbar kyphosis

Hypothyroidism, infant Partially absent vertebral body, hemivertebra

Immunodeficiency disorders Immune deficiency and short-limb dwarfism with platyspondyly; severe combined immunodeficiency and adenosine deaminase deficiency: platyspondyly, bone-in-bone vertebral bodies, beaked vertebral bodies

Incontinentia pigmenti Bloch-Sulzberger syndrome; optic atrophy, glioma, microphthalmia, recurrent encephalitis, meningitis, microcephaly, edema, atrophy, hydrocephalus, porencephaly, vertebral anomalies

Infantile multisystem inflammatory disease Prieur-Griscelli syndrome; macrocephaly, wormian bones, thick skull base, dilated ventricles and extracerebral spaces, osteoporosis, vertebral fractures, tall, narrow vertebra, gibbus with thoracolumbar kyphosis

Iron deficiency anemia Cranial diploic thickening, cranial and vertebral marrow hyperplasia

Jackson-Weiss syndrome Craniosynostosis

Jaffe-Campanacci syndrome Nonossifying fibromas, kyphoscoliosis

Jarcho-Levin syndrome Spondylothoracic dysostosis, hemivertebrae, widely bifid arches, absent vertebral bodies, cerebral polygyria

Johanson-Blizzard syndrome Microcephaly

Joubert syndrome Aplasia-hypoplasia cerebellar vermis with retrocerebellar fluid space, unsegmented tectum, occipital meningocele or encephalocele, microcephaly, coloboma, agenesis corpus callosum, sacral dermoid sinus

Juberg-Hayward syndrome Orocraniodigital syndrome; microcephaly, absent sella

Jugular foramen syndrome Cranial nerve palsies 9-12 due to skull base trauma, tumor, vascular occlusion, infection, etc

Kabuki make-up syndrome Niikawa-Kuroki syndrome; butterfly vertebra, sagitally cleft vertebra, scoliosis, narrow disk spaces

Kallmann's syndrome Microcephaly, hypoplasia or absent olfactory sulcus, brain calcifications, suprasellar cyst, choanal atresia

Kartagener's syndrome Situs inversus, absent or hypoplastic sinuses, nasal polyps, otitis

Kasabach-Merritt syndrome Hemangiomaas with thrombocytopenia, rare consumptive coagulopathy

Kaufman-McKusick syndrome Pituitary dysplasia, vertebral anomalies

Kawasaki syndrome Juvenile periarteritis nodosa; acute multisystem vasculitis; cerebral thromboses, stenoses, aneurysms, calcifications, infarction

KBG syndrome Vertebral anomalies

Kearns-Sayre syndrome Oculocraniosomatic syndrome; mitochondrial and muscle fiber abnormalities with white matter degeneration; microcephaly, calcifications (basal ganglia, thalami, cerebral), cerebellar hypoplasia, white matter abnormalities

Klippel-Trenaunay-Weber syndrome Angioosteohypertrophy syndrome; hemihypertrophy with visceral and peripheral vascular anomalies, spinal cord vascular malformations, Sturge-Weber syndrome, aplasia cervical internal carotid artery, circle of Willis anomalies, cerebral and cerebellar hemihypertrophy, scoliosis, kyphosis

Klüver-Bucy syndrome Temporal lobe atrophy from degenerative disease, encephalitis, surgery, epilepsy, hypoglycemia, trauma, hypoxia

Kousseff syndrome Sacral meningocele

Kugelberg-Welander syndrome Proximal spinal muscular atrophy; muscle replacement with fatty infiltration

Kuskokwim syndrome Multiple joint contractures, kyphoscoliosis, hypoplastic atlas or axis, L5 pedicle elongation and spondylolisthesis, flat thoracic vertebral bodies

Kyphomelic dysplasia Mild platyspondyly

Langer-Giedion syndrome Vertebral segmentation defects with scoliosis

Lead intoxication Acute cerebral edema; chronic atrophy, calvarial hyperdensity, and calcifications (cerebral, basal ganglia, vermian)

Lennox-Gastaut syndrome Childhood epileptic encephalopathy; cerebral atrophy

Lenz-Majewski hyperostotic dwarfism Delayed fontanelle closure, progressive craniofacial and vertebral sclerosis

Lenz's microphthalmos syndrome Microphthalmos, anophthalmos, microcephaly, kyphoscoliosis, lordosis

Leopard syndrome Cardiomyopathic lentiginosis; kyphoscoliosis, cervical fusion, spina bifida occulta

Lesch-Nyhan syndrome Uric acid metabolic disorder; microcephaly, brain atrophy

Levy-Hollister syndrome Lacrimoauriculodentodigital syndrome; lacrimal anomalies (absence), salivary gland anomalies (absence)

Lichtenstein syndrome Large foramen magnum, atlantoaxial subluxation, L5 spondylolysis

Lipodystrophy Lipoatrophy; calvarial thickening, falx calcifications, sinus and tympanomastoid overpneumatization, large cisterns and ventricles, dense transverse vertebral body bands, canal narrowing

Lipoid proteinosis Intracranial calcifications (hippocampal)

Lissencephaly syndrome *Type I* (Miller-Diecker syndrome, Norman-Roberts syndrome, isolated): lissencephaly with microcephaly; *Type II* (Walker-Warburg syndrome, cerebrooculomuscular syndrome): lissencephaly with hydrocephalus; Type I and Type II with craniofacial dysmorphia

Lowe's syndrome Oculocerebrorenal syndrome; buphthalmos, calvarial scalloping, ventricular dilatation, white matter abnormalities, basilar impression, occipitalization of the atlas, atlantoaxial subluxation, scoliosis, kyphosis, platyspondyly

Lumbocostovertebral sequence Scoliosis, hemivertebra, anterior meningocele

Maffucci's syndrome Multiple enchondromatoses with hemangiomata, skull base involvement, malignant degeneration to chondrosarcoma (15% to 20%), glioma, astrocytoma, pituitary adenoma, paraganglioma

Man-in-the-barrel syndrome Bilateral border–end zone infarction of temporooccipital and frontoparietal white matter from acute cerebral hypoperfusion with severe hypotension

Mandibuloacral dysplasia Craniomandibular dermatodysostosis; delayed suture closure and wormian bones

Mannosidosis Macrocephaly, calvarial thickening, partial craniosynostosis, communicating hydrocephalus, flat vertebral bodies, anterior thoracolumbar vertebral wedging or beaking, gibbus, osteoporosis

Maple syrup urine disease Acute brain edema in infants, cystic brain degeneration, gliosis, hypomyelination, global brain atrophy without treatment

Marden-Walker syndrome Microcephaly, cerebellar hypoplasia, kyphoscoliosis

Marfanoid hypermobility syndrome Scoliosis

Marinesco-Sjögren syndrome Kyphoscoliosis

Marshall's syndrome Calvarial thickening, dural calcifications, bullet-shaped vertebrae, platyspondyly with irregular end plates

Martsolf's syndrome Microcephaly

Maternal PKU fetal effects Cervical and sacral spinal anomalies

Mayer-Rokitansky-Kuster syndrome Klippel-Feil anomaly, vertebral wedging

McCune-Albright syndrome Precocious puberty, polyostotic fibrous dysplasia, café-au-lait spots, fibrous dysplasia involving cranium, pathological fractures, pituitary enlargement

Meckel's syndrome Gruber's syndrome; dyesencephalia splanchnocystica; microcephaly, anencephaly, occipital encephalocele, hydrocephalus, Chiari II malformation, micropthalmia, anophthalmia

Median cleft face syndrome Frontonasal dysplasia, anterior cranium bifidum, coloboma, microphthalmia, encephalocele, meningocele, callosal dysgenesis or agenesis, lipoma, dermoid, midline ossification, hydrocephalus, holoprosencephaly, choanal atresia

MELAS syndrome Mitochondrial myopathy, encephalopathy, lactic acidosis, calcifications, atrophy, recurring cerebral infarctions

Melnick-Needles osteodysplasty Skull base sclerosis, sinus hypoplasia, tall vertebra, anterior concave thoracic vertebral bodies, narrow lumbar disks, kyphoscoliosis

Melorheostosis Glomus tumors, cord lipoma, monostotic or polyostotic involvement of spine and skull

Membranous lipodystrophy Leukodystrophy, diffuse generalized atrophy, white matter sclerosis (especially frontal), brain atrophy, basal ganglia calcifications

Menkes' syndrome Kinky-hair syndrome; microcephaly, wormian bones, progressive brain atrophy, subdural hematoma/hygromas, multiple cerebral infarction, tortuous carotid-cerebral arteries and supernumerary branches, rounding of the thoracic and lumbar vertebral bodies

Mesomelic dysplasias Robinow type (vertebral anomalies), Maroteaux type (scaphocephaly, hypoplastic vertebrae), Campailla-Martinelli type (vertebral anomalies, scoliosis)

Metachondromatosis Thoracic and lumbar anterior vertebral body processes, irregular end plates

Metaphyseal chondrodysplasias Jansen type (skull base hypoplasia, brachycephaly, sinus hypoplasia, choanal atresia), McKusick type (hypoplastic vertebrae, end plate irregularities, lumbar lordosis, scoliosis, atlantoaxial subluxation)

Metaphyseal chondrodysplasia with exocrine pancreatic insufficiency and cyclic neutropenia Schwachman-Diamond syndrome; central pontine myelinolysis, focal pontine leukencephalopathy

Metaphyseal–sella turcica dysplasia, Rosenberg Thick dorsum sellae, vertebral wedging, vertebral end plate sclerosis, platyspondyly

Mevalonic aciduria Generalized brain atrophy

Minamata disease Cerebral and cerebellar atrophy

Mitral valve insufficiency–deafness–skeletal malformation syndrome Cervical fusion

Mitral valve prolapse syndrome Connective tissue disorder (Marfan's, Ehlers-Danlos), Klippel-Feil anomaly, scoliosis

Mixed sclerosing bone dysplasia Cranial sclerosis

Möbius sequence Early embryonic interruption of the subclavian-vertebral arterial supply, congenital facial diplegia, other cranial neuropathies, brain stem hypoplasia, Klippel-Feil anomaly

Mohr's syndrome Scoliosis

Morgagni-Stewart-Morel syndrome Hyperostosis frontalis interna; frontal calvarial thickening

Morning glory syndrome Optic nerve coloboma, agenesis corpus callosum, sphenoid encephalocele, other midline anomalies

Moulded baby syndrome Scoliosis, torticollis, craniofacial dysmorphia

Mucolipidosis II Leroy I-cell disease; macrocephaly, cranial thickening, beaked vertebral bodies T12-L3, narrow thoracolumbar vertebral bodies, thoracic canal narrowing, disk calcification

Mucolipidosis III PseudoHurler polydystrophy; craniosynostosis, J-shaped sella, vertebral beaking with gibbus upper lumbar region, dens hypoplasia, hydrosyringomyelia

MULIBREY nanism Hydrocephalus

Multiple endocrine neoplasia syndromes Pituitary tumors (adenomas)

Multiple epiphyseal dysplasia Fairbank's disease; vertebral end plate irregularity, anterior vertebral wedging, Schmorl's nodes

Multiple neuroma syndrome Scoliosis

Multiple synostosis syndrome Progressive bony fusions, including vertebral fusion, vertebral anomalies, Scheuermann's disease, auditory ossicular fusion

MURCS association Cervicothoracic vertebral defects (especially C5 to T1), Klippel-Feil anomaly (occasionally)

MYHRE syndrome Calvarial thickening, large, flat vertebral bodies and pedicles

Myotonic dystrophy Muscular atrophy, calvarial thickening, large sinuses

MZ twinning Sacrococcygeal teratoma, sirenomelia, Vater association

Nager's syndrome Acrofacial dysostosis; vertebral anomalies

Nail-patella syndrome Spina bifida, scoliosis

Nelson's syndrome ACTH-secreting pituitary tumor after total adrenalectomy for Cushing's syndrome with adrenal hyperplasia

Nemaline myopathy Kyphoscoliosis, hyperlordosis

Neu-Laxova syndrome Microcephaly, lissencephaly, callosal agenesis, cerebellar hypoplasia, spinal cord hypoplasia, kyphosis

Neurocutaneous melanosis sequence Rokitansky–van Bogaert syndrome; skin and leptomeningeal melanocytic proliferation, hydrocephalus, calcifications, melanoma, syringomyelia

Nevoid basal cell carcinoma syndrome Gorlin-Goltz syndrome; craniofacial keratocysts, fibrosarcomas, ameloblastomas; coloboma, medulloblastoma, meningioma, craniopharyngioma, Sotos' syndrome; scoliosis, kyphoscoliosis, spina bifida occulta, interspinous fusions, disk narrowing, square vertebral bodies, osteoporosis, craniocervical junction anomalies (dens hypoplasia, third occipital condyle), cervical spondylolisthesis, sacral lumbarization; falx and other dural calcification, pial and choroid plexus calcifications, cerebellar atrophy, callosal agenesis, septum pellucidum cyst, hydrocephalus

Niemann-Pick disease Sphingomyelin lipidoses; anterior notched thoracolumbar vertebral bodies; CNS demyelination and gliosis

Noonan's syndrome Microcephaly, macrocephaly, kyphosis, scoliosis, Klippel-Feil anomaly

Occipital horn syndrome Bilateral occipital exostosis, platyspondyly

Oculocerebrocutaneous syndrome Microphthalmia, orbital cyst, coloboma, callosal agenesis, cerebellar hemispheric defect, gray matter heterotopia, cranial defects, vertebral anomalies

Oculodentoosseous dysplasia Microphthalmia, basal ganglia calcifications, cord compression

Oculopalatoskeletal syndrome Spina bifida occulta, lambdoid synostosis

Opsoclonus-myoclonus syndrome CNS infection, hydrocephalus, intracranial tumor, thalamic hemorrhage, toxic encephalopathy, neuroblastoma, ganglioneuroblastoma, ganglioneuroma

Optic atrophy–spastic paraplegia syndrome Degenerative disorder; symmetrical putamen and caudate lesions, optic atrophy

Ornithine-transcarbamylase deficiency Cerebral edema, cerebral white matter and gray matter infarction or necrosis progressing to atrophy with cavitation, intracranial hemorrhage

Orofaciodigital syndromes I, II Hydranencephaly, callosal agenesis, cortical hypoplasia, septum pellucidum cyst, subdural hygroma, microcephaly, cerebellar encephalocele, microgyria, cysts, megalencephaly, polygyria, gray matter heterotopia, hydrocephalus, porencephaly, lipoma, Dandy-Walker syndrome

Osteoarthropathy, familial idiopathic Wide sutures, fontanelles, wormian bones

Osteogeophonic dysplasia Craniofacial dysostosis with fibrous metaphyseal defects; craniosynostosis, lumbar lordosis, platyspondyly, anterior vertebral processes, posterior lumbar vertebral scalloping

Osteomesopyknosis   Vertebral end plate sclerosis

Osteopathia striata with cranial sclerosis   Macrocephaly, calvarial and skull base sclerosis with foraminal involvement, sinus hypoplasia, vertebral sclerosis

Osteopetrosis   Albers-Schönberg disease; cranial vault and skull base thickening with foraminal involvement, sinus hypoplasia, petrous temporal abnormalities, macrocephaly, choanal atresia, basal ganglia calcifications, hydrocephalus, subdural collections, bone-in-bone vertebral bodies, vertebral arch fractures, compressive cervical myelopathy

Osteoporosis, idiopathic juvenile   Vertebral collapse

Osteoporosis-pseudoglioma syndrome   Microphthalmia, microcephaly, wormian bones, craniosynostosis, kyphoscoliosis, osteoporosis, fractures

Otopalatodigital syndrome   Taybi's syndrome; cranial thickening, sinus hypoplasia, delayed fontanelle closure, tympanomastoid hypoplasia, vertebral arch defects, wide thoracolumbar canal, small pedicles

Otospondylomegaepiphyseal dysplasia   Coronal vertebral clefts, large odontoid, platyspondyly, anterior vertebral wedging

Pallister-Hall syndrome   Hypothalamic hamartoblastoma and hypopituitarism, imperforate anus, postaxial polydactyly, microcephaly, narrow cervical vertebra, hemivertebra, and ventricular dilatation

Papillon-Lefèvre syndrome   Hyperkeratosis palmoplantaris and periodontoclasia; dural and choroid calcifications

Parastremmatic dysplasia   Platyspondyly, kyphoscoliosis

Parietal foramina–clavicular hypoplasia syndrome   Congenital parietal defects, macrocephaly, tympanomastoid anomalies

Paroxysmal nocturnal hemoglobinuria   Cerebral venous thrombosis and infarction

Partial trisomy 10q syndrome   Kyphoscoliosis, vertebral anomalies

Patterson syndrome   Psuedoleprechaunism; cranial vault and skull base thickening, odontoid hypoplasia, atlantoaxial subluxation, ovoid thoracolumbar vertebral bodies, kyphoscoliosis, cervical platyspondyly, deformed vertebral bodies with irregular dense end plates

Pena-Shokeir syndrome   Fetal akinesia deformation sequence; hydrocephalus, migrational anomalies, optic nerve hypoplasia, cerebellar hypoplasia, absent septum pellucidum, cavum septum pellucidum, hydranencephaly, absent olfactory nerves, spinal cord dysgenesis, thoracic kyphosis, scoliosis, vertebral segmentation anomalies

Pendred's syndrome   Goiter, Mondini cochlear anomaly

Pfeiffer's syndrome   Acrocephalosyndactyly, craniosynostosis, hydrocephalus, Chiari malformation, petrous temporal bone anomalies

Pick's disease   Dementia, symmetrical localized or lobar atrophy (frontal greater than temporal)

Pleonosteosis   Wide vertebral bodies, cervical posterior neural arch enlargement, narrow L2 and L3 vertebral bodies, cord compression

POEMS syndrome   Sclerotic and/or lytic ringlike cranial and vertebral lesions, ivory vertebrae, calvarial thickening

Poland syndrome   Vertebral anomalies including hemivertebra, scoliosis

Polycystic renal disease   Cerebral aneurysms, hemorrhage

Polyposis syndromes   Brain neoplasia

Popliteal pterygium syndrome   Spina bifida occulta, vertebral anomalies, scoliosis

Porencephaly, familial   Irregular ventriculomegaly (especially frontal) porencephaly

Porphyrias   Dural and calvarial calcification

Potter sequence   Oligohydramnios tetrad of craniofacial dysmorphia, limb anomalies, pulmonary hypoplasia, renal agenesis; microcephaly, migrational anomalies, cerebellar heterotopia

Prader-Willi syndrome   Microcephaly, wormian bones, wide sutures, small sella, ventricular dilatation, scoliosis, osteoporosis

Progeria   Calvarial thinning and irregular ossification, delayed suture and fontanelle closure, infantile ovoid vertebral bodies

Progressive familial encephalopathy   Microcephaly, basal ganglia calcifications

Progressive pseudorheumatoid chondrodysplasia   Platyspondyly, anterior end plate defects, kyphoscoliosis

Proteus syndrome   Congenital neurocutaneous hamartomatous disorder; craniofacial dysmorphia, macrocephaly, microphthalmos, scoliosis, kyphosis, cranial hyperostosis, tall and wide irregular vertebral bodies, disk abnormalities, megaspondylodysplasia, kyphoscoliosis

Prune belly syndrome   Microcephaly, myelomeningocele, scoliosis, torticollis

Pseudoachondroplasia   Lumbar hyperlordosis, scoliosis, kyphosis, platyspondyly, vertebral end plate grooves, biconcave vertebral bodies, atlantoaxial subluxation, anterior vertebral beaking, short pedicles

Pseudodiastrophic dysplasia   Platyspondyly, ovoid vertebral bodies, scoliosis

Pseudohypoparathyroidism and pseudopseudohypoparathyroidism (type I)   Calvarial thickening, intracranial calcifications (cerebral and basal ganglia); progressive posterior longitudinal ligamentous ossification with cord compression; anterior foramen magnum tubercle with cord compression

Pseudotumor cerebri syndrome   Intracranial hypertension (no evidence of mass or hydrocephalus), dural sinus thrombosis, sinus or tympanomastoid inflammatory disease, trauma, endocrine syndromes, metabolic disorders, allergic or toxic etiologies, cystic fibrosis, familial, systemic lupus erythematosis, empty sella syndrome, small ventricles and subarachnoid spaces, thickened optic nerves, periventricular edema

Pseudoxanthoma elasticum syndrome Grönblad-Strandberg syndrome; cerebrovascular malformations, vertebral dysplasia

Pterygium syndromes Associated with other syndromes; microcephaly, craniofacial dysmorphia, scoliosis, lordosis, vertebral anomalies

Pyknodysostosis Wormian bones, delayed fontanelle and suture closure, sinus and tympanomastoid hypoplasia, craniosynostosis, vertebral arch fractures, spondylolisthesis, scoliosis

Pyruvate dehydrogenase complex deficiency Lactic acidosis, acute brain edema, gross brain atrophy

Radial aplasia–thrombocytopenia syndrome Spina bifida

Radial ray aplasia–renal anomalies Tympanomastoid anomalies

Radial ray hypoplasia syndrome Choanal stenosis

Red-eyed shunt syndrome Carotid-cavernous fistula

Reiger's syndrome Coloboma, optic atrophy, scoliosis, kyphosis, hydrocephalus, syringomyelia, empty sella

Renal, genital, and ear anomalies Tympanomastoid anomalies

Rendu-Osler-Weber syndrome Hereditary hemorrhagic telangiectasia; CNS telangiectasias, arteriovenous malformations, aneurysms, hemorrhage, infarction

Rett's syndrome White matter degenerative disease, atrophy, scoliosis

Rickets/osteomalacia Kyphoscoliosis, scoliosis, craniosynostosis, basilar impression, wormian bones, abnormal cranial ossification

Rigid spine syndrome Progressive loss of motion of cervical spine, wide interlaminar separation between atlas and axis (alligator sign), scoliosis, loss of adipose tissue

Riley-Day syndrome Familial dysautonomia; subarachnoid hemorrhage, microcephaly, hydrocephalus, kyphoscoliosis

Riley-Smith syndrome Macrocephaly-pseudopapilledema-hemangiomata syndrome; cranial thickening

Robert's syndrome Coloboma, frontal encephalocele, hydrocephalus

Robin sequence Pierre Robin syndrome; associated with other syndromes; occipitoatlantal and atlantoaxial hypermobility with anterior and posterior atlas arch defects

Robinow-Sorauf syndrome Acrocephalosyndactyly, craniosynostosis

Robinow's syndrome Macrocephaly, hemivertebra, vertebral fusions, scoliosis, canal narrowing

Rokitansky sequence Vertebral anomalies

Romberg's syndrome Progressive hemifacial atrophy syndrome; porencephaly, occipital calcifications, parietal high densities on CT

Rothmund-Thomson syndrome Flat, elongated vertebral bodies

Rubinstein-Taybi syndrome Large foramen magnum, large anterior fontanelle, parietal foramina, callosal agenesis, vertebral anomalies, kyphoscoliosis, bifid posterior arch of the atlas

Ruvalcaba syndrome Microcephaly, craniostenosis, spinal osteochondrosis, kyphoscoliosis

Saethre-Chotzen syndrome Acrocephalosyndactyly, craniosynostosis, microcephaly, hydrocephalus

Sakati-Nyhan syndrome Acrocephalopolysyndactyly; craniosynostosis

Sarcoidosis Lytic calvarial defects, granulomatous meningitis and arachnoiditis with masses, hydrocephalus, white matter lesions, orbital masses, optic pathway masses

Scapuloiliac dysostosis Microphthalmia, coloboma, tympanomastoid anomalies, cranium bifidum, rounded vertebral bodies, lumbosacral lordosis

Schinzel-Giedion syndrome Choanal stenosis, short sclerotic skull base, wormian bones, wide sutures and fontanelles, vertebral sclerosis

Schwartz-Jampel syndrome Chondrodystrophic myotonia; kyphosis or kyphoscoliosis, compressive myelopathy, basilar invagination, platyspondyly

Schwarz-Lélek syndrome Macrocephaly, cranial hyperostosis (especially frontal and occipital), obliterated paranasal sinuses

Sclerosteosis Cranial sclerosis with foraminal obliteration, sclerotic vertebral end plates and pedicles

Seckel's syndrome Bird-headed dwarfism; microcephaly, craniosynostosis, kyphoscoliosis

Shapiro's syndrome Agenesis of corpus callosum

Sheehan's syndrome Postpartum pituitary necrosis, empty sella, small sella

Short rib syndrome—Beemer type Same as type II (Majewski); cerebral dysgenesis, arrhinencephaly

Short rib–polydactyly syndromes *Type I* (Saldino-Noonan syndrome): square vertebral bodies, coronal clefts; *Type II* (Majewski): cerebral dysgenesis, arrhinencephaly; *Type III* (Verma-Naumoff): cranial base shortening, short, thin vertebral bodies, irregular vertebral margins, wide disks

Shprintzen-Goldberg syndrome Craniosynostosis, scoliosis

Shy-Drager syndrome Progressive autonomic nervous system failure, hypothalamic and basal ganglia (caudate, putamen) lesions

Sialidosis Sialic acid metabolic disorder; platyspondyly, vertebral beaking, irregular vertebral end plates, calvarial thickening

Sickle cell anemia Major or distal carotid-cerebral arterial occlusion or stenosis, moyamoya, aneurysms, border zone infarction, intracranial hemorrhage, spinal cord infarction, cranial dyploic thickening (myeloid hyperplasia), cranial osteolysis or sclerosis, cranial bone infarcts, spine osteoporosis, depressed vertebral end plates, thoracic hyperkyphosis, lumbar hyperlordosis, persistent thoracic anterior vertebral vascular foramina

Silver-Russell syndrome Vertebral end plate irregularities

Simpson-Golabi-Behmel syndrome Sacral anomaly, coccygeal bony process

Sirenomelia sequence Vitelline arterial steal, absent sacrum and fused lower extremities with other vertebral defects, distinguished from caudal regression syndrome

Sjögren-Larsson syndrome Neurocutaneous syndrome with white matter abnormalities, cerebral cortical thickening, hydrocephalus, basilar impression, kyphosis

Smith-Lemli-Opitz syndrome Microcephaly, hydrocephaly, frontal lobe hypoplasia, callosal dysgenesis, cerebellar and brain stem hypoplasia, pachygyria

Sneddon's syndrome Atypical moyamoya; nonlupus cutaneous and ischemic cerebral lesions

Sotos' syndrome Cerebral gigantism, ventriculomegaly, cavum septum pellucidum and cavum septum velum interpositum, vertebra plana, disk protrusions, kyphosis, kyphoscoliosis, callosal agenesis

Spherocytosis Chronic hemolytic anemia, cerebral infarction, secondary hemochromatosis (marrow iron deposition) secondary to repeated transfusions, calvarial diploic thickening (myeloid hyperplasia), paraspinal extramedullary hematopoiesis

Sponastrime dysplasia Kyphoscoliosis, lumbar lordosis

Spondylocostal dysostosis Block vertebra, hemivertebra, butterfly vertebra, sagittal vertebral clefts, normal skull

Spondyloenchondrodysplasia Enchondromatosis with severe platyspondyly, thoracic kyphosis, lumbar lordosis, irregular end plates

Spondyloepimetaphyseal dysplasias *Irapa type:* platyspondyly, end plate irregularity; *Strudwick type:* platyspondyly, scoliosis, odontoid hypoplasia; *Joint laxity type:* newborn thoracic kyphoscoliosis, platyspondyly, end plate irregularity

Spondylomegaepiphyseal-metaphyseal dysplasia Absent vertebral body ossification

Spondyloperipheral dysplasia Mild platyspondyly, wedge vertebral deformity, biconcave vertebral bodies

Stickler syndrome Scheuermann-like vertebral changes, thoracic kyphosis, anterior vertebral wedging, scoliosis

Stiff-man syndrome Progressive muscle rigidity, spinal column hypertrophic arthropathy, cerebral atrophy

Straight back syndrome Sternospinal cardiac compression; thoracic hypokyphosis

Summitt syndrome Acrocephalosyndactyly, craniosynostosis

Thalassemia Chronic hemolytic anemia; craniofacial dysmorphia with cranial osteoporosis and diploic thickening (myeloid hyperplasia), calvarial lytic lesions, sinus hypoplasia, secondary hemochromatosis (posttransfusion) with iron deposition in marrow and pituitary gland, biconcave vertebral bodies, paraspinal extramedullary hematopoiesis, cord compression

Thanatophoric dysplasia Short narrow skull base with small foramen magnum, large cranial vault, craniosynostosis-cloverleaf deformity, severe platyspondyly, anterior rounded vertebral bodies, anterior vertebral spike, disk widening, canal narrowing, migrational anomalies of the brain

Thanatophoric variants Decreased skull base ossification, platyspondyly

13q syndrome Lumbar spinal agenesis

3-M syndrome Sagitally narrow lumbar vertebral bodies, irregular end plates, spina bifida oculta

Tolosa-Hunt syndrome Painful ophthalmoplegia; granulomatous inflammation in cavernous sinus or superior orbital fissure; rule out tumor or aneurysm; superior orbital venous occlusion with collaterals, obliterated cavernous sinus, cavernous internal carotid arterial narrowing

Treacher Collins' syndrome Mandibulofacial dysostosis; craniofacial dysmorphia, tympanomastoid anomalies, coloboma, microphthalmia, choanal atresia, otic capsule anomalies, vertebral anomalies

Trichodentoosseous syndrome Skull base and tympanomastoid sclerosis, calvarial sclerosis

Trichorhinophalangeal dysplasia *Type I:* scoliosis, lordosis, kyphoscoliosis; *Type II:* microcephaly, cerebral atrophy

Trichorrhexis nodosa syndrome tympanomastoid infection, sinusitis, axial osteosclerosis, kyphosis

Trigonocephaly, familial Metopic craniosynostosis, hemivertebra

Triploidy Hydrocephalus, coloboma, microphthalmia, callosal agenesis, myelomeningocele, holoprosencephaly, Chiari II malformation

Tubular stenosis dysplasia (Kenny-Caffey) Microphthalmia, macrocephaly

Turcot syndrome Glioma-polyposis syndrome; glioblastoma, medulloblastoma, colonic polyposis; reported also in some cases of Gardner's syndrome or familial polyposis

Usher's syndrome Congenital hearing loss and vestibular dysfunction with cerebellar atrophy

Velocardiofacial syndrome Shprintzen syndrome; microcephaly, coloboma, microphthalmia, holoprosencephaly

Vitamin A deficiency Brain edema

Vitamin A intoxication Brain edema, hydrocephalus, cranial osteopenia

Vitamin B₁ deficiency Beriberi; brain edema, extrapyramidal and white matter degeneration, brain atrophy

Vitamin B₁₂ deficiency Atrophy, white matter degeneration, reversible with treatment

Vitamin D intoxication Dural calcifications, dense vertebral end plates, calvarial thickening

von Willebrand's disease Rare intracranial hemorrhage, associated with hereditary hemorrhagic telangiectasia

Waardenburg's syndrome Sensory neural hearing loss with inner ear anomalies, supernumerary vertebral bodies and ribs, spina bifida, scoliosis

Waardenburg's syndrome Acrocephalosyndactyly, craniosynostosis

Walker-Warburg syndrome Hydrocephalus, agyria, retinal dysplasia, encephalocele, cerebellar dysplasia, callosal agenesis, white matter hypoplasia, Dandy-Walker syndrome, Chiari malformation, aqueductal stenosis

Wallenberg's syndrome Lateral medullary syndrome; vertebral artery branch occlusion with medullary infarction

Warfarin embryopathy Craniofacial dysmorphia, choanal stenosis, optic atrophy, microphthalmia, hydrocephalus, occipital meningocele, stippled vertebral calcifications

Waterhouse-Friderichsen syndrome Fulminant septicemia, especially meningococcal with disseminated intravascular coagulation; intracranial hemorrhage, edema, necrosis

Wegener's granulomatosis Angiitis, focal necrosis, granulomatous reaction; paranasal sinuses, orbit, and tympanomastoid destruction; cavernous sinus invasion, cerebral vasculitis, edema, hemorrhage

Weill-Marchesani syndrome Skull vault thickening, rounded vertebral bodies, spinal canal narrowing, narrow disks

Weismann-Netter syndrome Kyphoscoliosis, dural calcification

Weissenbacher-Zweymuller phenotype Vertebral coronal clefts

Werdnig-Hoffmann disease Spinal muscular atrophy; anterior horn cell–spinal cord degeneration, muscular atrophy with fatty replacement, osteoporosis

Wiedemann-Rautenstrauch syndrome Hydrocephalus, CNS demyelination, wide sutures and fontanelles

Wildervanck syndrome Cervicooculoacoustic syndrome; Klippel-Feil anomaly, cervical encephalocele, fused cervical or thoracic vertebrae, occipitalization of the atlas, occipital vertebra, spina bifida occulta, inner ear anomalies (Mondini)

Williams syndrome Idiopathic hypercalcemia-supravalvular aortic stenosis syndrome; craniofacial dysmorphia, craniosynostosis, basilar invagination, kyphoscoliosis

Wilson's disease Hepatolenticular degeneration, irregular square vertebral bodies, Schmorl's nodes, wedge vertebral bodies, kyphosis, narrow disks, osteoporosis, osteomalacia, basal ganglia cavitation, necrosis, atrophy

Winchester's syndrome Wide sutures and fontanelles (delayed closure), atlantoaxial subluxation, vertebral fractures, kyphoscoliosis

Wiskott-Aldrich syndrome Immunodeficiency, recurrent infections, thrombocytopenia, astrocytoma, lymphoma, histiocytosis, leukemia, intracranial abscess, intracranial hemorrhage or intracranial neoplasm, sinus and tympanomastoid infection

Wolcott-Rallison syndrome Platyspondyly

Wrinkly skin syndrome Microcephaly, kyphosis, lordosis, scoliosis

Yunis-Varon syndrome Dolichocephaly, wide fontanelles

Zellweger's syndrome Cerebrohepatorenal syndrome; cerebral dysgenesis with migration anomalies, callosal dysgenesis, cerebellar hypoplasia, leukoencephalomyelopathy, gliosis, macrocephaly, wide sutures and fontanelles, optic nerve hypoplasia

Zimmermann-Laband syndrome Kyphosis, scoliosis

REFERENCES

Jones K: *Smith's recognizable patterns of human malformations,* ed 4, Philadelphia, 1988, WB Saunders.
Magalini S, Scrasia E: *Dictionary of medical syndromes,* ed 2, Philadelphia, 1981, JB Lippincott.
Taybi H, Lachman R: *Radiology of syndromes, metabolic disorders, and skeletal dysplasias,* Chicago, 1990, Mosby–Year Book.

Index

Page numbers in *italics* indicate illustrations.
Page numbers followed by *t* indicate tables.